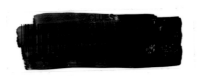
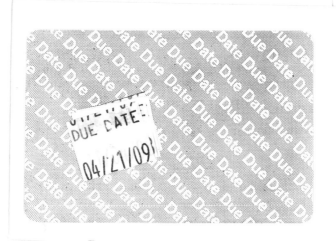

Alzheimer's Disease

CURRENT CLINICAL NEUROLOGY

Daniel Tarsy, MD, SERIES EDITOR

Alzheimer's Disease

A Physician's Guide
to Practical Management

Edited by

Ralph W. Richter, MD, FACP

Clinical Professor of Neurology and Psychiatry
The University of Oklahoma College of Medicine

Director, Alzheimer's Disease Research Unit
St. John Medical Center, Tulsa, OK

Brigitte Zoeller Richter, DiplPharm

Pharmacist, Publicist, Tulsa, OK

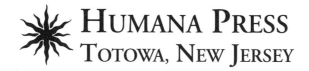
HUMANA PRESS
TOTOWA, NEW JERSEY

© 2004 Humana Press Inc.
999 Riverview Drive, Suite 208
Totowa, New Jersey 07512

www.humanapress.com

The content and opinions expressed in this book are the sole work of the authors and editors, who have warranted due diligence in the creation and issuance of their work. The publisher, editors, and authors are not responsible for errors or omissions or for any consequences arising from the information or opinions presented in this book and make no warranty, express or implied, with respect to its contents.

Due diligence has been taken by the publishers, editors, and authors of this book to assure the accuracy of the information published and to describe generally accepted practices. The contributors herein have carefully checked to ensure that the drug selections and dosages set forth in this text are accurate and in accord with the standards accepted at the time of publication. Notwithstanding, as new research, changes in government regulations, and knowledge from clinical experience relating to drug therapy and drug reactions constantly occurs, the reader is advised to check the product information provided by the manufacturer of each drug for any change in dosages or for additional warnings and contraindications. This is of utmost importance when the recommended drug herein is a new or infrequently used drug. It is the responsibility of the treating physician to determine dosages and treatment strategies for individual patients. Further it is the responsibility of the health care provider to ascertain the Food and Drug Administration status of each drug or device used in their clinical practice. The publisher, editors, and authors are not responsible for errors or omissions or for any consequences from the application of the information presented in this book and make no warranty, express or implied, with respect to the contents in this publication.

For additional copies, pricing for bulk purchases, and/or information about other Humana titles, contact Humana at the above address or at any of the following numbers: Tel.: 973-256-1699; Fax: 973-256-8341, E-mail: humana@humanapr.com; or visit our Website: www.humanapress.com.

Cover design: Patricia Cleary.
Production Editor: J. Morgan.

This publication is printed on acid-free paper. ∞
ANSI Z39.48-1984 (American National Standards Institute) Permanence of Paper for Printed Library Materials.

Printed in the United States of America. 10 9 8 7 6 5 4 3 2 1

E-ISBN 1-59259-661-4

Library of Congress Cataloging-in-Publication Data
   Alzheimer's disease : a physician's guide to practical management / edited by Ralph W. Richter, Brigitte Zoeller Richter.

         p. ; cm. — (Current clinical neurology)
   Includes bibliographical references and index.
   ISBN 0-89603-891-2 (alk. paper)
   1. Alzheimer's disease. 2. Alzheimer's disease—Treatment.
   [DNLM: 1. Alzheimer Disease. WT 155 A4756 2004] I. Richter, Ralph W. II. Zoeller Richter, Brigitte. III. Series.
   RC523.A3748 2004
   616.8'31—dc21
                                                              2003006948

Preface

Alzheimer's disease (AD) is a devastating and dehumanizing illness affecting increasingly large numbers of elderly and even middle-aged persons in a worldwide epidemic. *Alzheimer's Disease: A Physician's Guide to Practical Management* was written by selected clinicians and scientists who represent some of the world's leading centers of excellence in AD research. The editors are proud and grateful for their profound contributions.

This book is particularly designed to assist physicians and other health-care professionals in the evaluation, assessment, and treatment of individuals with AD. At the same time, by illuminating the basic scientific background, we hope to provide state-of-the art information about the disease and possible future therapeutic strategies. The recent psychiatric treatment aspects of AD are also clearly presented.

Because the early diagnosis of the dementia process is now considered of increasing importance, we focus particularly in several chapters on early changes and preclinical conditions, such as mild cognitive impairment and predementia AD.

The pathway toward reaching the goal of prevention of the disease is arduous and requires patience and fortitude. Patients and their families are not well served by overenthusiastic releases from companies or from scientists at a stage of research that can offer only experimental and animal data as grounds for optimism. Nevertheless, it is necessary to be informed about what might be coming up in the future. For this reason, comprehensive and timely information about potential future options for prevention and treatment of AD is included. A number of basic scientists discuss their areas of research in this volume. As a result, we have provided our readers with broad insight into such new therapeutic directions as stem cell therapy and other unique strategies.

AD imposes a tremendously painful burden on caregivers as well as friends. The consequences of providing this care are associated with deep feelings of isolation, loneliness, and despair. This has led us to include treatment of these aspects in this volume. We also provide some guidance for caregivers and medical providers on how to overcome the breakdown of communication that the illness creates.

It was our primary goal as editors to provide established scientific and clinical knowledge in comprehensible language and to touch upon more recent objects of research. As the reader may notice, we also cover aspects of the disease that have not yet been discussed in the available textbooks on AD.

We certainly hope that *Alzheimer's Disease: A Physician's Guide to Practical Management* will serve as a rich source of information that can be utilized by physicians in their daily practice of diagnosing and treating patients with AD. We must particularly bear in mind that the disease still appears to be underdiagnosed and undertreated *(1)*.

Supporting physicians in their management of AD is a way of helping patients and families to live better with the disease and to cope with the problems it poses. As we all know, dealing with an AD patient can be an extremely sad and frustrating task. Perhaps this book, by providing practical guidance, can make the task a little easier and help to "keep our hearts open in hell," as a caregiver once said *(2)*.

Ralph Walter Richter, MD, FACP
Brigitte Zoeller Richter, DiplPharm

1. Reichman, W.E.: Current pharmacologic options for patients with Alzheimer's disease. Ann Gen Hosp Psychiatry 2003; 2: 1.
2. Cited from: Thobaben, M.: Helping families understand and communicate with family members who suffer from dementia. Home Care Provid 1999; 4: 139–139,146.

Contents

Contributors

PIERO ANTUONO, MD • *Professor of Neurology and Pharmacology, The Medical College of Wisconsin, Milwaukee, WI*

ROBERT BARBER, MD, MRCPsych • *Centre for Health of the Elderly, Newcastle General Hospital, Newcastle upon Tyne, United Kingdom*

FRED BASKIN, PhD • *Associate Professor, Department of Neurology, University of Texas Southwestern Medical Center, Dallas, TX*

ROSE A. BEESON, DNSc, RN • *Assistant Professor, William F. Connell School of Nursing, Boston College, Cushing Hall, Chestnut Hill, MA*

JOHN P. BLASS, MD, PhD • *Director, Dementia Research Service, Burke Medical Research Institute; Professor of Neurology and Medicine, Weill Medical College of Cornell University, White Plains, NY*

HEIKO BRAAK, MD • *Professor, Institute for Clinical Neuroanatomy, Johann-Wolfgang-Goethe-University, Frankfurt/Main, Germany*

DAVID CASTRO-BLANCO, PhD • *Associate Professor, Doctoral Program in Clinical Psychology, Department of Psychology, Long Island University, Brooklyn Campus, New York, NY*

AMY S. CHAPPELL, MD • *Lilly Corporate Center, Indianapolis, IN*

CARL I. COHEN, MD • *Professor and Director, Division of Geriatric Psychiatry, Department of Psychiatry, SUNY Downstate Medical Center, Brooklyn, NY*

UMBERTO CORNELLI, MD, PhD, DrScHc • *Adjunct Professor of Pharmacology, Loyola University Stritch School of Medicine Chicago, Milan, Italy*

JEFFREY L. CUMMINGS, MD • *Professor of Neurology and Psychiatry, Reed Neurological Research Center, Department of Neurology, UCLA School of Medicine, Los Angeles*

KELLY DEL TREDICI, PhD • *Institute for Clinical Neuroanatomy, Johann-Wolfgang-Goethe-University, Frankfurt/Main, Germany*

RAMON DIAZ-ARRASTIA • *Associate Professor, Department of Neurology, University of Texas Southwestern Medical School, Dallas, TX*

DAVID A. DRACHMAN, MD • *Professor of Neurology, Department of Neurology, University of Massachusetts Medical School, Worcester, MA*

TIMO ERKINJUNTTI, MD, PhD • *Department of Neurology, University of Helsinki, Helsinki, Finland*

MARTIN R. FARLOW, MD • *Professor and Vice Chairman for Research in Neurology, Department of Neurology, Indiana University School of Medicine, IUPUI; Director, Clinical Care of Alzheimer Disease Care Center; Co-Director Alzheimer's Disease Clinic; Affiliated Scientist, Indiana University Center for Aging Research, Indianapolis, IN*

HOWARD FELDMAN, MD, FRCP(C) • *Professor and Head, Division of Neurology, University of British Columbia Hospital, Vancouver, BC, Canada*

NORMAN L. FOSTER, MD • *Professor, Department of Neurology, Senior Research Scientist, Institute of Gerontology, University of Michigan, Ann Arbor, MI*

MALGORZATA FRANCZAK, MD • *Assistant Professor of Neurology, The Medical College of Wisconsin, Milwaukee, Wisconsin*

PAUL E. GILBERT, PhD • *Department of Head and Neck Surgery, University of California San Diego, School of Medicine; Lifespan Human Senses Laboratory, San Diego, CA*

CHRISTINA A. GITTO, DDS • *Department of Dentistry and Maxillofacial Prosthetics, The Cleveland Clinic Foundation, Cleveland, OH*

GABRIEL GOLD, MD • *Hôpital de Gériatrie, Thônex-Genève, Switzerland*

VONDA K. GRAVELY, MD • *Chief Geriatric Psychiatry Fellow, Alzheimer's Research and Clinical Program, Medical University of South Carolina, Charleston, SC*

ANDREW R. GUSTAVSON, MD • *Fellow, Alzheimer's Disease Research Center, Department of Neurology, UCLA School of Medicine, Los Angeles, CA*

JOHN HARDY, PhD • *Chief, Laboratory of Neurogenetics, National Institute on Aging, National Institutes of Health, Bethesda, MD*

GING-YUEK ROBIN HSIUNG, MD, MHSc, FRCPC • *Division of Neurology, University of British Columbia, Vancouver, Canada*

M. SALEEM ISMAIL, MD • *Senior Instructor in Psychiatry, Department of Psychiatry; Program in Neurobehavioral Therapeutics, University of Rochester Medical Center, Rochester, NY*

MICHELLE KEHN, MA • *Doctoral Student, Department of Psychology, Long Island University, Brooklyn Campus, New York, NY*

DIANA KERWIN, MD • *Assistant Professor of Geriatrics, The Medical College of Wisconsin, Milwaukee, Wisconsin*

DANIELLE LAURIN, PhD • *Assistant Professor, Geriatric Research Unit, Centre de Recherche du CHA, Laval University, Quebec, Canada*

JOAN LINDSAY, MD • *Adjunct Professor, Department of Epidemiology and Community Medicine, Faculty of Medicine, University of Ottawa, Ottawa, ON, Canada*

IAN G. MCKEITH, MD, FRCPsych • *Professor, Institute for Aging and Health, Wolfson Unit, Newcastle General Hospital, Newcastle upon Tyne, United Kingdom*

SUSAN MCPHERSON, PhD, ABPP • *Private Practice, Golden Valley, MN*

JOSÉ R. MEDINA, MD, FACC, FACP • *Clinical Professor of Medicine, University of Oklahoma, Tulsa, Cardiologist, Heart Center of Tulsa, Tulsa, OK*

JEAN-PIERRE MICHEL, MD • *Professeur, Hôpital de Gériatrie, Thônex-Genève, Switzerland*

JACOBO MINTZER, MD • *Co-Director of Alzheimer's Research and Clinical Programs; Director of Geriatric Psychiatry; Professor of Psychiatry and Neurology; Director, Minority Training on Mental Health & Aging, Institute of Research; Associate Director for Alzheimer's Research, Neuroscience Institute, Medical University of South Carolina; Staff Physician, Ralph H. Johnson VA Medical Center, Charleston, SC*

HANS JÖRG MÖBIUS, MD, PhD • *Vice-President, Research & Development and DRA, General Manager, Merz Pharmaceuticals, Frankfurt am Main, Germany*

ANDREAS U. MONSCH, PhD • *Privat-Dozent, Director, Memory Clinic–Neuropsychology Center, Geriatric University Hospital, Basel, Switzerland*

MICHAEL J. MORONI, DDS • *Private Practice, Parker, CO*

CLAIRE MURPHY, PhD • *SDSU-UCSD Joint Doctoral Program in Clinical Psychology, San Diego State University; Department of Head and Neck Surgery, University of California San Diego, School of Medicine, San Diego, CA*

JANE NEWBY, MRCPsych • *Centre for Health of the Elderly, Newcastle General Hospital, Newcastle upon Tyne, United Kingdom*

BRIAN R. OTT, MD • *Professor of Clinical Neurosciences, Brown University School of Medicine, Providence, RI*

SOPHIE PAUTEX, MD • *Hôpital de Gériatrie, Thônex-Genève, Switzerland*

BEATRICE POLLOCK, BS • *Clinical Research Director, Department of Psychiatry and Neurology, Tulane University Health Sciences Center, New Orleans, LA*

DOMENICO PRATICÒ, MD • *Assistant Professor of Pharmacology, Center for Experimental Therapeutics, Department of Pharmacology, University of Pennsylvania School of Medicine, Philadelphia, PA*

JACOB RABER, PhD • *Departments of Behavioral Neuroscience and Neurology, Oregon Health & Science University, Portland, OR*

PAUL MICHAEL RAMIREZ, PhD • *Associate Professor, Doctoral Program in Clinical Psychology, Department of Psychology, Long Island University, Brooklyn Campus, New York, NY*

RALPH W. RICHTER, MD, FACP • *Clinical Professor of Neurology and Psychiatry, The University of Oklahaoma College of Medicine; Director, Alzheimer's Disease Research Unit, St. John Medical Center, Tulsa, OK*

KENNETH ROCKWOOD, MD, MPA, FRCPC • *Professor of Medicine (Geriatric Medicine and Neurology), Kathryn Allen Weldon Professor of Alzheimer Research, Dalhousie University, Halifax, Nova Scotia, Canada*

SATINDERPAL K. SANDU, MD • *Department of Geriatrics, MetroHealth Center for Skilled Nursing Care, Highland Hills, OH*

LON S. SCHNEIDER, MD, MS • *Professor of Psychiatry, Neurology and Gerontology, Keck School of Medicine, University of Southern California, Los Angeles, CA*

RAYMELLE SCHOOS, MD • *Resident Physician, Division of Geriatric Psychiatry, Department of Psychiatry, SUNY Downstate Medical Center, Brooklyn, NY*

CHRISTIAN SCHULTZ, MD, *Institute for Clinical Neuroanatomy, Johann-Wolfgang-Goethe-University, Frankfurt/Main, Germany*

BEN SELTZER, MD • *Professor of Neurology and Psychiatry; Director, Alzheimer's Disease and Memory Disorders Center, Tulane University School of Medicine, New Orleans, LA*

SCOTT A. SMALL, MD • *Assistant Professor of Neurology, Department of Neurology, Taub Institute for Research on Alzheimer's Disease and the Aging Brain, and Center for Neurobiology and Behavior, Columbia University College of Physicians and Surgeons, New York, NY*

HANNES B. STAEHELIN, MD • *Professor Internal Medicine and Geriatric Medicine, Geriatric Clinic University Hospital, Basel, Switzerland*

KIMINOBU SUGAYA, PhD • *Assistant Professor of Psychiatry, Assistant Professor of Physiology and Biophysics, Department of Psychiatry, University of Illinois at Chicago, Chicago, IL*

PIERRE N. TARIOT, MD • *Professor of Psychiatry, Neurology, Medicine, and Aging and Developmental Biology, Department of Psychiatry and Program in Neurobehavioral Therapeutics, University of Rochester Medical Center, Rochester, NY*

KIRSTEN I. TAYLOR, PhD • *Centre for Speech and Language, Department of Experimental Psychology, University of Cambridge, Cambridge, UK*

GEZA T. TEREZHALMY, DDS, MA • *Professor and Head, Division of Oral Medicine, Department of Dental Diagnostic Science, The University of Texas Health Science Center Dental School, San Antonio, TX*

MARK H. TUSZYNSKI, MD, PhD • *Professor of Neurosciences; Director, Center for Neural Repair, University of California San Diego, La Jolla, CA*

FRANK JOHN EMERY VAJDA, MD, FRCP, FRACP • *Professor, Director, Australian Centre for Clinical Neuropharmacology, Raoul Wallenberg Centre, St. Vincent's Hospital Melbourne, University of Melbourne, Victoria, Australia*

RENÉ VERREAULT, MD, PhD • *Professor, Department of Social and Preventive Medicine, Laval University, Hôpital du St-Sacrement, Quebec, Canada*

PIETER JELLE VISSER, MD, PhD • *Assistant Professor, Department of Psychiatry and Neuropsychology, University of Maastricht, Maastricht; Department of Neurology, VU Medical Centre, Amsterdam, The Netherlands*

LORNA WALCOTT-BROWN, MA • *Director of Social Services, Brooklyn Alzheimer's Disease Assistance Center, Department of Psychiatry, SUNY Downstate Medical Center, Brooklyn, NY*

MYRON F. WEINER, MD • *Dorothy L. and John P. Harbin Chair in Alzheimer's Disease Research, Professor of Psychiatry and Associate Professor of Neurology, University of Texas Southwestern Medical Center, Dallas, TX*

PETER J. WHITEHOUSE, MD, PhD • *Professor of Neurology, Case Western Reserve University School of Medicine; University Memory and Aging Center, University Hospitals of Cleveland; Cleveland, OH*

ANDERS WIMO, MD, PhD • *Associate Professor, Department of Clinical Neuroscience; Occupational Therapy and Elderly Care Research, NEUROTEC; Division of Geriatric Epidemiology, Karolinska Institute, Stockholm, Sweden*

BENGT WINBLAD, MD, PhD • *Professor, Department of Clinical Neuroscience; Occupational Therapy and Elderly Care Research, NEUROTEC; Aging Research Center, Karolinska Institute, Stockholm, Sweden*

MICHAEL M. WITTE, PhD • *Lilly Corporate Center, Eli Lilly and Company, Indianapolis, IN*

WEIMING XIA, PhD • *Assistant Professor of Neurology, Harvard Medical School; Center for Neurologic Diseases, Brigham and Women's Hospital; Harvard Institute of Medicine, Boston, MA*

DINA ZEKRY, MD • *Hôpital de Gériatrie, Thônex-Genève, Switzerland*

BRIGITTE ZOELLER RICHTER, DiplPharm • *Pharmacist, Publicist, Tulsa, OK*

GILBERT ZULIAN, MD • *Centre de Soins Continus, Thônex-Genève, Switzerland*

I Scientific Background of Alzheimer's Disease

Genetics of Alzheimer's Disease and Related Disorders

John Hardy

INTRODUCTION

The purpose of this chapter is to review the genetics of Alzheimer's disease (AD) and related neurodegenerative disorders, making three fundamental points. First, genetic analysis of kindreds with AD has unequivocally pointed to beta-amyloid (Aβ) as the initiating molecule in the disease. Second, genetic analysis of frontal temporal dementia (FTDP-17) has suggested that tau dysfunction is a proximal cause of neurodegeneration in that disorder and also in both progressive supranuclear palsy (PSP) and corticobasal degeneration (CBD), and by analogy, is also likely to be a proximal cause of neurodegeneration in AD. Third, genetic analysis of Parkinson's disease (PD) kindreds has shown that α-synuclein dysfunction is a proximal cause of degeneration in that disorder, and by analogy is also likely to be a proximal cause of neurodegeneration in AD, because Lewy bodies are a frequent part of the pathology in AD. The theme of this chapter is that genetic analysis—together with pathology investigation—has shown that these diseases share common mechanisms of neurodegeneration, and that they can be grouped into one broadly sketched pathway of pathogenesis.

THE ROLE OF THE APP GENE

The modern era of research into AD came with the identification of the sequence of the Aβ peptide and the recognition that this peptide was also deposited in trisomy 21, suggesting that the gene encoding this protein was likely to be on chromosome 21 (1,2). When the gene, APP, was cloned (3), this was shown to be the case and the Aβ section of the molecule was derived from the perimembranous section of the type 1 integral membrane protein (Fig. 1).

At the same time, genetic linkage to chromosome 21 markers was reported (4a), and this too led to increased suspicion that the APP gene might be the site of mutations leading to disease. Initially, genetic analysis ruled out this possibility (5,6). However, this analysis was flawed in two ways. First, the original report of linkage was an error, because all the pedigrees used in this report were later shown to have presenilin mutations (4b,7). Second, the analysis was based on the reasonable, but incorrect, supposition that the disease is genetically homogenous. The later demonstration that the disease is genetically heterogenous (8,9) subverted these analyses.

During this period, the relevance of analysis of hereditary cerebral hemorrhage with amyloidosis, Dutch type, to AD research became clear. This happens to be a stroke, not a dementing, disorder, but is characterized by Aβ deposition in cerebral blood vessels (10). Genetic analysis showed that this disease is caused by mutations at the APP locus (11) in the middle of the Aβ part of the molecule (12).

From: *Current Clinical Neurology,*
Alzheimer's Disease: A Physician's Guide to Practical Management
Edited by: R. W. Richter and B. Zoeller Richter © Humana Press Inc., Totowa, NJ

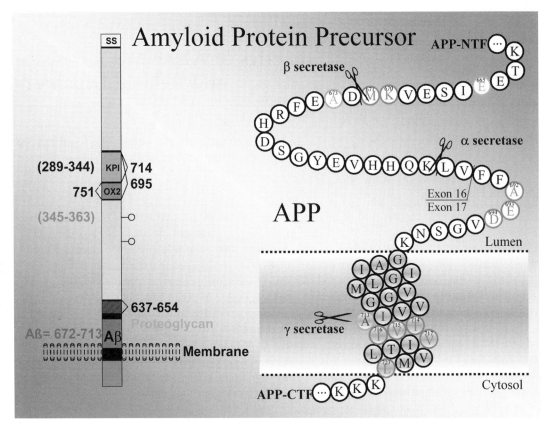

Fig. 1. Diagram of the APP molecule showing, in the expanded segment, the positions of major cleavages and mutations.

This combination of findings—the realization that previous analyses of chromosome 21 markers had been flawed, and the demonstration that APP mutations could lead to Aβ deposition, albeit not in the brain parenchyma—led to the reanalysis of the APP gene in selected families with AD, and the identification of pathogenic APP mutations *(13)*. The first mutations found were all to the same codon *(14,15)* leading to the prediction that they would alter APP processing in specific ways to make Aβ deposition more likely *(14)*. Work on APP processing showed that there were two pathways of APP metabolism *(16)* and that all the pathogenic mutations altered processing such that Aβ42 production was more likely (Fig. 2) *(17–19)*. This combination of genetic and biochemical data led to the formulation of the amyloid cascade hypothesis *(20,21;* Fig. 3), which suggested that Aβ deposition is the primary event in disease pathogenesis *(22)*.

THE AMYLOID CASCADE HYPOTHESIS

The name amyloid cascade hypothesis requires some explanation because it has been the subject of controversy. First, the name was coined by my then co-author *(20)*, but was based on the then name of Aβ—amyloid-β—and second, it has been correctly stated that early formulations of the hypothesis emphasized amyloid deposits as the key pathogenic lesions. Although this is indeed true, there has been the implicit criticism that the formulators of the amyloid cascade hypothesis have somehow cheated by changing the emphasis over the last period to discuss the toxicity of soluble oligomers of Aβ *(23)*. I regard this criticism as ridiculous. If we had been sure of the precise causes of AD in 1992, we would not have continued to experiment. Furthermore, the discussion of the precise name of the

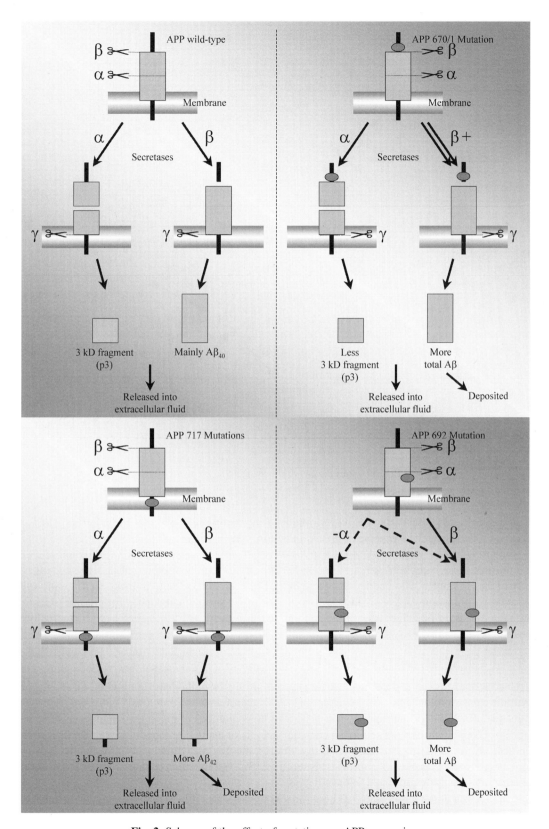

Fig. 2. Schema of the effect of mutations on APP processing.

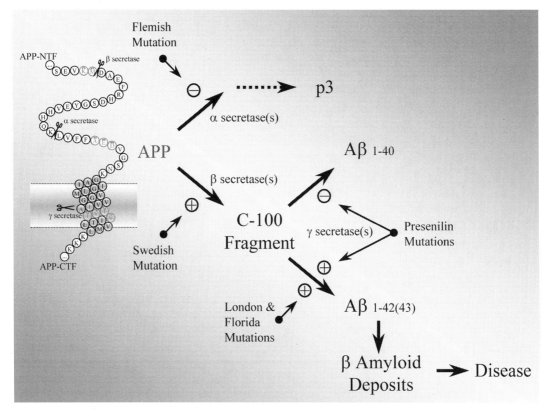

Fig. 3. A formulation of the amyloid cascade hypothesis.

hypothesis ignores the fact that the review articles were merely formulations encapsulating the work of others in isolating the Aβ peptide *(1)* and in cloning the gene *(3)*.

Mutations in APP were found to be responsible for a very small percentage of AD familial cases, and most of these had onset ages in the mid-50s. Clearly, there were other genes involved, particularly in those families who had an onset age in the 30s and 40s. Linkage in these families showed a locus on chromosome 14 *(24)*, which was soon confirmed as the major locus for disease *(4,25,26)*. With the benefit of hindsight it is interesting that the chromosome 14 locus had been correctly localized many years previously *(27)*.

FROM PRESENILIN TO γ-SECRETASE

Genetic analysis rapidly narrowed the region containing the pathogenic locus (Fig. 4), and the presenilin 1 gene was cloned by positional cloning *(7)*. The protein was a previously unknown one, whose immediate function was not known, but in which a large number of pathogenic mutations have subsequently been identified *(27)* (Fig. 5). Genetic analysis of a small number of pedigrees of Russian-German origin revealed a further locus on chromosome 1 *(28)*, which was immediately shown to correspond to the presenilin 1 homolog, presenilin 2 *(29–31)*, in which a small number of mutations, which cause AD, have also been found (Fig. 5).

The function of the presenilins was not immediately apparent. It was, however, quickly shown that the mutation altered APP processing in plasma and tissues from mutation carriers *(32)* as well as in transfected cells and transgenic animals which harbored the mutation *(33–35)*. Subsequent work has shown that the presenilins are probably γ-secretase *(36,37)* (Fig. 6).

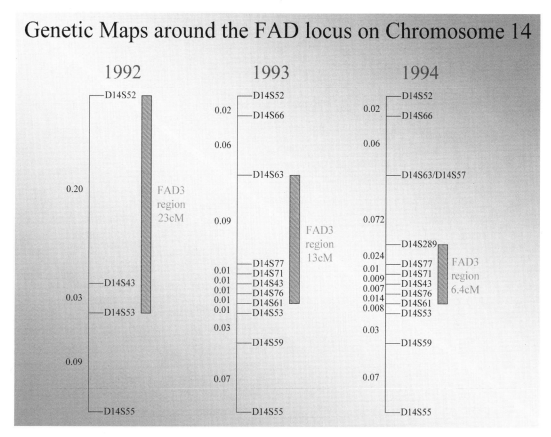

Fig. 4. The history, 1992–1994, of the positional cloning effort to clone the presenilin 1 gene showing how the analysis of more genetic markers and more linked families allowed the region to be narrowed down.

The identification of APP and presenilin mutations has allowed the production of increasingly useful transgenic models of amyloid depositions, based initially on APP mutations *(38,39)* and subsequently on APP/PS transgene crosses *(40,41)*. Although these mice are useful in developing plaque pathology, they develop no tangle pathology and little cell loss (Fig. 7).

These data provide convincing evidence that Aβ is indeed the initiating molecule in AD. However, these data relate directly only to the early-onset familial forms of the disease; it is less clear that they are relevant to late-onset disease. In addition, the fact that transgenic animals do not develop either tangles or cell loss has led to debate about the accuracy of the amyloid cascade hypothesis.

There are three lines of evidence that circumstantially support the notion that Aβ is central to the initiation of late-onset disease. First, the APP locus seems to contribute to risk for this form of the disease *(42,43)*. Second, transgenic animals, which lack their ApoE gene, do not deposit amyloid *(44)*. Finally, both high-plasma Aβ and late-onset AD show localization to the same region of chromosome 10 *(45,46)*. However, clearly the data for typical late-onset disease is less compelling than for the early-onset forms of the disease.

HOW TAU FITS IN THE CONCEPT

Genetic analysis of families with a wide variety of clinical presentations, including dementia and parkinsonism, showed linkage to chromosome 17 *(47,48)* in the same region as the tau gene (Fig. 8). Initially, sequencing of the tau gene failed to identify mutations, but careful examination of the brains

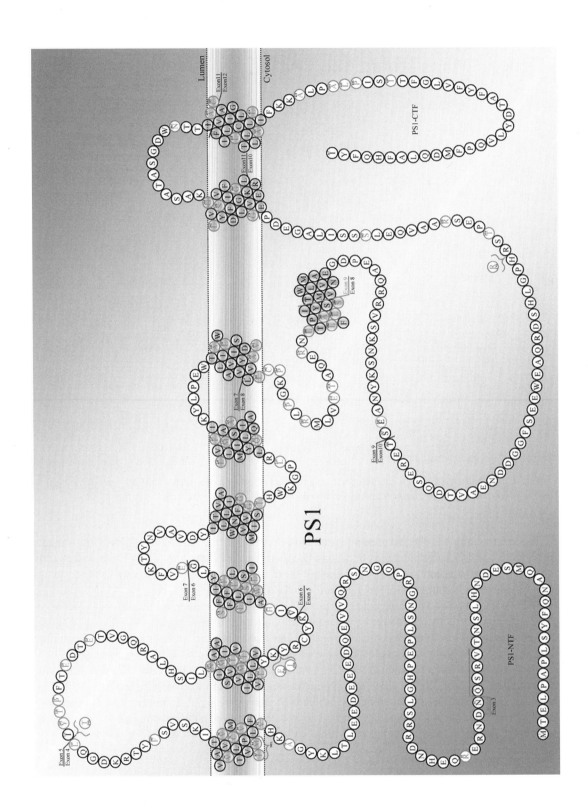

PS1

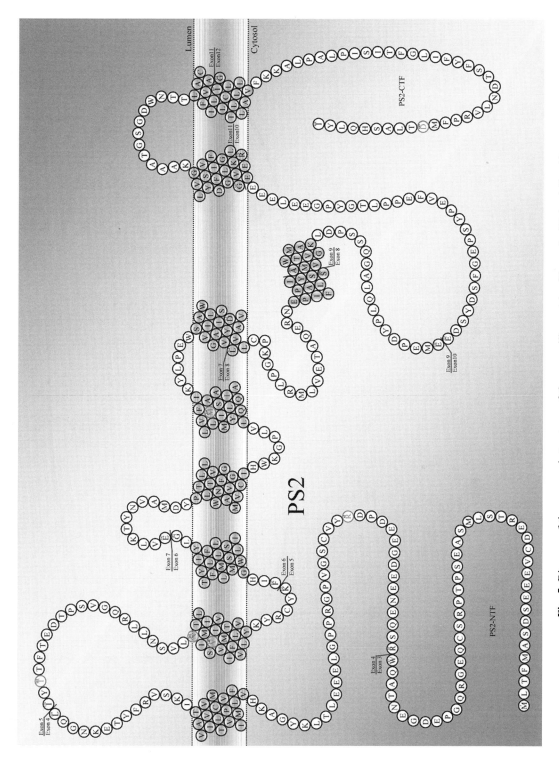

Fig. 5. Diagram of the proposed structures of the presenilin proteins (drawn by Richard Crook).

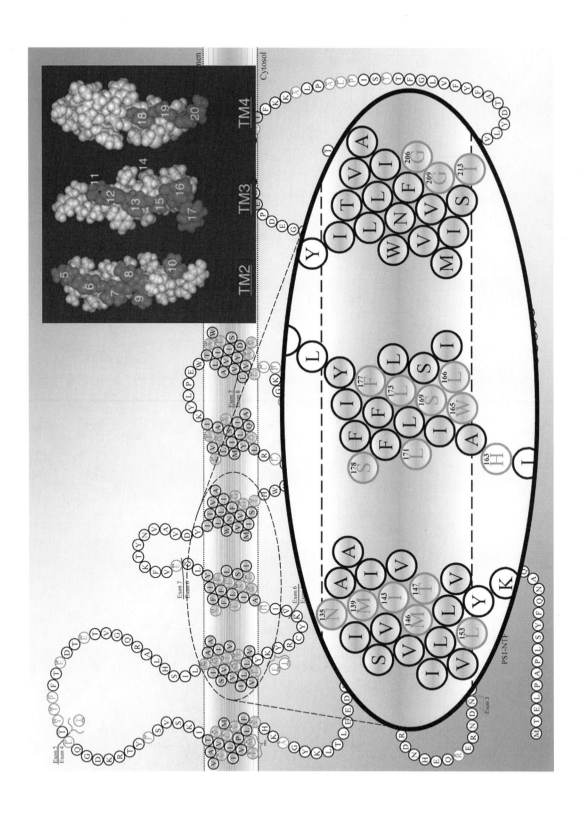

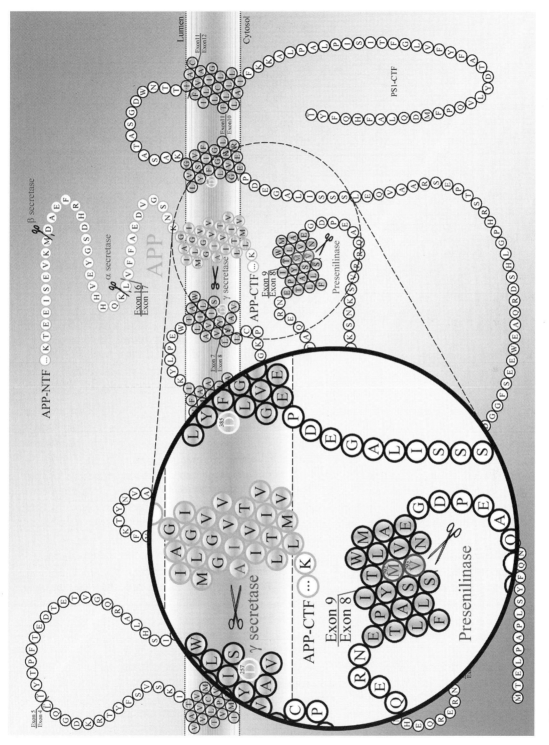

Fig. 6. Diagram of presenilin 1 showing APP in the proposed active site: this diagram omits the newly identified auxiliary protein to the γ-secretase complex and the alignment of mutations along helical faces.

11

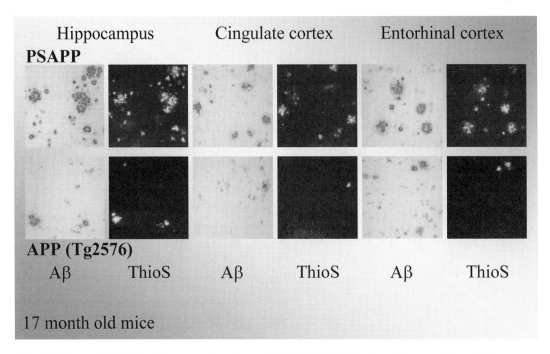

Fig. 7. Plaques in APP Swedish transgenic mice and APP/PS1 (M146V) mice (thanks to Eileen McGowan).

of patients dying of disease showed that all of them had some tau pathology, although in some cases it was very subtle *(49)*. The first sequence analyses failed to find mutations *(50)*, but occasional changes were found *(51)*. However, reanalysis of families in which tau mutations had not been identified showed that they had intronic changes that affected the alternate splicing of exon 10 (Figs. 8 and 9) *(52)* such that only 4-repeat tau was produced from the mutant allele. Subsequently, a large number of pathogenic mutations have been found (Fig. 9b), and there exists an extremely elegant general correspondence between the site of the mutation and the pathology. Those with the splice site mutations deposit normal, 4-repeat tau as wispy deposits. Those with mutations in exon 10 produce heavy deposits of mutant tau. Those with mutations in other exons deposit both 3 and 3-repeat tau as tangles indistinguishable from AD tangles, though some deposit only 3-repeat tau as Pick bodies.

The importance of this work is twofold. First, it is important for our understanding of FTDP-17. Second, however, is its more general importance to AD research. These data clearly show that tau dysfunction leads to both tangle formation and neurodegeneration, but does not appear to lead to amyloid deposition and AD. This puts the sequence of events in the diseases in a temporal one (Fig. 10): with Aβ upstream of tau dysfunction and with tau dysfunction and tangle formation proximal to cell death *(53)*.

Identification of these mutations also allowed the creation of mouse models of tangle formation *(54)*. In these mice, the tau P301L-transgene expression was driven by the prion promoter, and tangle formation and cell death was restricted essentially to the spinal cord and midbrain. When, however, these mice were crossed with APP mice *(39)*, tangle formation was precipitated in the cortex in addition to the midbrain (Fig. 11); amyloid pathology, in contrast, was not altered *(55)*. This provides experimental evidence that the schema sketched in Fig. 10 is approximately correct and provides the first experimental evidence that the amyloid cascade hypothesis is correct.

During the sequencing of the tau gene, it was noted that there are two tau haplotypes in Caucasian populations *(56,57)*. These did not differ in amino acid sequence but rather in wobble bases and intronic

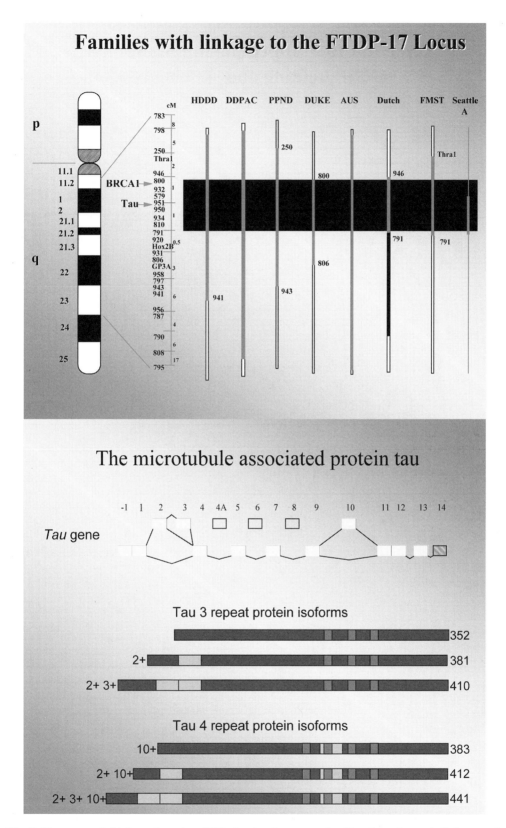

Fig. 8. Upper panel: Linkage data circa 1998 showing how many families showed genetic linkage to chromosome 17 in the vicinity of the tau gene. **Lower panel**: structure of the tau protein showing alternate splicing of exons 2 and 3 and of exon 10. This latter is extremely important and is discussed in the text.

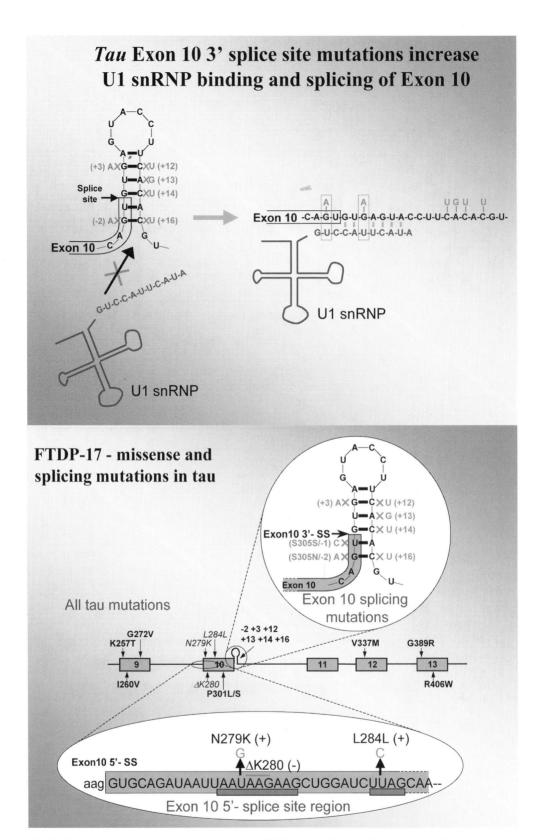

Fig. 9. Upper panel: the stem loop structure in hnRNA just 3 of exon 10 showing the disruption by pathogenic FTDP-17 mutations. **Lower panel**: an update on mutations in the tau gene that lead to disease.

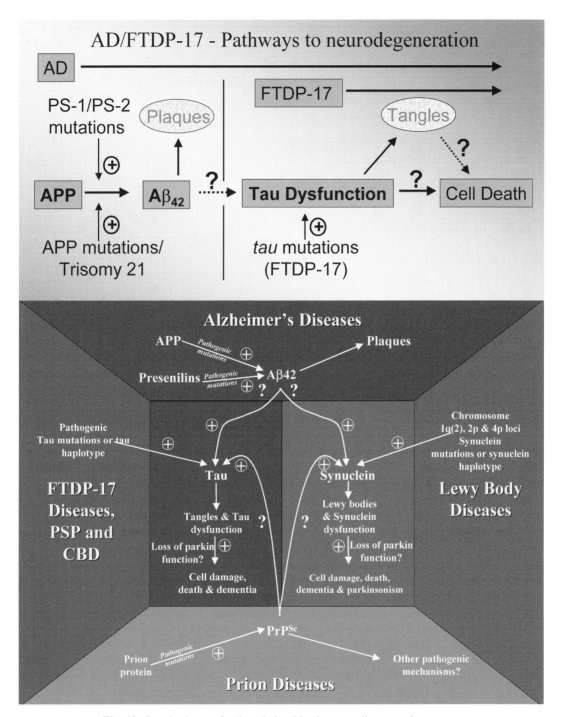

Fig. 10. Grand schemes for the relationships between disease pathogeneses.

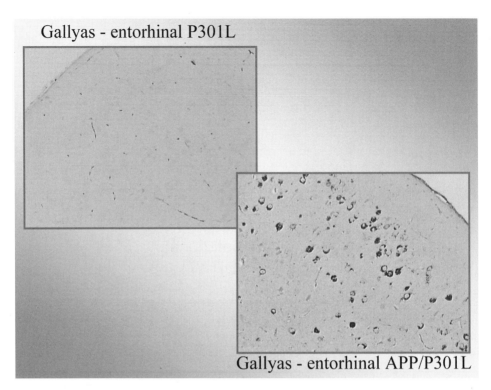

Fig. 11. Upper panel: silver stained cortex of a mouse with a mutant P301L tau gene. Tangles are essentially absent but were found in this mouse in the midbrain. **Lower panel**: P301L/APP Sw mouse cortex of the same age. Many tangles are seen in the cortex in addition to those that were found in the midbrain.

sequences. The H1 haplotype clade has a frequency of ~70% and the H2 has a frequency of ~30% in Caucasians (Fig. 12). In all other populations the H2 haplotype is essentially absent. Thus, in Caucasians, ~50% of individuals are H1 homozygotes. However, 95% of individuals with both progressive supranuclear palsy (PSP) and corticobasal degeneration (CBD) are H1 homozygotes *(57,58)*. Thus, tau is a risk factor locus for the sporadic tauopathies, PSP and CBD *(58,59)*.

FROM α-SYNUCLEIN TO LEWY BODIES

Although Parkinson's Disease (PD) was always considered a nongenetic disorder, in fact there have been many families in which the disease was clearly inherited *(60,61)*. In the most famous of these—the Contursi kindred—linkage to chromosome 4q markers was reported *(62)*, and a mutation in the α-synuclein gene was identified *(63)*. Subsequently, α-synuclein was identified as the primary component of Lewy bodies *(64)*. Mice made with α-synuclein transgenes develop some synuclein pathology *(65)*, and this pathology is accentuated by crossing these animals with APP transgenic mice *(66)*. This series of data concerning α-synuclein parallels the data presented above concerning tau. Thus, mutations in the cognate protein lead to hereditary disorder and to its deposition in the pathognomonic lesion. Overexpression of the protein in mice leads to a partial model of the disease, and crossing of these mice with APP-overexpressing mice accentuates the pathology. Finally, genetic analysis of the α-synuclein promoter in sporadic PD shows that the high-expressing promoter *(67)* is associated with risk for disease *(68,69)*, in an analogous fashion to the association between tau haplotypes and sporadic tauopathies.

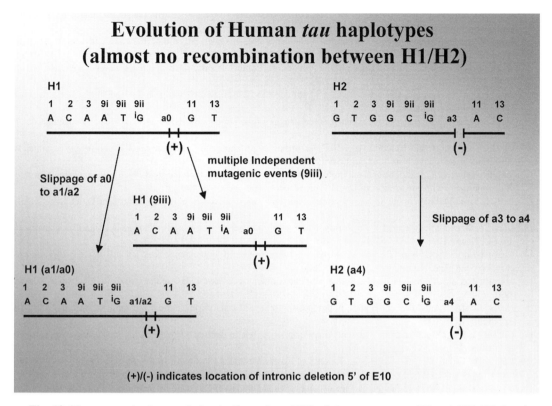

Fig. 12. The two *tau* haplotype clades: in Caucasians, 70% of chromosomes are H1 and 30% H2. In other populations H2 is essentially absent. Thus approx 50% of Caucasians are H1 homozygotes, but 95% of people with PSP are H1 homozygotes (*see* text).

STRONG LINKAGES BETWEEN PATHOLOGIES

This broad series of experimental and genetic observational data can be incorporated into a single framework linking these pathologies and diagnoses (Fig. 10) *(70)*. This roadmap sketches the relationships between the pathologies and the diagnostic categories. Clearly, much work still needs to be done. The relationships denoted by question marks indicate large areas of ignorance, and there are many genetic loci for Lewy body disease that still need to be found *(71)*. However, this framework should act as a guide for both determining the likely direction of interactions and for designing therapies.

REFERENCES

1. Glenner, G.G.; Wong C.W.: Alzheimer's disease: initial report of the purification and characterization of a novel cerebrovascular amyloid protein. Biochem Biophys Res Commun 1984; 120: 885–890.
2. Glenner, G.G.; Wong, C.W.: Alzheimer's disease and Down's syndrome: sharing of a unique cerebrovascular amyloid fibril protein. Biochem Biophys Res Commun 1984; 122: 1131–1135.
3. Kang, J. et al.: The precursor of Alzheimer's disease amyloid A4 protein resembles a cell-surface receptor. Nature 1987; 325: 733–736.
4a. St George-Hyslop, P.H. et al.: The genetic defect causing familial Alzheimer's disease maps on chromosome 21. Science 1987; 235: 885–890.
4b. St George-Hyslop, P. et al.: Genetic evidence for a novel familial Alzheimer's disease locus on chromosome 14. Nat Genet 1992; 2:330–334.

5. Van Broeckhoven, C. et al.: Failure of familial Alzheimer's disease to segregate with the A4-amyloid gene in several European families. Nature 1987; 329: 153–155.

6. Tanzi, R.E. et al.: The genetic defect in familial Alzheimer's disease is not tightly linked to the amyloid beta-protein gene. Nature 1987: 329: 156–157.

7. Sherrington, R. et al.: Cloning of a gene bearing missense mutations in early-onset familial Alzheimer's disease. Nature 1995; 375: 754–760.

8. Schellenberg, G.D. et al.: Absence of linkage of chromosome 21q21 markers to familial Alzheimer's disease. Science 1988; 241: 1507–1510.

9. St. George Hyslop, P. et al.: Genetic linkage studies suggest that Alzheimer s disease is not a single homogenous disorder. Nature 1990; 347: 194–197.

10. van Duinen, S.G. et al.: Hereditary cerebral hemorrhage with amyloidosis in patients of Dutch origin is related to Alzheimer disease. Proc Natl Acad Sci USA 1987; 84: 5991–5994.

11. Van Broeckhoven, C. et al.: The beta-amyloid precursor protein gene is tightly linked to the locus causing hereditary cerebral hemorrhage with amyloidosis of Dutch Type. Science 1990; 248: 488–490.

12. Levy, E. et al.: Mutation of the Alzheimer's disease amyloid gene in hereditary cerebral hemorrhage, Dutch type. Science 1990; 248: 1124–1126.

13. Goate, A.M. et al.: Segregation of a missense mutation in the amyloid precursor protein gene with familial Alzheimer's disease. Nature 1991; 349: 704–706.

14. Chartier-Harlin, M.C. et al.: Early onset Alzheimer's disease caused by mutations at codon 717 of the β-amyloid precursor protein gene. Nature 1991; 353: 844–846.

15. Murrell, J. et al.: A mutation in the amyloid precursor protein associated with hereditary Alzheimer's disease. Science 1991; 254: 97–99.

16. Haass, C. et al.: Amyloid beta-peptide is produced by cultured cells during normal metabolism. Nature 1992; 359: 322–325.

17. Citron, M. et al.: Mutation of the beta-amyloid precursor protein in familial Alzheimer's disease increases beta-protein production. Nature 1992; 360: 672–674.

18. Cai, X.D.; Golde, T.E.; Younkin, S.G.: Release of excess amyloid beta protein from a mutant amyloid beta protein precursor. Science 1993; 259: 514–516.

19. Suzuki, N. et al.: An increased percentage of long amyloid beta protein secreted by familial amyloid beta protein precursor (beta APP717) mutants. Science 1994; 264: 1336–1340.

20. Hardy, J.A.; Higgins, G.A.: Alzheimer s disease: the amyloid cascade hypothesis. Science 1992; 286: 184–185.

21. Selkoe, D.J.: The molecular pathology of Alzheimer's disease. Neuron 1991; 6: 487–498.

22. Hardy, J.; Allsop, D.: Amyloid deposition as the central event in the aetiology of Alzheimer's disease. Trends Pharm Sci 1991; 12: 383–388.

23. Hardy, J.; Selkoe, D.J.: The amyloid hypothesis of Alzheimer's disease: progress and problems on the road to therapeutics. Science 2002; 297: 353–356.

24. Schellenberg, G.D. et al.: Genetic linkage evidence for a familial Alzheimer's disease locus on chromosome 14. Science 1992; 258: 668–671.

25. Van Broeckhoven, C. et al.: Mapping of a gene predisposing to early-onset Alzheimer's disease to chromosome 14q24.3. Nat Genet 1992; 2: 335–339.

26. Mullan, M. et al.: A locus for familial early onset Alzheimer s disease on the long arm of chromosome 14, proximal to alpha1-antichymoreypsin. Nat Genet 1992; 2: 340–343.

27. Cruts, M.; Van Broeckhoven, C.: Presenilin mutations in Alzheimer's disease. Hum Mutat 1998; 11: 183–190.

28. Levy-Lahad, E., et al.: A familial Alzheimer's disease locus on chromosome 1. Science 1995; 269: 970–973.

29. Levy-Lahad, E. et al.: Candidate gene for the chromosome 1 familial Alzheimer's disease locus. Science 1995; 269: 973–977.

30. Rogaev, E.I. et al.: Familial Alzheimer's disease in kindreds with missense mutations in a gene on chromosome 1 related to the Alzheimer's disease type 3 gene. Nature 1995; 376: 775–778.

31. Clark, R.F. et al.: The structure of the presenilin 1 (S182) gene and identification of six novel mutations in early onset AD families. Nat Genet 1995; 11: 219–222.

32. Scheuner, D. et al.: Secreted amyloid β-protein similar to that in the senile plaques of Alzheimer's disease is increased in vivo by the presenilin 1 and 2 and APP mutations linked to familial Alzheimer's disease. Nat Med 1996; 2: 864–870.

33. Borchelt, D.R. et al.: Familial Alzheimer's disease-linked presenilin 1 variants elevate Abeta1-42/1-40 ratio in vitro and in vivo. Neuron 1996; 17: 1005–1013.

34. Citron, M. et al.: Mutant presenilins of Alzheimer's disease increase production of 42-residue amyloid beta-protein in both transfected cells and transgenic mice. Nat Med 1997; 3: 67–72.

35. Duff, K. et al.: Increased amyloid β42(43) in brains of mice expressing mutant presenilin 1. Nature 1996; 383: 710–713.

36. De Strooper, B. et al.: Deficiency of presenilin-1 inhibits the normal cleavage of amyloid precursor protein. Nature 1998; 391: 387–390.

37. Wolfe, M.S. et al.: Two transmembrane aspartates in presenilin-1 required for presenilin endoproteolysis and gamma-secretase activity. Nature 1999; 398: 513–517.

38. Games, D. et al.: Alzheimer-type neuropathology in transgenic mice overexpressing V717F beta-amyloid precursor protein. Nature 1995; 373: 523–527.

39. Hsiao, K. et al.: Correlative memory deficits, Abeta elevation, and amyloid plaques in transgenic mice. Science 1996; 274: 99–102.

40. Holcomb, L. et al.: Accelerated Alzheimer-type phenotype in transgenic mice carrying both mutant amyloid precursor protein and presenilin 1 transgenes. Nat Med 1998; 4: 97–100.

41. Borchelt, D.R. et al.: Accelerated amyloid deposition in the brains of transgenic mice coexpressing mutant presenilin 1 and amyloid precursor proteins. Neuron 1997; 19: 939–945.

42. Wavrant-De Vrieze, F. et al.: Genetic variability at the amyloid-beta precursor protein locus may contribute to the risk of late-onset Alzheimer's disease. Neurosci Lett 1999; 269: 67–70.

43. Olson, J.M. et al.: The amyloid precursor protein locus and very-late-onset Alzheimer disease. Am J Hum Genet 2001; 69: 895–899.

44. Bales, K.R. et al.: Lack of apolipoprotein E dramatically reduces amyloid beta-peptide deposition. Nat Genet 1997; 17: 263–264.

45. Myers, A. et al.: Susceptibility locus for Alzheimer's disease on chromosome 10. Science 2000; 290: 2304–2305.

46. Ertekin-Taner, N. et al.: Linkage of plasma Abeta42 to a quantitative locus on chromosome 10 in late-onset Alzheimer's disease pedigrees. Science 2000; 290: 2303–2304.

47. Wilhelmsen, K.C. et al.: Localization of disinhibition-dementia-parkinsonism-amyotrophy complex to 17q21-22. Am J Hum Genet 1994; 55: 1159–1165.

48. Foster, N.L. et al.: Frontotemporal dementia and parkinsonism linked to chromosome 17: a consensus conference. Conference participants. Ann Neurol 1997; 41: 706–715.

49. Spillantini, M.G.; Bird, T.D.; Ghetti, B.: Frontotemporal dementia and Parkinsonism linked to chromosome 17: a new group of tauopathies. Brain Pathol 1998; 8: 387–402.

50. Poorkaj, P. et al.: Tau is a candidate gene for chromosome 17 frontotemporal dementia. Ann Neurol 1998; 43: 815–825.

51. Baker, M. et al.: Localization of fronto-temporal dementia with parkinsonism in an Australian pedigree to chromosome 17q21-22. Ann Neurol 1997; 42: 794–798.

52. Hutton, M. et al.: Coding and splice donor site mutations in tau cause autosomal dominant dementia (FTDP-17). Nature 1998; 393: 702–705.

53. Hardy, J. et al.: Genetic dissection of Alzheimer's disease and related dementias: amyloid and its relationship to tau. Nat Neurosci 1998; 1: 95–99.

54. Lewis, J. et al.: Neurofibrillary tangles, amyotrophy and progressive motor disturbance in mice expressing mutant (P301L) tau protein. Nat Genet 2000; 25: 402–405.

55. Lewis, J. et al.: Enhanced neurofibrillary degeneration in transgenic mice expressing mutant tau and APP. Science 2001; 293: 1487–1491.

56. Lilius, L. et al.: Tau gene polymorphisms and apolipoprotein E epsilon4 may interact to increase risk for Alzheimer's disease. Neurosci Lett 1999; 277: 29–32.

57. Baker, M. et al.: Association of an extended haplotype in the tau gene with Progressive Supranuclear Palsy. Hum Mol Genet 1999; 4: 711–715.

58. Houlden, H. et al.: Corticobasal degeneration and progressive supranuclear palsy share a common tau haplotype. Neurology 2001; 56: 1702–1706.

59. Conrad, C. et al.: Genetic evidence for the involvement of tau in progressive supranuclear palsy. Ann Neurol 1997; 41: 277–281.

60. Golbe, L.I. et al.: The Contursi kindred, a large family with autosomal dominant Parkinson's disease: implications of clinical and molecular studies. Adv Neurol 1999; 80: 165–170.

61. Muenter, M.D. et al.: Hereditary form of parkinsonism—dementia. Ann Neurol 1998; 43: 768–781.

62. Polymeropoulos, M.H. et al.: Mapping of a gene for Parkinson's disease to chromosome 4q21-q23. Science 1996; 274: 1197–1199.

63. Polymeropoulos, M.H. et al.: Mutation in the alpha-synuclein gene identified in families with Parkinson's disease. Science 1997; 276: 2045–2047.

64. Spillantini, M.G. et al.: Alpha-synuclein in Lewy bodies. Nature 1997; 388: 839–840.

65. Masliah, E. et al.: Dopaminergic loss and inclusion body formation in alpha-synuclein mice: implications for neurodegenerative disorders. Science 2000; 287: 1265–1269.

66. Masliah, E. et al.: Beta-amyloid peptides enhance alpha-synuclein accumulation and neuronal deficits in a transgenic mouse model linking Alzheimer's disease and Parkinson's disease. Proc Natl Acad Sci USA 2001; 98: 12245–12250.

67. Chiba-Falek, O.; Nussbaum, R.L.: Effect of allelic variation at the NACP-Rep1 repeat upstream of the alpha-synuclein gene (SNCA) on transcription in a cell culture luciferase reporter system. Hum Mol Genet 2001; 10: 3101–3109.

68. Farrer, M. et al.: α-synuclein gene haplotypes are associated with Parkinson's disease. Hum Mol Genet 2001; 10: 1847–1851.
69. Kruger, R. et al.: Increased susceptibility to sporadic Parkinson's disease by a certain combined alpha-synuclein/apolipoprotein E genotype. Ann Neurol 1999; 45: 611–617.
70. Hardy, J. Pathways to primary neurodegenerative disease. Mayo Clin Proc 1999; 74: 835–837.
71. Gwinn-Hardy, K.: Genetics of parkinsonism. Mov Disord 2002; 17: 645–656.

2

Neuropathology of Alzheimer's Disease

Christian Schultz, Kelly Del Tredici, and Heiko Braak

INTRODUCTION

Alzheimer's disease (AD) is a progressive neurodegenerative and dementing disorder that can be detected clinically only in its end phase. AD is the most widespread type of dementia and affects about 10% of individuals older than 65 years and about 40% of individuals older than 80 years of age *(1,2)*. The earliest sign of AD is a subtle decline in memory functions in a state of clear consciousness. Mental capabilities gradually worsen and personality changes appear, followed by deterioration of language functions, impairment of visuospatial tasks, and, in the disease's final stages, dysfunction of the motor system in the form of a hypokinetic-hypertonic syndrome.

A definitive diagnosis of AD based on clinical observations is impossible and requires confirmation by postmortem examination. One of the neuropathological hallmarks of AD is comprised of extracellular precipitations of the β-amyloid peptide *(3,4)*, which is derived from the amyloid precursor protein (APP) by proteolytic cleavage.

The second acknowledged neuropathological hallmark of AD is the presence of neurofibrillary inclusions composed of an abnormally phosphorylated and aggregated microtubule-associated tau protein *(5–7)*. The lesions develop in the form of neurofibrillary tangles (NFTs, first described and depicted by Aloys Alzheimer) and neuropil threads (NTs). Such neurofibrillary pathology is not unique to AD, but is also seen in other diseases that are collectively designated as "tauopathies." These other disorders that make up this group are distinct from AD in that different brain areas are affected and abundant tau-positive inclusions in glial cells are present *(8,9)*. A heterogeneous group of hereditary tauopathies, referred to as "frontotemporal dementia" and "parkinsonism linked to chromosome 17 (FTDP-17)," is caused by dominant mutations in the tau gene *(10)*. This genetic link underscores the significance of tau dysfunction as a pathogenic factor that can cause neurodegeneration and dementia in humans. AD-related neurofibrillary changes are closely associated with neuronal cell loss and correlate well with the severity of clinical symptoms *(11–13)*. The destructive process that underlies the neurofibrillary pathology in AD commences in a few susceptible types of nerve cells in predisposed cortical induction sites and subsequently invades other portions of the cerebral cortex and specific sets of subcortical nuclei. The pathological changes evolve according to a predictable topographic sequence with little variation among individuals *(6,14–18)*.

ANATOMICAL CONSIDERATIONS

Understanding of the significance of Alzheimer-related lesions can be facilitated by using schematic diagrams of the major cortical pathways that become involved (Fig. 1). The human cerebral cortex is not a uniform entity; rather, it is composed of two divisions: an extensive neocortex and a small allocortex. The allocortex includes limbic system centers, such as the hippocampal formation and the entorhinal region, both of which are interconnected with the subcortical nuclear complex of the amyg-

From: *Current Clinical Neurology,*
Alzheimer's Disease: A Physician's Guide to Practical Management
Edited by: R. W. Richter and B. Zoeller Richter © Humana Press Inc., Totowa, NJo

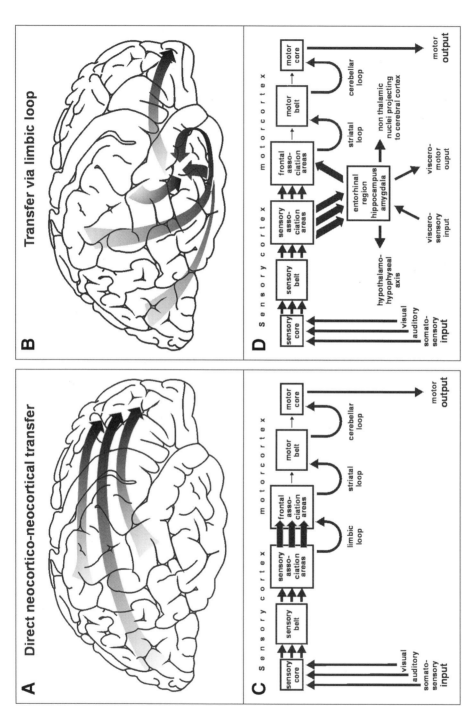

Fig. 1. Two pathways for transfer of somatosensory, visual, and auditory information to the prefrontal cortex are shown schematically in (**A**) and (**B**), and as block diagrams, including subsequent data flow through motor areas, in (**C**) and (**D**). The bulk of the sensory data is transferred directly via long cortico-cortical pathways, as depicted in (**A**) and (**C**), but data entering the prefrontal cortex following processing in the limbic loop in (**B**) and (**D**) are essential for endowing the sensory information with significance as well as vital for processes involving memory, motivation, and emotion. In both cases, data are transferred through primary and secondary areas of the neocortex to a variety of related association areas. From the prefrontal cortex, data flow to the secondary and primary motor fields occurs primarily by way of the striatal and cerebellar loops.

dala. The parietal, occipital, and temporal territories of the neocortex are each comprised of a primary area, a belt of secondary fields, and related higher-order association areas *(19,20)*. Visual, auditory, and somatosensory information proceeds through the respective primary and secondary fields to a variety of related association areas and is then conveyed by long cortico-cortical pathways to the prefrontal cortex (Fig. 1A,C). These data are then transferred through the premotor areas to the primary motor field. The major pathways for this continual data flow are the striatal and the cerebellar loops, which integrate the basal ganglia, many nuclei of the lower brainstem, and the cerebellum into the regulation of cortical output. Some of the exteroceptive data that flow from the sensory association areas to the prefrontal neocortex converge on the entorhinal region and amygdala by way of multiple cortical relay stations. These connections comprise the afferent trunk of the limbic loop, thereby making the neocortex the chief source of input to the human limbic system. The data are subsequently processed by the entorhinal region, amygdala, and hippocampal formation, which represent the principal governing entities within the limbic system. Projections from all components of the limbic loop supply the efferent trunk, which exerts important influence on the prefrontal cortex (Fig. 1B,D). The limbic loop centers play significant roles in memory functions as well as in the maintenance of emotional equilibrium. Notably, these centers are the sites that are most prone to develop Alzheimer-related neurofibrillary lesions.

INTRANEURONAL AGGREGATION OF ABNORMALLY PHOSPHORYLATED TAU PROTEIN

AD-related cytoskeletal alterations result from the formation of an abnormally phosphorylated and aggregated tau protein within a few susceptible classes of neurons. In healthy nerve cells, the tau protein stabilizes microtubular components of the neuronal cytoskeleton that are involved in transporting substances between cellular compartments. Destabilization of the microtubules and obstruction of axonal transport owing to the formation of abnormal tau protein probably result in inappropriate protein metabolism, synaptic malfunction, and impaired signaling by retrograde neurotrophic factors. Decline in these functions may contribute significantly to neuronal death *(21–23)*. The initial product of the pathological phosphorylation is a soluble nonargyrophilic tau protein. In this state, the protein is evenly distributed throughout the cytoplasm of the afflicted nerve cells (group 1 in Fig. 2), which do not yet exhibit any obvious morphological alterations *(24,25)*. Such neurons in the "pretangle" phase appear initially in the transentorhinal region, the site of the earliest cortical AD-related lesions. The later stages of tangle formation are characterized by an aggregation of the abnormal tau protein and the appearance of insoluble argyrophilic precipitates (groups 2 and 3 in Fig. 2). The distal dendritic segments of involved cells become abnormally curved, dilated, and probably detached from the proximal stem. Gracile NTs appear within the twisted dendrites and NFT formation begins in the soma. The argyrophilic fibrillary material accumulates gradually, fills large portions of the cytoplasm, and occasionally extends into the proximal dendrites. After deterioration of the parent cell, the pathological material remains visible in the tissue as an extraneuronal tangle ("ghost tangle"; groups 4 and 5 in Fig. 2).

STAGES IN THE DEVELOPMENT OF NEUROFIBRILLARY TANGLES AND NEUROPIL THREADS

Pathoarchitectonic analyses demonstrate that the destructive process begins in predisposed cortical induction sites, then infiltrates other portions of the cerebral cortex and specific subcortical nuclei in a consistent, predictable topographic sequence *(6,15,26)*. Specific projection cells of the transentorhinal region are the first cortical neurons to become involved in the pathological process. The lesions advance from the transentorhinal region and gradually appear in the entorhinal region proper, the hippocampal formation, amygdala, in higher-order multimodal association areas of the neocortex, and eventually in the primary motor area as well as primary sensory fields. This topographic sequence is remarkably consistent across cases. Through postmortem examination of the distribution pattern and

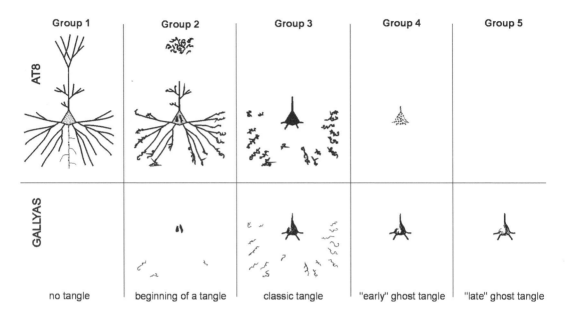

Fig. 2. Schematic drawing that summarizes AT8 immunostaining for abnormally phosphorylated tau protein with the corresponding Gallyas silver staining. The progression of pathological alterations of the neuronal cytoskeleton is shown from group 1 neuron to group 5 structure. Fine dots indicate granular AT8 immunostaining, whereas large dots represent degenerating terminals attached to the disintegrated cell body. Ghost tangles gradually lose anti-tau immunoreactivity (groups 4 and 5). Reprinted with permission from Heidelberg *(25)*. © Springer-Verlag GmbH & Co. KG.

severity of the cytoskeletal pathology, six stages in the evolution of the neurofibrillary changes have been differentiated *(6,27)*. Since 1997, these stages have been integrated into the consensus recommendations for the postmortem diagnosis of AD by the National Institutes on Aging and by the Reagan Institute Working Group *(28,29)*. In a biochemical study, the predictable sequence of AD-related neurofibrillary lesions was reproduced using Western blot detection of the abnormally phosphorylated and aggregated tau protein *(30)*.

Transentorhinal Stages I and II

The transentorhinal region, normally hidden in the depths of the rhinal sulcus, is the first cortical region to exhibit neurofibrillary changes. This region represents the portal for neocortical information that enters the limbic loop *(20)*. In stage I, the lesions are confined to a few projection cells at this site (Fig. 3A). Increased transentorhinal involvement, together with modest participation of the entorhinal region proper and the first Ammon's horn sector, are seen in stage II (Fig. 3B,C). This limited destruction does not yet manifest itself in the form of clinical symptoms. Accordingly, stages I and II represent the silent, preclinical phase of the disease *(31)*.

Limbic Stages III and IV

Severe affection of the transentorhinal and entorhinal regions is the central feature of stage III (Fig. 3D). Moderate alterations occur in the hippocampal formation, in temporal and insular proneocortical areas, and in a few subcortical nuclei. The mature neocortex remains virtually free of neurofibrillary changes. In stage IV, the destructive process progresses from the entorhinal territory into adjoining higher-order association areas of the neocortex (Fig. 3E,F). The lesions that typify both of these stages are capable of producing the first clinically detectable functional deficits, because they hamper the data exchange between the sensory association fields, the higher-order components of the limbic system, and the prefrontal cortex. Connections between components of the limbic loop are interrupted at multiple sites, and the influence of the limbic system on the prefrontal cortex becomes markedly reduced. Many patients with stage III or IV pathology exhibit mental deterioration and subtle personality aberrations, whereas in others, the appearance of symptoms still may be obscured by individual reserve capacities *(13)*. Because of the common occurrence of initial clinical symptoms and characteristic brain lesions, stage III or IV is regarded as representing the morphological counterpart of incipient AD *(11,32–35)*.

The Neocortical Stages V and VI

At present, the initial diagnosis of AD by physicians is usually made when patients are in the final phase of the illness, corresponding to stages V and VI (Fig. 3G–I). The hallmark of stage V is the widespread devastation of the neocortex (Fig. 3G). From inferior temporal areas, the lesions spread superolaterally, and large numbers of NFTs/NTs gradually infest the extended multimodal association areas of the neocortex. Only the acoustic system, the primary motor field, primary sensory areas, and unimodal secondary fields remain uninvolved or sustain only mild damage. In stage VI, the pathological process even penetrates into these fields. The end stages of AD are accompanied by a macroscopically detectable cortical atrophy, ventricular widening, and a notable loss in brain weight. With the degeneration of the neocortex, patients become severely demented *(13)*, and major autonomic dysfunctions reflect the far-reaching devastation of the limbic loop centers.

PREVALENCE OF AD-RELATED NEUROFIBRILLARY CHANGES IN NONSELECTED AUTOPSY BRAINS

Age continues to be acknowledged as the single most important risk factor for AD. The relationship between age and AD-related neurofibrillary changes was studied in a large number of nonselected brains at autopsy ($n = 2661$) *(27)*. By extending this previously published sample, the diagram in Fig. 4 summarizes the NFT stages of 5089 nonselected brains collected postmortally between 1986 and 2002. The columns show the percentage of cases in transentorhinal, limbic, or isocortical stages for the respective age groups. The diagram illustrates a continuum of lesions, beginning with the first NFT at stage I and going on to include the massive destruction seen in fully developed AD at stage VI. The fact that NFTs/NTs occur in a very large proportion of the aging population does not detract from their insidious nature, nor should it mislead us to view them as normal concomitants of aging *(10,28)*. There are considerable interindividual differences regarding the point at which the first "pretangle"-phase neurons begin to develop. The preclinical stages occasionally can be detected at a surprisingly young age. Approximately 23% of individuals in the age group from 30 to 39 years exhibit abnormal changes corresponding to stage I or II. The earliest lesions occur in young, otherwise healthy brains. Several decades elapse between the onset of histologically verifiable lesions and those phases of the illness in which the damage is extensive enough for clinical symptoms to become apparent *(36)*.

SELECTIVE VULNERABILITY IN ALZHEIMER'S DISEASE

The destructive process that underlies AD not only affects specific areas, layers, and subcortical nuclei but also targets only a few of the many types of nerve cells in the human brain *(26)*. It still is not known why some kinds of neurons tend to develop NFTs/NTs, whereas others do not do so until the last stages of the disease.

It has been postulated that neurofibrillary changes are a secondary phemomenon induced by the toxic influence of extracellular β-amyloid deposits designated as "plaques" (review in ref. *4*). Nonetheless, this hypothesis is fraught with inconsistencies. The brain regions, for example, that are most susceptible to the neurofibrillary changes are the ones that are relatively resistant to β-amyloid deposition. For instance, as detailed above, the entorhinal cortex and hippocampal formation are affected by neurofibrillary pathology in the early stages of AD. By contrast, these same regions

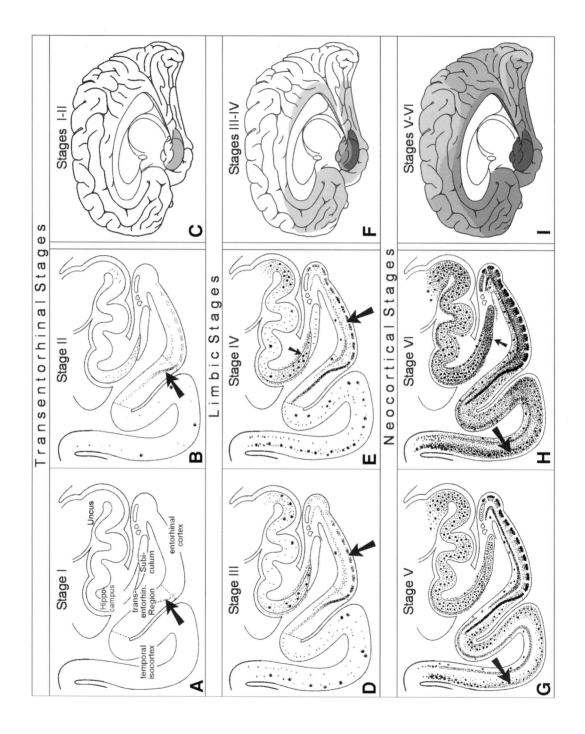

Transentorhinal Stages

A — Stage I
temporal isocortex
Uncus
Hippocampus
trans- entorhin. Region
Subiculum
entorhinal cortex

B — Stage II

C — Stages I-II

Limbic Stages

D — Stage III

E — Stage IV

F — Stages III-IV

Neocortical Stages

G — Stage V

H — Stage VI

I — Stages V-VI

26

develop amyloid plaques only in advanced stages of β-amyloid deposition *(37)*. In comparison to neurofibrillary changes the initial β-amyloid deposits evolve in a rather widespread, unpredictable manner and are capable of appearing in nearly any neocortical region *(31,38)*.

During the search for other putative pathogenic factors in AD, it was observed that most of the neuronal types with a propensity for succumbing to the neurofibrillary changes mature late during ontogenesis of the human brain *(39)*. In the cerebral cortex, all NFT-bearing nerve cells belong to the class of pyramidal neurons, and those with long ipsilateral cortico-cortical connections are particularly prone to become involved. In subcortical nuclei, most of the vulnerable cells are also characterized by a conspicuously lengthy axon *(40)*. Late-myelinating cortical areas and layers develop NFTs and NTs earlier and at higher densities than those that commence myelination early. As such, the pathological changes in AD develop in the inverse sequence of cortical myelination during early development of the brain *(39)*.

ANIMAL MODELS OF ALZHEIMER-RELATED NEUROPATHOLOGY

Because of the limitations imposed on experimental studies of the human brain, the question of whether AD-related changes can be investigated in experimental animals is of considerable importance. Amyloid plaques can be induced in transgenic mice that express APP mutations causing autosomal dominant forms of AD in humans (review in ref. *41*). These transgenic mice have provided insights into the pathogenesis and possible treatment of β-amyloid deposition *(41)*. Recent studies have succeeded in generating authentic NFTs in transgenic mice that express human FTDP-17-associated mutations *(42)*. The severity of neurofibrillary changes in FTDP-17 mice is augmented by cortical injections of fibrillar β-amyloid *(43)*. Likewise, the density of NFTs is increased in mice which are carriers of both FTDP-17 and AD-related APP mutations *(44)*. These murine models serve as a means for elucidating possible modulating effects of β-amyloid on the expression of NFTs.

All of the transgenic models are inherently limited by the large phylogenetic gap that exists between the murine brain and that of humans. Nonhuman primate models could help to narrow this gap. In this context, it is of interest to note that a conspicuous pattern of tau pathology was recently revealed in baboons *(45–47)*. The tau pathology in these nonhuman primates preferentially affects neurons and glial cells in the medial temporal lobe. In some of the older animals, a specific pattern of tau pathology was noted in the entorhinal cortex, resembling an early stage of AD-related pathology (Fig. 5A–C). Filamentous tau-positive inclusions accumulated in the dentate granule cells of a 30-year-old animal (Fig. 5D–G).

The aged baboon thus provides a potentially valuable nonhuman primate model for studies of the pathogenesis of selective neuronal tau pathology as it is characteristic of all human tauopathies, including AD. Experiments on both transgenic mice and nonhuman primates may complement one another, thereby helping to pinpoint pathogenic factors that underlie the neurofibrillary pathology in the aging human brain.

SUMMARY

The neuropathological hallmarks of AD are comprised of extracellular and intracellular precipitations of insoluble protein aggregates. Extracellular aggregates consist of the β-amyloid peptide, which is derived from amyloid precursor protein. Intracellular neurofibrillary inclusions are composed of abnormally phosphorylated and aggregated microtubule-associated tau protein. The intracellular lesions develop in the form of neurofibrillary tangles and neuropil threads. The overall amount of these

---

Fig. 3. *(see opposite page)* Distribution pattern of neurofibrillary changes in the course of AD. On the left and in the middle, typical lesions observed in cross sections of the hippocampus, entorhinal region, and temporal neocortex are shown schematically as they appear in appropriately stained sections for each of the six stages in the development of neurofibrillary tangles and neuropil threads. Arrows designate key features discussed in the text. On the right, locations and density of lesions are indicated by shading on medial views of a right hemisphere.

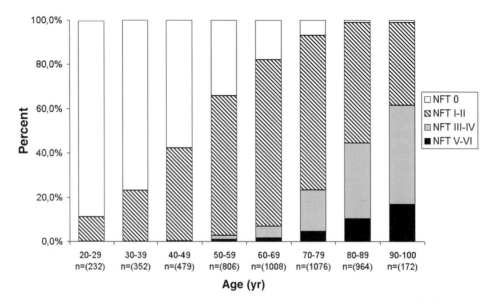

Fig. 4. Procentual frequency of the six stages in the development of AD-related neurofibrillary changes in 5089 nonselected autopsy cases (shown by 10-year age groups). Frequency and severity of the lesions increase with age. The early transentorhinal stages I/II are very common, whereas the symptomatic end stages V and VI are confined largely to elderly age groups. NFT, neurofibrillary tangles.

neurofibrillary changes correlates well with the severity of neuronal cell loss and clinical symptoms. Specific neuronal subsets of the limbic system are most prone to neurofibrillary changes. The lesions advance in a predictable manner from the transentorhinal region and gradually appear in the entorhinal region proper, the hippocampal formation, amygdala, and finally in higher-order association areas of the neocortex. Through postmortem examination, six stages in the evolution of neurofibrillary changes can be differentiated. Several decades elapse between the onset of histologically verifiable lesions and those stages of the illness in which the damage is extensive enough for clinical symptoms to become apparent. The causes underlying the selective vulnerability in AD are still undetermined. The recent identification of authentic tau pathology in transgenic mice and nonhuman primates may lead to experimental studies increasing our knowledge of these enigmatic changes.

ACKNOWLEDGMENTS

This study was supported by Deutsche Forschungsgemeinschaft, Bundesministerium für Bildung, Wissenschaft, Forschung und Technologie, and Degussa of Hanau. The skillful assistance of Miss I. Szász (drawings) is gratefully acknowledged.

Fig. 5. *(see facing page)* Tau pathology in baboons as detected by AT8-immunostaining (**A–D**) and by Gallyas silver staining (**E–G**) (100-μm-thick sections). (**A–C**) Tau pathology in a 25-year-old baboon. (**A**) Low-power view demonstrating AT8-ir changes in the basal medial temporal lobe (framed box). (**B**) The changes preferentially affect the fascia dentata (FD) and the projections neurons in the lamina II of the entorhinal cortex (EC). The subiculum (S) remains virtually untouched; mild involvement is seen in the first Ammon's horn sector (CA1). (**C**) Multipolar projection neurons of entorhinal layer II (Pre-α) with aberrant somatodendritic localization of abnormal tau protein. (**D–G**) Neurofibrillary changes in a 30-year-old male baboon. (**D**) A dense accumulation of AT8-positive cytoskeletal changes is noted in the hippocampal formation (framed). (**E**) Layer-specific accumulation of Gallyas-positive neurofibrillary tangles in the granule cell layer (traced out by arrowheads). (**F**) Typical crescent-shaped NFT located in the granule cell layer. (**G**) Large NFT in the hilus (arrow). Scale bar in (**A**) also applies for (**D**). (**A–C** reproduced with permission from *[46]* with permission from Elsevier Science, © 2000; **D–G** reproduced with permission from the *Journal of Neuropathology and Experimental Neurology [45]*.)

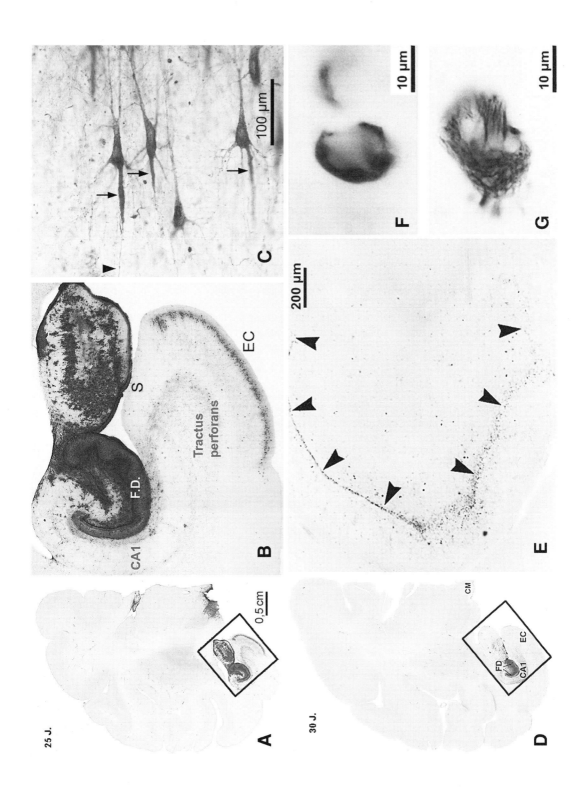

29

REFERENCES

1. Evans, D.A. et al.: Prevalence of Alzheimer's disease in a community population of older persons. Higher than previously reported. JAMA 1989; 262: 2551–2556.

2. McKhann, G. et al.: Clinical diagnosis of Alzheimer's disease: report of the NINCDS-ADRDA Work Group under the auspices of Department of Health and Human Services Task Force on Alzheimer's Disease. Neurology 1984; 34: 939–944.

3. Beyreuther, K.; Masters, C.L.: Amyloid precursor protein (APP) and beta amyloid-4 amyloid in the etiology of Alzheimer's disease: precursor product relationships in the derangement of neuronal function. Brain Pathol 1991; 1: 241–252.

4. Selkoe, D.J.: Alzheimer's disease: genes, proteins, and therapy. Physiol Rev 2001; 81: 741–766.

5. Arriagada, P.V. et al.: Neurofibrillary tangles but not senile plaques parallel duration and severity of Alzheimer's disease. Neurology 1992; 42: 631–639.

6. Braak, H.; Braak, E.: Neuropathological stageing of Alzheimer-related changes. Acta Neuropathol 1991; 82: 239–259.

7. Esiri, M.M. et al.: Aging and dementia. In: Graham, D.L.; Lantos, P.I. (eds.): Greenfield's neuropathology. Arnold, London, 1997: 153–234.

8. Feany, M.B., et al.: Neurodegenerative disorders with extensive tau pathology: a comparative study and review. Ann Neurol 1996; 40: 139–148.

9. Ikeda, K. et al.: Glial tau pathology in neurodegenerative diseases: their nature and comparison with neuronal tangles. Neurobiol Aging 1998; 19: S85–S91.

10. Hutton, M. et al.: Association of missense and 5'-splice-site mutations in tau with the inherited dementia FTDP-17. Nature 1998; 393: 702–705.

11. Bancher, C. et al.: Neuropathological staging of Alzheimer lesions and intellectual status in Alzheimer's and Parkinson's disease. Neurosci Lett 1993; 162: 179–182.

12. Price, J.L.; Morris, J.C.: Tangles and plaques in non-demented aging and "preclinical" Alzheimer's disease. Ann Neurol 1999; 45: 358–368.

13. Riley, K.P. et al.: Alzheimer's neurofibrillary pathology and the spectrum of cognitive function: findings from the Nun Study. Ann Neurol 2002; 51: 567–577.

14. Kemper, T.L.: Senile dementia: a focal disease in the temporal lobe. In: Nandy, E. (ed.): Senile dementia: a biomedical approach. Elsevier, Amsterdam, 1978: 105–113.

15. Hyman, B.T. et al.: Alzheimer's disease: cell-specific pathology isolates the hippocampal formation. Science 1984; 225: 1168–1170.

16. Hyman, B.T. et al.: Memory-related neural systems in Alzheimer's disease: An anatomic study. Neurology 1990; 40: 1721–1730.

17. van Hoesen, G.W.; Hyman, B.T.: Hippocampal formation: anatomy and the patterns of pathology in Alzheimer's disease. Progr Brain Res 1990; 83: 445–457.

18. van Hoesen, G.W. et al.: Entorhinal cortex pathology in Alzheimer's disease. Hippocampus 1991; 1: 1–8.

19. Braak, H.; Braak, E.: Architectonics as seen by lipofuscin stains. In: Peters, A.; Jones, E.G. (eds.): Cerebral cortex. Vol. 1: Cellular organization of the cerebral cortex. Plenum Press, New York, 1984: 59–104.

20. Braak, H.; Braak, E.: Temporal sequence of Alzheimer's disease-related pathology. In: Peters, A.; Morrison, J.H. (eds.): Cerebral cortex. Vol. 14, Neurodegenerative and age-related changes in structure and function of the cerebral cortex. KluwerPlenum, New York, 1999: 475–512.

21. Goedert, M.: Tau protein and the neurofibrillary pathology of Alzheimer's disease. Trends Neurosci 1993; 16: 460–465.

22. Iqbal, K. et al.: Mechanism of neurofibrillary degeneration in Alzheimer's disease. Molec Neurobiol 1994; 9: 119–123.

23. Mandelkow, E.; Mandelkow, E.M.: Microtubules and microtubule-associated proteins. Curr Opin Cell Biol 1995; 7: 72–81.

24. Bancher, C. et al.: Accumulation of abnormally phosphorylated tau precedes the formation of neurofibrillary tangles in Alzheimer's disease. Brain Res 1989; 477: 90–99.

25. Braak, E. et al.: A sequence of cytoskeleton changes related to the formation of neurofibrillary tangles and neuropil threads. Acta Neuropathol 1994; 87: 554–567.

26. Hyman, B.T.; Gomez-Isla, T.: Alzheimer's disease is a laminar, regional, and neural system specific disease, not a global brain disease. Neurobiol Aging 1994; 15: 353–354.

27. Braak, H.; Braak, E.: Frequency of stages of Alzheimer-related lesions in different age categories. Neurobiol Aging 1997; 18: 351–357.

28. Hyman, B.T.; Trojanowski, J.Q.: Editorial on consensus recommendations for the postmortem diagnosis of Alzheimer disease from the National Institutes of Aging and the Reagan Institute Working Group on diagnostic criteria for the neuropathological assessment of Alzheimer disease. J Neuropathol Exp Neurol 1997; 56: 1095–1097.

29. Hyman, B.T.: New neuropathological criteria for Alzheimer's disease. Arch Neurol 1998; 55: 1174–1176.

30. Delacourte, A. et al.: The biochemical pathway of neurofibrillary degeneration in aging and Alzheimer's disease. Neurology 2000; 52: 1158–1165.

31. Delacourte, A. et al.: Non-overlapping but synergetic tau and APP pathologies in sporadic Alzheimer's disease. Neurology 2002; 59: 398–407.

32. Jellinger, K., et al.: Alzheimer lesions in the entorhinal region and isocortex in Parkinson's and Alzheimer's diseases. Ann NY Acad Sci 1991; 640: 203–209.
33. Duyckaerts, C. et al.: Diagnosis and staging of Alzheimer's disease in a prospective study involving aged individuals. Neurobiol Aging 1994 (suppl. 1); 15: 140–141.
34. Dickson, D.W. et al.: Identification of normal and pathological aging in prospectively studied non-demented elderly humans. Neurobiol Aging 1991; 13: 179–189.
35. Hulette, C.M. et al.: Neuropathological and neuropsychological changes in "normal" aging: evidence for preclinical Alzheimer disease in cognitively normal individuals. J Neuropathol Exp Neurol 1998; 57: 1168–1174.
36. Ohm, T.G. et al.: Close-meshed prevalence rates of different stages as a tool to uncover the rate of Alzheimer's disease-related neurofibrillary changes. Neuroscience 1995; 64: 209–217.
37. Thal, D.R. et al.: Sequence of A beta-protein deposition in the human medial temporal lobe. J Neuropathol Exp Neurol 2000; 59: 733–748.
38. Thal, D.R. et al.: Phases of A beta-deposition in the human brain and its relevance for the Development of AD. Neurology 2002; 58: 1791–1800.
39. Braak, H.; Braak, E.: Development of Alzheimer-related neurofibrillary changes in the neocortex inversely recapitulates cortical myelogenesis. Acta Neuropathol 1996; 92: 197–201.
40. Braak, H.; Braak, E.: Pathology of Alzheimer's disease. In: Calne, D.B. (ed.): Neurodegenerative diseases. Saunders, Philadelphia, 1994: 585–613.
41. Hock, B.J.; Lamb, B.T.: Transgenic mouse models of Alzheimer's disease. Trends Genet 2001; 17: S7–S12.
42. Ishihara, T. et al.: Age-dependent induction of congophilic neurofibrillary tau inclusions in tau transgenic mice. Am J Pathol 2001; 158: 555–562.
43. Götz, J. et al.: Formation of neurofibrillary tangles in P301l tau transgenic mice induced by Abeta 42 fibrils. Science 2001; 293: 1491–1495.
44. Lewis, J. et al.: Enhanced neurofibrillary degeneration in transgenic mice expressing mutant tau and APP. Science (2001); 293: 1487–1491.
45. Schultz, C. et al.: Filamentous tau pathology in nerve cells, astrocytes, and oligodendrocytes of aged baboons. J Neuropathol Exp Neurol 2000; 59: 39–52.
46. Schultz, C. et al.: Age-related progression of tau pathology in brains of baboons. Neurobiol Aging 2000; 21: 905–912.
47. Schultz, C. et al.: The brain of the aging baboon: a non-human primate model for neuronal and glial tau pathology. In: Erwin, J.M.; Hof, P.R. (eds.): Aging in non-human primates. Interdiscipl Top Gerontol, Vol. 31. Karger, Basel, 2002: 118–129.

3

Oxidative Stress in the Development
of Alzheimer's Disease and Other Dementias

Domenico Praticò

INTRODUCTION

Alzheimer's disease (AD) is the most common, complex, and challenging form of neurodegenerative disease associated with dementia in the elderly. As people live to older ages, AD is becoming a major medical and social concern. It affects approximately 4 million individuals in the United States and 16 million worldwide, with an incidence that doubles every 5 years, beyond the age of 65 *(1,2)*. A search of the National Institutes of Health database (Medline/PubMed) in December 2002 using the term "Alzheimer's disease" produced 34,800 citations. This finding clearly indicates the enormous amount of basic science, animal, and human research that has been devoted in recent years to the understanding of this devastating disease.

Although the initiating events are still unknown, it is clear that AD, at least in its sporadic form, results from the combination of genetic risk factors with different epigenetic events. Besides the pathological hallmarks of the disease, which include the accumulation of protein deposits in the brain as extracellular amyloid beta (Aβ) plaques and as neurofibrillary tangles (NFT) inside neurons, AD brains exhibit evidence of reactive-oxygen species (ROS)-mediated injury *(3,4)*. ROS are formed under normal conditions, and although they are chemically unstable and highly reactive, their levels are kept relatively low by efficient antioxidant systems. However, in some situations their generation can exceed the endogenous ability of the body to destroy them. As a consequence, the oxidative homeostasis is altered and oxidative stress is the final result *(5)*.

The brain is highly sensitive to oxidative stress because it is very rich in easily peroxidizable fatty acids, has a high request for oxygen, and a relative paucity of antioxidant systems. Further, it has a high content of transition metals and high ascorbate levels, which together act as potent pro-oxidants *(6)*. Depending on the substrate attacked by ROS, oxidative stress will manifest as protein oxidation, DNA oxidation, or lipid peroxidation. All of these signature markers of oxidative stress have been described in the AD brain, and a role for it has been widely discussed in the pathogenesis of AD *(5,7–9)*.

In general, oxidative damage in the central nervous system manifests predominantly as lipid peroxidation, because the brain has a very high lipid content and in particular high levels of polyunsaturated fatty acids that are easily susceptible to ROS attack *(7)*. In this chapter, I will review recent data supporting a role for oxidative stress in AD and other forms of dementia, with particular emphasis on lipid peroxidation.

LIPID PEROXIDATION

Lipid peroxidation is the mechanism by which lipids are attacked by ROS that have sufficient reactivity to abstract a hydrogen atom from a methylene carbon in their side chain. The greater the number

From: *Current Clinical Neurology,*
Alzheimer's Disease: A Physician's Guide to Practical Management
Edited by: R. W. Richter and B. Zoeller Richter © Humana Press Inc., Totowa, NJ

of double bonds in the molecule, the easier is the removal of the hydrogen atom. This explains why polyunsaturated fatty acids (PUFA) are particularly susceptible to oxidation. In the last 20 years, lipid peroxidation has become probably one of the most extensively investigated processes in biochemistry, and measurement of it is the evidence most frequently cited to support the involvement of oxidative stress in biology and medicine *(10)*.

Unfortunately, considerable confusion about the role of lipid peroxidation in human disease has been caused by lack of sensitivity, specificity, and inappropriate application to human material of assays that do not usually measure what they are supposed to measure *(11)*. A wide range of techniques is available to measure the rate of this process and the level of products of lipid peroxidation, but all of them have specific advantages and disadvantages *(12)*.

Isoprostanes are members of a complex family of lipids, isomers of conventional enzymatically derived prostaglandins, which are produced by ROS-catalyzed peroxidation of polyunsaturated fatty acids *(13)*. Most of the work has focused on a group of isomers of prostaglandin $F_{2\alpha}$, called F_2-isoprostanes (F_2-iPs), and abundant literature has established that their measurement provides a reliable marker of in vivo lipid peroxidation and oxidative stress *(14)*. F_2-iPs are present in detectable levels in all healthy animal and human biological fluids and tissues. This indicates a level of ongoing lipid peroxidation in the normal state, which is incompletely suppressed by the elaborate system of antioxidant defenses that have evolved to prevent oxidative stress. Several approaches have been employed to the measurement of F_2-iPs *(15)*. We developed assays for specific F_2-iP isomers using gas chromatography-mass spectrometry (GC/MS) assays and determined that the isoprostane $8,12$-iso-iPF$_{2\alpha}$-VI is the most abundant F_2-iP in humans as well as in animals *(16–18)*.

OXIDATIVE STRESS AND AD

There are a considerable number of published studies on lipid peroxidation in AD. Most of them have been performed on postmortem brain tissues, some using quantitative (biochemical) and some qualitative (histological) assays to demonstrate it. I will focus my presentation only on the quantitative analyses.

Historically, malonaldehyde (MDA) and the thiobarbituric acid-reactive substances (TBARS) assays have been the first techniques employed to quantitate biochemically lipid peroxidation in AD. The majority of these investigations have shown higher MDA and/or TBARS levels in AD than in control brains *(19–21)*. Several studies have attempted to measure serum and plasma levels of MDA in living patients with AD, but conflicting results were reported *(22,23)*. Another by-product of the oxidation of PUFA that has been quantified is 4-hydroxy-2-nonenal (4-HNE). Its levels have been reported elevated in AD brain tissue as well as in ventricular cerebrospinal fluid (CSF) *(24,25)*. However, its use in biological systems has been relatively limited, because its levels are generally low and there is a need for large quantities of sample in order to measure it.

Initially, we investigated levels of two distinct isoprostane isomers—iPF$_{2\alpha}$-III and iPF$_{2\alpha}$-VI—in postmortem brain tissue from AD patients and compared them with tissues of patients with other neurological diseases or neurologically healthy controls *(26)*. We found that the levels were markedly higher in both frontal and temporal poles, as well as in ventricular CSF of AD subjects compared with the other groups. Remarkably, no such difference was observed in cerebellum, an area traditionally devoid of the pathological hallmarks of the disease.

This study confirmed that oxidative stress is a feature of AD, and it localizes in areas specifically affected by the disease. However, it did not address the question of whether oxidative imbalance and subsequent lipid peroxidation are early components or final common steps of the neurodegenerative process. For this reason we collected urine, plasma, and CSF from subjects with clinical diagnosis of AD and age-matched controls *(27)*. We found that—compared with controls—AD patients had increased CSF, plasma, and urinary levels of $8,12$-iso-iPF$_{2\alpha}$-VI. Urinary and circulating plasma levels of this isoprostane correlated directly with the levels in CSF of AD patients, suggesting a common mechanism of formation: brain oxidative stress. Interestingly, we observed a direct correlation between CSF 8,12-iso-iPF$_{2\alpha}$-VI levels and CSF tau and an inverse correlation with the percentage of CSF Aβ_{1-42} in AD patients. Further, we found a significant correlation between 8,12-iso-iPF$_{2\alpha}$-VI CSF levels and the severity of the dementia in AD patients, as measured by two of the most common cognitive tests, the mini-mental state examination (MMSE) and the dementia severity rating (DSR) scale *(27)*.

Taken together, these findings suggest that elevation of this isoprostane not only is reflecting brain oxidative stress, but also correlates with the progression of the disease. In summary, our study supports the hypothesis that this phenomenon occurs early in the course of this dementing disorder, thereby implying that it might be a potential contributor to brain degeneration in AD. Further, the fact that urine correlated with CSF levels offers—for the first time—the potential for using a noninvasive tool to investigate brain oxidative damage and monitor therapeutic responses in AD. These findings were recently confirmed by another research group *(28)*.

To further confirm that brain oxidative imbalance is an early event in AD, we assayed levels of 8,12-iso-iPF$_{2\alpha}$-VI in young patients with Down's syndrome. These subjects exhibit increased concentration of Aβ in the brain and a precocious AD-like pathology and dementia later in life *(29)*. We found elevated 8,12-iso-iPF$_{2\alpha}$-VI levels in urine samples of subjects with Down's syndrome, correlating with the duration of the disease, compared with those of matched controls *(30)*.

It is well known that AD has a long mute stage of neuropathological changes and cognitive decline before it is diagnosed. In recent years, it has been shown that the onset of AD is often preceded by an interim phase, known as mild cognitive impairment (MCI). Despite a potential heterogeneity of an MCI diagnosis, some studies have suggested that this condition is associated with an up to 50% probability of progressing to symptomatic AD within a 4-year period *(31)*. Because MCI individuals are considered to be at high risk for progression to overt AD, we have investigated whether they already show signs of brain oxidative stress, measured as levels of this specific F$_2$-iP.

For this purpose we compared levels of 8,12-iso-iPF$_{2\alpha}$-VI in urine, plasma, and CSF of AD patients, MCI subjects, and age-matched controls *(32)*. First, we confirmed that AD patients had the highest levels of this marker among the three groups. However, we found that patients who meet standardized clinical criteria for MCI also have increased CSF, plasma, and urinary levels of 8,12-iso-iPF$_{2\alpha}$-VI, compared with cognitive normal elderly controls. In accordance with previous reports, we found that among the three groups studied, AD had the highest values for CSF tau and the lowest percentage of CSFβ_{1-42}. No significant difference was observed between MCI subjects and age-matched controls for both CSF markers. By contrast, MCI subjects had CSF 8,12-iso-iPF$_{2\alpha}$-VI levels significantly higher than controls. Taking into account that CSF tau and the percentage of CSF Aβ_{1-42} levels are considered to be good markers of pathological changes and disease progression *(33)*, this observation would further support the hypothesis that brain oxidative stress is present before the detection of the typical neuropathological changes of early AD.

Remarkably, in our study we found that MCI subjects are different from elderly controls with respect only to this marker of oxidative stress. This suggests that measurement of 8,12-iso-iPF$_{2\alpha}$-VI may provide a reliable biochemical marker that could help in identifying those MCI subjects who present with early brain oxidative stress. This subset of individuals could be at increased risk for progression to AD, and also the most responsive to antioxidant treatment. However, future longitudinal studies measuring this marker in MCI subjects are needed in order to test these hypotheses.

OXIDATIVE STRESS AND NON-AD DEMENTIA

There is a large group of neurodegenerative diseases associated with dementia that are histopathologically different from AD, and can be grouped under the general term of non-AD dementias. Among them, frontotemporal dementia (FTD) is probably the most representative. FTD is a heterogenous group of neurodegenerative conditions that accounts for 3–10% of all cases of dementia. Typically, all FTDs are characterized by a striking and profound degeneration of the frontal and temporal lobe, which is similar to the findings in AD *(34)*. However, while these brain regions are affected in most FTDs, several FTD subtypes have been proposed depending on the pathological involvement of other cortical, subcortical, white matter, and brainstem regions *(35–37)*. One of the most common sporadic FTD subtypes is known as dementia lacking distinctive histopathology (DLDH). Others include progressive supranuclear palsy (PSP), FTD with parkinsonism linked to chromosome 17 (FTD-17), and Pick's disease *(38)*. Despite this phenotypic heterogeneity, there are reports suggesting a role for oxidative stress in most cases of FTDs *(39,40)*, suggesting that, similar to AD, oxidative stress may be a common disease pathway or a final common step of the neurodegenerative process *(40)*.

Even though dementia in both AD and FTD is of neurodegenerative nature, their neuropathology appears to be significantly different. For instance, abundant NFT and amyloid plaques are diagnostic for AD, while some FTD variants have disease specific tau lesions (e.g., Pick's disease, Pick's bodies). Others again are not associated with tau or any other specific lesions (DLDH). All FTDs present several characteristic aspects of neurodegenerative disorders (e.g., neuronal loss, reactive astrocytosis, and microglia proliferation), which are considered to be common responses of the brain to different insults, such as oxidative stress and inflammation. However, conflicting results have been reported regarding the notion that oxidative stress also plays a role in most FTDs.

A possible explanation for these contrasting findings is that some of these studies used markers of lipid peroxidation known to lack specificity and sensitivity, such as MDA and TBARS assays *(41,42)*. For example, a study reported immunocytochemical and biochemical evidence for lipid peroxidation, but not protein oxidation or glycoxidation *(43)*. By contrast, another group, using an antiserum against 4-HNE pyrrole adducts, failed to show any positive immunostaining in PSP, and only a minimal reaction in one case of Pick's disease *(44)*.

To investigate whether an increase in brain lipid peroxidation is part of a generic response to neurodegeneration, we recently compared levels of 8,12-iso-iPF$_{2\alpha}$-VI in different brain regions from patients assigned a postmortem diagnosis of FTD, or AD, or age-matched normal elderly. In this study we demonstrated that brain levels of 8,12-iso-iPF$_{2\alpha}$-VI are significantly increased in AD, but not in any of the FTD subtypes considered, and no difference in the levels of this marker was found between FTD and controls. This was true when we analyzed each FTD subtype alone, and also when we divided all the subgroups into cases with and without tau deposition and abnormalities *(45)*.

These findings support the hypothesis that oxidative stress to the brain is highly specific for AD. It is not a uniform phenomenon across neurodegenerative diseases, even among those associated with similar clinical and pathological features, such as FTD. This suggests that mechanisms of diseases underlying FTD are not able to induce an increase in brain oxidative stress.

CONCLUSIONS

The fact that age is a risk factor for dementia has provided the initial basis for the involvement of oxidative stress in this disease. Although an increase in lipid peroxidation has been widely and extensively demonstrated in AD, conflicting results have been reported for non-AD dementias. This is because for many years our understanding of the role of oxidative stress in neurodegeneration has been hampered by the lack of sensitivity and specificity of many of the assays used for measurements. However, although some traditional views maintain that oxidative stress is the simple result of neurodegeneration, the contribution of ROS-mediated reactions to neuronal loss in AD and non-AD dementias is now beginning to be elucidated. F$_2$-isoprostanes are a new class of lipids derived from the peroxidation of PUFA. Consistent data have been accumulated that clearly pinpoint the measurement of these molecules as a reliable and noninvasive approach for studying oxidative stress in vivo.

Today we have consistent evidence to support the concept that oxidative stress to the brain is not a general and final common pathway of the neurodegenerative process. It may, in contrast, involve specific mechanism(s) characteristic of the disease process, which are present in AD but not in other forms of dementia. Thus, oxidative stress is an early damaging event during the evolution of AD, and it might play a more important role in the pathogenesis of AD than in non-AD dementias. This new concept provides a rational basis for therapeutic intervention with potent antioxidants in AD patients at the earliest stage of the disease.

SUMMARY

As people worldwide live to an older age, dementia, whose best-known risk factor is aging, has become a serious growing public health problem. Although AD is the most frequent cause of dementia, other progressive neurodegenerative disorders can be responsible for it. For these reasons they are grouped as non-AD dementias. There is evidence that reactive-oxygen species-mediated reactions, particularly of neuronal lipids, are present in brains of both kinds of dementing disorders. Traditional views claim that oxidative-mediated brain injury in these diseases is the mere result of neurodegeneration. Although numerous investigations have shown that oxidative stress is increased in AD, conflicting results exist for the heterogeneous group of non-AD dementias. The availability of specific and sensitive markers to monitor in vivo oxidative stress, in combination with studies performed in living patients, are helping us to elucidate these issues. In this chapter, I have summarized some of the most recent research on the relevance that oxidative stress and lipid peroxidation have in AD and non-AD dementias. The evidence accumulated so far clearly indicates that oxidative stress is an early and specific aspect of AD but not other forms of dementia. This new concept implies that this phenomenon is not a general and common pathway of the neurodegenerative process, but it may play a more important role in AD than in non-AD dementias.

ACKNOWLEDGMENTS

Part of the work described in this chapter has been supported by grants from the National Institutes of Health and the American Heart Association.

REFERENCES

1. Clark, C.M.: Clinical manifestations and diagnostic evaluation of patients with Alzheimer s disease. In: Clark, C.M.; Trojanowski, J.Q. (eds.): Neurodegenerative dementias: clinical features and pathological mechanisms. McGraw-Hill, New York, 2000: 95–114.
2. Zabar, Y.; Kawas, C.H.: Epidemiology and clinical genetics of Alzheimer's disease. In: Clark, C.M.; Trojanowski, J.Q. (eds.): Neurodegenerative dementias: clinical features and pathological mechanisms. McGraw-Hill, New York, 2000: 79–94.
3. Khachaturian, Z.S.: Diagnosis of Alzheimer's disease. Arch Neurol 1985; 42: 1097–1105.
4. Praticò, D.; Trojanowski, J.Q.: Inflammatory hypotheses: novel mechanisms of Alzheimer's neurodegeneration and new therapeutic targets? Neurobiol Aging 2000; 21: 441–445.
5. Praticò, D.; Delanty, N.: Oxidative injury in diseases of the central nervous system: focus on Alzheimer's disease. Am J Med 2000; 109: 577–585.
6. Floyd, R.A.: Antioxidants, oxidative stress, and degenerative neurological disorders. Proc Soc Exp Biol Med 1999; 222: 236–245.
7. Praticò, D.: Alzheimer's disease and oxygen radicals: new insights. Biochem Pharmacol 2002; 63: 563–567.
8. Smith, M.A. et al.: Oxidative stress in Alzheimer's disease. Biochim Biophys Acta 2000; 1502: 139–144.
9. Christen, Y.: Oxidative stress and Alzheimer's disease. Am J Clin Nutr 2000; 71: 621S–629S.
10. Halliwell, B.; Chirico, S.: Lipid peroxidation: its mechanism, measurement, and significance. Am J Clin Nutr 1993; 57: 715S–725S.
11. Halliwell, B.; Gutteridge, J.M.C.: Free radicals in biology and medicine, 3rd ed. Oxford University Press, Oxford, 1999.
12. Praticò, D.: Lipid peroxidation and the aging process. SAGE KE 50/re5, 2002.
13. Praticò, D.: F_2-isoprostanes: sensitive and specific non-invasive indices of lipid peroxidation in vivo. Atherosclerosis 1999; 147: 1–10.
14. Praticò, D. et al.: The isoprostanes in biology and medicine. Trends Endocrinol Metab 2001; 12: 243–247.
15. Morrow, J.D. et al.: A series of prostaglandin F_2-like compounds are produced in vivo in humans by a non-cyclooxygenase, free radical-catalyzed mechanism. Proc Natl Acad Sc USA 1990; 87: 9383–9387.
16. Praticò, D.; Lawson, J.A.; FitzGerald, G.A.: Cyclooxygenase-dependent formation of the isoprostane 8-epi $PGF_{2\alpha}$. J Biol Chem 1995; 270: 9800–9808.

17. Praticò, D. et al.: IPF$_{2\alpha}$-I: a novel index of lipid peroxidation in humans. Proc Natl Acad Sci USA 1998; 95: 3449–3454.
18. Lawson, J.A. et al: Identification of two major F$_2$ isoprostanes, 8,12-iso and 5-epi-8,12-iso-isoprostane F$_{2\alpha}$-VI, in human urine. J Biol Chem 1998; 273: 29295–29301.
19. Subbarao, K.V.; Richardson, J.S.; Ang, L.C.: Autopsy samples of Alzheimer's cortex show increased peroxidation in vitro. J Neurochem 1990; 55: 342–345.
20. Balazs, L.; Leon, M.: Evidence of an oxidative challenge in the Alzheimer's brain. Neurochem Res 1994; 19: 1131–1137.
21. Lovell, M.A. et al.: Elevated thiobarbituric acid-reactive substances and antioxidant enzyme activity in the brain in Alzheimer's disease. Neurology 1995; 45: 1594–1601.
22. Jeandel, C. et al.: Lipid peroxidation and free radical scavengers in Alzheimer's disease. Gerontology 1989; 35: 275–282.
23. Bourdel-Marchyasson, I. et al.: Antioxidant defenses and oxidative markers in erythrocytes and plasma from normally nourished elderly Alzheimer patients. Age Ageing 2001; 30: 235–241.
24. Markesbery, W.R.; Lovell, M.A.: Four-hydroxynonenal, a product of lipid peroxidation, is increased in the brain in Alzheimer's disease. Neurobiol Aging 1998; 19: 33–36.
25. Lovell, M.A. et al.: Elevated 4-hydroxynonenal in ventricular fluid in Alzheimer's disease. Neurobiol Aging 1997; 18: 457–461.
26. Praticò, D. et al.: Increased F$_2$-isoprostanes in Alzheimer's disease: evidence of enhanced lipid peroxidation in vivo. FASEB J 1998; 12: 177–178.
27. Praticò, D. et al.: Increased 8,12-iso-iPF$_{2\alpha}$-VI in Alzheimer's disease: correlation of a noninvasive index of lipid peroxidation with disease severity. Ann Neurol 2000; 48: 809–812.
28. Tuppo, E.E. et al.: Sign of lipid peroxidation as measured in the urine of patients with probable Alzheimer's disease. Brain Res Bull 2001; 54: 565–568.
29. Coyle, J.T. et al.: The neurobiologic consequences of Down's syndrome. Brain Res Bull 1986; 16: 773–787.
30. Praticò, D. et al.: Down's syndrome is associated with increased 8,12-iso-iPF$_{2\alpha}$-VI levels: evidence for enhanced lipid peroxidation in vivo. Ann Neurol 2000; 48:795–798.
31. Petersen, R.C.: Normal aging, mild cognitive impairment, and early Alzheimer's disease. Neurologist 1995; 1: 326–344.
32. Praticò, D. et al.: Increase of oxidative stress in mild cognitive impairment: a possible predictor of Alzheimer's disease. Arch Neurol 2002; 59: 972–976.
33. Andreasen, N. et al.: Evaluation of CSF-tau and CSF-Abeta42 as diagnostic markers for Alzheimer's disease. Arch Neurol 2001; 58: 373–379.
34. McKhann, G.M. et al.: Clinical and pathological diagnosis of frontotemporal dementia: report of work group on frontotemporal dementia and Pick's disease. Ann Neurol 2001; 58: 1803–1809.
35. Knopman, D.S.: Overview of dementia lacking distinctive histology: pathological designation of a progressive dementia. Dementia 1993; 4: 132–136.
36. Giannakopoulos, P.; Holf, P.R.; Bouras, C.: Dementia lacking distinctive histopathology: clinicopathological evaluation of 32 cases. Acta Neuropathol 1995; 89: 346–355.
37. Mann, D.A. et al.: Dementia of the frontal lobe type-neuropathology and immunohistochemistry. J Neurol Neurosurg Psychiatry 1993; 56: 605–614.
38. Arnold, S.E.: Cellular and molecular pathology of the frontal dementias. In: Clark, C.V.M.; Trojanowski, J.Q. (eds.): Neurodegenerative dementias: clinical features and pathological mechanisms. McGraw-Hill, New York, 2000: 291–301.
39. Castellani, R.J. et al.: Evidence for oxidative stress in Pick's disease and corticobasal dgeneration. Brain Res 1995; 696: 268–271.
40. Gerst, J.L. et al.: Role of oxidative stress in frontotemporal dementia. Dement Geriatr Cogn Disord 1999; 10(S): 85–87.
41. Albers, D.S. et al.: Evidence for oxidative stress in the subthalamic nucleus in progressive supranuclear palsy. J Neurochem 1997; 73: 881–884.
42. Albers, D.S. et al.: Frontal lobe dysfunction in progressive supranuclear palsy: evidence for oxidative stress and mitochondrial impairment. J Neurochem 2000; 72: 878–881.
43. Odetti, P. et al.: Lipoperoxidation is selectively involved in progressive supranuclear palsy. J Neuropathol Exp Neurol 2000; 59: 393–397.
44. Montine, K.S. et al.: 4-Hydroxy-2-nonenal pyrrole adducts in human neurodegenerative disease. J Neuropathol Exp Neurol 1997; 56: 866–871.
45. Clark, C.M. et al.: A urine measure of oxidative damage distinguishes patients with frontotemporal dementia from those with Alzheimer's disease. Neurobiol Aging 2003; 23: S234.

4

Metabolism and Alzheimer's Disease

John P. Blass

INTRODUCTION

Many abnormalities have been described in the brains of patients with Alzheimer's disease (AD), particularly in tissue obtained at autopsy. AD patients usually die in late stages of the disease, although sometimes other illnesses or accidents lead to death in early AD. Abnormalities in autopsy brain can be the result of agonal and postmortem artifacts. A major issue has therefore been to try to decide which abnormalities in AD brain are primary and which are secondary to the disease or to the terminal state.

The dominant although still controversial opinion in early 2003 is that the most important, seminal alteration in AD is abnormal metabolism of amyloid (1,2). This view has been called the amyloid cascade hypothesis. In its most recent form this hypothesis states that soluble fragments of amyloid precursor protein (APP) interfere directly with synaptic function and thereby interfere with information processing by the AD brain (1). The popular amyloid cascade hypothesis has led to many elegant biological studies. It has fostered many attempts to develop diagnostic tests or treatments focusing on amyloid, and these attempts continue. Up to now, however, studies of AD amyloidosis have not led to practical developments that have been widely incorporated into clinical practice.

Of perhaps greater interest to clinicians and to patients and their families is whether abnormalities found in AD brain lead to better treatments. An outstanding success in this regard has been the recognition of a deficiency in systems that use acetylcholine (ACh) as a neurotransmitter. The discovery of the cholinergic lesion in AD brain has led to the use of at least three medications for AD that have been approved in the United States, as well as several others in other countries. The clinically useful drugs inhibit cholinesterase (ChE)—the enzyme that breaks down and thereby inactivates ACh. As discussed elsewhere in this volume, there is now no serious question about the utility of cholinesterase inhibitors in AD.

Other abnormalities found in AD brain have led to clinical interventions whose usefulness is less clear. These include the noncellular, complement-mediated inflammatory reaction that has led to trials of anti-inflammatory medications including prednisone; oxidative stress, which has led to trials of vitamin E and other free-radical scavengers; and animal data as well retrospective epidemiological studies that have led to attempts to reduce the incidence of AD by postmenopausal hormone replacement therapy. All these abnormalities and the results of attempts to treat them in AD are discussed elsewhere in this volume.

IMPAIRMENTS OF CEREBRAL METABOLISM AS DIRECT CAUSE OF THE DISEASE

Impairments in cerebral metabolism are robustly characteristic of AD. However, they may well not be the primary events in the development of the neuropathological damage that by definition characterizes this disease. Numerous studies have established that the neuropathological evidence of AD—

From: *Current Clinical Neurology,*
Alzheimer's Disease: A Physician's Guide to Practical Management
Edited by: R. W. Richter and B. Zoeller Richter © Humana Press Inc., Totowa, NJ

specifically, amyloid plaques—precedes the development of clinical signs and symptoms of dementia. This observation suggests that a distinction be made between two overlapping entities: Alzheimer's disease (AD) and Alzheimer's dementia (dementia of Alzheimer type, DAT) *(3)*.

AD has been proposed to refer to the neuropathological entity, independent of the clinical findings, whereas DAT refers to clinical dementia occurring in a person who has concomitant AD by neuropathology. Abundant evidence implicates the decrease in cerebral metabolism in the development of the disabilities that characterize the clinical disorder. In other words, available evidence is consistent with the view that the cerebrometabolic lesion is a direct cause of DAT if not of AD. As discussed below, recent data suggest that the cerebrometabolic deficiency results at least in part as a consequence of amyloid accumulation. Thus, the cerebrometabolic lesion in AD is consistent with the widely held amyloid cascade hypothesis. Data gathered in the last few years provide preliminary evidence that treatments directed at the cerebrometabolic abnormality can benefit patients with AD *(4–7)*.

The cerebrometabolic lesion in AD has been extensively reviewed, including recent reviews *(3,8–12)*. The reader is referred to those reviews for more detailed discussions and for original references supporting the statements made in the following paragraphs. The discussion below deals with a series of questions that are likely to be relevant to clinical practice. (1) Is the evidence for a cerebrometabolic lesion in AD robust? (2) What causes this lesion? (3) Is there significant evidence that the cerebrometabolic deficiency contributes to the signs and symptoms of this disease? (4) Is knowledge of this lesion useful for diagnosis? (5) Is knowledge of this lesion useful for treatment?

EVIDENCE FOR THE CEREBROMETABOLIC LESION IN AD

It is fair to describe the evidence for the cerebrometabolic lesion in AD as overwhelming. The metabolic lesion is characteristic of AD in vivo in functional imaging studies and in vitro in biochemical analyses of brain obtained at autopsy. It includes evidence of damage to mitochondrial markers and of disordered metabolism of free radicals (reactive oxygen species, ROS). Metabolic abnormalities have also been found in non-neural tissues from AD patients. Quantitatively, the extent of the cerebrometabolic lesion correlates well, both in vivo and in vitro, with the extent of the clinical disability.

In Vivo Studies

The profound decrease in the rate at which the brains of older people with dementia oxidize glucose—the main substrate of the brain—were first recognized and measured by invasive methods in the late 1940s and 1950s. The decrease was evident whether metabolic rate was measured by utilization of glucose (CMR_{glu}) or of oxygen (CMR_{O2}) or by cerebral blood flow (CBF). Very extensive subsequent studies have confirmed these findings by more advanced imaging techniques, including regional cerebral blood flow (rCBF), PET (positron emission tomography) scanning, SPECT (single photon electron tomography) scanning, and most recently, functional magnetic resonance imaging (fMRI). There are essentially no contradictory reports.

The reduction in cerebral metabolism in AD cannot be attributed to brain atrophy or to slower thinking, despite earlier attempts to do so. The reductions precede any evidence of brain atrophy by detailed imaging studies or any evidence of difficulties with thinking on sensitive neuropsychological tests. Quantitative considerations indicate that the decreases in cerebral metabolism are too great to be accounted for by the rather mild slowing of electrical activity found in AD brain by EEG. Loss of brain mass is also an inadequate reason for the decreases in cerebral metabolism in AD. CMR is calculated per unit remaining brain tissue. Decreases in CMR occur in areas that do not show significant neuropathology in AD. Nor are the differences in metabolic activity between neurons and glia great enough for the selective neuronal loss to account for the decreases in CMR found in neuropathologically affected areas *(8–12)*.

In Vitro Studies

Extensive studies of AD brain obtained at autopsy have documented the existence of an inherent defect in the apparatus for oxidation of glucose, specifically in mitochondria. These studies have measured the activities of mitochondrial marker enzymes—specifically, enzyme complexes that carry out dehydrogenase reactions and electron transport. At least four independent laboratories have reported deficiencies in the activities of the pyruvate dehydrogenase complex (PDHC) and of the α-ketoglutarate dehydrogenase complex (KGDHC). There are no contravening reports.

Activities are reduced in both histologically normal brain regions as well as in regions with the plaques, tangles, and synaptic and neuronal loss that characterize AD neuropathologically. This observation suggests that the defects in PDHC and KGDHC are not simply consequences of tissue damage visible under the light microscope. PDHC catalyzes the reaction by which carbons from glucose enter the Krebs tricarboxylic acid cycle. KGDHC catalyzes a key step in that cycle, which is also a step in glutamate metabolism. Both PDHC and KGDHC are found in the inner mitochondrial compartment (i.e., in mitoplasts). Both have relatively low activity in human brain compared to other enzymes of energy metabolism; both have been suggested to be control steps.

Several laboratories have reported decreased activity in AD brain of complex IV of the electron transport chain (also known as cytochrome oxidase). There are also contravening reports. Reductions in complex IV activity in AD brain were limited to regions of obvious neuropathological damage. The activity of complex IV depends on neuronal activity, making reductions in its activity in damaged tissue hard to interpret unequivocally. Complex IV catalyzes the step in energy metabolism that uses molecular oxygen (O_2) as a substrate. The activity of complex IV in human brain is rather high compared to that of several other enzymes of energy metabolism. In rat brain, activity has to be reduced proportionately more than it is in AD brain before there is an effect on overall brain metabolism. Impairment of complex IV activity leads to an increase in the production of oxygen free radicals (ROS) by earlier steps in mitochondrial electron transport. The diminution in complex IV activity in AD brain, like other mitochondrial abnormalities, might contribute to damage by impairing the metabolism of free radicals. This possibility is discussed in more detail below.

Oxidative Stress

Many studies have described abnormal metabolism of free radicals in AD brain. Generally these have indicated increased damage by ROS, leading to the now widely accepted view that the AD brain is under oxidative stress. Quantitatively, the increased damage by ROS has been very small in absolute terms, even if impressive in relative terms. For instance, in AD brain the proportion of guanosine in DNA that has been oxidized to the 8-hydroxy derivative is only 0.01–0.1% of the total. The distribution of the oxidized base is so random in both nuclear DNA and mitochondrial DNA (mtDNA) as to make it unlikely that any single site of damage leads to functional consequences. This has led to the proposal that the reported changes in AD brain are a marker of oxidative stress rather than a direct cause of cerebral dysfunction.

Within the last two decades it has become clear that the signaling functions of mitochondria are as important to cells as is mitochondrial production of ATP (adenosine triphosphate). Damage to mitochondria can lead to cell death, even when ATP levels are initially maintained—for instance, by triggering cell death programs through the release of proteins, such as cytochrome c and apoptosis-inducing factor (AIP). Murad and others have pointed out that free radicals including ROS have important signal functions. This suggests that the most important mechanisms by which oxidative stress damages AD brain may be by alterations in signaling, with resulting dysregulation of cell functions including intermediary metabolism *(6)*.

Non-Neural Tissues

Extensive reports have documented the existence of abnormalities in AD tissues other than brain, including such readily available tissues as cultured skin fibroblasts and blood cells. These have included reports of deficiencies in KGDHC or complex IV activity in fibroblasts and of oxidative stress in white blood cells. PDHC activity does not appear to be reduced in AD skin fibroblasts. The existence of abnormalities have led to the proposal that at the molecular and cellular levels, although not the clinical level, AD is a systemic disease, but at the clinical level it is best thought of as a brain disease. The importance of the abnormalities in non-neural tissues is that they indicate that these metabolic abnormalities are an intrinsic part of the biology of AD. These metabolic abnormalities occur in AD tissues in which there is no accumulation of amyloid and no more than subtle abnormalities in the metabolism of amyloid precursor protein (APP), such as a small increase in the ratio of β-amyloid (Aβ) $A\beta_{42}/A\beta_{40}$.

Proportionality of Metabolic Impairments and Clinical Disability

The decreases in cerebral metabolic rate in AD correlate well with the degree of clinical disability, in living patients as well as in AD brain obtained at autopsy.

In vivo, i.e., in living AD patients, the extent of the decreases in cerebral metabolism in AD correlates so well with the degree of cognitive impairment that measurements of brain metabolism have been used to follow the progression of the disease. The decreases in metabolism affect the whole brain but are quantitatively most marked in the areas of brain damage. Thus, AD patients whose language is more impaired than their spatial skills tend to have more profound cerebrometabolic defects in their dominant left (speech) hemispheres than in their right hemispheres. Patients in whom language is relatively spared, compared to practice, tend to have more profound reductions in metabolism in their nondominant right hemispheres. As discussed below, attempts have been made to use the pattern of decreased brain metabolism in AD on functional imaging as an aid to the diagnosis of AD.

In vitro studies of autopsy AD brain have also shown a relationship between the degree of mitochondrial damage (as measured by KGDHC activity) and clinical disability. Gibson and co-workers measured KGDHC activity in autopsy brain tissue from AD patients at Mount Sinai Medical School, who were closely followed neuropsychologically until death. The decrease in KGDHC activity correlated as well with disability as did the count of neurofibrillary tangles; both correlated better with disability than did estimates of dense amyloid (i.e., plaque counts). Gibson and co-workers found that the relation between decreases in the mitochondrial marker and disability was due to a surprisingly tight correlation in the subgroup of patients who carried a specific genetic risk factor for AD, namely the ε4 allele of the apolipoprotein E (ApoE) gene. (The relationship of this gene to AD is discussed in detail elsewhere in this volume.) For this genetic subgroup, ρ was 0.7, implying that about half of the clinical variance could be accounted for by variations in KGDHC activity. A close relationship between disability and this specific mitochondrial marker was not found in patients negative for ApoE4, but other mitochondrial markers were not extensively evaluated.

CAUSES OF THE CEREBROMETABOLIC ABNORMALITY IN AD

The causes of the cerebrometabolic abnormality in AD are not known. Available evidence supports their being both an effect and a contributing cause of free-radical damage. Alzheimer amyloid can be a source of such damage. An argument can be made that aging plays a role, because ROS damage appears to increase as age advances. Preliminary evidence suggests that environmental toxins may contribute. Other mechanisms, including inactivation by transglutaminase, may also play a role. Evidence for a genetic cause is weak. The data argue against loss of mitochondria or other nonspecific mitochondrial damage.

Free radicals (ROS) can impair mitochondrial markers whose activity is reduced in AD brain. Specifically, KGDHC is readily inactivated by ROS. Bunik and co-workers have shown that purified KGDHC can itself generate free radicals. They have proposed that free-radical inactivation is a mechanism by which KGDHC regulates its own activity. Gibson and co-workers have shown that free-radical inactivation of KGDHC readily occurs in intact cultured cells and other more physiological systems. Free radicals can also inactivate other enzymes, including PDHC and complex IV. Indeed, high enough concentrations of free radicals such as hydrogen peroxide can inactivate most proteins.

Alzheimer amyloid can be a source of free radicals and specifically of ROS that can damage mitochondria. A specific methionine residue in Aβ amyloid peptides readily oxidizes to form a free radical, and amyloid damage to cultured cells can be prevented by free-radical quenchers. Extensive evidence indicates that amyloid peptide can damage mitochondria and mitochondrial function. In other words, the amyloid cascade hypothesis could explain the cerebrometabolic lesion in AD. That explanation is supported by direct experimental data involving free-radical mechanisms.

Aging appears to increase oxidative stress. Denman Harmon and others have proposed that ROS damage is an important general mechanism of aging. This proposal has aroused widespread interest and received much experimental support. Experimentally, evidence of free-radical damage tends to increase with the passage of time in most tissues including brain. Age is the most important risk factor for AD. The connection between age and AD may arise in part because of increased action of ROS on KGDHC and other enzymes of intermediary metabolism during aging, as well as on dysregulation of intermediary metabolism because of altered free-radical signaling.

Environmental pollutants may also play a role in generating the cerebrometabolic lesion characteristic of AD. Cooper and Gibson and their co-workers have shown that mitochondrial enzymes and specifically KGDHC are sensitive to the effects of halogenated hydrocarbons. Epidemiological studies have not yet implicated environmental pollution as a cause of AD, although it does seem to be a contributing cause of Parkinson's disease (PD). Further studies in this area are clearly warranted.

Transglutaminases (TGases) can inactivate many proteins by cross-linking them covalently to other proteins, through glutamine–lysine linkages. Mitochondrial constituents including KGDHC are among the proteins on which transglutaminases act. Recent studies by Kim and co-workers have provided evidence for the existence of a mitochondrial form of TGase. TGase activity is stimulated by calcium, and calcium tends to accumulate in the mitochondria of injured cells, including neurons exposed to hypoxia. Convincing data for a role of TGases in the cerebrometabolic lesion of AD is not yet available, however.

Genetic contributions to the cerebrometabolic lesion in AD brain have not been convincingly identified, despite extensive studies. Early reports of an association between AD and the gene encoding the core of KGDHC, namely, the DLST gene, have been followed by refutations. DLST was studied intensively because it is in the same region as the PS1 gene that accounts for much but not all of early-onset, familial AD. The other group of genes of energy metabolism that have been extensively examined in relation to AD are genes encoded on the mitochondrial genome, i.e., on mtDNA. Although mutations have sometimes been found in patients with AD, no clear pattern of an association with any single mutation or with a pattern of mutations in mtDNA has emerged.

Nonspecific damage to mitochondria does not seem to be a cause of the cerebrometabolic lesion in AD. The activity of a number of mitochondrial constituents that have been examined is normal. That includes other components of the Krebs tricarboxylic acid cycle, specifically, fumarase; other components of the electron transport chain, specifically complexes I, II, and III; and other components of mitochondria, specifically glutamate dehydrogenase. The damage to mitochondria in AD is therefore selective, even though it involves more than one mitochondrial component.

Decreased brain mass or activity cannot be the cause of the reduced cerebral metabolism in AD. This idea was proposed in the 1950s and widely accepted for some years. Two pieces of data disprove it. A definitive proof is that the cerebrometabolic abnormality precedes both loss of brain substance as detected by sensitive modern imaging techniques and any sign of cognitive difficulty detectable on sensitive neuropsychological testing. The identification of decreases in brain metabolism before any clinical evidence of disease was made possible by the identification of patients who were highly likely on genetic grounds to develop the clinical disabilities of AD, and eventually did so.

CEREBROMETABOLIC DEFICIENCY AND CLINICAL DEFICIENCIES IN AD

Extensive evidence supports the view that the cerebrometabolic lesion can be the proximate cause of the clinical disabilities in AD *(8,12)*. Much of the data were gathered over a decade ago, and are so firmly ensconced in medical literature that they can be described in simple declarative sentences. These data are from in vivo studies of humans and animals and in vivo and in vitro studies of animals and cultured cells.

Reduced rates of cerebral metabolism essentially always accompany clinically significant acquired cognitive impairment. Psychoses are usually not classified as causes of cognitive impairment, even if they interfere with judgment and performance on neuropsychological tests. Psychoses are not generally associated with impairments in cerebral intermediary metabolism, with some exceptions. The impairment of cerebral metabolism described above for AD also occurs in other types of dementia, including those caused by strokes, diffuse Lewy body disease, and other conditions. It also occurs in delirium, another clinical form of cognitive impairment. Both invasive techniques and PET, SPECT, and fMRI have documented decreased cerebral metabolism in those other forms of cognitive impairment. Thus, the analogy to one of Koch's postulates on how to establish a relation between a biological abnormality and a disease is met: the biological abnormality occurs in the clinical disorder.

Impairing cerebral metabolism leads to cognitive changes similar to those of AD, in humans and experimental animals. Cognitive impairments can be induced by reducing cerebral metabolic rate by any form of hypoxia—hypoxic, histotoxic, or anemic. They can be induced by reducing the availability of glucose (hypoglycemia) or by damaging the metabolic apparatus for utilizing substrates—for instance, by thiamine deficiency. In humans, the cognitive impairments are evident on neuropsychological testing. In animals, performance tests demonstrate analogous cognitive problems. If the metabolic impairment is relatively brief, the consequences for mental function are transient. The condition is then called delirium. If the metabolic impairments are relatively long-lasting, the consequences for mental function are at least in part irreversible. The condition is then called dementia. It is now customary in general medicine to conceptualize delirium and dementia as two different conditions. However, neurologists and psychiatrists have long recognized them as related, both biologically and clinically. For instance, dementia predisposes to delirium even if the dementia is subclinical. Engel and Romano proposed in the 1950s that delirium and dementia are best thought of as poles on a spectrum of brain failure.

Impairing cerebral metabolism also leads in experimental animals to molecular and cellular changes similar to those observed in AD brain. Gary Gibson and colleagues have studied this issue intensively in relation to inter- and intracellular signaling. Impairing cerebral metabolism leads to proportional impairment in synthesis and release of the neurotransmitter acetylcholine. Deficiency of cholinergic function, we know, is a major mechanism of impaired cognition in AD. Impairing cerebral metabolism also increases the release of potentially neurotoxic neurotransmitters including glutamate. Impairing metabolism also leads to alterations in the regulation of intracellular second messengers, including cAMP (cyclic adenosine monophosphate), cGMP (cyclic guanosine monophosphate), calcium, and the inositol phosphate cascade. Of interest in this regard is redundant evidence of altered activity of in AD tissues including extraneural tissues of enzymes involved in the inositol phosphate signaling pathway. Impairing cerebral metabolism also leads to the accumulation of materials that react with antibodies to the abnormal tau proteins that occur in AD brain. It also leads to altered metabolism of the Alzheimer APP. Accumulations of altered tau proteins and of amyloid are, of course, the characteristic neuropathological findings in AD.

Impairments of cerebral metabolism including hypoxias and hypoglycemia are a classic cause of damage to synapses and neuronal cell death, both of which are also characteristic neuropathological findings in AD. Synaptic function including specifically cholinergic transmission is more sensitive to impairment of energy metabolism than are neuronal cell bodies. With adequately prolonged impairment of energy metabolism, cells themselves die; neurons are more sensitive than other brain cells to metabolic impairment. Depending on the intensity of the insult, cell death can be apoptotic, necrotic, or somewhere on the spectrum between these poles.

The relationship of cerebrometabolic impairment to the clinical manifestations of AD therefore meets another of Koch's postulates on establishing the relation of a biological to a clinical abnormality: causing the biological abnormality causes the clinical disorder. This statement holds true for both behavioral and cell-biological abnormalities in AD.

THE CEREBROMETABOLIC LESION AND DIAGNOSIS OF AD

Measurements of the cerebrometabolic lesion by functional imaging techniques are among the most widely used laboratory aids to the diagnosis of AD. They include PET and SPECT scanning, as well as fMRI. The use of these techniques to aid diagnosis is relatively limited, however, for several reasons. These techniques are less widely available than are the anatomic imaging techniques of CT (computed tomography) and MRI. PET and fMRI remain relatively expensive, with SPECT less so. The need for specific laboratory aids for the diagnosis of AD is relatively small. Careful clinical evaluation and neuropsychological assessment can make the diagnosis of AD with 90–100% accuracy, particularly if additional information is made available by the master diagnostician, time. Confirmation of the diagnosis by functional imaging is necessary only in special cases, for very early diagnosis or in confusingly atypical clinical presentations.

The diagnostically characteristic feature of AD on functional imaging has been proposed to be a biparietal pattern of reduction in metabolic rate. Reduction in the overall rate of cerebral metabolism or blood flow does not distinguish AD from a number of other conditions that impair cognition. Imaging of the hippocampus and associated structures in AD is becoming of great interest, with accumulating evidence that damage in these regions is an early and functionally very important part of AD.

None of the attempted diagnostic aids based on detection of metabolic abnormalities in non-neural tissues has become significantly useful clinically. Most are cumbersome, technically demanding, and robust only in research laboratories devoted to their development. This includes abnormalities described in cultured skin fibroblasts. The discovery of abnormalities in non-neural AD tissues has been more important for what it tells us about the mechanisms of the disease than because of diagnostic utility.

Nevertheless, the main laboratory aids to AD diagnosis that are now in use depend on measuring the extent of the cerebrometabolic lesion by functional imaging. These techniques are in much wider use than are, for instance, kits to measure amyloid or tau fragments in spinal fluid. Perhaps future developments in imaging or in in vitro analytical techniques will lead to an adequately cheap and robust biological technique to confirm the diagnosis of AD.

THE CEREBROMETABOLIC LESION AND TREATMENT OF AD

If the cerebrometabolic lesion is a proximate cause of the clinical disabilities of AD, then treatment directed to this lesion might be hoped to benefit the patients. Preliminary data do not contradict this hope.

At least two groups have reported that elevating blood glucose improved cognitive function in AD patients *(4,5)*. Neuropsychological function was measured with and without clamping of blood glucose in the low diabetic range (about 240 mg/dL). Robust, statistically significant neuropsychological improvements were found with glucose infusion. The theory behind these studies was to improve cerebral glucose metabolism. Subsequently, Craft and co-workers presented evidence that the improvement in memory is mediated by hormonal changes stimulated by the increase in blood glucose, including specifically an increase in blood insulin *(4)*. The hormonal alterations are thought to increase glucose metabolism in critical regions of the brain, including the hippocampus. Of interest, there is a poorly documented, anecdotal clinical observation that one way to calm agitated AD patients is to give them a piece of candy rich in sugar. (Also, sugar craving is one of the early signs observed in patients who are in the process of developing AD.) The normal controls in the studies described above showed neuropsychological improvements of about the same magnitude as the AD patients, but the improvements did not reach statistical significance over the much higher baseline function of the normal subjects. The notion that ingesting sugar has rapid effects on the alertness of normal people is so widespread that candy companies use it in their advertising. However, scientific evidence for such an effect on normal human physiology is essentially absent. Those anecdotal observations are mentioned here to emphasize the possibility that an effect of elevated blood glucose on attention or cognition might be nonspecific rather than related specifically to AD.

The author of this chapter and his co-workers have treated AD patients with a nutritional cocktail that contains not only glucose but also an antioxidant and a metabolic intermediate to prime the Krebs tricarboxylic acid cycle *(6)*. Results from a 3-month, prospective, double-blind, placebo-controlled, single-center trial have been encouraging. After 3 months, the treated patients performed better than the placebo patients on both of two standard, robust neuropsychological tests: plus 2.05 points on the Mini-Mental State Examination (MMSE) and minus 3.48 points on the cognitive subset of the Alzheimer Disease Assessment Scale (ADAS-cog). (Improvement on the MMSE is an increase and on the ADAS-cog a decrease in score.) Both results were statistically significant ($p < 0.001$ by Z-test). These data suggest that ingesting the nutritional supplement may have tended to retard the progress of the disease. The results were consistent with an earlier, small open study *(6)*. Independent double-blind studies to check the validity of these preliminary results are being set up.

The preliminary data available at this time are therefore consistent with the cerebrometabolic lesion meeting another analogy of a Koch postulate relating a biological abnormality to a clinical syndrome: treating the biological abnormality ameliorates the clinical illness. If these preliminary data hold up, then increased knowledge of the cerebrometabolic lesion may prove useful not only to those interested in investigating it but also, and much more importantly, to AD patients and their families.

CONCLUSION

Claude Bernard, one of the pioneers of modern biomedical investigation, wrote that scientific hypotheses are not more or less true but more or less useful. This maxim seems particularly apt for clinicians. The clinically interesting question about an abnormality in patients is whether knowing about it helps diagnosis, treatment, or other aspects of management. The cerebrometabolic lesion in AD already appears to have some utility in diagnosis, through modern imaging techniques. Preliminary therapeutic trials raise a rational hope that understanding the metabolic lesion might even end up being useful for treatment. Further studies of this approach are warranted.

REFERENCES

1. Selkoe, D.J.: Alzheimer's disease is a synaptic failure. Science 2002; 298: 1789–1791.
2. Obrenovich, M.E. et al.: Amyloid-beta: a (life) preserver for the brain. Neurobiol Aging 2002; 23: 1097–1099.
3. Blass, J.P.: Alzheimer's disease and Alzheimer's dementia: distinct but overlapping entities. Neurobiol Aging 2002; 23:1077–1084.
4. Craft, S. et al.: Insulin effects on glucose metabolism, memory, and plasma amyloid precursor protein in Alzheimer's disease differ according to apolipoprotein-E genotype. Ann NY Acad Sci 2000; 903:222–228.
5. Manning, C.A.; Ragozzino, M.E.; Gold, P.E.: Glucose enhancement of memory in patients with probable senile dementia of the Alzheimer's type. Neurobiol Aging 1993; 14: 523–528.
6. Blass, J.P.: Metabolic enhancement for the treatment of Alzheimer disease. Res Practice Alz Dis Cognit Decline 2002; 6: 282–287.
7. Blass, J.P. et al.: A nutritional supplement in Alzheimer disease. Neurosci Abstr, in press.
8. Blass, J.P.: The mitochondrial spiral. An adequate cause of dementia in the Alzheimer's syndrome. Ann NY Acad Sci 2000; 924:170–183.
9. Gibson, G.E.: Interactions of oxidative stress with cellular calcium dynamics and glucose metabolism in Alzheimer's disease. Free Radic Biol Med 2002 ; 32: 1061–1070.

10. Blass, J.P.; Sheu, R.K.; Gibson, G.E.: Inherent abnormalities in energy metabolism in Alzheimer disease. Interaction with cerebrovascular compromise. Ann NY Acad Sci 2000; 903: 204–221.
11. Mattson, M.P. et al.: Cellular and molecular mechanisms underlying perturbed energy metabolism and neuronal degeneration in Alzheimer's and Parkinson's diseases. Ann NY Acad Sci 1999; 893: 154–175.
12. Blass, J.P.; Gibson, G.E.; Hoyer, S.: The role of the metabolic lesion in Alzheimer's disease. J Alz Dis 2002; 4: 225–232.

II Epidemiology

5

Alzheimer's Disease

Epidemiological and Statistical Data

Brigitte Zoeller Richter and Ralph W. Richter

INTRODUCTION

Alzheimer's disease (AD) today represents a major worldwide public health concern. AD has become the most common form of late-life dementing illness and requires an enormous amount of human, medical, and financial resources. The true burden of this disease for societies is only now emerging, considering the steadily increasing life expectancy and the growing number of people reaching a high age, particularly in developing countries. This, of course, is then paralleled by a dramatic increase in prevalence.

PROJECTIONS

By 2030, the number of people in the United States over age 65 is expected to double, from today's 35 million to 70 million, and then increase to 82 million by 2050. Today's 4.3 million people 85 years or older are estimated to be at almost 9 million by 2030, and at more than 19 million by 2050 (Table 1; *1*). As age is an independent risk factor for AD, people in this age group of 85 or older are at highest risk for AD.

The number of incident cases is expected to double, from 377,000 in 1995 to 959,000 in 2050 *(2)*. To date, 4–5 million people in the United States suffer from AD. This number is projected to rise to about 14 million by 2050—unless methods of primary prevention are attained. If interventions could delay the onset of the disease by 2 years, after 50 years there would be nearly 2 million fewer cases than projected; if the onset could be delayed by 1 year, nearly 800,000 prevalent cases could be avoided *(3)*.

Some years ago, Jorm and colleagues documented the exponential rise of dementia with age in a number of prevalence studies *(4)*. Roughly 7% of the population aged 65 and over has AD *(5)*. From the age of 65 years the prevalence doubles every 5 years and may well exceed 50% after the age of 85.

U.S. society spends at least $100 billion a year on AD *(6)*. Neither Medicare nor most private health insurance covers the long-term care most patients require. Almost 75% of the home care for patients with AD still is being provided by family and friends. Half of all nursing home residents suffer from AD or a related disorder. The average cost for nursing home care amounts to $42,000 per year, but can exceed $70,000 in some areas of the country. The average lifetime cost per patient reaches $174,000 *(2)*.

Prevalence Rates

The incidence of AD appears to be similar in most industrialized countries. The published prevalence rates show considerable variations among different countries. The prevalence rate of dementia (with AD as most prevalent cause) in persons aged 65 and older has been reported to be 3.6–10.3%

From: *Current Clinical Neurology,*
Alzheimer's Disease: A Physician's Guide to Practical Management
Edited by: R. W. Richter and B. Zoeller Richter © Humana Press Inc., Totowa, NJ

Table 1
Statistics of AD in the United States

Number of deaths per year:	44,536
Age-adjusted death rate:	16.5 per 100,000 persons
Cause of death rank:	8th

Source: *National Vital Statistics Report for 1999*, Vol. 49, No. 8.

in Western countries, 1.8–4.6% in China, 8.5% in Japan, 9.5–10.8% in Korea *(7,8)*. As dementia in some countries—such as India—still is a largely hidden problem *(9)*, the total worldwide picture of the disease remains from the epidemiological point of view somewhat blurred.

The above data correspond to hospital-derived figures. The prevalence of dementia among patients discharged from a general hospital in the region of Baltimore was 3.9% (2.6% in the age group 60–64; 8.9% in the age group 85 years and above) *(10)*. Not surprisingly, the mean length of stay was longer in the demented patients than in those without dementia (10.4 vs 6.5 days).

Are Women at Greater Risk than Men?

It has long been hypothesized that women are at greater risk for the development of AD than men, and that female gender is a risk factor *(11)*. According to the findings of a pooled analysis of four European population-based cohort studies with 28,768 person-years of follow-up, a significant gender difference in the incidence of AD after the age of 85 years exists. There was, however, no gender difference documented for the rates and risk for vascular dementia *(12)*. The cumulative risk for 65-year-old women to develop AD at the age of 95 years was 0.22, compared with 0.09 for men. These gender differences could not be discovered in cohort studies in the United States *(13)*. Edland and colleagues, in their most recent study of the population of Rochester, Minnesota, could not find a substantial difference between men and women in the incidence of AD *(14)*.

SURVIVAL AFTER THE ONSET OF DEMENTIA AND MORTALITY DATA

There is no question that dementia shortens life expectancy, and that dementing disorders are a major risk factor for death. The median survival time after the onset and diagnosis of dementia, however, appears to be shorter than hitherto believed. Previous estimates ranged from 5 to 9.3 years. A group of epidemiologists in Montreal reported an adjusted mean survival time of only 3.3 years after the onset of symptoms *(15)*. The results from a prospective French community-based cohort study found the median survival time of patients with dementia (over 65 years of age) to be 4.5 years *(16)*. Significant predictors for early mortality were elements of mobility, difficulty in dressing, gait abnormalities, history of falls, and abnormal motor strength *(17)*.

Carriers of the e4-allele of the apolipoprotein E (ApoE) gene have a higher mortality risk for AD as well as for ischemic heart disease, whereas the e2/e3-genotype seems to be protective (relative risk 0.84) *(18)*. Near the age of 50, the e3/e4-genotype is associated with a relative risk of death of 1.81. Over the age of 100 years, the ApoE genotype has little influence on the death risk.

Predictors of survival in African American patients with AD have been investigated recently by Freels and colleagues in Chicago. Patients with AD who were older and had a lower Barthel score were at higher risk for death *(19)*.

A Swedish group of researchers at the Stockholm Gerontology Research Center/Karolinska Institute reviewed prognostic factors in very old demented subjects. In their investigation, older age, male gender, low education, co-morbidity, and functional disability predicted shorter survival *(20)*. Other factors, such as type of dementia, severity, and duration of the illness, did not turn out to be significant. Type of dementia (AD in particular) and higher baseline cognitive function, however, predicted a faster decline. The average rate of cognitive decline in the mildly to moderately demented subjects in this Swedish survey who survived 3 years was 2.4 points on the Mini-Mental State Examination (MMSE) per year.

The most frequent immediate cause of death of patients with AD is a life-threatening infection, such as pneumonia, usually related to aspiration, malnutrition, immobility, and incontinence—consequences of the progressive functional impairment *(21)*. A very common cause of death—as in the general population—is cardiovascular disease. Cardiac causes of death and especially cardiac failure are more frequent in vascular dementia (VaD) than in AD or mixed dementia *(22)*.

ALZHEIMER'S DISEASE IN NATIVE AMERICANS

Although the elder population of Native Americans continues to grow, very little is known to date about how dementia and Alzheimer's disease affect this group *(23)*. Population-based studies have not yet been performed. Very little is also known on the clinical picture of AD in Native Americans, on patient profiles, and on family caregiving as well as care facilities.

Prevalence of AD in Native Americans

Available prevalence data suggest a significantly lower AD prevalence for Native Americans compared to Caucasians. In Cree aged 65 years and older, registered in Northern Manitoba, the prevalence was reported at 0.5% for AD and 4.2% for all forms of dementia *(24)*. This is in contrast to an age-adjusted prevalence of 3.5% for AD and 4.2% for all dementias in Caucasians.

Risk Factors and Genetic Features

Little is known about the actual risk factors for AD and dementia in Native American populations. Differences are seen regarding the frequency of co-morbid cardiovascular conditions, such as diabetes, hypertension, and obesity, all more prevalent in Native Americans than in Caucasian Americans. Hypertension in particular, but diabetes as well, is considered to be an independent risk factor for vascular dementia (VaD) and AD.

Native Americans suffer disproportionately from diabetes. Particularly between 1990 and 1997, a huge increase in diabetes prevalence (29%) among all age groups of Native Americans was documented, compared to an increase of 14% in the general population *(25)*. It is believed that lifestyle changes strongly contributed to this still-growing epidemic of diabetes, and that these lifestyle changes, characterized by diminished physical activity and increased calorie and fat intake, have interacted with genetic susceptibility.

Some information is available about the genetic background. Observational data indicate that as the genetic degree, for example, of Cherokee ancestry increases, the representation of AD decreases *(26)*.

This inverse relationship between the genetic degree of Cherokee ancestry and AD—independent of the status of ApoEe4-allele—however, diminishes with increasing age, suggesting an age-related protective effect of being Cherokee. For a decrease of 10% in Cherokee ancestry, the odds of developing AD are estimated to be 9.00 times greater at age 65, but only 1.34 times greater at age 80 years *(26)*. This finding is not yet explained. One explanation might be that the older Cherokees maintain a more traditional, healthier lifestyle.

Compared with Caucasians both, the ApoEe4-allele and the tau H2 haplotype frequency were reported to be low among Choctaw, suggesting a lesser genetic predisposition for AD and degenerative dementia *(27)*.

ApoE data from Cherokees are also of interest. The ApoEe4-allele was reported in only 13% of cases with a more then 50% Native American heritage. In Caucasians, in contrast, this allele is found with a frequency of 66% *(28)*.

It is possible that Native Americans carry some not-yet-revealed protective factor against the development of AD. Even though greater Native American heritage in the study of Weiner and colleagues was associated with significantly lower education and a history of vascular co-morbidities, Cherokee

Table 2
Allele Frequencies in Cherokee Patients with AD (*n* = 28)

ApoE genotype	> 50% Cherokee	< 50% Cherokee
ApoEe2	1.8%	8.9%
ApoEe3	23.2%	42.9%
ApoEe4	7.1%	16.1%

Table 3
Allele Frequencies in Cherokee Controls (*n* = 36)

ApoE genotype	> 50% Cherokee	< 50% Cherokee
ApoEe2	—	2.8%
ApoEe3	65.3%	23.6%
ApoEe4	4.2%	4.2%

Indians had fewer memory problems in their families, higher MMSE scores, and a later age of AD onset, compared to Caucasians *(28)*.

The influence of lifestyle, particularly of nutrition, on the occurrence of AD in Native Americans has not yet been studied. From cancer studies, however, it is known that the major changes in nutrition that have been experienced by American Indians have been paralleled by an increased risk for nutrition-related cancers (such as colon and prostate cancer) *(29)*. Diets of American Indians today are similar to the modern average American diet, that is, high in fat and relatively low in fruits and vegetable.

DEMENTIA STUDIES AMONG CHEROKEES IN OKLAHOMA

Among the 3.15 million residents of Oklahoma, Native Americans comprise 8%. The Cherokee Nation represents the largest of the 37 tribes in Oklahoma, and the second largest in the United States. We studied the relationship between genetic degree of being Cherokee, ApoEe4-allele frequency, and the development of AD in subjects 65 years and older. Results: Initially an inverse relationship was observed between the allelic frequency of ApoEe4 and the genetic degree of Cherokee (Tables 2 and 3). When controlled for the presence or absence of the e4-allele, a significant protective effect appears to be provided by higher-degree Cherokee. This effect diminishes with age *(30)*.

CONCLUSION

Issues of ethnicity, minority, and culture, particularly in their relationship to diseases of later life such as AD, are widely neglected and understudied *(31)*. Particularly with regard to AD, it is of utmost importance to study family dynamics, caregiving processes, and the meaning and acceptance of old age as well as dementia. Cultural values and perceptions should be investigated and the findings incorporated in future models of research and practice. Communication barriers have to be recognized and overcome.

Clinical trials should be designed to include minorities and implemented to investigate the distinct cultural ways of living and believes of illness. The recruitment of Native Americans, for example, in clinical trials, however, requires special sensitivity and recognition of their own cultural values and beliefs. Such research must not exploit individuals for mere scientific merits but should always provide enhanced medical care as a major humanitarian component.

REFERENCES

1. American Medical Association: News Release, June 7, 2001.
2. Hebert, L.E. et al.: Annual incidence of Alzheimer disease in the United States projected to the year 2000 through 2050. Alz Dis Assoc Disord 2001; 15: 169–173.
3. Brookmeyer, R. et al.: Projections of Alzheimer's disease in the United States and the impact of delaying disease onset. Am J Public Health 1998; 88: 1337–1342.
4. Jorm, A.F. et al.: The prevalence of dementia: A quantitative integration of the literature. Act Psych Scand 1987; 76: 464–479.
5. McDowell, I.: Alzheimer's disease: insights from epidemiology. Aging (Milano) 2001; 13: 143–162.
6. Alzheimer's Association: Media News Release January 9, 2003.
7. Lee, D.Y. et al.: The prevalence of dementia in older people in an urban population of Korea: the Seoul Study. J Am Geriatr Soc 2002; 50: 1233–1239.
8. Meguro, K. et al.: Prevalence of dementia and dementing diseases in Japan: the Tajiri Project. Arch Neurol 2002; 59: 1109–1114.
9. Shaji, K.S. et al.: Revealing a hidden problem. Int J Geriatr Psychiatry 2002; 17: 222–225.
10. Lyketsos, C.G. et al.: Dementia in elderly persons in a general hospital. Am J Psychiatry 2000; 157: 704–707.
11. Launer, L.J. et al.: Rates and risk factors for dementia and Alzheimer's disease: results from EURODEM pooled analyses. Neurology 1999; 52: 78–84.
12. Andersen, K. et al.: Gender differences in the incidence of AD and vascular dementia: The EURODEM studies. Neurology 1999; 53: 1992–1997.
13. Kawas, C. et al.: Age-specific incidence rates of Alzheimer's disease: the Baltimore Longitudinal Study of Aging. Neurology 2000; 54: 2072–2077.
14. Edland, S.D. et al.: Dementia and Alzheimer disease incidence rates do not vary by sex in Rochester, Minn. Arch Neurol 2002; 59: 1589–1593.
15. Wolfson, C. et al.: A reevaluation of the duration of survival after the onset of dementia. N Engl J Med 2001; 344: 1111–1116.
16. Helmer, C. et al.: Mortality with dementia: results from a French prospective community-based cohort. Am J Epidemiol 2001; 154: 642–648.
17. Koutsavlis, A.T.; Wolfson, C.: Elements of mobility as predictors of survival in elderly patients with dementia: findings from the Canadian Study of Health and Aging. Chronic Dis Can 2000; 21: 93–103.
18. Ewbank, D.C.: Mortality differences by ApoE genotype estimated from demographic synthesis. Genet Epidemiol 2002; 22: 146–155.
19. Freels, S. et al.: Predictors of survival in African American patients with AD, VaD, or stroke without dementia. Neurology 2002; 59: 1146–1153.
20. Aguero-Torres, H. et al.: Prognostic factors in very old demented adults: a seven-year follow-up from a population-based survey in Stockholm. Am Geriatr Soc 1998; 46: 444–452.
21. Volicer, L. et al.: Infections in advanced dementia. In: Volicer, L.; Hurley, A. (eds.): Hospice care for patients with advanced progressive dementia. Springer-Verlag, New York, 1998: 29–47.
22. Kammoun, S. et al.: Immediate causes of death of demented and non-demented elderly. Act Neurol Scand Suppl 2000; 176: 96–99.
23. Jervis, LL; Manson, S.M.: American Indians/Alaska natives and dementia. Alz Dis Assoc Disord 2002; 16 (suppl 2): S89–S95.
24. Hendrie, H.C. et al.: Alzheimer's disease is rare in Cree. Int Psychogeriatr 1993; 5: 5–14.
25. Rios Burrows, N. et al.: Prevalence of diabetes among Native Americans and Alaska natives. Diabetes Care 2000; 23: 1786–1790.
26. Rosenberg, R.N.; et al.: Genetic factors for the development of Alzheimer disease in the Cherokee Indian. Arch Neurol 1996; 53: 997–1000.
27. Henderson, J.N. et al.: Apolipoprotein E4 and tau allele frequencies among Choctaw Indians. Neurosci Lett 2002; 324: 77–79.
28. Weiner, M.F. et al.: A comparison of Alzheimer's disease in Native Americans and Caucasians. Int Psychogeriatrics, 2003, accepted for publication.
29. Byers, T.: Nutrition and cancer among American Indians and Alaska Natives. Cancer 1996; 78 (7 suppl): 1612–1616.
30. Richter, R.W. et al.: Studies of dementia within the Cherokee Nation of Oklahoma (Abstr.) Neurobiol Aging 1996; 17 (4S): S56.
31. Dilworth-Anderson, P.; Gibson, B.E.: The cultural influence of values, norms, meanings and perceptions in understanding dementia in ethnic minorities. Alz Dis Assoc Disord 2002; 16 (suppl 2): S56–S63.

6

The Economic Burden of Alzheimer's Disease and Dementia

Anders Wimo and Bengt Winblad

INTRODUCTION

The societal consequences of dementia disorders in general, and Alzheimer's disease (AD) in particular, are among the most important issues when discussing the situation of the health and social sectors *(1)*. Dementia is regarded by the Organization for Economic Cooperation and Development (OECD) as one of the most important health and social policy issues in its member states *(2)* and the World Health Organisation (WHO) has regarded dementia as one of the major reasons for disability *(3)*. Our research group at the Karolinska Institute in Stockholm, Sweden, has estimated that today, there are about 25 million people in the world suffering from dementia *(4)*. Dementia disorders are costly and, combined with an economic crisis in many public health-care systems, raise fundamental questions that are included in any health economical analysis. Since we also have drugs that influence the symptomatology and also resource utilization and costs, issues of cost-effectiveness are of great importance. The economic and social burden of dementia disorders, particularly AD, is therefore the focus of this chapter. However, it must be stated that there are several methodological issues that need to be highlighted *(5)*.

THE PERSPECTIVE

Any health economical analysis must define its perspective. The societal perspective includes all relevant costs (direct costs within the health sector, indirect costs due to production losses, and costs of informal care) and outcomes *(6)*. However, the analysis is often done from a specific payer's point of view. This can be a municipality, a county council, an insurance company, a health maintenance organization (HMO), a caregiver, or a patient (out-of-pocket costs). Depending on the chosen perspective, the results of the analysis are different. The societal perspective is recommended, but in many analyses it may be an advantage if the results can be interpreted from several perspectives (but with the broad societal perspective as the basic option).

COSTING

The costing process can in a simple way be divided into two steps: The first step, resource utilization, is quantified in physical units (e.g., hours, days). The second step, in which costs are calculated by multiplying the physical units by a per-item figure (e.g., the cost of a nursing home bed is US$100 per day). We have developed an instrument for the first step, resource utilization in dementia (RUD), which

From: *Current Clinical Neurology,*
Alzheimer's Disease: A Physician's Guide to Practical Management
Edited by: R. W. Richter and B. Zoeller Richter © Humana Press Inc., Totowa, NJ

Table 1
Components of the Resource Utilization Battery in RUD *(7)*

Patient	Caregiver
Accommodation/long-term care	Informal care time (for patient)
Work status[a]	Work status[a]
Respite care	Respite care
Hospital care	Hospital care
Out clinic visits	Out clinic visits
Social service	Social service
Home nursing care	Home nursing care
Day care	Day care
Drug use	Drug use

[a]For persons who have a job in the labor market.

aims at serving as a source for cost calculations from a societal perspective *(7)*. In RUD, the resource utilization by caregivers is also included. The main components of RUD are shown in Table 1.

One important issue is to judge the external validity and generalizability of health economic studies. Even if resource utilisation data are collected prospectively and in the next step are used for cost calculations, the question is whether such figures can be generalized for a general dementia population. This, of course, is of particular interest for those who pay for the care, regardless of whether the payer is the state, a local authority (e.g., a municipality), or a private company. Moreover, it is also important to analyze how costs are distributed among payers of different social sectors, and how intervention might cause a reallocation of resources and costs, in both the short and long term.

Basic facts are necessary to answer these questions. Longitudinal, population-based studies that include information about resource utilization are the best sources of information. The Kungsholmen Project in Sweden, which started in 1987, is an example of such a longitudinal, population-based cohort study *(8)*. All persons in the target area (Kungsholmen, in Stockholm) who were born in 1912 or earlier were invited to participate. A new cohort from a rural area (Nordanstig) has also been included in the project. After the initial phase, there has been a follow-up every third year, and the project has produced a great amount of scientific data on the elderly, which can also be used for health economic studies.

The close relationship between decreasing cognitive capacity (in terms of Mini-Mental State Examination [MMSE]) *(9)* and living situation of the elderly was nicely documented in the Kungsholmen project *(10)*. The most striking correlation was recognizable between MMSE performance and home care, while the comparison patterns between MMSE performance and different forms of institutional living seemed to be more complicated.

Because institutional care is the major cost driver in dementia care, it is important to clarify that there are different kinds of institutions with different resources and costs. An institution can be a huge building with hundreds of patients, but it can also be a small, homelike unit with six to nine residents and staffing around the clock *(11)*.

DIFFERENT TYPES OF HEALTH ECONOMIC STUDIES

Although this chapter focuses on the economic burden of AD and dementia, the principles for other types of health economic studies will also be described briefly *(12)*. Health economic studies are of two major types, descriptive and evaluation (normative) studies.

Descriptive Studies

In cost description (CD), costs are presented without any comparison with alternative treatments, nor are outcomes analyzed. Therefore CD is not a complete health economic analysis, but the basis for such analyses, since the cost components that are included in any health economic study are based on the principles of CD.

From a theoretical health economy point of view, costs should be presented in terms of opportunity cost *(13)*, which is based on the assumption that any resource has an alternative use to a certain cost. The opportunity cost should in theory reflect the market value of a resource. For example, for an informal caregiver of working age, the opportunity cost equals the value of the work on the market that this caregiver has given up.

There are different ways to categorize types of costs. It is common to present spending as direct costs and as indirect costs (although this is under debate). Simplified, direct costs are derived from resources used, such as costs in the formal health care and social service systems (e.g., hospital care, nursing home care, medications, home support), while indirect costs reflect resources lost (e.g., loss of production due to morbidity and mortality).

Cost-of-Illness Studies

Cost-of-illness (COI) studies are descriptive (such as the costs of illness of dementia in Sweden in Swedish crowns [SEK], 38 billions per year). Such results cannot be used in priority discussions, but they describe how costs are distributed among different players (such as 80% of the costs of dementia are the municipalities' responsibility). COI results can also be used to compare the burden of different diseases (the latter may, however, be problematic; it is necessary to know how the calculations are made of the diseases that are compared).

In theory, a COI should describe opportunity costs: the cost of the illness in question is equal to what these resources would have been used for, if there had been no case of illness. Two approaches can be used, an incidence approach or a prevalence approach. In the incidence approach, the costs for new cases that occur during the year are estimated, and both annual costs and future (discounted) costs are included. In the prevalence approach, the costs for all dementia cases during the year are estimated— both for those already suffering from dementia and for new cases occurring during the year in question *(14)*. The choice of approach depends on the purpose of the study. If the aim is to illustrate the economic consequences of various interventions, it is logical to use the incidence approach. If the idea is to estimate the economic burden during a specific year, the prevalence approach is the option.

Another methodological issue is whether to analyze the data using a top-down or a bottom-up approach. In the top-down approach, the total national cost for a specific resource is distributed over different diseases: for example, the total number of bed-days in nursing homes is classified according to use by demented people and use by people with other diagnoses. The "bottom-up" method starts from a defined subgroup with the disease and registers all costs related to this subgroup. The cost for the subpopulation is then extrapolated to the total population with the disease.

One problem with COI studies is the difficulty of compensating for, e.g., co-morbidity and hotel costs (e.g., costs of housing and food in an institution, which a person will have even without the disease). If the costs for all demented are analyzed without compensating for co-morbidity and hotel costs, a gross cost is presented, while a net cost should include only costs that are linked to the disease of interest.

In any COI study, clarification is needed regarding the method of calculating the costs and what cost categories are included, together with facts about how a dementia population is distributed in a specific country's care organization. Demographic and epidemiological figures about the prevalence of dementia are also necessary.

Since many of the basic facts in a COI may vary (different prevalence and incidence figures, gross costs or net costs, informal care costs included or not, opportunity costs or replacement approach in the costing of informal care, top-down or bottom-up approach, incidence or prevalence approach), the resulting COI can vary and comparisons between countries can be confusing. This is illustrated in Table 2 *(15)*, showing COI figures from several countries *(16–25)*. It is obvious that the costs of dementia are high, but it is also clear that the range of costs also depends on methodological factors. The most

Table 2
Cost-of-Illness Studies *(15)*, Expressed as US$2000[a]

Country	Annual costs per patient, 2000 (US$)	Cost categories included[b]	Source
USA	53,300	D, IC	Ernst and Hay *(16)*
England	6,500	D	Smith et al. *(17)*
Canada	13,500	D, IC	Ostbye and Crosse *(18)*
Sweden	24,400	D	Wimo et al. *(19)* (gross costs)
Sweden	15,900	D	Wimo et al. *(19)* (net costs)
Germany	13,800	D	Schulenberg et al. *(20)*
Denmark	8,900	D	Kronborg-Andersen et al. *(22)*
Italy	59,700	D, IC	Cavallo et al. *(23)*
Netherlands	10,400	D	Koopmanschap et al. *(21)*
Ireland	11,900	DC, IC	O'Shea and O'Reilly *(24)*

[a]Currency conversions to US$ by PPP (Purchasing Power Parities), time transformations by CPI (consumer price index); source for PPP and CPI: OECD, data on file: www.oecd.org.
[b]D, directs costs, IC, costs of informal care.

critical issue is whether costs of informal care are included or not, and, if included, how informal care is calculated.

SEVERITY-RELATED COSTS

Costs of dementia can also be described in terms of severity of dementia. In such studies, costs are described in relation to some kind of measure of severity, such as cognition, stage of dementia, or the capacity to perform activities of daily living (ADL). Most frequently used are different levels of MMSE. One example is seen in Table 3 *(15)*, in which costs for formal home care, informal care, long-term care, sheltered living, and drugs are included. This table covers about 96% of the costs in an update of a previous COI study of dementia in Sweden *(26)*, although some cost components are not included (costs of day care, patients' productivity losses, costs of diagnostic procedures, hospital and ambulant care). A similar study by Hux et al. from Canada, which also includes costs of informal care (Table 3), shows a similar pattern *(27)*, with a strong relationship between costs and severity of dementia, although the Swedish figures are higher. This can partly be explained by the fact that the Swedish figures represent overall dementia costs, while the Canadian figures refer to AD. Overall dementia includes costs of vascular dementia, which are higher than those of AD *(28)*.

Results such as those presented in Table 3 can be used in the discussion of intervention effects. However, it is not as easy to say that the difference between two stages of severity represents a true saving, if an evaluation can postpone or prevent deterioration from one stage of dementia to another. Such effects must be proven in controlled comparison studies. Nevertheless, the strong correlation between costs on the one hand and cognitive and functional capacity on the other hand supports the view that delaying progression may result in cost savings.

EVALUATION STUDIES

Evaluation studies are normative, that is, they aim at supporting policy discussions and decisions. At least two different treatment strategies should be compared, but a do-nothing alternative (such as placebo in randomized controlled trials) may also be a comparator. In cost analyses (CA), the costs of different therapies are compared, but not the effects or outcomes. A CA therefore does not represent a complete evaluation study, which includes measurements of both costs and outcomes. There

Table 3
Annual Costs per MMSE Range (Swedish Crowns, SEK)[a]

	Annual costs	
Severity	Sweden *(15)*	Canada *(41)*
MMSE 21–26	11,400	8,000
MMSE 15–20	27,400	13,400
MMSE 10–14	31,600	21,600
MMSE 0–9	41,900	30,900

[a]Figures are rounded and expressed as US$ (2000).

should also be a comparison between at least two treatment alternatives. In a cost-minimization analysis (CMA), the effects of different treatments are shown or assumed to be equal (although it sounds easy in theory, this may be difficult in practice). Thus, in a CMA, the analysis is focused on finding the therapy that results in the lowest costs.

In cost–effectiveness analysis (CEA), the effect is expressed in terms of a nonmonetary but quantifiable outcome, such as the cost per nursing home admission averted or the cost to prevent a shift to a more severe stage of illness. In a cost–benefit analysis (CBA), costs and outcomes are expressed in the same unit (usually monetary). Although early CBA studies were based mostly on the human capital approach, the modern theory of CBA appears to be more complex, including willingness to pay and willingness to accept approaches *(29)*. So far, few attempts have been made to apply CBA to dementia. In a cost–utility analysis (CUA), the effect is expressed in terms of utilities, mostly as outcomes linked to the concept of quality of life. In CUA, the concept of QALYs (quality-adjusted life years) is frequently used *(30)*. In a cost–consequence analysis (CCA), cost and outcomes are analyzed and presented separately. There is no direct mathematical connection between these two components in a health economical analysis. The value of CCA is under discussion, since it includes a risk of a strategic and perhaps retrospective selection of outcomes *(31)*.

INFORMAL CARE

Informal care is of great interest from two points of view. First, informal caregivers (in most cases spouses or children of demented patients) are part of a dementia family. In this sense, their situation is often very stressing and can be described in terms of burden, coping, or morbidity *(32–34)*. Second, informal caregivers deliver unpaid care, which is also a very important part of the total costs of dementia from a societal perspective. The amount of informal care is huge. In a Swedish study we found that the ratio between informal and formal care is about 4–5 : 1 in terms of support in personal and instrumental ADL *(35)*. If the need for supervision and surveillance is included, the ratio ranges about 8–9 : 1. Informal caregivers spend about 10 hours a day on caregiving. This amount of informal care has been highlighted in many other studies *(23,36–39)*

Calculating informal care is, however, a complicated topic *(40)*. The replacement cost approach and the opportunity cost approach, which are two frequently used methods, have drawbacks when they are applied to dementia *(6)*. As mentioned earlier, from a theoretical point of view, the opportunity cost approach is preferable. The replacement cost approach means that if informal care had not been provided, professional help would be needed. For informal caregivers of working age, the opportunity cost is the value of the work on the market that these caregivers have given up. However, leisure time and the work offered by retired people may be more problematic to describe in terms of opportunity costs. In most cases, the replacement cost approach results in higher costs of informal care than use of the opportunity cost approach. In many parts of the world, where several generations live together (e.g., a family with children plus grandparents), it is not easy to separate caring activities from family life, particularly in terms of instrumental ADL.

Another important point is that many caregivers, although tired and even exhausted, do not regard their informal care as a burden. On the contrary, some regard it as a natural part of life, like marriage, and describe it in positive terms, making it more complicated to describe it in terms of lost benefits or similarly.

CONCLUSION

In contrast to the great impact that dementia in general and AD in particular have on the public health budgets, the health economics database, which is supposed to be a support in care planning, is limited. However, there is great interest in these issues among policy makers, reimbursement authorities, clinical researchers, drug companies, and patient/caregiver organizations. We therefore think that the economic burden of dementia and AD will be more strongly highlighted in the future. The need for research, however, is crucial, and it is vital that the resources and funding for research reach the proportion that is represented by public health costs.

REFERENCES

1. Johnson, N.; Davis,T.; Bosanquet, N.: The epidemic of Alzheimer's disease. How can we manage the costs? Pharmacoeconomics 2000; 18 (3): 215–223.
2. OECD: Policy issues in dementia care in OECD countries. OECD; Paris, 2002.
3. WHO: World Health Report, 1999. World Health Organization (WHO), Geneva, 1999.
4. Wimo, A.; Winblad, B.; Aguero-Torres, H.; von Strauss, E.: The magnitude of dementia occurrence in the world. Alzheimer Dis Assoc Disord 2003; 17: 63–67.
5. Winblad, B. et al.: What are the costs to society and to individuals regarding diagnostic procedures and care of patients with dementia? Acta Neurol Scand Suppl 1996; 168: 101–104.
6. Jonsson, B. et al.: Cost of dementia. In: May, M.; Sartorius, N. (eds.): Dementia. WPA series evidence and experience in psychiatry. Wiley, London, 2000: 335–363.
7. Wimo, A. et al.: Evaluation of the resource utilisation and caregiver time in anti-dementia drug trials—a quantitative battery. In: Wimo, A. et al. (eds.): The health economis of dementia. Wiley, London, 1998.
8. Fratiglioni, L. et al.: Occurrence of dementia in advanced age: the study design of the Kungsholmen Project. Neuroepidemiology 1992; 11 (suppl 1): 29–36.
9. Folstein, M.F.; Folstein, S.E.; McHugh, P.R.: "Mini-mental state." A practical method for grading the cognitive state of patients for the clinician. J Psychiatr Res 1975; 12: 189–198.
10. Wimo, A. et al.: Treatment of Alzheimer's disease with tacrine: a cost-analysis model. Alzheimer Dis Assoc Disord 1997; 11: 191–200.
11. Wimo, A. et al.: Cost-utility analysis of group living in dementia care. Int J Technol Assess Health Care 1995; 11: 49–65.
12. Drummond, M.F. et al.: Methods for the economic evaluation of health care programmes. Oxford University Press, Oxford, 1997.
13. Karlsson, G. et al.: Methodological issues in health economics of dementia. In: Wimo, A. et al. (eds.): Health economics of dementia. Wiley, London, 1998: 161–169.
14. Lindgren, B.: Costs of illness in Sweden 1964–1975. Liber, Lund, 1981.
15. Wimo, A.; Winblad, B.: Pharmacoeconomics of dementia: impact of cholineesterase inhibitors. In: Gauthier, S.; Cummings, J. (eds.): Alzheimer's disease and related disorders, annual 2002. Martin Dunitz, London, 2002.
16. Ernst, R.L.; Hay, J.W.: The US economic and social costs of Alzheimer's disease revisited. Am J Public Health 1994; 84: 1261–1264.
17. Smith, K.A.; Shah, A.: The prevalence and costs of psychiatric disorders and learning disabilities. Br J Psychiatry 1995; 166: 9–18.
18. Ostbye, T.; Crosse, E.: Net economic costs of dementia in Canada. Can Med Assoc J 1994; 151: 1457–1464.
19. Wimo, A. et al.: Cost of illness due to dementia in Sweden. Int J Geriatr Psychiatry 1997; 12: 857–861.
20. Schulenberg, J.; Schulenberg, I.: Cost of treatment and cost of care for Alzheimer's disease in Germany. In: Wimo, A. et al. (eds.): The health economics of dementia. Wiley, London, 1998.
21. Koopmanschap, M.A. et al.: Costs of dementia in the Netherlands. In: Wimo, A. et al. (eds.): The health economics of dementia. Wiley, London, 1998.
22. Kronborg Andersen, C. et al.: The cost of dementia in Denmark: the Odense Study. Dement Geriatr Cogn Disord 1999; 10: 295–304.
23. Cavallo, M.C.; Fattore, G.: The economic and social burden of Alzheimer's disease on families in the Lombardy region of Italy. Alzheimer Dis Assoc Disord 1997; 11: 184–190.
24. O'Shea, E.; O'Reilly, S.: The economic and social cost of dementia in Ireland. Int J Geriatr Psychiatry 2000; 15: 208–218.

25. Wimo, A.; Winblad, B.: Pharmacoeconomics of dementia: impact of cholineesterase inhibitors. In: Gauthier, S.; Cummings, J. (eds.): Alzheimer's disease and related disorders, annual 2002. Martin Dunitz, London, 2002: 145–167.

26. Wimo, A.; Jonsson, L.: Demenssjukdomarnas samh llskostnader (The societal costs of dementia) (in Swedish). Socialstyrelsen (National Board of Wealth and Health Care), Stockholm, 2001.

27. Hux, M.J. et al.: Relation between severity of Alzheimer's disease and costs of caring. CMAJ 1998; 159: 457–465.

28. Wimo, A.; Jonsson, L.; Winblad, B.: Social burden and pharmacoeconomics of vascular dementia. In: Erkinjuntti, T.; Gauthier, S. (eds.): Vascular cognitive impairment. Martin Dunitz, London, 2002: 629–639.

29. Olsen, J.A.; Smith, R.D.: Theory versus practice: a review of "willingness-to-pay" in health and health care. Health Econ 2001; 10: 39–52.

30. Siegel, J.E. et al.: Guidelines for pharmacoeconomic studies. Recommendations from the Panel on Cost Effectiveness in Health and Medicine. Panel on Cost Effectiveness in Health and Medicine. Pharmacoeconomics 1997; 11: 159–168.

31. Winblad, B. et al.: Issues in the economic evaluation of treatment for dementia. Position paper from the International Working Group on Harmonisation of Dementia Drug Guidelines. Alzheimer Dis Assoc Disord 1997; 11 (suppl 3): 39–45.

32. Grafstrom, M. et al.: Health and social consequences for relatives of demented and non-demented elderly. A population-based study. J Clin Epidemiol 1992; 45: 861–870.

33. Jansson, W.; Grafstrom, M.; Winblad, B.: Daughters and sons as caregivers for their demented and non-demented elderly parents. A part of a population-based study carried out in Sweden. Scand J Soc Med 1997; 25: 289–295.

34. Schulz, R.; Beach, S.R.: Caregiving as a risk factor for mortality: the Caregiver Health Effects Study. JAMA 1999; 282: 2215–2219.

35. Wimo, A. et al.: Time spent on informal and formal care giving for persons with dementia in Sweden. Health Policy 2002; 61: 255–268.

36. Stommel, M.; Collins, C.E.; Given, B.A.: The costs of family contributions to the care of persons with dementia. Gerontologist 1994; 34: 199–205.

37. Clipp, E.C.; Moore, M.J.: Caregiver time use: an outcome measure in clinical trial research on Alzheimer's disease. Clin Pharmacol Ther 1995; 58: 228–236.

38. Rice, D.P. et al.: The economic burden of Alzheimer's disease care. Health Aff (Millwood) 1993; 12: 164–176.

39. Albert, S.M. et al.: Hourly care received by people with Alzheimer's disease: results from an urban, community survey. Gerontologist 1998; 38: 704–714.

40. McDaid, D.: Estimating the costs of informal care for people with Alzheimer's disease: methodological and practical challenges. Int J Geriatr Psychiatry 2001; 16: 400–405.

41. Challis, D. et al.: Dependency in older people recently admitted to care homes. Age Ageing 2000; 29: 255–260.

7

Potential and Established Risk Factors for Alzheimer's Disease

Brigitte Zoeller Richter

INTRODUCTION

As long as the exact cause of Alzheimer's disease (AD) has not been identified, it will not be possible to name and address the actual risk factors with certainty. On the basis of epidemiological data and rather stable associations to date, some risk factors are considered established, whereas others still are discussed or remain controversial.

AGE, GENETIC DISPOSITION, AND GENDER

The most powerful risk factors for the development of AD are age and genetic susceptibility for dementia, which also means genetic predisposition for familial AD (FAD). Dementia becomes increasingly more common with increasing age. Approximately 1 in 10 people 65 years and older suffers from AD, and by the age of 85 years and older up to 30% will be affected (1). Additionally, there is at least a threefold greater mortality associated with dementia, compared to nondemented subjects (2). The scientific community, however, is still not sure whether dementia occurs simply because the brain is getting older, or whether the disease is caused by other events, which occur more commonly as a result of aging.

The second most important risk factor for AD is family history or genetic predisposition. Several gene mutations are associated with autosomal-dominant familial forms of the disease. These familial forms of early-onset AD are caused by heterozygous mutations in the genes encoding the amyloid precursor protein (APP) and the presenilins PS1 and PS2. The etiology of the more prevalent forms of late-onset AD, however, is still unknown. The neuropathological alterations of FAD are usually indistinguishable from those of sporadic AD. Apolipoprotein E (ApoE) genotype appears to contribute to the effect of family history on the overall risk of developing AD.

The clinical manifestations of trisomy 21, Down's syndrome, is another genetically based risk factor for AD, with occurrence of neuropathological changes by the fifth or sixth decade of life. The most likely mechanism is the overproduction of amyloid precursor protein (APP), regulated by a gene located on chromosome 21. For more information on genetics and ApoE, see Chapter 1, p. 3.

The gender issue, with women more likely to develop AD, follows a trans-Atlantic division line. Studies in Europe claim female gender to be a risk factor, but such an association has not been verified in the United States (3,4).

HEAD TRAUMA, HEAD CIRCUMFERENCE, AND BODY TEMPERATURE

Head trauma in early adulthood has been found to increase the risk of AD in later life (5). This relation seems to be established. The association of a lower than normal body temperature and the risk

From: *Current Clinical Neurology,*
Alzheimer's Disease: A Physician's Guide to Practical Management
Edited by: R. W. Richter and B. Zoeller Richter © Humana Press Inc., Totowa, NJ

for AD, however, is based mainly on anecdotal observations and findings in patients with Down's syndrome and dementia *(6)*. It is based on the belief that a low temperature influences the biomechanics of the disease and promotes its development. Still controversially discussed is (small) head circumference as a possible risk factor for AD.

EDUCATION, OCCUPATION, AND MARITAL STATUS

Low educational level, social, and economic status, are suggested to be risk factors for the development of AD. According to a national survey in Scotland, late-onset dementia is associated with lower mental ability scores in childhood *(7)*. A community-based cohort study conducted in Sweden shows an increased incidence of clinical AD or dementia in subjects with a low level of education compared to those with a higher level (less than eight formal school years vs more than eight) *(8)*. The same association has been documented in several other studies *(9,10)*.

Of particular interest, because of biological plausibility, could be the finding of occupational exposure to defoliants and fumigants as a significant risk factor for AD. Even after adjusting for age, education, and gender, the relative risk was still very high (4.35) *(10)*.

Being single or living alone places one at significantly higher risk for developing AD than being married *(11)*. The risk is twofold higher for dementia, and threefold higher for AD. The same positive correlation has been found between AD and social isolation or avoidance of social activities as well as unproductive job and lack of physical activity.

ENVIRONMENTAL INFLUENCES AND TOXINS

There is longstanding discussion of whether exposure to neurotoxicants can in the long run cause progressive declines in the function of the central nervous system beyond what is expected with normal aging.

Aluminum clearly is a powerful neurotoxicant, but convincing scientific evidence for an association with exposure to aluminum and the development of AD or dementia is still missing. Whether the link is causal is still open to debate. T. P. Flaten in Norway reviewed the epidemiological evidence linking aluminum and AD. Nine of 13 published studies of aluminum in drinking water and AD have consistently shown statistically significant positive relations, as the author states *(12)*.

Among putative neurotoxicants, lead is relatively well studied. Whereas lead exposure early in life is associated with cognitive and behavioral consequences in early adulthood, no convincing information existed concerning late-life neurobehavioral effects. A rather recent publication suggests for the first time with clear data that cognitive function, particularly functions such as learning and memory, can progressively decline due to past occupational exposure to lead *(13)*.

A Canadian group of researchers studied the influence of environmental pesticide exposure on the development of AD in 1924 randomly selected subjects 70 years of age and older. The results of this study failed to show a significant risk of AD with exposure to herbicides, insecticides, and pesticides *(14)*.

Pilot data from a recently published experimental study suggest the possibility of increased clearance of beta-amyloid (Aβ) from the brain, identified as increased blood levels, among cholesterol-fed rabbits administered distilled water instead of tap water *(15)*. These findings suggest a previously unrecognized role of dietary water quality in the severity of neuropathology induced by elevated cholesterol. Increased circulating cholesterol is known to promote the production and accumulation of Aβ deposited in the so-called senile plaques. The agents in tap water that are excluded by distillation, promoting accumulation of neuronal Aβ immunoreactivity, are yet undisclosed. The neuronal accumulation of Aβ induced by increased concentrations of circulating cholesterol in rabbits was in this study attenuated when the animals received distilled water.

OXIDATIVE STRESS AND HEME DEFICIENCY

Oxidative stress (with the formation of free oxygen radicals) can cause irreversible damage to the brain, especially when it affects the structures chronically. In the brains of AD patients, significantly increased levels of aluminum and of iron have been found in the regions susceptible for degeneration. These metals may be the source of chronic oxidative stress, but the definite mechanisms in the pathogenesis are still under investigation.

Heme is a major functional form of iron in the cell. It is synthesized in the mitochondria by ferrochelatase inserting ferrous iron into protoporphyrin IX. Heme deficiency in brain cells decreases mitochondrial complex IV, activates nitric oxide synthase, alters amyloid precursor protein (APP), and corrupts iron and zinc homeostasis. As Atamna and colleagues point out, the metabolic consequences resulting from heme deficiency seem similar to dysfunctional neurons in patients with AD *(16)*. Common causes of heme deficiency include aging, iron and vitamin B6 deficiencies, as well as exposure to toxic metals such as aluminum.

The rate-limiting enzyme for the degradation of heme (a pro-oxidant) to iron and biliverdin (which is converted into bilirubin) is heme oxygenase (HO). This enzyme is increased in AD, suggesting an increased turnover as a source of redox-active iron. At the same time, the number of mitochondria appears to be decreased in AD, indicating an accelerated mitochondria turnover *(17)*. The role of mitochondria is relevant mainly as a source of redox-active iron. Studies on redox-competent copper and iron indicate that redox activity in AD resides exclusively within the cytosol of vulnerable neurons. These recent findings taken together suggest that mitochondrial dysfunction could be seen as a potentially inseparable component of the initiation and progression of AD *(17)*.

LIFESTYLE FACTORS

Chronic alcoholism may lead to dementia, as observed in Wernicke-Korsakoff syndrome. Dementia in this syndrome relates also to nutritional deficiencies. Epidemiological studies, however, have not yet found strong evidence for a clear relationship between alcoholism and risk of dementia *(18)*. Some AD patients, however, compound their disease with sequelae from chronic alcoholism.

It was once believed from case-control studies that smoking might protect against AD. This can no longer be considered to be true. More recent cohort studies have suggested that smoking may even increase the risk of dementia *(19)*.

Diet obviously plays an important role, not only in terms of general health and well-being. Caloric restriction (reduced calorie intake), for example, can increase the resistance of neurons in the brain to dysfunction and death in experimental models of Alzheimer's and other diseases *(20)*. Higher intake of calories and fats, on the other hand, may be associated with higher risk of AD *(21)*. A recent survey revealed that high intake of unsaturated, unhydrogenated fats may be protective against AD, whereas the intake of saturated or trans-unsaturated (hydrogenated) fats might increase the risk of incident AD *(22)*.

MEMORY PERFORMANCE AND OLFACTORY DEFICITS

Are memory complaints predictive for dementia, or should they always be considered benign consequences of aging? According to a large review of clinical and population-based studies, memory complaints should be taken not only seriously, but as a possible early sign of dementia *(23)*. The prevalence of memory complaints shows a large variation, ranging from 25% to 50% in elderly individuals. Memory complaints were predictive of dementia in this review, particularly in subjects with mild cognitive impairment (defined as >23 on the Mini-Mental State Examination [MMSE]). In highly educated persons memory complaints appear to be predictive of dementia even when there is yet no apparent indication of cognitive impairment *(23)*.

Individuals with increased genetic risk for familial AD not only perform poorly on neuropsychological performance but also have early chemosensory impairments (for example, smell) that predate the onset of the disease compared to those not at risk *(24)*. Early olfactory impairment may be of predictive utility and is already used as diagnostic marker for AD (*see* Chapter 18, p. 165). Compared to healthy subjects, olfaction scores are lower in patients with mild cognitive impairment *(25)*. This helps support the belief that mild cognitive impairment indeed is a precursor of AD (see following).

MILD COGNITIVE IMPAIRMENT

Recent epidemiological studies suggest a screening and diagnostic classification of dementia into three groups: individuals who are demented; individuals who are not demented; and a third group, individuals who can be classified as neither normal nor demented, but who are cognitively (mostly memory) impaired. The latter are characterized as having mild cognitive impairment (MCI). These subjects are considered at increased risk for developing dementia or AD, and they, in order possibly to alter the course or the rate of progression to dementia, should be paid increased attention in terms of being offered treatment *(26)*. Controlled studies of MCI patients are already underway. If this concept receives final validation, it would represent one of the very few opportunities for potentially preventing dementia *(27)*. Whereas the conversion rate to AD in normal age-matched controls is not higher than 1–4% (depending on age), it is increased up to 15% on average in cases of MCI.

MCI is not easy to diagnose. One structural correlate of the condition, however, could be identified. Patients with MCI appear to have a measurably reduced hippocampal volume, which means smaller hippocampi, probably due to an atrophic process. MCI patients do not yet fulfill the actual clinical criteria for the diagnosis of AD. Essential features, however, are memory complaints, normal general cognition, intact activities of daily living, but with abnormal memory function *(28)*.

MEDICAL CONDITIONS

Several medical conditions can influence and alter cognition and mental status. Cancer patients, for example, often have multiple causes of delirium, many of which are treatable—with usually rapid improvement in their cognitive status.

A new and important finding is the possible association with a history of migraines and a significantly increased risk of AD *(10)*.

Major depression and depressive symptoms have been found to be a risk factor for AD. Depression can be considered an early manifestation of dementia, before cognitive symptoms become apparent *(29)*.

A relationship also was reported recently between cerebral white matter lesions (periventricular and subcortical) and subjective cognitive failures *(30)*. The white matter hyperintensities may contribute to specific neurological and neuropsychiatric manifestations but not to global cognitive impairment, which is more closely associated with brain atrophy, as the authors conclude. The white matter changes in AD seem to represent superimposed phenomena of vascular origin *(30)*.

Down's syndrome is now considered a clear risk factor for AD. As many as 50% of persons with Down's syndrome may develop clinical manifestations of AD, usually in the age group over 30 years.

Subclinical hyperthyroidism in the elderly is suggested to increase the risk of dementia and AD. The risk of dementia and of AD is more than threefold (relative risk 3.5) in subjects with reduced thyroid-stimulating hormone (TSH) levels at baseline compared to those with normal levels (<0.4 or >4.0 U/L), as was shown in the first prospective study on this relationship *(31)*. Also noted, elevated TSH levels (hypothyroidism) carried a risk for dementia in population-based studies *(32)*.

INFECTIONS AND INFLAMMATION

As in the field of cardiology for coronary heart disease, infection of the nervous system with *Chlamydia pneumoniae* now is considered by some researchers to be a risk factor for sporadic AD.

The organism was found in high frequency in glial cells within the brains of AD patients *(33)*. The hypothesis behind this reflects the fact that AD is a chronic condition in which inflammation has been shown to contribute to the neurodegenerative process.

The relationship between brain inflammation and neuropathological disorders has recently been confirmed by Weaver and colleagues in Boston. In a prospective cohort study, they investigated the effect of elevated levels of interleukin-6 (IL-6) on cognitive function. Result: High levels of IL-6 were indeed associated with poorer baseline cognitive function and predicted increased risk for cognitive decline for older men and women who had relatively higher functioning at the beginning of the study *(34)*.

HOMOCYSTEINE

Elevated plasma levels of homocysteine may be a risk factor not only for arteriosclerosis but also for dementia and AD *(35)*. Homocysteine enhances accumulation of DNA damage by impairing DNA-repair capacity. In mitotic cells such DNA damage can lead to cancer, while in postmitotic cells such as neurons it promotes cell death *(36)*. According to the recently published analysis by Miller and colleagues, elevated plasma homocysteine in patients with AD appears to be related to vascular disease and not AD pathology. Low vitamin B_6 status, however, is prevalent in AD patients *(37)*. It remains to be determined if elevated plasma homocysteine or low vitamin B_6 status directly influences AD pathogenesis or progression *(37)*.

The increase in homocysteine levels usually is caused by a (dietary) deficiency in folic acid (folate). It is generally considered that homocysteine potentiates endothelial and neuronal oxidative injury in vascular dementia and AD.

Unrecognized vitamin B_{12} deficiency, common particularly in the elderly, may produce significant neurpsychiatric symptoms, including memory and cognitive impairment *(38)*.

VASCULAR DISEASES AND HYPERTENSION

Cerebrovascular diseases may predispose for dementia. The association between AD and vascular factors may reflect some of the shared pathogenic pathways, such as ApoE4, oxidative stress, apoptosis, disturbance in the renin–angiotensin system, and psychological stress. AD, on the other hand, causes or stimulates vascular diseases.

Among cardiovascular diseases, diabetes mellitus and hypertension are positively associated with cognitive decline *(39)*. Both are considered risk factors for AD and vascular dementia (VaD). When both hypertension and diabetes are present, the risk for developing VaD is sixfold higher, according to recent data generated in the New York region *(40)*.

In the Rotterdam study, subjects taking antihypertensive medication at baseline had a reduced incidence of dementia (adjusted relative risk 0.76) *(41)*.

New and important data on the association between low blood pressure and AD was derived from the Swedish Kungsholmen project *(42)*. Both very low diastolic (≤65 mmHg) and high systolic pressure (>180 mmHg) in this study, examining an elderly population, were associated with an increased risk of AD and dementia. High diastolic blood pressure (>90 mmHg), in contrast, was not associated with dementia incidence *(42)*. This result certainly will have some clinical appreciation and implication, particularly with regard to the low blood pressure goals recommended in recent guidelines for antihypertensive therapy in diabetic patients.

Type 2 diabetes is a risk factor for AD and VaD. The association appears to be particularly strong among carriers of the apolipoprotein E (ApoE) e4-allele *(43)*. Individuals in the Honolulu–Asia aging study with both diabetes and ApoEe4-genotype had a relative risk of 5.5 for AD compared to those with neither risk factor. Pathologically, they showed an increased number of hippocampal neuritic plaques and neurofibrillary tangles in the cortex and hippocampus. They also had a higher risk of cerebral amyloid angiopathy, thus reflecting the very neuropathology of AD *(43)*.

Taken together, the data concerning diabetes and risk for AD are conflicting. There are studies in which an association could not be proven, even though diabetes was associated with incident vascular cognitive impairment *(44)*.

These findings nevertheless allow for the assumption that modification of vascular risk factors could have significant impact on prevention, successful treatment, and delay of AD.

The group of Jaakko Tuomilehto in Finland also regards hypercholesterolemia during midlife as a risk factor for AD in later life and recommends timely pharmacological intervention for lowering elevated lipid levels *(45)*.

POTENTIALLY PROTECTIVE FACTORS

Several variables appear to follow an inverse association with the presence of dementia or symptoms of AD. This suggests some potential for protection. These variables include the ApoE2-allele, higher educational level, use of anti-inflammatory agents, as well as the use of statins. In a large prospective study, researchers in the Netherlands found that the risk of developing AD decreased with increasing intake of nonsteroidal antiinflammatory agents (NSAIDs) *(46)*.

Past exposure to vaccines against diphtheria or tetanus, poliomyelitis, and influenza may also protect against subsequent development of AD. This observation resulted from an analysis conducted by René Verreault and collegues in Quebec *(47)*.

Neuroprotective mechanisms may be bolstered by dietary and behavioral modifications (caloric restriction; intellectual and physical activity). The risk for the development of AD may be reduced by the intake of antioxidant vitamins (C and E) or carotenes. In a recently published investigation, however, Luchsinger and colleagues concluded that neither dietary, supplemental, nor total intake of carotenes and vitamins C and E was associated with a decreased risk of AD *(48)*.

REFERENCES

1. Alzheimer's Disease International: Global perspective. November 2001: 7.
2. Aronson, M.K. et al.: Dementia. Age-dependent incidence, prevalence, and mortality in the old old. Arch Intern Med 1991; 151: 989–992.
3. Letenneur, L. et al.: Education and the risk for Alzheimer's disease: sex makes a difference. EURODEM pooled analyses. Am J Epidemiol 2000; 151: 1064–1071.
4. Edland, S.D. et al.: Dementia and Alzheimer disease incidence rates do not vary by sex in Rochester, Minn. Arch Neurol 2002; 59: 1589–1593.
5. Plassman, B.L. et al.: Documented head injury in early adulthood and risk of Alzheimer's disease and other dementias. Neurology 2000; 55: 1158–1166.
6. Holtzman, A.; Simon, E.W.: Body temperature as a risk factor for Alzheimer's disease. Med Hypotheses 2000; 55: 440–444.
7. Whalley, L.J. et al.: Childhood mental ability and dementia. Neurology 2000; 55: 1455–1459.
8. Qiu, C. et al.: The influence of education on clinically diagnosed dementia incidence and mortality data from the Kungsholmen project. Arch Neurol 2001; 58: 2034–2039.
9. Letenneur, L. et al.: Are sex and educational level independent predictors of dementia and Alzheimer's disease? Incidence data from the PAQUID project. J Neurol Neurosurg Psychiatry 1999; 66: 177–183.
10. Tyas, S.L. et al.: Risk factors for Alzheimer's disease: a population-based longitudinal study in Manitoba, Canada. Int J Epidemiol 2001; 30: 590–597.
11. Bernhardt, T. et al.: Psychosocial risk factors and dementia—a review. Fortschr Neurol Psychiatr 2002; 70: 283–288.
12. Flaten, T.P.: Aluminum as a risk factor in Alzheimer's disease, with emphasis on drinking water. Brain Res Bull 2001; 55: 187–196.
13. Schwartz, B.S. et al.: Past adult lead exposure is associated with longitudinal decline in cognitive function. Neurology 2000; 55: 1144–1150.
14. Gauthier, E. et al.: Environmental pesticide exposure as a risk factor for Alzheimer's disease: a case-control study. Environ Res 2001; 86: 37–45.
15. Sparks, D.L. et al.: Water quality has a pronounced effect on cholesterol-induced accumulation of Alzheimer amyloid beta (Abeta) in rabbit brain. J Alzheimers Dis 2002; 4: 523–529.
16. Atamna, H. et al.: Heme deficiency may be a factor in the mitochondrial and neuronal decay of aging. Proc Natl Acad Sci USA 2002; 99: 14807–14812.

17. Perry, G. et al.: Adventiously-bound redox active iron and copper are at the center of oxidative damage in Alzheimer's disease. Biometals 2003; 16: 77–81.
18. Tyas, S.L.: Alcohol use and the risk of developing Alzheimer's disease. Alcohol Res Health 2001; 25: 299–306.
19. Almeida, O.P. et al.: Smoking as a risk factor for Alzheimer's disease: contrasting evidence from a systematic review of case-control and cohort studies. Addiction 2002; 97: 15–28.
20. Mattson, M.P.: Neuroprotective signaling and the agin brain: take away my food and let me run. Brain Res 2000; 886: 47–53.
21. Luchsinger, J.A. et al.: Caloric intake and the risk of Alzheimer disease. Arch Neurol 2002; 59: 1258–1263.
22. Morris, M.C. et al.: Dietary fats and the risk of incident Alzheimer disease. Arch Neurol 2003; 60: 194–200.
23. Jonker, C. et al.: Are memory complaints predictive for dementia? A review of clinical and population-based studies. Int J Geriatr Psychiatry 2000; 15: 983–991.
24. Schiffman, S.S. et al.: Taste, smell and neuropsychological performance of individuals at familial risk for Alzheimer's disease. Neurobiol Aging 2002; 23: 397–404.
25. Devanand, D.P. et al.: Olfactory deficits in patients with mild cognitive impairment predict Alzheimer's disease at follow-up. Am J Psychiatry 2000; 157: 1399–1405.
26. Petersen, R.C. et al.: Practice parameter: early detection of dementia: mild cognitive impairment (an evidence-based review). Neurology 2001; 56: 1133–1142.
27. Burns, A.; Zaudig, M.: Mild cognitive impairment in older people. Lancet 2002; 360: 1963–1965.
28. Petersen, R.C.: Mild cognitive impairment: transition from aging to Alzheimer's disease. In: Iqbal, K.; Sisodia, S.S.; Winblad, B. (eds.): Alzheimer's disease: advances in etiology, pathogenesis and therapeutics. Wiley, New York, NY, 2001: 141–151.
29. Geerlings, M.I. et al.: Depression and risk of cognitive decline and Alzheimer's disease. Results of two prospective community-based studies in the Netherlands. Br J Psychiatry 2000; 176: 568–575.
30. Hirono, N. et al.: Impact of white matter changes on clinical manifestation of Alzheimer's disease: a quantitative study. Stroke 2000; 31: 2182–2188.
31. Kalmijn, S. et al.: Subclinical hyperthyroidism and the risk of dementia. The Rotterdam study. Clin Endocrinol 2000; 53: 733–737.
32. Ganguli, M. et al.: Association between dementia and elevated TSH: a community based study. Biol Psychiatry 1996; 40: 714–725.
33. Balin, B.J.; Appelt, D.M.: Role of infection in Alzheimer's disease. J Am Osteopath Assoc 2001; 101: S1–S6.
34. Weaver, J.D. et al.: Interleukin-6 and risk of cognitive decline. Neurology 2002; 59: 371–378.
35. Seshadri, S. et al.: Plasma homocysteine as a risk factor for dementia and Alzheimer's disease. N Engl J Med 2002; 348: 476–483.
36. Mattson, M.P. et al.: Folic acid and homocysteine in age-related disease. Ageing Res Rev 2002; 1: 95–111.
37. Miller, J.W. et al.: Homocysteine, vitamin B6, and vascular disease in AD patients. Neurology 2002; 58: 1471–1475.
38. Healton, E.B. et al.: Neurologic aspects of cobalamin deficiency. Medicine (Baltimore) 1991; 70: 229–245.
39. Knopman, D. et al.: Cardiovascular risk factors and cognitive decline in middle-aged adults. Neurology 2001; 56: 42–48.
40. Posner, H.B. et al.: The relationship of hypertension in the elderly to AD, vascular dementia, and cognitive function. Neurology 2002; 58: 1175–1181.
41. In't Veld, B.A. et al.: Antihypertensive drugs and incidence of dementia. The Rotterdam Study. Neurobiol Aging 2001; 22: 407–412.
42. Qiu, C. et al.: Low blood pressure and risk of dementia in the Kungsholmen project. A 6-year follow-up study. Arch Neurol 2003; 60: 223–228.
43. Peila, R. et al.: Type 2 diabetes, ApoE gene, and the risk for dementia and related pathologies: the Honolulu-Asia aging study. Diabetes 2002; 51: 1256–1262.
44. MacKnight, C. et al.: Diabetes mellitus and the risk of dementia, Alzheimer's disease and vascular cognitive impairment in the Canadian study of health and Aging. Dement Geriatr Cogn Disord 2002; 14: 77–83.
45. Kivipelto, M. et al.: Hypertension and hypercholesterolemia as risk factors for Alzheimer's disease: potential for pharmacological intervention. CNS Drugs 2002; 16: 435–444.
46. In't Veld, B.A. et al.: Nonsteroidal antiinflammatory drugs and the risk of Alzheimer's disease. N Engl J Med 2001; 345: 1515–1521.
47. Verreault, R. et al.: Past exposure to vaccines and subsequent risk of Alzheimer's disease. CMAJ 2001; 165: 1495–1498.
48. Luchsinger, J.A. et al.: Antioxidant vitamin intake and risk of Alzheimer disease. Arch Neurol 2003; 60: 203–208.

III Clinical Assessment

8

Medical Diagnosis and Workup of Alzheimer's Disease

Ralph W. Richter

INTRODUCTION

In 1907, Dr. Aloys Alzheimer, a German neuropsychiatrist, described a dementing syndrome with newly recognized neuropathological features. The clinical symptoms included memory loss, speech disorders, apraxia, and paranoid delusions. At autopsy, neurofibrillary changes and abnormal miliary foci were identified. Aloys Alzheimer provided a clinical and pathological basis for the disease that bears his name.

For a number of years, Alzheimer's disease (AD) was artificially divided into two entities: presenile dementia in individuals under the age of 65 years, and senile dementia of the Alzheimer's type for those over 65 years of age. This distinction is no longer viable since the best authoritative studies have found no major clinical difference between early- and late-onset forms of the disease.

DEFINITION

AD was originally defined in terms of the clinical and neuropathological pattern. Both elements are still required for definitive diagnosis. The accuracy of clinical diagnosis in reality is measured in the ability of the clinician to predict the presence or absence of the typical neuropathological lesions at autopsy.

AD is a progressive degenerative disorder, characterized by impairments of memory (particularly recent memory) and disturbances in at least one other cognitive domain (Table 1).

The clinical diagnosis of AD is based on a combination of thorough clinical testing—physical and neurological examination, neuroimaging techniques, and laboratory tests—and use of validated neuropsychological assessment tools (1). Previously it was considered a disease recognized after exclusion of other possible forms of dementia. Now AD can be considered a diagnosis of inclusion, with specific defining characteristics. Selected criteria for diagnosis of AD (NINCDS-ADRDA [2]) are listed in Table 2.

The course of AD tends to be slowly progressive, with a loss of 3–4 points per year on the Mini-Mental State Examination (MMSE) or an average yearly change on the Alzheimer's disease assessment scale—cognitive subscale (ADAS-cog) of between 7 and 9 points (3).

The disease is associated with various patterns of deficits: early impairment of recent memory, personality changes or increased irritability, sleep disturbances—day/night reversal, with so-called sundowning phenomenon—(in the early stages), gait and motor disturbances (in the later stages).

The diagnosis of AD can be suspected even in the presence of another potentially dementing disorder. The following discussion describes a basis for the workup of a person with possible AD, in terms of a series of questions.

From: *Current Clinical Neurology,*
Alzheimer's Disease: A Physician's Guide to Practical Management
Edited by: R. W. Richter and B. Zoeller Richter © Humana Press Inc., Totowa, NJ

Table 1
DSM-IV Diagnostic Criteria for AD

Multiple cognitive deficits
    Short- and long-term memory impairment
    One or more of the following:
        Aphasia (language disturbance)
        Apraxia (impaired ability to carry out familiar tasks)
        Agnosia (failure to recognize familiar objects)
        Disturbances in executive functioning (planning, organizing, abstract thinking)
    Gradual onset, significant functional impairment, and continuous decline
    Decline from a previously higher level of function
    Exclusion of other possible causes
    No evidence for delirium.

Source: Adapted from DSM-IV™, 1994.

Table 2
Selected NINCDS-ADRDA Criteria

Probable Alzheimer's disease
    Dementia
    Deficits in two or more cognitive domains
    Progressive worsening of memory and other cognitive functions
    No disturbance of consciousness
    Onset between 40 and 90 years of age
    Absence of other systemic disorders
    Progressive worsening of specific cognitive functions
    Impaired activities of daily life (ADL)
    Associated behavioral abnormalities
Possible Alzheimer's disease
    Dementia syndrome in the absence of other neurological, psychiatric, or systemic disorders sufficient to
    cause dementia, and in the presence of variations in the onset, in the presentation, or in the clinical course
Uncertain/unlikely Alzheimer's disease
    Sudden onset
    Focal neurological findings
    Early seizures or gait disturbances

Source: Modified from ref. 2.

Is the Patient Demented?

Dementia disorders include conditions in which multiple cognitive deficits occur (including memory impairment) as a consequence of the direct neurophysiological effects of a general medical condition, persisting effects of a toxic substance, or multiple etiologies.

Dementia must be distinguished from delirium, which is by definition transient and potentially reversible, and from depression, which leads to poor performance on mental status examination or formal neuropsychological testing.

Global cognitive impairment means, in practice, that the patient has difficulty with memory and with at least two other areas of cognitive function.

For the primary-care physician, a number of office tests are available that can be given by nurses or other paraprofessionals after minimal extra training and are potentially reimbursable. A review of rating scales used in clinical trials is provided in Chapter 38, pp. 337 ff. The most consistently used of these tests is the MMSE, developed by M. Folstein and colleagues *(4)*. Although brief, this test is in fact a neuropsychologically sophisticated instrument, which has been widely used and standardized. The MMSE evaluates, albeit not in depth, a variety of important functions including short- and long-term memory, calculation, orientation, and constructional ability. Age-related norms have been published *(5)*. In ordinary use, a patient who scores less than 24 (out of 30) is usually classified as having dementia or some other condition impairing cognitive function. A patient who scores 20 or less is likely to be clearly impaired, even if relatively mildly, in activities of daily living (ADL).

There is an educational curve in the MMSE. People who have not been to school consistently do more poorly than those with at least a sixth-grade education *(5)*. Researchers debate whether that is inherent in the nature of the test (which relies on language) or in fact indicates that lack of any education is a risk factor for dementia in later life.

For the primary-care physician, the use of the MMSE within an office practice provides a robust, simple, economical addition to the ability to diagnose and follow patients with cognitive impairments. It is particularly useful to reveal deficits in patients whose social skills are preserved and who are skillful at disguising their mental impairments. If the physician feels that further specification of the patient's mental state is needed, a specialist such as a geriatric neurologist or psychiatrist should be consulted.

Clock drawing may also provide a quick measure of cognitive function. The clinician or office staff member asks the patient for a free drawing of a clock. The accuracy of the drawing can be a valid measure of the patient's cognitive state. Kirsten I. Taylor and Andreas U. Monsch review clock drawing and dementia in Chapter 11, pp. 109 ff.

Is the Patient Delirious?

The changes in mental state in delirium are very similar to those in dementia, except that delirium is variable in time and manifestation. Delirium, unlike dementia, is in principle reversible. Table 3 outlines conditions, that may cause delirium.

The delirious patient tends to have fluctuating levels of awareness, which the alert physician recognizes by the patient's inability to pay consistent attention to the physician. This effect is often described as reduced vigilance. Visual and auditory hallucinations are said to be more prominent in delirium than in dementia, but they can certainly be seen in advanced demented patients as well. Delirious patients tend to have more tremor and other motor manifestations, as in delirium tremens, but these need not be present. In fact, delirium is often associated with alternating periods of excitation and stupor, and the patient with a stuporous delirium may easily be mistaken for a demented patient. Medical illnesses and seizures frequently accompany delirium, but can be seen in dementia as well. And, to make the diagnostic difficulties even more intense, patients with dementia are typically susceptible to conditions that cause delirium.

The neurologist's term for delirium is metabolic-toxic encephalopathy. This terminology is both mechanistic and etiological. Mechanistically, it indicates that delirium is classically associated with impairment of oxidative metabolism in the brain. Indeed, hypoxia is a classical cause of delirium. "Toxic" calls attention to how often neurotoxins can cause delirium. A wide spectrum of drugs may cause delirium, hostility, agitation, uncontrollable crying, confusion, and severe depression *(6)*. These include over-the-counter (OTC) drugs as well as those that require prescription and those that are typically obtained illicitly. Such drugs can lead to a misdiagnosis if the physician is not careful about recording the patient's drug history, especially when obtained from the family members. In elderly patients, higher doses of normally prescribed medications may lead to adverse reactions. In other instances, symptoms may not appear until after cessation of therapy, especially if cessation occurs abruptly.

Older patients may have premorbid pathologies such that the symptoms may be caused either by the disease or by the drug. For example, respiratory insufficiency can cause thought disorder. The addition of a drug that further depresses respiration will further complicate the mental symptoms.

Table 3
Conditions That Cause Delirium

Infections
    Septicemia
    Bronchopneumonia
    Severe urinary infection
    Chronic fungal meningitis
    HIV encephalitis
Head injury
    Acute or chronic subdural hematoma
    Postconcussion syndrome
Decreased cerebral perfusion
    Chronic pulmonary insufficiency
    Chronic hypoxemia
    Severe cardiac output defect
    Transient ischemic attacks (TIA)
    Acute myocardial infarction
Metabolic encephalopathy
    Hypoglycemia, hyperinsulinemia
    Diabetic acidosis
    Severe hypothyoidism
    Thyroid storm
    Severe vitamin B_{12} deficiency
    Electrolyte imbalance
        Hyponatremia or hypernatremia
        Hypocalcemia or hypercalcemia
    Renal insufficiency
    Hepatic encephalopathy
Toxic effects of drugs
    Mind-altering and addictive drugs
    Antipsychotics and antidepressants
    Antiparkinsonian drugs
    Cardiovascular drugs and antihypertensives
    Anticancer drugs
    Anesthetics
    Antimicrobial drugs
    Stimulants
    Muscle relaxants
    Anticholinergics

Advanced age is an important risk factor for delirium, particularly in patients who have become frail. In frail elderly patients, any medical illness has the potential to precipitate delirium. Indeed, altered state of consciousness is a typical presentation of acute myocardial infarction, dehydration with electrolyte imbalance, pneumonia, urosepsis, and other infections in this age group.

Delirium and dementia are not opposites: they fall in a spectrum. Romano and Engel pointed out that for any organ system, organ failure can be due to fixed anatomical damage or reversible functional damage *(7)*. In general, anatomical damage makes an organ more susceptible to functional insults, and functional impairment can often lead to fixed anatomical damage. Romano and Engel point out that dementia and delirium are both manifestations of brain failure. Dementia is evidence of anatomical brain damage, and delirium is a sign of functional impairment. The two conditions often interact. Patients with preexisting dementia or any prior cognitive impairment are at greater risk for prolonged delirium *(8)*.

For the primary-care physician, an altered state of consciousness, particularly in an elderly patient, presents a diagnostic problem analogous to fever of unknown origin. It presents the physician with the opportunity to use his or her full diagnostic abilities. There is no experience more gratifying than the restoration of an elderly person to active life and to his or her family by the recognition and appropriate treatment of an unrecognized and correctable illness.

Is the Patient Depressed? Is the Patient Psychotic?

An extensive literature discusses the difficulty of distinguishing dementia from depression, particularly in elderly subjects. The term "pseudodementia" was originally used by Madden to describe elderly individuals with depression and other psychiatric complaints, who had associated symptoms of cognitive impairment, which cleared when their depression was treated appropriately *(9)*. This condition has since been renamed the dementia of depression, to indicate that there is a real cognitive impairment. That latter term is itself misleading, however, because the depression is not clearly linked to fixed, anatomical brain damage.

In fact, the distinction between primary depression and primary dementia can usually be made by a careful examination by a sensitive clinician. Utilization of the Hamilton depression scale may also be of value *(10)*. Anyone who has taken a test on a day when he or she is "down" knows that affect can impair cognitive performance. For the patient who meets the criteria for true psychiatric depression, this problem is much worse. These patients do poorly if rushed or stressed. On the other hand, formal testing by procedures such as the MMSE normally does not indicate impairment adequate to diagnose dementia if the patient is not rushed and is induced to cooperate in the testing process.

The situation is complicated by the well-documented observation that depression is a common accompanying manifestation of dementing illnesses, including AD. Indeed, depression can be the presenting manifestation of what later turns out to be a dementing illness. Presumably, in these cases the damage involves structures in the brain that are involved in the regulation of mood. Thus the diagnosis of depression does not rule out the diagnosis of dementia, and vice versa. Furthermore, it should be emphasized that depression can be successfully treated in a patient who also has dementia.

Schizophrenia was originally described as dementia praecox *(11)*. It is commonly held, although it has not been extensively documented by current criteria, that a proportion of patients with schizophrenia and other psychoses go on to develop true dementia. In fact, it has been suggested in the literature that the following negative symptoms of schizophrenia are associated with structural brain disease *(12)*: (1) a loss or decline in normal psychological functioning; (2) problems in relating emotionally with other persons; and (3) inability to express emotions appropriately. Recognition that a patient with dementia has long-standing schizophrenia is usually made by an accurate history.

There is a syndrome of late-onset psychosis, termed in the European literature paraphrenia, whose etiology is unclear. Some of these patients, however, have AD presenting primarily as psychosis rather than primarily as a disorder of memory and other aspects of cognition. Alzheimer's own first index patient with this disease was, in fact, a woman in her 50s, whose first symptom was noted as pathological jealousy, although she soon thereafter developed memory problems.

For the primary-care physician, a careful history and appropriately performed MMSE will usually distinguish a dementia even in the presence of depression. Psychiatric manifestations of a dementing disorder can be extremely unpleasant for the patient and very troubling for the family or other caregivers, including nursing home staff. Judicious use of antidepressants or antipsychotics can be considered. For more complicated problems, consultation with a geriatric psychiatrist or neurologist may be recommended.

Table 4
Hachinski Ischemia Scale

For each item, circle the number if present.

1. Abrupt onset	2
2. Stepwise deterioration	1
3. Fluctuating course	2
4. Nocturnal confusion	1
5. Relative preservation of personality	1
6. Depression	1
7. Somatic complaints	1
8. Emotional incontinence	1
9. History or presence of hypertension[a]	1
10. History of strokes	2
11. Evidence of atherosclerosis	1
12. Focal neurological symptoms	2
13. Focal neurological signs	2
TOTAL _____	

[a]Defined as either a history of present or previous hypertensive therapy or a current and consistent blood pressure of 170/110 mmHg or more.

Source: Developed from Hachinski, V.C. et al.: Cerebral blood flow in dementia. Arch Neurol 1975; 32: 632–637. Rosen, W.G. et al.: Pathological verification of ischemic score in differentiation of dementias. Ann Neurol 1980; 7: 486–488.

What Further Evaluation Does the Patient Need?

In a landmark paper, Larson and co-workers showed that the amount of workup appropriate for a patient with cognitive problems depended on how well the patient was known to the examining physician *(13)*. In practice, an accurate history is always critical. Family physicians who know their patients may have a diagnostic advantage in being better able to recognize subtle or early cognitive changes as well as recent sudden changes that might indicate new associated conditions. Utilizing the Hachinski ischemia scale (Table 4) may help to identify patients at risk for cardiovascular problems including strokes (score above 5), but this is not a good predictor of the presence or absence of changes caused by AD *(14)*.

Complete historical data from relatives and previous caregivers is extremely useful when it can be obtained. However, a large number of elderly urban dwellers developing dementia live alone. They may have relatives who live some distance away and who are in denial of these changes. When the demented person's welfare appears endangered, concerned neighbors may have to come to their rescue by requesting help from municipal resources, such as an adult protection agency or police.

Intervention may also be precipitated by an acute illness or injury, necessitating admission to the urban hospital setting. Here also, demented patients are often seen for whom no history (i.e., no informant) is available. Considerable effort by social workers or other health-care personnel may be required to unravel these difficult patient situations.

PHYSICAL AND NEUROLOGICAL EXAMINATION

As discussed above, confusion can be the presenting sign of a wide variety of relatively acute medical and neurological conditions in the elderly. There is no recipe for how to conduct the physical and neurological evaluation of such a patient, except the invariant need to be careful and thorough.

If the physician knows the patient, he or she should look for new signs. The new onset of focal weakness might indicate a superimposed stroke or even early signs of evolving subdural hematoma. If the physician does not know the patient, then he or she should plan to focus even more on potentially abnormal neurological exam findings.

CLINICAL LABORATORY WORKUP

Appropriate laboratory studies again vary with how well the patient is known by the physician. A titer for Lyme disease may be appropriate in areas such as the Northeast, where Lyme disease is endemic. If there is any evidence of risk factors, an HIV (human immune deficiency virus) titer also seems advisable. Recently, in some U.S. retirement communities, a number of sexually promiscuous elderly persons have become HIV-positive.

If there is evidence of chronic fatigue, measuring Epstein-Barr viral titer may be useful. Administering antinuclear antibodies (ANA) or C-reactive protein to patients may help identify with unrecognized medical disorders leading to cerebral damage, such as cerebral vasculitis. Sedimentation (SED) rate is more useful in younger than in elderly patients, in whom it can be nonspecifically elevated.

If a patient is not well known to the physician, a more extensive clinical laboratory examination is recommended, including but not necessarily limited to SMAC 25, etc. Vitamin B_{12} levels should be determined routinely in the study of older patients. Unrecognized B_{12} deficiency may produce significant neuropsychiatric symptoms *(15)*. Cognitive and behavioral correlates of low vitamin B_{12} levels in patients with progressive dementia were recently reviewed *(16)*. Thyroid deficiency must be considered. In a population-based study, elevated thyroid-stimulating hormone (TSH) levels carried an increased risk for dementia *(17)*.

IMAGING TECHNIQUES

Computerized tomography (CT) or nuclear magnetic resonance imaging (MRI) is now part of standard U.S. practice, even though the yield of treatable illness is still low. Brain scans will detect subdural hematomas and tumors, and, along with isotope cisternography, may help identify the rare patient with normal pressure hydrocephalus. Structural imaging will also reveal brain atrophy. Certain structural correlates appear to be predictive for AD, such as progressive decrease in hippocampal volume on serial MRI.

Functional imaging takes pictures of brain activity at a particular moment. These images are created with functional MRI (fMRI), single photon emission computer tomography (SPECT), and positron emission tomography (PET). Neuroimaging techniques are reviewed by Norman L. Foster in Chapter 9, pp. 89 ff.

CARDIOLOGICAL ASPECTS

Cardiological studies, cardiovascular and cerebrovascular evaluation, such as Holter or event monitoring and echocardiogram (ECG), may raise suspicions of cardiogenic factors in inducing dementia in certain patients. It is very gratifying to see reversal of a dementing process in a person whose myocardial neural conduction defect has been recognized and treated with a pacemaker implant, thereby restoring adequate brain vascular perfusion. A search for cerebrovascular factors contributing to dementia would include duplex scanning of the carotid and vertebral arteries. José Medina reviews cardiological aspects of dementia in Chapter 26, pp. 225 ff.

OTHER NEUROLOGICAL CONDITIONS THAT CAN CAUSE DEMENTIA

Dementia can be caused by many other neurological conditions, some of which are extremely rare (Table 5). One must keep in mind that the dementia syndrome can have more than one etiological basis in the older patient.

Table 5
Differential Diagnosis of Dementia

Alzheimer's disease (AD)
Vascular dementia (VaD)
    Multi-infarct dementia (MID)
    Vascular cognitive impairment
    Binswanger's disease (BD)
Lewy body dementia (DLB)
    Diffuse Lewy body disease
    Lewy body variant of AD
Parkinson's disease (PD)
Other dementias
    Frontotemporal dementias (FTD)
    Progressive supranuclear palsy
    Down's syndrome
    Huntington's disease
    Normal pressure hydrocephalus
    Creutzfeldt-Jakob disease
    Infection-related dementias
    Alcoholism and drug abuse-related dementias

Vascular Dementia

Besides AD—which accounts for more than 60% of all cases of dementia—another very frequent form of dementia is vascular dementia (VaD, 10–20%). As AD and VaD share many symptoms, it is not always easy to distinguish between those two forms. AD and VaD frequently appear in a mixed form, as do AD and Lewy body dementia.

There are, however, several features to help distinguish both forms of dementia, AD and VaD, e.g., onset, disease progression, or gait (Table 6). VaD encompasses cases in which the pathology is associated with ischemic, hemorrhagic, and/or hypoxic-ischemic cerebral lesions. The underlying risk factors for cerebrovascular disease (CVD) include hypertension, diabetes, coronary artery disease, atrial fibrillation, hypercholesterolemia, smoking, and heavy alcohol drinking.

The clinical picture of VaD usually includes abrupt deterioration in cognitive functions or fluctuating stepwise progression of cognitive defects. Focal signs and symptoms are frequently present in VaD. Brain imaging—CT or MRI (including diffusion-weighted imaging)—are likely to demonstrate cerebrovascular insults. Large-vessel lesions of the dominant hemisphere or bilateral large-vessel hemispheric strokes may suddenly produce VaD.

Bilateral thalamic vascular lesions, strokes in the association areas (parietal temporal, temporooccipital territories), and bilateral anterior cerebral artery strokes are also frequently associated with VaD. Progressive and extensive small-vessel disease with multiple lacunes may produce more gradual stepwise deterioration.

For more information, see Chapter 12, pp. 121 ff.

Cardiac disease can be an independent risk factor for AD as well as for VaD. This topic is reviewed in Chapter 26, pp. 225 ff. There is also active interest in the possibility of microvascular lesions in AD, possibly related to cerebrovascular amyloidosis.

Binswanger's Disease

Binswanger's disease (BD) is considered to be of vascular origin, related to chronic hypertension. The pathological changes are greatest in the cerebral white matter, particularly in the territory of the long penetrating arteries. Clinical features include dementia with gait apraxia, hyperreflexia, and per-

Table 6
How to Distinguish AD and VaD—Diagnostic Differences

Feature	VaD	AD
Onset	Sudden or gradual	Gradual
Progression	In steps, fluctuations	Continuously
Gait	May be disturbed early	Normal until severe stage
CV conditions	Cardiovascular risk factors, previous stroke, or transient ischemic attacks	Less common (prevalent in mixed form)
Neurological	Focal deficits	Signs may not be present
Findings/imaging	Multiple infarcts	None but atrophy

sonality changes. BD patients show evidence of fluctuating dementia, with memory disorders in combination with a variety of focal motor impairments *(18)*.

Lewy Body Dementia

Lewy body dementia was previously referred to as diffuse Lewy body disease, Lewy body variant of AD, cortical Lewy body disease, or senile dementia of the Lewy body type. In 1996 Ian McKeith chaired a workshop that established guidelines for the clinical and pathological diagnosis of dementia with Lewy bodies (DLB). It is now recognized as the second most common cause of degenerative dementias.

Lewy bodies are neuronal inclusion bodies consisting of neurofilament material, found in neuronal cytoplasm. The presence of Lewy bodies in the neocortex is the finding necessary to arrive at diagnosis. Lewy bodies are found most often in the temporal lobe, in the cingular gyrus, in the amygdala, and in the insula.

The memory loss in patients with DLB may be more subtle than in those with AD. Patients mostly exhibit rather spontaneously Parkinsonian-type symptoms, hallucinations, delusions, disorders of executive function, and show progressive illness with fluctuation, leading to very severe dementia. Robert Barber, Jane Newby, and Ian McKeith present a review of DLB in Chapter 13, pp. 127 ff.

Parkinson's Disease

As many as 25–40% of elderly patients with advanced Parkinson's disease (PD) develop dementia *(19)*. Impairment in verbal memory and executive function appears to be associated with the early development of dementia in PD patients *(20)*. Visuospatial deficits and difficulties in inhibiting irrelevant stimuli may also be observed *(21)*. One recent study of 180 PD patients concluded that development of dementia was associated with a twofold increase in mortality risk *(22)*.

Clinical and histopathological overlap between AD and PD is common. Individuals with clear-cut clinical manifestations of PD and a progressive dementia, who have Lewy bodies in the brainstem, plus the presence of sufficient senile plaques and neurofibrillary tangles to meet the diagnostic criteria for AD, are to be diagnosed with combined PD and AD.

Frontotemporal Dementia

Frontotemporal dementia (FTD) is another relatively frequent degenerative cause of dementia. Alzheimer pathology is not present. FTD has been considered to be a presenile dementia, because many patients may become symptomatic in their 50s and 60s. Three possible subtypes are based on where the pathological process appears to originate. Initial symptoms may include loss of language functions, and/or personality changes including disinhibited or aggressive behavior. Malgorzata Franszak, Diane Kerwin, and Piero Antuono review FTD in Chapter 14, pp. 137 ff.

Progressive Supranuclear Palsy

Dementia occurs in about 60–80% of patients with progressive supranuclear palsy (PSP), though it is not an obligate part of the syndrome, which includes parkinsonism and ophthalmoparesis *(23)*. Frontal lobe deficits are common in PSP, and are recognized with functional imaging techniques.

Dementia in Down Syndrome

The localization of the APP gene on chromosome 21q is utilized as an explanation of the finding that patients with Down syndrome or trisomy 21 develop dementia with the classical neuropathological features of AD around the age of 30 years and slightly higher *(24)*. Because of the characteristic features of Down syndrome, there should be no difficulty in differential diagnosis.

Huntington's Disease

Huntington's disease (HD) may rarely occur late in life, with chorea and dementia. It is inherited as an autosomal dominant trait through a trinucleotide expansion mutation in a gene located on chromosome 4 *(25)*. Clinical features include changes in personality and deterioration in cognitive ability. Severe depressive symptoms may develop in up to 40% of patients, and suicide risk is substantial *(26)*.

Normal Pressure Hydrocephalus

Normal pressure hydrocephalus (NPH) or occult hydrocephalus may present with symptoms of memory loss, ataxia, and apraxia of gait, as well as urinary incontinence. Changes in mental status occur as a result of impaired cerebrospinal fluid (CSF) flow.

Isotope cisternography is utilized primarily for the demonstration of some types of hydrocephalus. Isotope is injected into the subarachnoid space in the lumbar region. Serial images are obtained to monitor the uptake, flow, and absorption of the isotope within the ventricular system over a 72-hour period. A delay of reabsorption of the isotope from the dilated ventricles is characteristic of NPH.

There has been considerable discussion pertaining to shunting procedures once NPH has been demonstrated *(27)*. In our experience, those who are identified early, before irreversible brain damage has occurred, may show gratifyingly beneficial results from placement of a ventriculo-peritoneal shunt.

Creutzfeldt-Jakob Disease

A rapidly progressing, rare dementia with pyramidal, extrapyramidal, and cerebellar signs as well as myoclonus suggests the presence of Creutzfeldt-Jakob disease (CJD), which is caused by prions. Onset usually occurs in the sixth or seventh decade of life. Symptoms of irritability and unusual somatic sensations are common. Characteristic changes are present on the EEG, with a periodic discharge pattern of 1–2 Hz. Familial forms have also been identified (Gerstmann-Straussler-Scheinker disease).

Harrington and colleagues demonstrated that the cerebrospinal fluid of CJD patients contain abnormal protein fractions *(28)*. The amino acid sequence matched a brain protein known as 14-3-3. A radioimmunoassay was developed and proved 14-3-3 to be a sensitive and relatively specific marker for prion diseases in humans and in animals *(29)*.

Infection-Related Dementias

Many neuropsychiatric manifestations of AIDS, including confusion, disorientation, memory loss, depression, and agitation, as well as neuropathological findings, have been observed *(30)*. Other subacute or chronic infectious diseases may cause memory loss and other symptoms of dementia. Among these are chronic fungal meningitis, viral encephalitis, and its sequelae, Creutzfeldt-Jakob disease, neurosyphilis, and early tuberculous meningitis.

Table 7
Recommendations for the Disease and Patient Management

Assessment

    The following abilities should be assessed and documented:

        Cognitive status (using MMSE)

        Daily and executive functions (eating/cooking, personal hygiene, dressing, continence, toileting; handling finances, planning, decisions)

        Behavioral changes (personality, mood, psychoses)

        Medical status/conditions (vigilance, nutrition, gait)

    Include family and caregiver, legal guardian, as well as support groups

    Discuss job situation/further employment, safe workplace

    Identify expectations, cultural beliefs and values of the patient and family

    Advise for long-term planning decisions (legal, financial, insurance, day care, nursing home, will), as well as environmental changes/adaptations, task simplification

    Address the issue of driving with the patient and the family

    Recommend and help with nursing-home placement in time

Treatment

    Develop treatment plan and define treatment goals, discuss with family

        Use approved and efficacy-proven drugs for AD, monitor tolerance

        Treat co-morbidities appropriately

        Include structured activities (e.g., memory training, physical exercise)

        Treat mood disorders and behavioral problems adequately

        Monitor eating abilities, nutrition/malnutrition

Caregiver/family support

    Discuss diagnosis and explain disease progression in a family conference with caregiver and relatives of the patient

    Provide written information about AD and material (phone numbers, websites) of support groups, Alzheimer's organizations, special-interest groups, local services

Monitoring

    Keep good documentation records of every single measure taken; monitor the patient consistently medically; observe caregiver and identify his/her needs and health status (exhaustion, loneliness, depression), advise for recreation periods and social support.

Source: Modified from ref. *32.*

Alcoholism and Drug Abuse as Causes of Dementia

Many elderly individuals with alcohol use disorders (AUD) or drug abuse are in denial of their problem. A recent survey indicated that primary-care physicians may underdetect AUD among older patients *(31)*. Some AD patients compound their disease with sequelae from chronic alcoholism. Dementia in Wernicke-Korsakoff syndrome relates to alcohol abuse and nutritional deficiencies. Heroin addicts who experience coma from overdose reaction may develop dementia. Adverse reactions to crack cocaine and various hallucinogens may also lead to permanent brain changes *(6)*.

FOLLOW-UP

If a patient is diagnosed with possible or probable AD, he should be scheduled for a continuous follow-up. Follow-up evaluations will document the mostly gradual, progressive worsening of the disease over the stages (mild, moderate, severe), as well as of the neuropsychiatric symptoms. The diagnosis as well as the progression must be discussed with the family of the patient and the caregiver consistently. Local services and support groups should be involved in the long-term management of a patient with AD. Table 7 offers short recommendations for the disease and patient management (Table 7).

CONCLUSIONS

Early identification of the patient who is developing AD or another form of dementia is of paramount importance and is the major goal of the clinical examination and assessment. A thorough clinical workup is particularly important also for the identification of potentially reversible, treatable medical or surgical conditions.

Medications for the treatment of AD are already available, which have produced improvement in cognitive functioning as well as activities of daily living. There are also data available to support the assumption that these medications have the potential to delay progression of the disease.

A number of promising new agents, with different mechanisms of action—for example, cognition-enhancing and neuroprotective compounds—have entered testing phases. New therapeutic methods, such as stem cell therapy, also are under evaluation. Nobody knows if these efforts will produce the urgently needed breakthroughs in order to modify the course of the disease.

SUMMARY

To evaluate a patient with cognitive impairment, a careful history from at least one and if possible more than one reliable informant is necessary. A careful physical and focused neurological examination are needed to determine if there are medical or neurological conditions that could account for the patient's memory complaints or impairments. Of particular importance is the state of vigilance of the patient, in order to differentiate between delirium and dementia. Mental status testing should be done for each of these patients, using the MMSE. Laboratory evaluation also is indicated, as is a CT or MRI scan. Manifestations should be managed clinically, and follow-up visits should be planned.

REFERENCES

1. Knopman, D.S. et al.: Practice parameter: diagnosis of dementia (an evidence-based review). Report of the Quality Standards Subcommittee of the American Academy of Neurology. Neurology 2001; 56: 1143–1153.
2. McKhann, G. et al.: Clinical diagnosis of Alzheimer's disease: report of the NINCDS-ADRDA Work Group under the auspices of Department of Health and Human Services Task Force on Alzheimer's Disease. Neurology 1984; 34: 939–944.
3. Mohs, R. et al.: Neuropathologically validated scales for Alzheimer's disease. In: Crook, T.; Ferris, S.; Bartus, R. (eds.): Assessment in geriatric psychopharmacology. Mark Powley, New Canaan, CT, 1983.
4. Folstein, M. et al.: Mini-Mental State: a practical method for grading the cognitive state of patients for the clinician. J Psychiatr Res 1975; 12: 189–198.
5. Crum, R.M. et al.: Population-based norms for the mini-mental state examination by age and educational level. JAMA 1993; 69: 2420–2421.
6. Richter, R.W. et al.: Neurotoxic syndromes. In: Rosenberg, R.N.; Pleasure, D.E. (eds.): Comprehensive neurology. 2nd edition. Wiley, New York, 1998: 851–887.
7. Engel, G.L.; Romano, J.: Delirium, a syndrome of cerebral insufficiency. J Chron Dis 1959; 9: 260–272.
8. Fick, D.M.; Agostini, J.V.; Inouye, S.K.: Delirium superimposed on dementia. A systematic review. J Am Geriatr Soc 2002; 50: 1723–1732.
9. Madden, J.J. et al.: Non-dementing psychoses in older persons. JAMA 1952; 150: 1567–1570.
10. Hamilton, M.: A rating scale for depression. J Neurol Neurosurg Psychiatry 1960; 23: 56–62.
11. Kraepelin, E,: Dementia praecox and paraphrenia [from the 8th German edition]. Textbook in psychiatry. Robert E. Krieger, Huntington, NY; Vol. III, 1971: vii–xix.
12. Klausner, J.D. et al.: Clinical correlates of cerebral ventricular enlargement in schizophrenia. Further evidence for frontal lobe disease. J Nervous Mental Dis 1992; 180: 407–412.
13. Larson, E.B. et al.: Diagnostic tests in evaluation of dementia: a prospective study of 200 elderly outpatients. Arch Intern Med 1986; 146: 1917–1922.
14. Moroney, J.T. et al.: Meta-analysis of the Hachinski ischemia score in pathologically verified dementias. Neurology 1997; 49: 1096–1105.
15. Lindenbaum, J. et al.: Neuropsychiatric disorders caused by cobalamin deficiency in the absence of anemia or macrocytosis. N Engl J Med 1988; 318: 1720–1727.
16. Whyte, E.M. et al.: Cognitive and behavioral correlates of low vitamin B12 levels in elderly patients with progressive dementia. Am J Geriatr Psychiatry 2002; 10: 321–327.
17. Ganguli, M. et al.: Association between dementia and elevated TSH: a community-based study. Biol Psychiatry 1996; 40: 714–725.

18. Babikian, V.; Kopper, A.H.: Binswanger's disease: a review. Stroke 1987; 18: 2–12.

19. Marder, K. et al.: The frequency and associated risk factors for dementia in patients with Parkinson's disease. Arch Neurol 1995; 52: 695–701.

20. Levy, G. et al.: Memory and executive function impairment predict dementia in Parkinson's disease. Movement Disord 2002; 17: 1221–1226.

21. Mahieux, F. et al.: Neuropsychological prediction of dementia in Parkinson's disease. J Neurol Neurosurg Psychiatry 1998; 64: 178–183.

22. Levy, G. et al.: The association of incident dementia with mortality in PD. Neurology 2002; 59: 1708–1713.

23. Litvan, I. et al.: Accuracy of the clinical criteria for the diagnosis of progressive supranuclear palsy (Steele-Richardson-Olszewski syndrome). Neurology 1996; 46: 922–930.

24. Lai, F.: Clinicopathologic features of Alzheimer disease in Down syndrome. In: Nadel, L.; Epstein, C.S. (eds.): Down syndrome and Alzheimer disease. Wiley-Liss, New York, 1992: 15–34.

25. Young, A.B.: Huntington's disease and other trinucleotide repeat disorders. In: Martin, J.B. (ed.): Molecular neurology. Scientific American, New York, 1998: 35–54.

26. Folstein, S.E. et al.: The association of affective disorder with Huntington's disease in a case series and in families. Psychol Med 1983; 13: 537–542.

27. Vanneste, J. et al.: Shunting normal pressure hydrocephalus: the predictive value of combined clinical and CT data. J Neurol Neurosurg Psychiatry 1993; 56: 251–256.

28. Harrington, M.G. et al.: Abnormal proteins in the cerebrospinal fluid of patients with Creutzfeldt-Jakob disease. N Engl J Med 1986; 315: 279–283.

29. Hsich, G. et al.: The 14-3-3 brain protein in cerebrospinal fluid as a marker for transmissible spongiform encephalopathies. N Engl J Med 1996; 335: 924–930.

30. Navia, B.A. et al.: The AIDS dementia complex. I. Clinical features. Ann Neurol 1986; 19: 517–524.

31. Reid, M.C. et al.: Physician awareness of alcohol use disorders among older patients. J Gen Intern Med 1998; 13: 781–782.

32. Cummings, J. L. et al.: Guidelines for managing Alzheimer's disease. Part I. Assessment. Am Fam Physician 2002; 65: 2263–2272.

9

Neuroimaging Techniques

CT, MRI, SPECT, PET

Norman L. Foster

INTRODUCTION

Even with current clinical diagnostic methods, there continues to be considerable difficulty in diagnosing neurodegenerative diseases with confidence. Neuroimaging has the potential to improve dementia diagnosis further by going beyond its traditional role of simply excluding mass lesions and stroke and helping to distinguish specific dementing diseases. Considerable research indicates that magnetic resonance imaging (MRI) can identify early structural changes caused by Alzheimer's disease (AD). MRI also can identify Creutzfeldt-Jakob disease (CJD) and frontotemporal dementia (FTD). Furthermore, molecular neuroimaging techniques reveal characteristic focal abnormalities in neurodegenerative diseases that are unrecognized by other methods. Although further research is needed to understand how the clinical potential of imaging can be optimally exploited, there is now sufficient experience to suggest ways in which neuroimaging can be incorporated into everyday diagnostic and treatment decisions about dementia.

STRUCTURAL IMAGING: CT AND MRI

Mass Lesions

The most obvious use of brain imaging is to identify a mass lesion. Brain tumors, subdural hematomas, and brain abesses all can cause dementia and are easily recognized with computed tomography (CT) and MRI. Although a few mass lesions will be identified during routine dementia evaluations, these days, most are found when a brain scan is obtained to evaluate focal neurological deficits rather than dementia. The most conspicuous exception is in elderly individuals in whom evaluations are delayed or incomplete. In our referral practice, we occasionally find unsuspected brain tumors and subdural hematomas with neuroimaging when previous physicians inappropriately presumed that an elderly patient had AD without considering other possibilities or incorrectly assumed that a scan must have been done previously. Fortunately, such diagnostic errors are becoming less common as physicians have learned that age is not an appropriate criterion for deciding whether to order brain imaging.

Mass lesions also may be recognized with neuroimaging first during a routine dementia evaluation, when a patient's initial symptoms are misinterpreted as psychiatric. Frontal mass lesions may cause few obvious focal neurological signs, so brain imaging might not have been considered necessary. This error can be avoided by always obtaining a CT or MRI scan when disruptive behavioral and personality changes occur *de novo* in middle or late adulthood.

Mass lesions are especially likely when dementia has developed over less than a year. Although it may seem obvious that brain tumors, such as glioma or central nervous system lymphoma, can cause

From: *Current Clinical Neurology,*
Alzheimer's Disease: A Physician's Guide to Practical Management
Edited by: R. W. Richter and B. Zoeller Richter © Humana Press Inc., Totowa, NJ

rapidly progressive dementia, it is sometimes very difficult to obtain a consistent or accurate history about the timing of symptom onset. When there is any reason to suspect a rapidly progressive dementia, a particularly diligent review of image results is warranted.

Vascular Lesions

Cerebral infarcts are a common cause of dementia, and like AD, the incidence of vascular dementia increases with age. Although stroke usually causes obvious clinical symptoms, imaging has demonstrated that stroke often can be asymptomatic (1,2). Furthermore, by the time of a dementia evaluation, patients with stroke may have substantial motor and sensory recovery, so that focal deficits are no longer apparent. In addition, the severity of dementia may preclude a detailed neurological examination, making it impossible to identify subtle deficits by clinical examination alone. For all of these reasons, structural imaging should be used routinely to look for evidence of cerebral infarcts causing or contributing to dementia.

Structural imaging is quite sensitive in identifying stroke, so the major clinical challenge in this use of neuroimaging is to interpret the significance of lesions that are found and whether they represent stroke (Fig. 1). White matter abnormalities are common in the elderly and do not always represent stroke (3). Increased signal on MRI may be caused by enlarged perivascular spaces, and AD itself can cause white matter changes, perhaps due to Wallerian degeneration. On the other hand, the presence of extensive white matter abnormalities is associated with diminished cognitive performance in otherwise healthy individuals (4,5). Dementia also can be seen in individuals with clear-cut, but silent, infarcts. One of the ways to determine the significance of white matter lesions is to assess their extent and location, and to consider the imaging results in the context of the patient history. The more extensive the white matter abnormalities are, the more likely it is that they are contributing to the dementia. The location is also important. Even small thalamic infarcts often cause cognitive impairment (6). Furthermore, if the location of infarcts and white matter changes corresponds to the localization suggested on the mental status exam, they are the likely explanation for the change in cognition (for example, preponderant left hemisphere lesions in a demented patient with prominent language disturbance). Finally, a sudden onset and stepwise decline in cognition suggests the diagnosis of vascular dementia, which imaging can confirm (7,8).

White matter abnormalities and even clear stroke on neuroimaging alone is insufficient to exclude AD. Lacunar and silent cortical infarcts are very common in the elderly, occurring in approximately 30% (9). In most cases, these strokes do not cause dementia. However, they may contribute to the severity of dementia in those with AD. Careful studies that have examined the combined effects of abnormal white matter, brain infarction, and measures of cerebral atrophy including hippocampal size consistently show stronger relations between brain atrophy measures and cognition than vascular factors. This supports the notion that AD pathology is often the primary factor for cognitive decline in older individuals with concurrent cerebrovascular injury (10). The phenomenon of mixed AD and vascular dementia is well recognized and stroke is found in approximately 30% of patients with AD at autopsy (11). One approach to identifying AD in patients who also have extensive vascular lesions is to document a slow, progressive cognitive decline while demonstrating with neuroimaging that vascular lesions have remained unchanged.

CT or MRI?

Although mass lesions are well visualized by both CT and MRI, MRI is preferable. It is more sensitive in identifying focal structural abnormalities, especially in the temporal cortex, provides better tissue contrast, and permits increased imaging flexibility by offering protocols that emphasize different tissue properties. For example, diffusion-weighted imaging can suggest that a vascular lesion is recent, and fluid attenuated inversion recovery (FLAIR) imaging can highlight otherwise indistinct white matter lesions. MRI also has some advantages in identifying particular dementing disorders, as

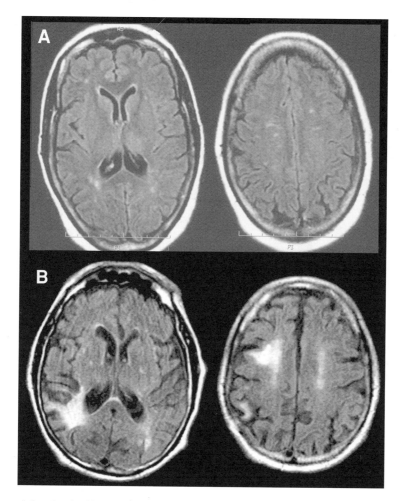

Fig. 1. Determining the significance of presumed vascular lesions identified by MRI. FLAIR-MRI images at the level of the caudate nucleus (left) and through the centrum semiovale (right) are shown from two patients with dementia. The radiographic interpretation of both reported extensive white matter abnormalities consistent with chronic ischemic changes. Treating physicians reading only these reports might conclude that both had vascular dementia. However, the clinical history and visual inspection of the images reveal significant differences. In the first patient (**A**), the family reported a memory predominant dementia that developed gradually over 2 years and was moderately severe at the time of the initial dementia assessment (MMSE score 18). The patient had a history of hypertension, myocardial infarction, and a behavioral episode without focal features, which was attributed to a TIA. She had a nonfocal neurological examination and cognitive deficits typical of Alzheimer's disease. Nevertheless, following this scan the patient was told she definitely did not have AD and her symptoms were due to "strokes." Despite the radiologist's report, on close inspection the MRI scan shows only mild abnormalities. Approximately a dozen areas of increased signal are seen in the white matter. They are very small, insufficient to account for the patient's cognitive impairments, and can be adequately explained by enlarged perivascular spaces and gliosis associated with aging.

In the other patient (**B**), symptoms also reportedly began gradually and were progressive, but had suddenly worsened. This patient also had significant stroke risk factors of atrial fibrillation and a TIA characterized by expressive aphasia that resolved completely after several hours. His dementia also was moderately severe at the time of assessment (MMSE score 13), and he appeared to have a nonfocal examination. In this case, however, despite the similarity of the radiologist's interpretation, there are several significant white matter abnormalities on MRI. There are two distinct cerebral infarcts. At the level of the caudate nucleus, there is an extensive area of increased signal in the right parietal lobe extending from the posterior horn of the lateral ventricle to the cerebral cortex. In more superior images a second, separate area of increased signal is evident in the right superior frontal lobe. In addition, multiple smaller white matter abnormalities are also seen at both brain levels. The physician was initially uncertain whether to rely on the history of gradual onset or of sudden worsening, and reviewing the MRI helped the physician confirm that strokes were contributing significantly to the patient's dementia.

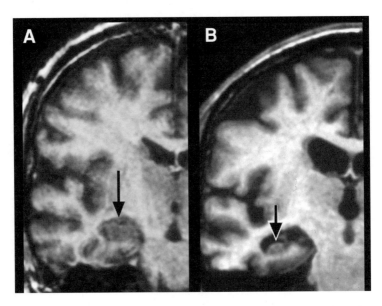

Fig. 2. Hippocampal atrophy in Alzheimer's disease. Coronal MRI shows atrophy of the hippocampus (arrows) and corresponding enlargement of the temporal horn in a patient with Alzheimer's disease (**A**) as compared to a normal individual of similar age (**B**).

detailed later. Unfortunately, expense, patient claustrophobia, and metal implants or medical devices common in older individuals can limit the use of MRI. As a result, CT scans will continue to have an important role in dementia care.

Quantifying Neurodegeneration With MRI

Recently MRI has been used to measure medial temporal volume loss in AD. Atrophy of medial temporal cortex has good sensitivity and specificity in distinguishing AD from normal aging, not only with laborious quantitative morphometry, but also using standardized visual interpretation methods *(12)*. Medial temporal lobe atrophy measured by MRI also may be useful in identifying which patients with mild cognitive impairment (MCI) will progress to dementia *(13)*. The ability of MRI to easily visualize the hippocampus with coronal slices clearly is a factor in the success of this technique (Fig. 2).

Further research will be needed to establish the most reliable and practical methods to use in clinical practice, but even now coronal MRI images should be obtained and examined for an estimate of hippocampal atrophy during the evaluation of dementia. Focal atrophy of the frontal and anterior temporal cortex can be seen with MRI and is useful in recognizing FTD. Although such focal volume loss can also be seen on CT, the superior ability to visualize areas of the temporal lobe in close proximity to the skull again favors MRI.

Rapidly Progressive Dementia and Creutzfeldt-Jakob Disease

The evaluation of rapidly progressive dementia is a situation in which MRI is clearly preferable to CT. The superior sensitivity and flexibility of MRI is often extremely valuable to detect multiple, small, disseminated lesions due to metastases and vasculitis and emboli following open-heart surgery, endocarditis, cardiac ventricular thrombus, or a peripheral venous thrombus through a patent foramen ovale. The recognition of these conditions is very important, because early treatment can often improve or stabilize the dementia.

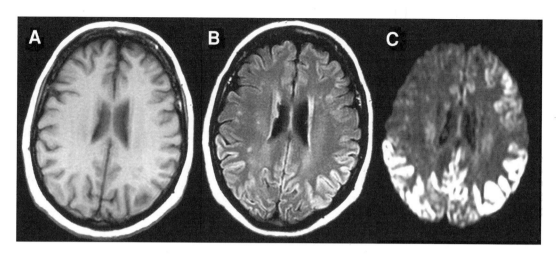

Fig. 3. MRI abnormalities in Creutzfeldt-Jakob disease. These MRI scans were obtained in a 57-year-old woman with a 3-month history of progressive memory loss and other cognitive symptoms mild enough to permit her to live alone. Mental status was the only abnormality on her examination. Diagnosis was delayed because her scan was initially interpreted as consistent with stroke. However, signal abnormalities are restricted to the cerebral cortical ribbon in a pattern not consistent with a specific vascular territory. While no abnormalities were seen on the T1-weighted scan (**A**), increased signal is apparent on both the FLAIR (**B**) and diffusion-weighted images (**C**). A brain biopsy confirmed the presence of spongiform encephalopathy and protease-resistant prion protein immunoreactivity.

Another extremely useful advantage of MRI is its ability to detect prion diseases early. CJD and other prion diseases very commonly cause focal increased signal on diffusion-weighted, FLAIR, and proton-weighted MRI, and to a lesser extent, on T2-weighted imaging *(14,15)*. It is not yet clear which scanning sequence is most sensitive, but it is important to recognize that CJD causes no abnormalities on CT scan or routine T1-weighted MRI images. It therefore may be necessary to specifically request diffusion-weighted and FLAIR images and to focus the attention of the radiologist to the suspected regions of interest, since many radiologists may not recognize the typical abnormalities of prion disease because of its low prevalence.

The most common MRI abnormality in typical, sporadic CJD is bilateral, symmetric, increased signal in the putamen and caudate *(16)*. There also can be focal abnormalities in the cerebral cortex (Fig. 3). The location of MRI changes in CJD reflects the distribution of prion pathology and correlates with patient symptoms *(17,18)*. In acquired new variant CJD, increased signal typically occurs in the pulvinar of the thalamus, so-called pulvinar sign *(19)*. This abnormality has not been reported in sporadic or familial prion disease. The cause of these MRI abnormalities is unclear, but they are probably due to diffusion changes caused by gliosis or microscopic spongiform vacuolization.

MOLECULAR IMAGING: SPECT AND PET

Molecular imaging techniques provide pictures of the brain that reflect the distribution of radioactive-labeled drugs (radioligands or tracers), chosen because they participate in biochemical reactions, interact with enzymes and transporters, or bind cellular receptors. Because changes in these processes do not require or often alter brain anatomy, single photon emission computed tomography (SPECT) and positron emission tomography (PET) complement rather than replace CT and MRI in the clinician's armamentarium. Indeed, the information provided by structural imaging methods is critical for accurately interpreting molecular imaging results, because the concentration of biochemical markers is affected when the cerebral cortex thins or the cellular composition of the brain changes.

Each SPECT and PET tracer has its own properties and must be separately studied and modeled for clinical application. Thus, a substantial initial research effort of a decade or more is needed before a radioligand is ready for clinical use. Many agents are in various stages of development, but clinical applications of SPECT have primarily involved measurement of cerebral blood flow. SPECT tracers for blood flow include inhaled ^{133}Xenon, *N*-isopropyl-*p*-^{123}I-iodoamphetamine (IMP), [^{99m}Tc]hexa-methyl-propyleneamine oxime (HM-PAO), and [^{99m}Tc] *N*,*N*′-1,2-ethylene-di-ylbis-L-cysteine diethyl ester (ethylene cysteine dimer, ECD). The properties of these agents differ and have their own advantages and disadvantages, but technetium tracers are more widely used because of their favorable emission characteristics and ease of use.

Most PET studies have measured glucose metabolism with the tracer ^{18}F-fluorodeoxyglucose (FDG). A tracer kinetic model for FDG allows quantitative measurement of local cerebral metabolic rate for glucose that primarily mirrors local synaptic activity (*20*). Use of this model requires an estimate of arterial glucose concentration, but this is not necessary for clinical purposes, when only regionally preferential reductions in glucose metabolism are of interest.

SPECT or PET?

PET is similar to but has several advantages over SPECT. High-energy positron emissions provide greater localizing information than low-energy single-photon (γ) emissions, permitting superior spatial resolution and correction for radiation attenuation. Positron-emitting isotopes are also more likely than γ-emitting isotopes to be inserted into naturally occurring substances or drugs without altering their biological activity. This has made it easier to develop tracer kinetic models that permit quantification.

When PET measurements of cerebral glucose metabolism were compared directly to SPECT measurements of cerebral perfusion in differentiating AD from vascular dementia, PET demonstrated superior diagnostic accuracy regardless of dementia severity (*21*). SPECT has been less expensive and more widely available than PET over the past two decades. This has made it more accessible. However, PET now is becoming widely available, particularly in the United States, since Medicare's recent decision to reimburse PET for some clinical indications. Because of its recognized advantages, it is likely that PET will gradually replace SPECT, if clinical PET studies for dementia are reimbursed.

Mass Lesions and Vascular Disease

Mass lesions and vascular disease cause focal SPECT and PET abnormalities that are easily predicted by their pathophysiology. However, PET is less sensitive at detecting mass lesions than CT and MRI, and the changes they cause in PET may be impossible to distinguish from those caused by nonstructural lesions. The major use of SPECT and PET, when there are known structural lesions, is to determine their effect—if any—on cognition. Molecular imaging abnormalities may be more extensive than suggested by structural imaging. Because FDG-PET primarily reflects synaptic activity, it may show metabolic changes remote from the structural lesion due to loss of efferent nerve terminals. If cerebral vessels are normal, this also applies to blood flow measured with SPECT. Thus, accurate interpretation of SPECT and PET scans requires knowledge of neurological pathways.

For example, a stroke localized only to the thalamus on MRI can show hypoperfusion and hypometabolism in the ipsilateral cerebral cortex because of damage to thalamocortical projections. These remote changes have significant implications. Recent studies have shown that cerebral cortical glucose hypometabolism on PET is the best predictor of whether subcortical lacunar stroke will cause dementia (*22*). Thus, SPECT and PET can help determine whether focal structural lesions detected by CT and MRI have cognitive consequences.

Stroke can be implicated as the cause of dementia when focal changes in molecular imaging correspond to the location of the stroke or its afferent projections and to the expected localization of observed clinical cognitive deficits.

Neurodegenerative Dementing Diseases

A unique contribution of molecular imaging techniques is their ability to demonstrate specific imaging abnormalities in neurodegenerative disorders that may be difficult to distinguish accurately on clinical examination alone. In most neurodegenerative diseases, blood flow closely parallels glucose metabolism and SPECT measures generally parallel PET measures of glucose metabolism. Therefore, to simplify the discussion, I will refer only to findings with FDG-PET. Although other PET ligands show abnormalities in neurodegenerative dementing diseases, the vast majority of clinical studies have used FDG-PET, and it is the only PET ligand widely available outside research centers. A review of research using other molecular imaging ligands is available elsewhere *(23)*.

FDG-PET shows different focal patterns of glucose hypometabolism in several dementing disorders (Table 1, Fig. 4). The same patterns are seen with SPECT blood flow ligands. In AD, FDG-PET has a consistent sequential pattern of reduced glucose metabolism that reflects the location of synaptic loss and patient symptoms. The metabolic changes begin in the posterior cingulate gyrus, then affect parietal and temporal association cortex, and eventually involve prefrontal cortex and the whole brain *(24)*. Posterior association cortex begins and remains the most hypometabolic region in the lateral cortex. The relative decrease in metabolism in posterior as compared to anterior association cortex remains a consistent finding throughout the course of AD, although it becomes harder to recognize as the frontal association cortex becomes progressively more affected. This visually apparent increase in the ratio of anterior to posterior association glucose metabolism can be helpful in distinguishing AD from trontotemporal dementia (FTD) *(25)*. The primary sensorimotor cortex surrounding the central sulcus is relatively preserved in AD, so that it becomes evident as surrounding cortex becomes progressively more hypometabolic. The occipital lobe, including the primary visual cortex, characteristically is also relatively spared. Interestingly, even though in AD neuronal loss is greatest in the hippocampus and medial temporal lobe, the synaptic consequences of this change are greater in the posterior cingulate cortex and lateral temporal cortex *(26,27)*.

The specific pattern of glucose hypometabolism in AD seen in an individual patient corresponds to his or her symptoms. This helps explain the variability in disease expression and means that FDG-PET can clarify the diagnosis in atypical cases. While the overall pattern of predominant posterior association cortex hypometabolism is unchanged in all AD patients, right/left hemispheric asymmetry often occurs *(28)*. When nondominant hemisphere hypometabolism is most severe, visuospatial abnormalities are clinically most prominent. When the dominant hemisphere is most hypometabolic, language dysfunction is particularly evident *(29,30)*. The degree of frontal hypometabolism also appears to reflect the appearance of behavioral symptoms.

Dementia with Lewy bodies (DLB) and dementia in Parkinson's disease demonstrate occipital hypometabolism in addition to temporal, parietal, and lesser frontal deficits that are otherwise similar to AD *(31,32)*. FDG-PET in FTD is characterized by predominant frontal and anterior temporal deficits that become more pervasive as symptoms progress *(33)*. The pattern of temporal hypometabolism in FTD is generally easy to distinguish from that seen in AD, in which lateral rather than inferior and anterior hypometabolism is characteristic. FDG-PET can help differentiate several different phenotypic variants of FTD *(34)*. Some have predominant right-hemisphere involvement associated with severe behavior disturbances, while others with progressive aphasia exhibit more hypometabolism in the dominant hemisphere. Some have hypometabolism mostly in the anterior temporal cortex, while in others hypometabolism is limited almost entirely to the frontal cortex. The reason for these individual variations is not yet understood.

Distinctive patterns of glucose hypometabolism also have been identified in Huntington's disease, progressive supranuclear palsy, and corticobasal degeneration, although FDG-PET is usually not needed to establish these diagnoses. Huntington's disease exhibits caudate and less prominent frontal deficits *(35)*. Progressive supranuclear palsy shows glucose hypometabolism in the caudate nucleus, putamen, thalamus, pons, and cerebral cortex, but not in the cerebellum as compared to normal sub-

Table 1
Typical Regional Abnormalities in Metabolism Detected by FDG-PET
in Common Dementing Disorders

Disease	Pattern of abnormality	Comments
Alzheimer's disease	Symmetric or asymmetric bilateral temporoparietal and posterior cingulate hypometabolism	Frontal association cortex may also be hypometabolic to a lesser extent, sparing of primary sensorimotor cortex
Multi-infarct dementia	Multifocal in cases of large cortical infarcts; variable pattern in cases of multiple subcortical infarction	Correlates with structural imaging studies, but may be more extensive than areas of infarction; common variety of subcortical infarction may disconnect cortical brain regions
Parkinson's disease with dementia	Symmetric or asymmetric bilateral temporoparietal hypometabolism	Frontal association cortex may also be hypometabolic, sparing of primary sensorimotor cortex
Dementia with Lewy bodies	Symmetric or asymmetric bilateral temporoparietal, posterior cingulate and occipital hypometabolism	Frontal association cortex may also be hypometabolic to a lesser extent, sparing of primary sensorimotor cortex
Frontotemporal dementia	Frontal, anterior cingulate and anterior temporal hypometabolism	May be asymmetric; left hemisphere mostly affected in progressive aphasia and semantic dementia forms; basal ganglia may also be hypometabolic in those with extrapyramidal symptoms
Huntington's disease	Hypometabolism of the caudate nucleus	Frontal association cortex may also be hypometabolic to a lesser extent
Progressive supranuclear palsy	Caudate nucleus, putamen, thalamus, pons, and primarily superior and anterior frontal cortex	Cerebellum spared; in patients with very mild or no dementia, there may be little or no change in cerebral cortical metabolism
Corticobasal degeneration	Asymmetric frontal, temporal and parietal hypometabolism with ipsilateral thalamic hypometabolism	Striatum relatively spared; most prominent limb symptoms occur contralateral to the hemisphere most hypometabolic

Table 2
Major Concerns about Potential Misuse of Neuroimaging

Overuse—cost of needlessly repeated studies
Overdependence—using imaging results to decide whether there is dementia, when clinical assessment is
    reliable; using imaging results to make a diagnosis without utilizing other relevant clinical data
Overinterpretation—assigning cause of dementia to clinically insignificant imaging findings
Misinterpretation—diagnostic errors in recognizing the presence of clinically significant lesions, mistakes in
    radiographic diagnosis
Omission—failure to incorporate significant imaging findings in diagnosis

jects *(36)*. Declines of glucose metabolism are most prominent in the superior and anterior portions of the frontal cortex in a pattern that is now better understood as causing a frontal dementia typical of tauopathies. Corticobasal degeneration is characterized by significant metabolic hemispheric asymmetry, just as clinical symptoms are typically very asymmetric. Nearly the entire affected hemisphere, including frontal, temporal, and parietal regions, is involved. However, in addition to the asymmetry in the cerebral cortex, ipsilateral thalamic hypometabolism occurs, while the striatum, somewhat surprisingly, seems relatively spared *(37)*.

USING NEUROIMAGING TECHNIQUES
TO ANSWER SPECIFIC CLINICAL QUESTIONS

As with any other diagnostic test, there should be a specific reason for ordering an imaging study. If the indications for the study are unclear, imaging can confuse rather than aid diagnosis. It is also important that the imaging results are put in appropriate context and not relied upon alone to arrive at a diagnosis. There is now general agreement that structural imaging studies should be obtained routinely in the evaluation of dementia *(38)*. Use of FDG-PET is properly reserved for answering specific diagnostic questions, particularly when symptoms are unusual, present diagnostic difficulties, or reflect diagnostic uncertainties between AD and FTD. Consideration of these issues can avoid most of the concerns raised about imaging by experts and insurers (Table 2).

Imaging is not infallible, and sensitivity and specificity need to be considered. The value of imaging depends on the accurate interpretation of the scan. This is improved by giving the radiologist appropriate information about the diagnostic question to be answered and the differential diagnosis being considered. If imaging does not confirm the suspected diagnosis, it may be worth looking at the film itself or consulting the radiologist directly. Many radiology and nuclear medicine training programs have not emphasized neuroimaging for dementing diseases, and there seems to be more variability in expertise than in other areas of imaging. Fortunately, a relatively short period of training focused on the interpretation of images in dementia leads to good interrater reliability, and professional organizations are beginning to address these concerns *(25,39)*.

The sensitivity and specificity of CT and MRI are widely understood, but studies of FDG-PET are more recent. Visual interpretation of PET scans has higher diagnostic accuracy than clinical evaluation alone when autopsy diagnosis is used as the gold standard *(40–42)*. The diagnostic sensitivity (93–94%) and specificity (73–79%) of PET is better than that of clinical evaluation alone (sensitivity 79–85% and specificity between 50% and 70%).

Deciding Whether Dementia Is Present

The available data indicate that FDG-PET is a useful biomarker for dementia. Patients with dementia due to neurological disease almost uniformly have abnormal FDG-PET scans, while those with cognitive complaints for other reasons often have normal scans *(22,41,42)*. FDG-PET scans are abnor-

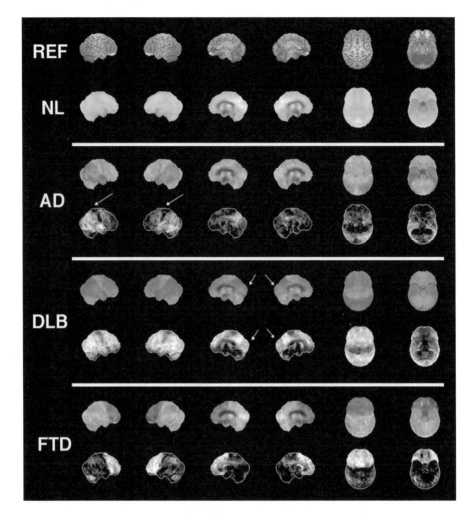

Fig. 4. Typical patterns of glucose hypometabolism in dementing neurodegenerative diseases. Images of FDG-PET scans are displayed using the three-dimensional stereotactic surface projection (3-D SSP) method of Minoshima *(24)*. This method summarizes in six images the results of scans typically consisting of 15 to 128 transaxial images, depending on the PET instrument used. The surface of the cerebral cortex is displayed (from left to right) as right lateral, left lateral, right medial, left medial, superior, and inferior views of the brain.

The first row (REF) shows anatomic views of the brain surface for reference. The second row (NL) shows mean glucose metabolism in 33 elderly normals relative to pons (used for comparison because it is little affected in most neurodegenerative diseases). Values of the picture elements (pixels) represent relative rates of glucose metabolism, with lighter shades representing higher metabolic rates. Subsequent images are from individual patients, each patient represented by two rows of images. The first row for each patient shows the relative rate of glucose metabolism using the same scale as used for the normal. The second row for each patient shows the results of the statistical comparison of that patient with the normal (*t*-score maps). Black areas of these images are not significantly different from normal. Statistically significant pixel values are gray, with lighter shades representing greater differences relative to normal.

In the patient with AD, metabolism is reduced particularly in the posterior temporoparietal association cortex and posterior cingulate gyrus with relative preservation in the primary sensorimotor cortex, which in the lateral views of the statistical map is apparent as a dark strip (arrows). In the patient with DLB, the same pattern of hypometabolism is observed, with the exception that occipital cortex has nearly as much hypometabolism as other areas of cortex (arrows). In the patient with FTD, the pattern is reversed, with frontal, anterior temporal, and anterior cingulate cortex most hypometabolic and posterior association regions relatively preserved.

mal even when symptoms of AD are mild. Thus, FDG-PET may be useful in differentiating neurological disease from other causes of behavioral and cognitive dysfunction, when the clinical history and examination are confusing or not definitive.

A few examples can illustrate this application. Drugs and seizures can cause cognitive impairments, but not the typical symmetric bilateral temporoparietal hypometabolism seen in AD. Thus, a typical AD pattern on FDG-PET in an elderly patient with a seizure disorder and cognitive impairment suggests that AD, rather than anticonvulsants or subclinical seizures with post-ictal confusion, is the cause of dementia. Likewise, significant frontal hypometabolism in a patient with behavior disturbance beginning in late life suggests FTD rather than senile psychosis or bipolar disorder. AD can also be pinpointed earlier when bilateral temporoparietal hypometabolism is identified in a patient with a long history of depression and presumed to be the cause of cognitive impairment.

Conversely, a normal MRI and FDG-PET scan will help confirm malingering in a prisoner unable to perform his daily care and performing very poorly on clinical examination and neuropsychological testing.

Determining the Cause of Dementia in Difficult Cases

If dementia is clearly present, it is often possible to be highly confident of a clinical diagnosis using clinical criteria and without relying on imaging results. For example, a patient who has the insidious onset of dementia and develops typical, spontaneous parkinsonian features within a year, has prominent visual hallucinations, and has a history of rapid-eye-movement sleep behavior disorder, is very likely to have DLB. Once structural imaging studies have excluded structural lesions contributing to the dementia, no further imaging may be warranted.

For other patients, however, the history and examination may not be so clear-cut. For example, in the previously described case, if behavior symptoms had been prominent early in the course of the illness, treatment with neuroleptics may have been started before the initial dementia evaluation. It might be necessary to continue neuroleptic treatment and thus it would be impossible to establish that the parkinsonism was spontaneous. Then the diagnosis of DLB would be less certain and this constellation of symptoms might well raise the possibility of FTD. A PET scan showing bilateral temporoparietal and visual cortex hypometabolism greater than frontal hypometabolism would then be valuable in establishing the diagnosis of DLB.

FUTURE USES OF NEUROIMAGING

Several other neuroimaging methods await further research and development. Magnetic resonance spectroscopy shows abnormalities in several neurodegenerative diseases, and it may also make a significant contribution to dementia diagnosis *(43)*. A few studies have also used functional MRI (fMRI) to evaluate differences in normal elderly and those with MCI and dementia *(44)*. Many additional PET probes have been developed.

Of particular interest in AD are cholinergic ligands that can determine the effect of cholinesterase inhibitors in the brain *(45)*. Particularly exciting is the development of small-molecule probes for the in vivo assessment of neurofibrillary tangles and neuritic plaques *(46,47)*. Additional studies also are needed to determine if hippocampal atrophy or FDG-PET can serve as reliable measures of impending dementia, as some preliminary studies suggest *(48–50)*. Some of these methods soon may be used as outcome measures in clinical drug trials.

It even is possible now to envision a future in which neuroimaging techniques could identify individual biochemical signatures in patients with dementia and use this information to tailor therapy. Overall, the future of neuroimaging in dementia appears bright, and ripe for further development.

SUMMARY

Neuroimaging has become an essential aid in dementia care. The advent of computed tomography (CT) for the first time provided clinicians a detailed view of brain anatomy, revealing previously unsuspected brain lesions causing dementia. Magnetic resonance imaging (MRI) has added further nuances, permitting recognition of some specific diseases and the quantification of neurodegeneration in others. Entirely different information is provided by single photon emission computed tomography (SPECT) and positron emission tomography (PET)—molecular imaging techniques that probe brain biochemistry. These techniques can improve the accuracy and specificity of diagnosis, sparing patients and their families the expense and frustration of unnecessary diagnostic odysseys. They also can guide management and assess response to treatment. The clinician's challenge is to utilize these tools optimally. The rapid development of new technology suggests that neuroimaging will have an increasing role in future dementia care.

ACKNOWLEDGMENTS

This work was supported in part by the Michigan Alzheimer's Disease Research Center (NIH grant P50-AG08671). I thank Douglas Quint, Robert Koeppe, Satoshi Minoshima, and Virginia Rogers for their assistance in preparing the figures.

REFERENCES

1. Price, T.R. et al.: Silent brain infarction on magnetic resonance imaging and neurological abnormalities in community-dwelling older adults. The Cardiovascular Health Study. CHS Collaborative Research Group. Stroke 1997; 28: 1158–1164.
2. Vermeer, S.E. et al.: Prevalence and risk factors of silent brain infarcts in the population-based Rotterdam Scan Study. Stroke 2002; 33: 21–25.
3. Chimowitz, M.I. et al.: Periventricular lesions on MRI. Facts and theories. Stroke 1989; 20: 963–967.
4. De Groot, J.C. et al.: Cerebral white matter lesions and cognitive function: The Rotterdam Scan Study. Ann Neurol 2000; 47: 145–151.
5. DeCarli, C. et al.: Cerebrovascular and brain morphologic correlates of mild cognitive impairment in the National Heart, Lung, and Blood Institute Twin Study. Arch Neurol 2001; 58: 643–647.
6. Mungas, D. et al.: MRI predictors of cognition in subcortical ischemic vascular disease and Alzheimer's disease. Neurology 2001; 57: 2229–2235.
7. Rosen, W.G. et al.: Pathological verification of ischemic score in differentiation of dementia. Ann Neurol 1980; 7: 486–488.
8. Román, G.C. et al.: Vascular dementia: diagnostic criteria for research studies. Report of the NINDS-AIREN International Workshop. Neurology 1993; 43: 250–260.
9. Longstreth, W.T. et al.: Lacunar infarcts defined by magnetic resonance imaging of 3660 elderly people: the Cardiovascular Health Study. Arch Neurol 1998; 55: 1217–1225.
10. Fein, G. et al.: Hippocampal and cortical atrophy predict dementia in subcortical ischemic vascular disease. Neurology 2000; 55: 1626–1635.
11. Gearing, M. et al.: The Consortium to Establish a Registry for Alzheimer's Disease (CERAD). Part X. Neuropathology confirmation of the clinical diagnosis of Alzheimer's disease. Neurology 1995; 45: 461–466.
12. Scheltens, P. et al.: Structural magnetic resonance imaging in the practical assessment of dementia: beyond exclusion. Lancet Neurol 2002; 1: 13–21.
13. Visser, P.J. et al.: Medial temporal lobe atrophy predicts Alzheimer's disease in patients with minor cognitive impairment. J Neurol Neurosurg Psychiatry 2002; 72: 491–497.
14. Finkenstaedt, M. et al.: MR imaging of Creutzfeldt-Jakob disease. Radiology 1996; 199: 793–798.
15. Na, D.L. et al.: Diffusion-weighted magnetic resonance imaging in probable Creutzfeldt-Jakob disease: a clinical-anatomic correlation. Arch Neurol 1999; 56: 951–957.
16. Schroter, A. et al.: Magnetic resonance imaging in the clinical diagnosis of Creutzfeldt-Jakob disease. Arch Neurol 2000; 57: 1751–1757.
17. Mittal, S. et al.: Correlation of diffusion-weighted magnetic resonance imaging with neuropathology in Creutzfeldt-Jakob disease. Arch Neurol 2002; 59: 128–134.
18. Kropp, S. et al.: The Heidenhain variant of Creutzfeldt-Jakob disease. Arch Neurol 1999; 56: 55–61.

19. Zeidler, M. et al.: The pulvinar sign on magnetic resonance imaging in variant Creutzfeldt-Jakob disease. Lancet 2000; 355: 1412–1418.

20. Phelps, M.E. et al.: Tomographic measurement of local cerebral glucose metabolic rate in humans with (F-18) 2-fluoro-2-deoxy-D-glucose: validation of method. Ann Neurol 1979; 6: 371–388.

21. Messa, C. et al.: High-resolution technetium-99m-HMPAO SPECT in patients with probable Alzheimer's disease: comparison with fluorine-18-FDG PET. J Nuclear Med 1994; 35: 210–216.

22. Kwan, L.T. et al.: Effects of subcortical cerebral infarction on cortical glucose metabolism and cognitive function. Arch Neurol 1999; 56: 809–814.

23. Foster, N.L.; Minoshima, S.; Kuhl, D.E.: Brain imaging in Alzheimer disease. In: Terry, R.D. et al. (eds.): Alzheimer Disease. 2nd ed. Raven Press, New York, 1999: 67–93.

24. Minoshima, S. et al.: Metabolic reduction in the posterior cingulate cortex in very early Alzheimer's disease. Ann Neurol 1997; 42: 85–94.

25. Foster, N.L. et al.: Inter-rater reliability and diagnostic accuracy of FDG-PET is superior to clinical history and examination in dementia. Neurobiol Aging 2002; 23: S353.

26. Meguro, K. et al.: Neocortical and hippocampal glucose hypometabolism following neurotoxic lesions of the entorhinal and perirhinal cortices in the non-human primate as shown by PET. Implications for Alzheimer's disease. Brain 1999; 122: 1519–1531.

27. Meguro, K. et al.: Relations between hypometabolism in the posterior association neocortex and hippocampal atrophy in Alzheimer's disease: a PET/MRI correlative study. J Neurol Neurosurg Psychiatry 2001; 71: 315–321.

28. Koss, E. et al.: Differences in lateral hemispheric asymmetries of glucose utilization between early- and late-onset Alzheimer-type dementia. Am J Psychiatry 1985; 142: 638–640.

29. Foster, N.L. et al.: Cortical abnormalities in Alzheimer's disease. Ann Neurol 1984; 16: 649–654.

30. Haxby, J.V. et al.: Longitudinal study of cerebral metabolic asymmetries and associated neuropsychological patterns in early dementia of the Alzheimer type. Arch Neurol 1990; 47: 753–760.

31. Imamura, T. et al.: Regional cerebral glucose metabolism in dementia with Lewy bodies and Alzheimer's disease: a comparative study using positron emission tomography. Neurosci Lett 1997; 235: 49–52.

32. Albin, R.L. et al.: Fluoro-deoxyglucose positron emission tomography in diffuse Lewy body disease. Neurology 1996; 47: 462–466.

33. Ishii, K. et al.: Regional cerebral glucose metabolism in dementia with Lewy bodies and Alzheimer's disease. Neurology 1998; 51: 125–130.

34. Miller, B.L. et al.: Progressive right frontotemporal degeneration: clinical, neuropsychological and SPECT characteristics. Dementia 1993; 4: 204–213.

35. Mazziotta, J.C. et al.: Reduced cerebral glucose metabolism in asymptomatic subjects at risk for Huntington's disease. N Engl J Med 1987; 316: 357–362.

36. Foster, N.L. et al.: Cerebral hypometabolism in progressive supranuclear palsy studied with positron emission tomography. Ann Neurol 1988; 24: 399–406.

37. Eidelberg, D. et al.: The metabolic landscape of cortico-basal ganglionic degeneration: regional asymmetries studied with positron emission tomography. J Neurol Neurosurg Psychiatry 1991, 54: 856–862.

38. Knopman, D.S. et al.: Practice parameter: diagnosis of dementia (an evidence-based review). Report of the Quality Standards Subcommittee of the American Academy of Neurology. Neurology 2001; 56: 1143–1153.

39. Hoffman, J.M. et al.: Interpretation variability of 18FDG-positron emission tomography studies in dementia. Invest Radiol 1996; 31: 316–322.

40. Lim, A. et al.: Clinico-neuropathological correlation of Alzheimer's disease in a community-based case series. J Am Geriatr Soc 1999; 47: 564–569.

41. Hoffman, J.M. et al.: FDG-PET imaging in patients with pathologically verified dementia. J Nuclear Med 2000; 41: 1920–1928.

42. Silverman, D.H.S. et al.: Positron emission tomography in evaluation of dementia: regional brain metabolism and long-term outcome. JAMA 2001; 286: 2120–2127.

43. Hsu, Y.Y. et al.: Magnetic resonance imaging and magnetic resonance spectroscopy in dementias. J Geriatr Psychiatr Neurol 2001; 14: 145–166.

44. Bookheimer, S.Y. et al.: Patterns of brain activation in people at risk for Alzheimer's disease. N Engl J Med 2000; 343: 450–456.

45. Kuhl, D.E. et al.: Limited donepezil inhibition of acetylcholinesterase measured with positron emission tomography in living Alzheimer cerebral cortex. Ann Neurol 2000; 48: 391–395.

46. Shoghi-Jadid, K. et al.: Localization of neurofibrillary tangles and beta-amyloid plaques in the brains of living patients with Alzheimer disease. Am J Geriatr Psychiatr 2002; 10: 24–35.

47. Mathis, C.A. et al.: A lipophilic thioflavin-T derivative for positron emission tomography (PET) imaging of amyloid in brain. Bioorg Med Chem Lett 2002; 12: 295–298.

48. Fox, N.C. et al.: Presymptomatic hippocampal atrophy in Alzheimer's disease. A longitudinal MRI study. Brain 1996; 119: 2001–2007.
49. Small, G.W. et al.: Cerebral metabolic and cognitive decline in persons at genetic risk for Alzheimer's disease. Proc Natl Acad Sci USA 2000; 97: 6037–6042.
50. Reiman, E.M. et al.: Preclinical evidence of Alzheimer's disease in persons homozygous for the e4 allele for apolipoprotein E. N Engl J Med 1996; 334: 752–758.

10

Biological Markers in Alzheimer's Disease

Ramon Diaz-Arrastia and Fred Baskin

INTRODUCTION

The recently completed "decade of the brain" witnessed fundamental advances in many areas of basic and clinical neurosciences, but few fields saw greater progress than investigations on Alzheimer's disease (AD). Mutations in the amyloid precursor protein (APP), presenilin-1, and presenilin-2 genes that result in autosomal dominant familial AD were identified in the early part of the decade *(1)*. These discoveries made possible the development of transgenic animals, which provide the best available experimental models to study AD neuropathology and therapeutics *(2)*. More recently, the enzymes involved in processing APP—β-secretase and γ-secretase—have been identified. Specific inhibitors of these proteases have been developed and are nearing or undergoing clinical trials. Further, much has been learned about inflammatory reactions in brain tissue during the course of AD, and both epidemiologically and animal model-based experimental observations suggest that anti-inflammatory or immunological strategies may be effective in ameliorating this devastating disease *(3–6)*. Clinical trials testing these therapies are under development.

It is an exciting time in AD research. Whether the current trials will result in effective treatments will be determined in due time. What is clear is that the age of AD therapeutics is here, and neurologists will need better tools than those currently available to use these therapies with optimal effectiveness. Although the clinical diagnosis of AD is not difficult once the disease is established, it is likely that many therapies will be most useful in the early stages of the illness, and may not significantly reverse dementia once it is overt. Thus, there is a great need for a technique to detect neurodegeneration in the early or preclinical stages. It is also likely that a particular treatment will not work in all patients. Thus there is a need for sensitive tools that will allow us to monitor the effectiveness of therapy. Such assessments will be essential as surrogate markers in clinical trials, and will likely significantly accelerate the development of effective therapies. Active research is ongoing to develop psychometric, neuroimaging, and biochemical assays to meet these important clinical needs.

This chapter deals with biochemical assays of molecules found in accessible biological fluids that have been reported to be reliable either diagnostically or as markers of disease severity. We have followed the recommendation of the Working Group on AD Biomarkers, and considered only those markers with high sensitivity and specificity (each over 80%) *(7)*. Table 1 lists some of the more thoroughly evaluated putative biological markers for AD and their published estimates of sensitivity (false negatives among probable AD patients) and specificity (false positives among age-matched controls, or in some cases, false positives among patients with other dementing illnesses).

CSF AMYLOID BETA

The pathological hallmarks of AD are senile plaques (SP) and neurofibrillary tangles (NFT). The major component of SP are the amyloid beta-peptides (Aβ), a group of 39 to 42 amino acid peptides

From: *Current Clinical Neurology,*
Alzheimer's Disease: A Physician's Guide to Practical Management
Edited by: R. W. Richter and B. Zoeller Richter © Humana Press Inc., Totowa, NJ

Table 1
Specificity and Sensitivity of Biological Markers in AD

Marker	Direction of change	Fluid	Specificity	Sensitivity	Reference
Tau	+	CSF	0.86	0.93	Andreasen et al. *(41)*
Tau	+	CSF	0.97	0.89	Kurz et al. *(42)*
Tau	+	CSF	0.94	0.31	Shoji et al. *(43)*
Tau	+	CSF	0.89	0.63	Khale et al. *(24)*
Phospho-tau (231)	+	CSF	0.80	0.90	Buerger et al. *(15)*
Phospho-tau (199)	+	CSF	0.85	0.85	Itoh et al. *(12)*
$A\beta_{1-42}$	−	CSF	0.82	0.51	Shoji et al. *(43)*
Tau and $A\beta_{1-42}$		CSF	0.88	0.69	Shoji et al. *(43)*
Tau and $A\beta_{1-42}$		CSF	0.86	0.85	Hulstaert et al. *(11)*
AD7c-NTP	+	CSF	0.87	0.70	Kahle et al. *(24)*
Tau and AD7c-NTP	+	CSF	0.93	0.63	Khale et al. *(24)*
Tau and sIL-6RC	+	CSF	0.90	0.92	Hampel et al. *(44)*
Platelet APP 120-130/ 110 kDa	−	Blood	0.63	0.80	Rosenberg et al. *(19)*
Platelet APP 120-130/110 kDa	−	Blood	1.00	1.00	Baskin et al. *(22)*
Tau and AD7c-NTP	+	CSF	0.93	0.63	Khale et al. *(24)*
Tau and sIL-6RC	+	CSF	0.90	0.92	Hampel et al. *(44)*
Platelet APP 120-130/110 kDa	−	Blood	0.63	0.80	Rosenberg et al. *(19)*
Platelet APP 120-130/110 kDa	−	Blood	1.00	1.00	Baskin et al. *(22)*
Platelet APP 120-130/110 kDa	−	Blood	0.88	0.89	Padovani et al. *(21)*
F_2-iso-prostanes	+	CSF	1.00	1.00	Praticò et al. *(30)*

produced by ragged C-terminal proteolysis. Aβ1-40 represents the major species produced by cells (accounting for approximately 70% of total Aβ), while Aβ1-42 comprises 15%, with a variety of other minor species constituting the remainder *(8)*. Of these, $A\beta_{1-42}$ is believed to be the most important in AD pathogenesis, as it has a higher tendency to form fibrils than the other peptides, and it is the most abundant species found in SP.

$A\beta_{1-42}$ is the only peptide that is diagnostically altered in cerebrospinal fluid (CSF) *(9)*. About 70–90% of AD patients have significantly decreased levels of $A\beta_{1-42}$, including those with mild dementia *(10,11)*. There is a weak inverse correlation between $A\beta_{1-42}$ levels and severity of dementia. Nondemented subjects, even those with other neurological diseases, rarely have decreased $A\beta_{1-42}$ levels. However, 30–40% of individuals with dementia other than AD (such as vascular dementia or frontotemporal dementia) may have decreased $A\beta_{1-42}$ levels, particularly those with the apolipoprotein E (ApoE) e4-allele *(10,11)*. Thus, as a diagnostic biomarker for AD, $A\beta_{42}$ (or Aβ 42/40 ratios) has good sensitivity but weaker specificity.

CSF TAU

Neurofibrillary tangles are the other neuropathological hallmark of AD. Their major component is the microtubule associated protein tau, which is found primarily in an insoluble and hyperphosphorylated form. Tau is elevated in 65–90% of AD patients, and does not correlate with age, sex, severity of dementia, or ApoE phenotype *(9–11)*. Tau is elevated early in the disease, and studies of patients with mild cognitive impairment (MCI) find increased levels in 70–85% of subjects. Levels remain stable for up to 2 years. Though reasonably sensitive, CSF tau elevations are not specific for AD, as high tau levels are found in patients with Creutzfeld-Jakob disease, encephalitis, acute stroke, amyotrophic lateral sclerosis, and Guillain-Barré syndrome *(11)*. Although most of these conditions can readily be distinguished from AD on clinical grounds, CSF tau is also elevated in 20–40% of patients with vascular dementia or frontotemporal dementia, conditions for which a confirmatory laboratory test would be a useful complement to clinical diagnosis *(10,11)*.

More recent studies have looked at phosphorylated tau, in the hope that it will be a more specific marker that measurements of total tau. Tau is phosphorylated at multiple sites, and it has proven difficult to implicate a phosphorylation at a particular site as specific for AD. Assays using antibodies specific for phosphorylation at ser199, threo231, and threo181 have revealed increased levels of phosphorylation at all three sites in AD relative to controls *(12–16)*. Preliminary evidence suggests that it may be a more specific marker than total tau. Combined analysis of total or phosphorylated tau with Aβ may produce modest improvements in sensitivity and specificity *(10,11,17,18)*.

PLATELET APP ISOFORMS

The APP (amyloid precursor protein) gene is expressed in all tissues, although its physiological role is not clear in any. Platelets are a particularly rich source of APP, which is readily accessible to clinical analysis. Two groups found independently that the ratio of two differentially processed APP proteins in blood platelets was significantly lower in AD subjects *(19,20)*. This difference is apparent early in the course of AD, as subjects with early AD and mild cognitive impairment (MCI) had a decreased platelet APP ratio *(21)*. Although the pathophysiological significance of altered platelet APP isoform ratios is unclear, Baskin et al. *(22)*, showed that the ratio decreased as the dementia progressed *(22)*. There was also a good correlation between the change in APP ratios and the decrease in Mini-Mental State Examination (MMSE) scores over a 3-year period. There was no overlap between ratios of elderly controls and moderate to severely affected AD patients, whereas the same subjects showed modest overlap when assayed 3 years earlier *(19)*. The usefulness of this assay to follow disease progression or responsiveness to therapy is currently under investigation.

NEURONAL THREAD PROTEIN

AD7c-neuronal thread protein (NTP) is a recently discovered protein that may be involved in neuritic sprouting. AD7c-NTP immunoreactivity is increased in the brains of patients dying from AD, primarily in association with the early stages of neurofibrillary degeneration. CSF levels of AD7c-NTP are elevated in AD, and appear to correlate with severity of dementia *(23)*. A recent study of 60 demented and nondemented subjects found that elevations of AD7c-NTP in CSF had a specificity of 87% and a sensitivity of 70% for AD *(24)*. Combined evaluation of AD7c-NTP and CSF tau levels only slightly improved the specificity of this test.

ISOPROSTANES

Isoprostanes are prostaglandin-like compounds produced by the nonenzymatic free-radical-catalyzed peroxidation of arachidonic acid in membrane phospholipids *(25)*. Although they comprise a complex family, several isoprostanes are stable in biological fluids, and have been used as a measure of in vivo lipid oxidation. Montine and co-workers have found elevated levels of F_2-isoprostanes in CSF of AD patients *(26,27)*. Montine and colleagues, combining total F_2-isoprostane measurements with $A\beta_{1-42}$ and tau levels, distinguished probable AD patients from age-matched controls and patients with non-AD dementias with 84% sensitivity and 89% specificity *(28)*.

One study looked at patients with MCI and found elevations in CSF F_2-isoprostanes roughly comparable to those found in subjects with probable AD *(29)*. Praticò and co-workers reported increased F_2-isoprostane levels in urine and plasma from AD patients, in addition to CSF, although the sensitivity was greater for CSF measurements *(29,30)*. However, Montine and co-workers, using somewhat different analytical techniques, were unable to find differences between AD and controls in plasma and urine *(31,32)*. The utility of these measurements is limited by the fact that the analytical techniques required to assay these compounds in CSF are complex and not widely available.

OTHER BIOMARKERS

Several other potentially important biological markers have not yet been sufficiently evaluated for sensitivity and specificity in AD diagnoses to be included in Table 1. For example, 8-hydroxyguanosine (8-OHG) is produced by hydroxyl radical damage to RNA. It has been useful as an in vivo marker of oxidative stress. Recent analytical advances have made it possible to measure this compound in CSF. In a relatively small study, 8-OHG levels in lumbar CSF were elevated fivefold in AD subjects compared to neurologically normal individuals *(33)*.

The ratio of 24S-hydroxycholesterol/cholesterol is reduced in patients with probable AD as well as in vascular dementia *(34)*. This reduction is proportional to the severity of cognitive loss. Nerve growth factor (NGF) levels were markedly higher in AD patients than in controls or in patients with major depression *(35)*. Human kallikrein-6 levels were increased threefold in the CSF of AD subjects as compared to normal controls ($p < 0.001$) and were 10 times higher in whole blood ($p < 0.002$) *(36)*.

The specificity and sensitivity of these biomarkers has not yet been determined on large samples of patients with AD and other non-AD dementias. It is likely, as in the case of markers of free-radical stress, that alterations in several of these biomarkers may also be found in other neurodegenerative diseases *(37)*. This would not make these measures less useful as a tool to monitor therapy, but it would make it important to have corroboration of the diagnosis. Finally, it must be determined whether these markers change in parallel with progression of dementia. There is a need for more research on these promising measures.

Table 1 indicates which investigations have differentiated patients with probable AD from age-matched controls and which have increased the difficulty by including patients with MCI or early AD, and which have contrasted AD patients with patients with other dementing illnesses. In this regard, only Padovani and co-workers have differentiated small groups of MCI patients from age-matched controls and from patients with mild or moderate AD with statistical significance *(21)*. Riemenschneider and co-workers have attempted the most difficult discrimination, differentiating patients with frontotemporal degeneration from those with probable AD (85% sensitivity, 85% specificity) and from age-matched controls (90% sensitivity, 77% specificity) *(38)*.

CLINICAL USEFULNESS OF BIOMARKERS

The diagnosis of AD remains one that is established on clinical grounds *(39)*. The combination of a careful medical, neurological, and psychiatric history and physical examination, with the addition of neuroimaging studies and selected blood tests for endocrine, metabolic, or nutritional disorders, is accurate and reliable in establishing the diagnosis of AD. It also helps to exclude treatable conditions that may explain or contribute to the prevalent cognitive problem *(40)*.

We agree with the practice guideline promulgated by the Quality Standards Subcommittee of the American Academy of Neurology that there are no CSF or other biomarkers recommended for routine use in determining the diagnosis of AD at this time *(40)*. Nonetheless, we believe that this situation will change over the next couple of years. The impetus for this change will come from the need to develop and test therapies for AD, which is already upon us. We expect that validation of effective therapies will only increase the need for biochemical markers as adjuncts in diagnosis, as well as for monitoring effectiveness of therapy.

Over the past three decades, neurology has moved from a primarily descriptive and diagnostic discipline to one actively involved in dissecting the pathophysiology of brain diseases. These pathophysiological studies are now bearing fruit. Therapeutics lies just over the horizon for many of the diseases we manage, prominently AD. Our patients and their families can hardly wait.

ACKNOWLEDGMENTS

Ramon Diaz-Arrastia is supported by grants RO1AG17861 and RO3MH64889 from the National Institutes of Health, and H133A02052601 from the U.S. Department of Education. Fred Baskin is supported by grants P30AG12300 from the National Institues of Health, IIRG-98-044 from the Alzheimer's Association, and the M. B. Rudman Foundation, Dallas, Texas.

SUMMARY

Recent progress in understanding the pathophysiology of AD has identified molecules that are convincingly associated with features of the disease. Several of these can be measured in biological fluids, such as cerebrospinal fluid (CSF), plasma, or urine, and thus are potentially useful in clinical management. The significance of these biological markers is threefold. First, they may provide clues to the pathogenesis of AD, and thus may be valuable in developing novel therapies. Second, they may assist in distinguishing AD from other neurodegenerative disorders, particularly early in the course of the illness, when therapy is likely to be most effective. Finally, they may be helpful in following disease progression and monitoring therapeutic interventions. The first of these goals has been fulfilled by several of these molecules. For the second, only a few biological markers have reached utility, and none has yet found acceptance as a marker of disease severity. However, as new potentially disease-modifying therapies enter the clinical arena, precise early diagnosis will become increasingly important, as will measures to assess disease progression. This chapter reviews several of the biomarkers that can be measured in accessible biological fluids. Although few of these have clinical utility at present, it is likely that these and several others will become familiar to clinicians dealing with AD and related dementias over the next decade.

REFERENCES

1. Levy-Lahad, E.; Bird, T.D.: Genetic factors in Alzheimer's disease: A review of recent advances. Ann Neurol 1996; 40: 829–840.
2. Emilien, G. et al.: Alzheimer disease. Mouse models pave the way for therapeutic opportunities. Arch Neurol 2000; 57: 176–181.
3. Xia, M.; Hyman, B.T.: Chemokines/chemokine receptors in the central nervous system and Alzheimer's disease. J Neurovirol 1999; 5: 32–41.
4. Stewart, W.F. et al.: Risk of Alzheimer's disease and duration of NSAID use. Neurology 2000; 48: 626–632.
5. Lim, G.P. et al.: Ibuprofen suppresses plaque pathology and inflammation in a mouse model for Alzheimer's disease. J Neurosci 2000; 20: 5709–5714.
6. Schenck, D. et al.: Immunization with amyloid-beta attenuates Alzheimer-disease-like pathology in the PDAPP mouse. Nature 1999; 400: 173–177.
7. Alzheimer's Association and National Institute on Aging Working Group. Consensus Report of the Working Group on Molecular and Biochemical Markers in Alzheimer's Disease. Neurobiol Aging 1998; 19: 109–116.
8. DeStrooper, B.; Annaert, W.: Proteolytic processing and cell biological functions of the amyloid precursor protein. J Cell Sci 2000; 113: 1857–1870.
9. Galasko, D.: Biological markers and the treatment of Alzheimer's disease. J Molec Neurosci 2001; 17: 119–125.
10. Galasko, D. et al.: High cerebrospinal fluid tau and low amyloid beta42 levels in the clinical diagnosis of Alzheimer disease and relation to apolipoprotein E genotype. Arch Neurol 1998; 55: 937–945.
11. Hulstaert, F. et al.: Improved discrimination of AD patients using beta-amyloid (1-42) and tau levels in CSF. Neurology 1999; 52: 1555–1562.
12. Itoh, N. et al.: Large-scale, multicenter study of cerebrospinal fluid tau protein phosphorylated at serine 199 for the antemortem diagnosis of Alzheimer's disease. Ann Neurol 2001; 50: 150–156.
13. Ishiguro, K. et al.: Phosphorylated tau in human cerebrospinal fluid is a diagnostic marker for Alzheimer's disease. Neurosci Lett 1999; 270: 91–94.

14. Buerger, K. et al.: Differential diagnosis of Alzheimer disease with cerebral fluid levels of tau protein phosphorylated at threonine-231. Arch Neurol 2002; 59: 1267–1272.

15. Buerger, K. et al.: CSF tau protein phosphorylated at threonine-231 correlates with cognitive decline in MCI subjects. Neurology 2002; 59: 627–629.

16. Vanmechelen, E. et al.: Quantification of tau phosphorylated at threonine 181 in human cerebrospinal fluid: a sandwich ELISA with a synthetic phosphopeptide for standardization. Neurosci Lett 2000; 285: 49.

17. Andreasen, N. et al.: Evaluation of CSF-tau and CSF-Abeta42 as diagnostic markers for Alzheimer disease in clinical practice. Arch Neurol 2001; 58: 373–379.

18. Blennow, K.; Vanmechelen, E.; Hampel, H.: Abeta42 and phosphorylated tau protein as biomarkers for Alzheimer's disease. Molec Neurobiol 2001; 24: 87–97.

19. Rosenberg, R.N. et al.: Altered amyloid protein processing in platelets of patients with Alzheimer's disease. Arch Neurol 1997; 54: 139–143.

20. Di Luca, M. et al.: Differential level of platelet amyloid beta precursor protein isoforms: an early marker for Alzheimer disease. Arch Neurol 1998; 55: 1195–1200.

21. Padovani, A. et al.: Abnormalities in the pattern of platelet amyloid precursor protein forms in patients with mild cognitive impairment and Alzheimer disease. Arch Neurol 2002; 59: 71–75.

22. Baskin, F. et al.: Platelet APP isoform ratios correlate with declining cognition in AD. Neurology 2000; 54: 1907–1909.

23. De la Monte, S.M. et al.: Characterization of AD7c-NTP cDNA expression in Alzheimer's disease and measurement of a 41-kD protein in cerebrospinal fluid. J Clin Invest 1997; 100: 3093–3104.

24. Kahle, P.J. et al.: Combined assessment of tau and neuronal thread protein in Alzheimer's disease CSF. Neurology 2000; 54: 1498–1504.

25. Greco, A.; Minghetti, L.; Levi, G.: Isoprostanes, novel markers of oxidative injury, help understanding the pathogenesis of neurodegenerative diseases. Neurochem Res 2000; 25: 1357–1364.

26. Montine, T.J. et al.: Cerebrospinal fluid F2-isoprostane levels are increased in Alzheimer's disease. Ann Neurol 1998; 44: 410–413.

27. Montine, T.J. et al.: Increased CSF F2-isoprostane concentration in probable AD. Neurology 1999; 52: 562–565.

28. Montine, T.J. et al.: Cerebrospinal fluid Abeta, tau, and F2-isoprostane concentrations in patients with Alzheimer disease, other dementia, and in age-matched controls. Arch Pathol Lab Med 2001; 125: 510–512.

29. Praticò, D. et al.: Increase of brain oxidative stress in mild cognitive impairment. Arch Neurol 2002; 59: 972–976.

30. Praticò, D. et al.: Increased 8,12-iso-iPF2alpha-VI in Alzheimer's disease: correlation of a noninvasive index of lipid peroxidation with disease activity. Ann Neurol 2000; 48: 809–812.

31. Montine, T.J. et al.: No difference in plasma or urinary F2-isoprostanes among patients with Huntington's disease or Alzheimer's disease and controls. Ann Neurol 2000; 48: 950

32. Montine, T.J. et al.: Peripheral F2-isoprostanes and F4-neuroprostanes are not increased in Alzheimer's disease. Ann Neurol 2002; 52: 175–179.

33. Abe, T. et al.: Remarkable increase in the concentration of 8-hydroxyguanosine in cerebrospinal fluid form patients with Alzheimer's disease. J Neurosci Res 2002; 70: 447–450.

34. Pappassotiropoulos, A. et al.: Plasma 24S-hydroxycholesterol: a peripheral indicator of neuronal degeneration and potential state marker for Alzheimer's disease. NeuroReport 2000; 11: 1959–1962.

35. Hock, C. et al.: Increased CSF levels of nerve growth factor in patients with Alzheimer's disease. Neurology 2000; 54: 2009–2011.

36. Diamandis, E.P. et al.: Human kallikrein 6 as a biomarker of Alzheimer's disease. Clin Biochem 2000; 33: 663–667.

37. Markesbery, W.R.: The role of oxidative stress in Alzheimer disease. Arch Neurol 2000; 56: 1449–1452.

38. Riemenschneider, M. et al.: Tau and Abeta42 protein in CSF of patients with frontotemporal degeneration. Neurology 2002; 58: 1622–1628.

39. Weiner, M.F.; Lipton, A.M.; Diaz-Arrastia, R.: Medical Evaluation. In: Weiner, M.F.; Lipton, A.M. (eds.): The demetias: diagnosis, treatment, and research. 3rd ed. American Psychiatric Publishing, Washington, DC, 2003: 77—101.

40. Knopman, D. et al.: Practice parameter: diagnosis of dementia (an evidence-based review). Report of the Quality Standards Subcommittee of the American Academy of Neurology. Neurology 2001; 56: 1143–1153.

41. Andreasen, N. et al.: Sensitivity, specificity, and stability of CSF-tau in AD in a community-based patient sample. Neurology 1999; 53: 1488–1494.

42. Kurz, A. et al.: Tau protein in cerebrospinal fluid is significantly increased at the earliest clinical stage of Alzheimer disease. Alz Dis Assc Disord 1998; 12: 372–377.

43. Shoji, M. et al.: Combination assay of CSF tau, A beta 1-40 and a beta 1-42(43) as a biochemical marker of Alzheimer's disease. J Neurol Sci 1998; 158: 134–140.

44. Hampel, H. et al.: Discriminant power of the combined cerebrospinal fluid tau protein and of the soluble interleukin-6 receptor complex in the diagnosis of Alzheimer's disease. Brain Res 1999; 823: 104–112.

11

The Neuropsychology of Alzheimer's Disease

Kirsten I. Taylor and Andreas U. Monsch

INTRODUCTION

Neuropsychology is the study of the higher-order cerebral functioning, that is, of the relationship between the brain and cognitive and affective behavior. The neuropsychological examination is thus essential in the diagnosis of Alzheimer's disease (AD), whose cardinal symptom is an impairment of memory. The focus of current neuropsychological research is early detection of the AD patient. The primary goal is to implement symptomatic treatments at an early stage in the disease process in order to achieve the greatest possible benefit. Great strides have been made in delineating the earliest cognitive changes associated with AD and in developing tools and methods for their detection. These can be implemented in a two-step approach composed of screening of suspected AD patients by the general practitioner (to be considered as step 1) and referral to a specialist center for an interdisciplinary diagnostic workup (step 2).

THE MEMORY DEFICIT IN AD IS SPECIFIC

The cardinal symptom of AD is the insidious and progressive loss of memory. The type of memory deficit in AD is specific: patients have difficulty acquiring new information and rapidly forget the information they were able to learn. In contrast, older memories are spared, with the oldest memories remaining intact for the longest (temporal gradient). Although occasional forgetfulness is a normal, albeit exasperating, human trait, AD patients forget

Much more frequently,
More frequently with time, and
To such an extent that these incidents interfere significantly with daily life.

Forgetfulness is apparent in everyday interactions with patients. They may repeat the same questions or stories, misplace objects, and forget the names of especially recently made acquaintances. Neuropsychological research has consistently shown that a failure to store new information is the first detectable cognitive deficit to occur in AD (1). Hence, learning and memory tests of new information remain the cornerstone not only of formal neuropsychological assessments but also of current screening instruments for dementia.

BUT IT IS NOT FORGETFULNESS ALONE

Memory impairment alone does not fulfill the diagnostic criteria for dementia (Table 1). According to the *Diagnostic and Statistical Manual of Mental Disorders*, 4th ed. (DSM-IV) of the American Psychiatric Association (2), the diagnosis of dementia also requires impairment in at least one other cognitive domain: language, praxia, gnosis, or executive functioning. Besides poor memory, a typi-

From: *Current Clinical Neurology,*
Alzheimer's Disease: A Physician's Guide to Practical Management
Edited by: R. W. Richter and B. Zoeller Richter © Humana Press Inc., Totowa, NJ

Table 1
Neuropsychological Diagnostic Criteria for Dementia
of Alzheimer's Type According to DSM-IV (2)

A. The development of multiple cognitive deficits manifested by both
   1. Memory impairment, and
   2. One (or more) of the following cognitive disturbances:
      a. Aphasia (language disturbance);
      b. Apraxia (impaired ability to carry out motor activities despite intact motor function);
      c. Agnosia (failure to recognize or identify objects despite intact sensory function);
      d. Disturbance in executive functioning (i.e., planning, organizing, sequencing, abstracting).
B. The cognitive deficits in criteria A1 and A2 each cause significant impairment in social or occupational
   functioning and represent a significant decline from a previous level of functioning.

cal early sign of AD is a disturbance in language, particularly the inability to recall the names of objects (anomia). In conversations, patients may have word-finding difficulties and resort either to protracted descriptions of the object they are unable to name (circumlocutions) or simply identify the object as "that thing." They may also commit paraphasic errors (i.e., misnamings), either substituting the intended word with one similar in sound (phonemic paraphasias, e.g., "house" for "mouse") or meaning (semantic paraphasias, e.g., "cat" for "mouse"). Impaired executive functions include difficulties with planning, organizing, sequencing, and abstracting. These may be presenting signs of AD and are thought to rely on dorsolateral frontal lobe structures. Work performance may suffer, and previously mastered complex tasks may take much longer than they used to (e.g., paying the bills). It may also become difficult to follow complex conversations with abstract content. Higher-order motor (apraxic) and perceptual (agnostic) deficits usually occur later in the course of AD. These include the inability to pantomime meaningful gestures upon command (e.g., waving hello and goodbye; motor, or ideomotor apraxia) as well as difficulties recognizing objects, especially from atypical perspectives (object agnosia). Although the clinical impression is fundamental to detecting AD patients, a formal neuropsychological assessment identifies and quantifies the individual cognitive impairments.

DIAGNOSIS IS BASED ON A DISTINCTIVE PATTERN OF NEUROPSYCHOLOGICAL PERFORMANCE

The formal neuropsychological examination assesses the cognitive functions of attention, memory, language, praxis, gnosis, and executive functions with a wide variety of mainly paper-and-pencil tests. The diagnosis and the generation of differential diagnoses are based on the pattern of neuropsychological performance, which is distinctive in AD and other neurological diseases. Moreover, neuropsychological assessments provide critical measures to document disease progression and response to treatment, and are often employed to help develop therapeutic and management strategies for the patient (Table 2).

Normal Cognitive Aging

The initial and indeed greatest challenge for the neuropsychologist examining an older individual with suspected early-stage dementia is to determine whether the individual's cognitive performance is pathological or normal given the individual's age, gender, education, and cultural background. This is an especially difficult task in AD, as the earliest signs are subtle, insidious, and may vary among patients.

Cognitive changes occur with aging, presumably independent from but exacerbated by physiological decrements in hearing or vision (3) (see also Chapter 15). The most well accepted change in cognitive functioning with age is a decline in the speed of central (i.e., cognitive) information processing,

Table 2
The Goals of Neuropsychological Testing

Quantify cognitive performance (diagnostics): dementia? Yes/No
Contribute to differential diagnosis
Document disease progression
Document treatment response
Establish areas of preserved function for milieu therapy and care

a capacity that influences and indeed may reflect intellectual functioning in general *(4)*. Information processing speed is often a main component in tests of executive functioning; thus, it is not surprising that considerable debate continues to surround findings of age-related declines in executive functioning. A recent review found no support for the theory that the frontal lobes, substrates of executive functions, are more affected during the aging process than other brain regions (the so-called frontal aging hypothesis *[5]*).

Performance on memory tests assessing very old memories (remote memory) and information acquired within the past few minutes (short-term memory) remain stable with age *(6)*. Age-associated declines have been documented in the ability to store new information (long-term memory), specifically, in the ability to transfer material from short-term to long-term memory *(7)*. However, it is far from clear that these findings reflect genuine age-related memory impairments: a primary deficit in central processing speed could also account for the impaired transfer into long-term memory *(8)*. Indeed, memory impairments in the elderly documented with tasks that require the manipulation of different sets of information within a short amount of time diminish greatly when more time is allotted or fewer elements are provided.

Delays in speed may be compensated for by an increase in task efficiency, such that ". . . healthy older people may take a little longer to answer, but their answers may make wonderful sense when they do appear" *(9*, p. 210). Some nonspeeded neuropsychological measures of language, abstract reasoning and visuospatial abilities remain stable or may indeed improve with age *(8,9)*.

Do these changes in cognitive functioning with age reflect actual, mild pathology? As such, they may occur as a consequence of the normal biological aging process itself or as a result of the increasing amount of time during which an individual has been exposed to a number of harmful influences *(10)*. One important attempt to shed light on these issues divided cognitive changes into those that we would all be willing to accept and those that would compromise our productivity beyond retirement. These groups have been termed optimal and typical agers, respectively *(11)* (Fig. 1).

Optimal agers do not suffer from the medical conditions known to compromise cognitive functioning and may function normally up to the 10th decade of life and beyond *(12)*. This small, yet potentially growing segment of our population remains non-demented and shows no noticeable decrements in neuropsychological functioning when measured annually for 15 years up to the age of 90 *(3,13)*. Moreover, some cohorts of optimally aging elderly individuals show constant and minimal brain volume changes up to the 11th decade, which are no greater in magnitude than the changes in younger brains, and may evidence little or no neocortical pathology upon autopsy *(14,15)*.

The second and much larger group of typical agers exhibits significant cognitive impairments compared with younger persons, which, however, are not severe enough to fulfill the diagnostic criteria for dementia *(11)*. Characteristically, these individuals suffer from medical conditions that interfere significantly with their cognitive functioning. For example, a recent review of the factors that affect cognitive functioning in the elderly concluded that numerous demographic (e.g., education) and somatic (e.g., blood pressure, cardiovascular or cerebrovascular disease) variables negatively influence cognitive functioning during the aging process *(16)*. Thus, typically aging individuals may well exhibit minor cognitive changes as a consequence of their suboptimal somatic aging process. Cognitive function, however, will not necessarily continue to decline until the individual develops AD. Indeed,

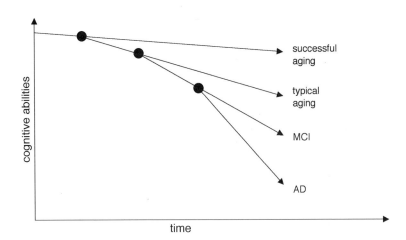

Fig. 1. Cognitive aging. A hypothetical depiction of the course of cognitive functioning in optimal and typical aging, mild cognitive impairment (MCI), and AD.

a central feature to the concept of typical aging is that these individuals, unlike demented patients, theoretically retain the capacity to improve their cognitive functioning and thus at any point join the group of optimal agers.

The term "typical" unfortunately implies that nothing should or can be done to improve cognitive function. Mild decrements in cognitive functioning with age in the past have indeed been neglected by patients as well as by clinicians; they were considered a normal, harmless consequence of the aging process, requiring no treatment. The diagnostic concept of "mild cognitive impairment" (MCI) challenged this assumption (*see* Chaper 16). The initial hope was to identify clinical subgroups among the group of typical agers, to create diagnostic criteria for these syndromes and to embark on clinical pharmacological treatment trials. More than 20 different diagnostic criteria for MCI exist today, criteria that share two central features:

1. MCI subjects are cognitively inferior to non-MCI subjects, usually in the domain of memory, yet still
2. Do not fulfill the diagnostic criteria for dementia.

Importantly, the criteria for MCI require that cognitive deficits remain stable with time, a criterion that necessitates longitudinal neuropsychological assessments *(17)*. One major aim of current neuropsychological research is to investigate the utility of some MCI diagnostic criteria to identify dementia patients in the preclinical stages of the disease *(18)*.

The current consensus in neuropsychology is that normality should be defined as what is desirable, or optimal, and not as what is most common or a statistical norm. Any deviation from the optimum should be identified and—if possible—treated. Normative data for neuropsychological tests are thus collected from optimally healthy individuals. A crucial component of any normative study is the collection of demographic data. Demographic factors, such as age, gender, and education, are known to influence performance on neuropsychological tests independent of any pathological process. Thus, only when demographic factors are taken into consideration (e.g., by demographic stratification or statistical correction of the normative data) can a judgment of "normal" or "pathological" neuropsychological test performance be made (Fig. 2).

COGNITIVE IMPAIRMENTS CONSISTENT WITH AD

As noted earlier (Table 1), the neuropsychological diagnosis of AD requires the documentation of a memory impairment and a deficit in at least one other domain of cognition. Moreover, the deficits

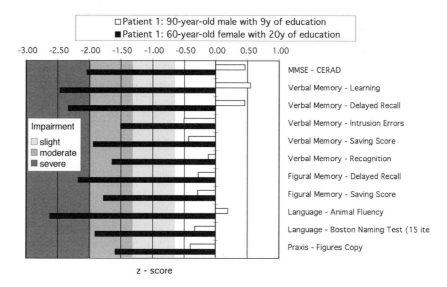

Fig. 2. Effects of the demographic variables age, gender, and education on the German version of the Consortium to Establish a Registry for Alzheimer's Disease—Neuropsychological Assessment Battery (CERAD-NAB; [35]) performance. Two hypothetical patients achieved exactly the same test scores. Their raw scores were then corrected for the effects of age, gender, and education. The corrected scores are shown as z-scores, i.e., in terms of the number of standard deviations of healthy subjects' performances. While patient 1's cognitive performance is within normal limits, patient 2's is clearly impaired.

must impinge on everyday functioning and represent a decline from a former higher level. The latter criterion implies that a follow-up neuropsychological examination is required to make a definite neuropsychological diagnosis of AD. In practice, a thorough interdisciplinary diagnostic workup—including interviewing the patient's caregiver—may provide grounds for a tentative diagnosis and thus treatment.

Long-term memory is consistently impaired in AD patients. Decrements in other domains of cognitive functioning are equally important, but vary among patients and thus will not be discussed here. The type of memory that is already affected early in the course of AD is episodic memory, i.e., memories for past events in an individual's life, an individual's autobiography (19,20). Episodic memory is typically assessed by requiring an individual to recall words (i.e., verbal episodic memory) or figures (i.e., nonverbal episodic memory) from previously learned materials. Delayed recall refers to the number of items recalled from the original learning list after a delay typically lasting from several minutes to 1 hour.

The delayed recall measure, however, is confounded with subjects' learning abilities. Clearly, the number of items recalled after a delay depends on the number of items that were learned (poor learning performances *per se* may indicate a primary deficit in executive functioning). The savings score takes the amount of learned material into consideration by quantifying memory performance as the proportion of recalled to learned items. Measures of forgetting (delayed recall, savings scores) on verbal episodic memory tasks have been shown to be the most sensitive in detecting AD patients in the early stages of the disease (21).

Poor recall performance could reflect either an inability to encode new material (i.e., the information never reached the memory store) or an inability to retrieve successfully encoded material.

Following the delayed recall task, subjects are therefore typically presented with items that had actually been part of the learning list mixed together with novel items and asked to identify the original items (recognition task). If the primary deficit is in retrieving information that was in fact successfully stored, patients will be able to recognize the original items. Since AD patients' primary deficit is in storing, not retrieving, information, their recognition discriminability (i.e., the ability to distinguish between the original and novel items) is also impaired.

When healthy individuals learn a list of words, they typically recall more stimuli from the end (recency region) than the beginning (primacy region) of the list—a phenomenon termed the serial position effect. The recall of words from the recency region is taken to reflect short-term memory abilities (recency effect), whereas the recall of words from the primacy region is thought to depend on their successful storage in episodic long-term memory (primacy effect)—a more difficult task. Consistent with their theorized impairment in long- and not short-term memory, AD patients recall significantly fewer words from the primacy region but just as many words from the recency region compared to healthy control subjects *(22)*.

Another important aspect of memory assessment is the analysis of errors. The errors committed by subjects in recall portions of episodic memory tasks can be grouped into two general categories: perseverations and intrusions. Perseverations are repetitions of response items, either following relatively few or following many intervening responses (proximal and distal perseverations, respectively). These errors are interpreted as an impaired response inhibition due to frontal lobe dysfunction. Intrusions are generally defined as the production of responses not on the target list and purportedly reflect a subject's difficulty in discriminating relevant from irrelevant responses. Counterintuitively, AD patients in the early stages of the disease do not commit more perseverative errors than healthy controls. However, compared to healthy individuals, even patients with mild AD commit substantially more intrusion errors *(23)*.

Semantic memory refers to knowledge of the world, such as facts, concepts, and vocabulary, the storehouse of information which supplies an individual with the necessary material for thought. Indirectly, episodic memory measures also reflect semantic memory capacity, as these two functions depend on one another *(24)*. Thus, findings of impaired episodic memory performance warrant the further investigation of semantic memory functioning in possible AD patients. Measures of semantic memory include vocabulary, confrontation naming, and information (general knowledge), that is, tests that also strongly depend on language skills. Semantic fluency, another test of semantic memory, may be less burdened by this confound. This task requires subjects to name as many exemplars from a predefined semantic category as possible within a given time period. Since the generation of, e.g., types of animals depends on knowledge of the attributes that define the concept "animal," any loss of these defining characteristics should result in fewer correct exemplars being produced *(25)*.

To control for search and retrieval strategies, so-called letter fluency (also known as phonemic or lexical fluency) tasks are commonly administered along with semantic fluency tasks. The letter fluency task requires the patient to produce as many words as possible beginning with a predefined letter within a given time period. It can be performed without taxing semantic memory by employing phonemic and/or lexical cues to guide production. AD patients indeed evidence greater impairments in semantic compared to letter fluency tasks, indicating a primary deficit in semantic memory and not search and retrieval processes *(26)*. This finding, among others, has led to the hypothesis that AD patients suffer from a breakdown in their structures of semantic knowledge *(27,28)*.

THE SPECIFICITY OF NEUROPSYCHOLOGY: AN EXAMPLE

One general diagnostic taxonomy that has been proposed for the group of dementias is the cortical (e.g., AD) and subcortical (e.g., Huntington's disease, Parkinson's disease) distinction. Today it is clear that this classification does not adequately identify the primary sites of neuroanatomical

Table 3
Neuropsychological Testing and Differential Diagnosis

Cognitive domain	Cortical dementia (e.g., Alzheimer's disease)	Subcortical dementia (e.g., Huntington's disease)
Memory deficit	Storage	Retrieval
Retrograde amnesia	Severe	Relatively mild
Forgetting	Fast	Normal
Intrusion errors	Many	Few
Recognition discriminability	Impaired	Normal
Semantic structure	Impaired	Normal
Psychomotor functioning	Normal	Slowed
Skill learning	Normal	Impaired

Neuropsychological testing contributes to the differential diagnosis, as different types of dementia are characterized by different profiles of cognitive performance, as illustrated with cortical and subcortical dementias.

pathology in dementia syndromes. It has, however, proven useful as a triage concept in neuropsychology, i.e., to broadly classify patterns of neuropsychological performance and to generate differential diagnoses.

The primary memory deficit in cortical dementia is presumably one of storage, and in subcortical dementia it is one of retrieval. Thus, cortical, but not subcortical dementia patients have difficulties acquiring new information (retrograde amnesia). They will rapidly forget what they were able to learn (forgetting) and will commit more intrusion errors, thus reflecting their difficulties in deciding whether what comes to mind during a delayed recall task was actually on the list. Recognition tasks will help to alleviate the subcortical dementia patients' retrieval difficulties, whereas individuals with a cortical dementia evidence poor recognition discriminability. The memory impairment in cortical dementia extends to semantic memory, such that these patients will evidence greater impairments in semantic fluency compared to letter fluency tasks. The combination of impaired retrieval and spared semantic memory in subcortical dementia patients, on the other hand, will lead to equally poor performance on both fluency tasks. Finally—in contrast to subcortical dementia patients who present with psychomotor slowing and impaired skill learning abilities, AD patients converse and work at a normal pace and may even be able to acquire new skills (as measured by, e.g., continuous improvements in mirror-reading speed with practice) (Table 3).

DETECTING THE ALZHEIMER PATIENT

Preclinical AD

The progressive neuropathological processes in AD—loss of synapses, deposition of tangles and plaques—are manifested by a progressive deterioration in cognitive functioning. Clearly, the diagnosis of AD is based on the documentation of these clinical symptoms and thus necessarily occurs when significant pathological changes have already taken place (29) (Fig. 3). Major efforts are currently underway to identify patients in the preclinical phase of the disease, that is, at a stage in which some pathological changes have taken place but social or occupational functioning is not yet impaired. This is the time point at which currently available symptomatic pharmacotherapies with their documented 1-year delay in disease progression would be most beneficial (30).

The knowledge gained from the search for preclinical cognitive markers for AD has helped develop new or helped refine existing neuropsychological tools for the earliest possible detection of AD. These may be employed in practice in a two-step approach, the cooperative effort of

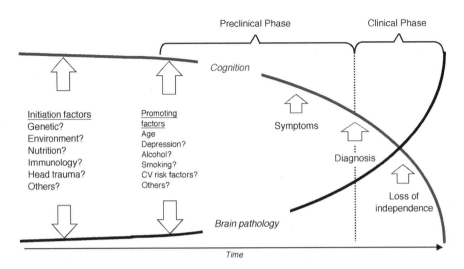

Fig. 3. A conceptual model of the development and course of AD (adapted from *29*).

1. The primary-care physician, who screens patients with a suspected dementia, and
2. Specialist centers, who conduct further interdisciplinary diagnostic examinations and provide treatment recommendations *(31)*.

Screening in the Two-Step Approach

Early detection of the AD patient is a challenging endeavor. The earliest cognitive symptoms of the disease are subtle and difficult to differentiate from the typical aging processes, demographic status, and changed demands of life. Moreover, an adequate diagnostic workup of an individual with suspected AD is time-consuming and costly. A well-structured and cost-effective approach for both the primary-care physician and specialist centers is therefore critical. In a first step, the early detection of AD requires a valid and efficient screening strategy suited for systematic or opportunistic screening at patient–physician encounters. The specialist or Alzheimer's disease center conducts the second step, the interdisciplinary diagnostic procedure including a formal neuropsychological assessment described above (Fig. 4).

Screening for AD is recommended for every patient over 60 years of age and when dementia is suspected. This screening is based on clinical judgment, the histories obtained from both the patient and his or her significant other, as well as findings from the physical examination. Since the insidious onset of AD may escape detection without an explicit quantitative assessment, a cognitive screening must be performed. Besides good screening properties (i.e., high sensitivity and specificity), it is important that the cognitive screening instruments are acceptable to the patient and easy to administer, score, and interpret. Among the many scales introduced for this purpose, the Mini-Mental State Examination (MMSE) enjoys the most widespread use *(32)*.

Our understanding of normal and pathological aging has improved significantly since the introduction of the MMSE in 1975. Indeed, by today's standards, the patient sample in the 1975 study may be conceived of as moderately, not mildly, demented, and the healthy population may have included typical, instead of exclusively optimal agers. Consequently, the MMSE cutoff score of 23/24 then proposed by Folstein et al. may no longer be appropriate.

This hypothesis was supported by the results of a study by Thalmann and colleagues *(33)*, who studied 176 mildly impaired dementia patients and 88 optimally healthy individuals matched for age, gender, and education *(33)*. They all were assessed using the MMSE. The optimal cutoff score was

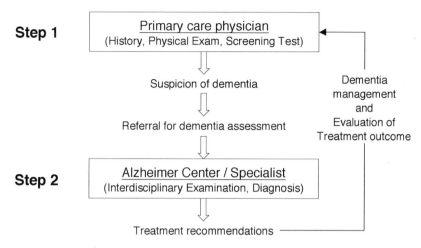

Fig. 4. The two-step dementia screening and diagnostic procedure.

defined as the one that maximized sensitivity (i.e., the percentage of accurately diagnosed dementia patients) and specificity (i.e., the percentage of accurately identified healthy individuals). As shown in Fig. 5, the optimal MMSE cutoff score for these samples was 26/27—three points higher than the one originally published. The 26/27 cutoff score identified 47/176 more patients but only 8/88 fewer healthy controls than the original 23/24 cutoff score.

The MMSE has also been criticized on the grounds that it is too dependent on verbal functioning and does not adequately assess executive functioning, a possible presenting symptom in early AD. In order to compensate for these drawbacks, Thalmann et al. analyzed the utility of administering an additional test, the clock drawing test (CDT), along with the MMSE *(34)*. The CDT is simple to administer. Patients are presented with a circle on a piece of paper and instructed to "draw a clock, fill in all the numbers and hands." When the patient indicates that the drawing is finished, he is asked to "write down the time your clock shows as if it were in a train schedule or TV guide." Thalmann et al. analyzed the 36 published scoring criteria for the CDT with a stepwise logistic regression analysis in the 176 early-stage dementia patients and 88 normal control subjects described above *(33)*. This procedure isolated four criteria with optimal sensitivity (77%) and specificity (75%) with a cutoff score of 4/5 out of a possible 7 points:

1. Twelve numbers are present (1 point).
2. The number "12" is placed correctly (2 points).
3. The hands have the correct proportions (2 points).
4. The subject wrote the time correctly (2 points).

The diagnostic accuracy of the combined MMSE (cut-off score 26/27) and CDT was not statistically superior to that of the MMSE alone. It is recommended, however, that both instruments be routinely administered to screen for AD in order to identify those patients who present with secondary executive system dysfunction (Fig. 6).

SUMMARY

The neuropsychological assessment generates profiles of cognitive functioning which are essential to the diagnostic and differential diagnostic process in AD. It may also be employed to track dis-

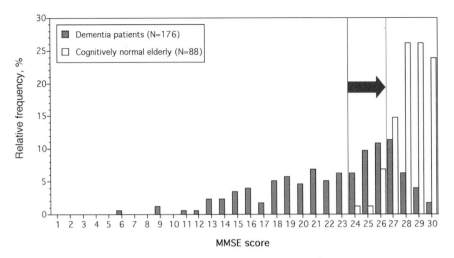

Fig. 5. Distribution of MMSE scores in dementia patients and healthy elderly individuals *(33)*. The more accurate cutoff score of 26/27 identified 47 more dementia patients than the originally published cutoff score of 23/24 *(32)*.

ease progression and treatment response, and to develop behavioral management strategies. One of the greatest challenges faced in the neuropsychology of dementia is to differentiate the typical seque-lae of the aging process from the earliest signs and symptoms of a dementing illness. This is an especially critical issue in light of currently available treatment options. Clearly, it would be desirable to implement these at a stage in the disease process in which the least amount of neurodegeneration has taken place. The earliest sign of AD is poor (episodic) memory performance, that is, difficulties in learning new material and quickly forgetting the information that was learned. The neuropsychological diagnosis of AD further requires an impairment in at least one other domain of cognitive functioning (language, praxia, gnosis, or executive function). These dysfunctions must show a decline from a previous level of functioning and interfere significantly with daily life. The insidious nature of the disease onset and the difficulty of differentiating pathological cognitive functioning from the changed demands of life necessitate a highly sensitive and standardized screening procedure to identify the AD patient as early as possible. Neuropsychological research has identified cognitive screening methods suited for routine use in persons over 60 years of age or those in whom dementia is suspected. The Mini-Mental State Examination (MMSE) has been identified as a cognitive screening instrument of high diagnostic accuracy when a cutoff score of 26/27 (and not the originally published 23/24) is employed. It is recommended that the MMSE be administered in conjunction with the clock drawing test to identify patients presenting with largely nonverbal or executive system dysfunction. Patients with a suspected dementia based on clinical judgment or poor screening performance should be referred to a specialist center for an interdisciplinary workup in the second of this two-stage approach.

ACKNOWLEDGMENTS

We gratefully acknowledge the generous support of the Betty and David Koetser Foundation for Brain Research (K. I. Taylor), the Hartmann-Müller Foundation (K. I. Taylor), and the Swiss National Science Foundation, grant 3200-049107 (A. U. Monsch).

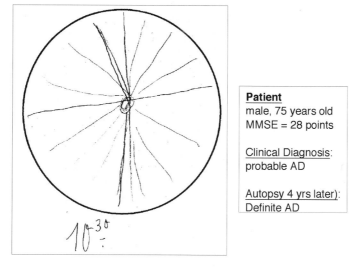

Patient
male, 75 years old
MMSE = 28 points

Clinical Diagnosis:
probable AD

Autopsy 4 yrs later):
Definite AD

Fig. 6. The figure depicts the importance of additionally administering the clock drawing test (CDT) in the cognitive dementia screening examination. Although the patient obtained a MMSE score of 28, he obviously failed the CDT. An intensive diagnostic workup at our Memory Clinic resulted in a diagnosis of probable AD, a diagnosis confirmed at autopsy 4 years later. Thus, the combined MMSE and CDT may better detect those patients who initially present with largely intact verbal abilities but impaired executive functioning than the MMSE alone.

REFERENCES

1. Almkvist, O.; Brane, G.; Johanson, A.: Neuropsychological assessment of dementia: state of the art. Acta Neurol Scand Suppl 1996; 168: 45–49.
2. American Psychiatric Association: Diagnostic and Statistical Manual of Mental Disorders. 4th ed. American Psychiatric Association, Washington, DC, 1994.
3. Rowe, J.W.; Katzman, R.: Principles of geriatrics as applied to neurology. In: Katzman, R. Rowe, J.W. (eds.): Principles of geriatric neurology. FA Davis, Philadelphia, 1992: 3–17.
4. Salthouse, T.A.: The processing-speed theory of adult age differences in cognition. Psychol Rev 1996; 103: 403–428.
5. Greenwood, P.M.: The frontal aging hypothesis evaluated. J Int Neuropsychol Soc 2000; 6: 705–726.
6. Rabbitt, P.M.A.: Aging of memory. In: Tallis, R.C.; Fillit, H.M.; Brocklehurst, J.C. (eds.): Brocklehurst's textbook of geriatric medicine and gerontology. 5th ed. Churchill Livingstone, London, 1998: 123–152.
7. Petersen, R.C. et al.: Memory function in normal aging. Neurology 1992; 42: 396–401.
8. Small, S.A. et al.: Selective decline in memory function among healthy elderly. Neurology 1999; 52: 1392–1396.
9. Blass, J.P.: Age-associated memory impairment and Alzheimer's disease. J Am Geriatr Soc 1996; 44: 209–211.
10. Luszcz, M.A.; Bryan, J.: Towards understanding age-related memory loss in late adulthood. Gerontology 1999; 45: 2–9.
11. Rowe, J.W.; Kahn, R.L.: Human aging: usual and successful. Science 1987; 237: 143–149.
12. Shah, Y.; Tangalos, E.G.; Petersen, R.C.: Mild cognitive impairment. When is it a precursor to Alzheimer's disease? Geriatrics 2000; 55: 62, 65–68.
13. Morris, J.C.: Is Alzheimer's disease inevitable with age? Lessons from clinicopathologic studies of healthy aging and very mild Alzheimer's disease. J Clin Invest 1999; 104: 1171–1173.
14. Morris, J.C. et al.: Cerebral amyloid deposition and diffuse plaques in "normal" aging: evidence for presymptomatic and very mild Alzheimer's disease. Neurology 1996; 46: 707–719.
15. Mueller, E.A. et al.: Brain volume preserved in healthy elderly through the eleventh decade. Neurology 1998; 51: 1555–1562.
16. Anstey, K.; Christensen, H.: Education, activity, health, blood pressure and apolipoprotein E as predictors of cognitive change in old age: a review. Gerontology 2000; 46: 163–177.
17. Burns, A.; Zaudig, M.: Mild cognitive impairment in older people. Lancet 2002; 360: 1963–1965.
18. Almkvist, O. et al.: Conversion from preclinical to clinical stage of Alzheimer's disease as shown by decline of cognitive function in carriers of the Swedish APP-mutation. J Neural Transm 2002; 62 (Suppl): 117–125.

19. Squire, L.R.: Mechanisms of memory. Science 1986; 232: 1612–1619.

20. Tulving, E.: How many memory systems are there? Am Psychologist 1985; 40: 385–398.

21. Monsch, A.U. et al.: Clinical validity of the Mattis Dementia Rating Scale in detecting dementia of the Alzheimer type. A double cross-validation and application to a community-dwelling sample. *Arch Neurol 1995; 52: 899–904.*

22. Massman, P.J.: Does impaired primacy recall equal impaired long-term storage? Serial position effects in Huntington's disease and Alzheimer's disease. Developmental Neuropsychol 1993; 9: 1–15.

23. Hart, S.; Smith, C.M.; Swash, M.: Intrusion errors in Alzheimer's disease. Br J Clin Psychol 1986; 25: 149–150.

24. Tulving, E.: Concepts of human memory. In: Squire, L.R. et al. (eds.): Memory: organization and locus of change. Oxford University Press, New York, 1991: 3–32.

25. Martin, A.: Representation of semantic and spatial knowledge in Alzheimer's patients: implications for models of preserved learning in amnesia. J Clin Exp Neuropsychol 1987; 9: 191–224.

26. Monsch, A.U. et al.: Comparisons of verbal fluency tasks in the detection of dementia of the Alzheimer type. Arch Neurol 1992; 49: 1253–1258.

27. Butters, N. et al.: Episodic and semantic memory: a comparison of amnesic and demented patients. J Clin Exp Neuropsychol 1987; 9: 479–497.

28. Martin, A.; Fedio, P.: Word production and comprehension in Alzheimer's disease: the breakdown of semantic knowledge. Brain Lang 1983; 19: 124–141.

29. Katzman, R.: Education and the prevalence of dementia and Alzheimer's disease. Neurology 1993; 43: 13–20.

30. Giacobini, E.: Is anti-cholinesterase therapy of Alzheimer's disease delaying progression? Aging (Milano) 2001; 13: 247–254.

31. Staehelin, H.B.; Monsch, A.U.; Spiegel, R.: Early diagnosis of dementia via a two-step screening and diagnostic procedure. Int Psychogeriatr 1997; 9 (Suppl 1): 123–130.

32. Folstein, M.F.; Folstein, S.E.; McHugh, P.R.: "Mini Mental State"—A practical method for grading the cognitive state of patients for the clinician. J Psychiatr Res 1975; 12: 189–198.

33. Thalmann, B. et al.: Dementia screening in general practice: optimized scoring for the Clock Drawing Test. Brain Aging 2002; 2: 36–43.

34. Freedman, M. et al.: Clock drawing: a neuropsychological analysis. Oxford University Press, New York, 1994.

35. Morris, J.C. et al.: The Consortium to Establish a Registry for Alzheimer's Disease (CERAD). Part I. Clinical and neuropsychological assessment of Alzheimer's disease. Neurology 1989; 39: 1159–1165.

12

Vascular Cognitive Impairment in Clinical Practice

Kenneth Rockwood and Timo Erkinjuntti

INTRODUCTION

Why do we use the term "vascular cognitive impairment" (VCI)? This term has a fairly recent history. Although it was long held that "senility" arose from cerebral arteriosclerosis, this view began to be undermined about 30 years ago, with the promulgation of the doctrine that dementia in the setting of cerebrovascular illness was a matter of small or large cerebral infarcts *(1,2)*. With this view of vascular dementia (VaD) being a matter of strokes large and small, the term multi-infarct dementia (MID) became synonymous with VaD. In the early 1990s, however, the term MID was seen as inadequate. Specifically, it did not include many patients with clinically important cognitive impairment, especially those who, while impaired, did not meet traditional criteria for dementia *(3)*. The latter, modeled on the dementia of Alzheimer's disease (AD), excluded, for example, patients in whom memory complaint was not dominant, or in whom functional impairment might be due simply to the motoric effects of stroke. Initially, MID was replaced with VaD, which was conceptualized in two widely promulgated sets of consensus-based criteria *(4,5)*.

Later, these criteria, and others like them, were criticized as being unwieldy, incompatible with each other, and having poor interrater reliability *(6)*. By the late fall of 2001 a consensus conference, held under the auspices of the International Psychogeriatrics Association, proposed that the term VCI replace VaD *(7)*. This is the current situation, which has some implications for how we understand the burden of cerebrovascular disease on cognition, function, and behavior.

THE POPULATION BURDEN OF CEREBROVASCULAR DISEASE

VCI is an important contributor to the cost of managing illnesses associated with cognitive impairment *(8)*. On a per-patient basis, the natural history costs are equal to that of caring for AD *(9)*. In the Canadian Study of Health and Aging (CSHA), it was estimated that about 5% of the elderly population suffers from VCI. VCI was defined there as consisting of three groups: patients who meet the criteria for dementia (VaD—prevalence 1.5%); people who have cognitive impairment but who nevertheless do not meet dementia criteria (vascular cognitive impairment, no dementia [Vasc CIND] prevalence 2.4%), and people with mixed AD and VaD (prevalence 0.9%) *(8)*.

In general, VaD, as traditionally defined, is the second most common single cause of dementia *(10)*. The incidence of VaD has varied between 6 and 12 cases per year per 1000 persons aged 70 years and older, and increases with increasing age *(11,12)*. Patients with VaD have substantially impaired cognition (as bad as AD), but demonstrate a higher mortality rate *(8,13)*. In the above-mentioned CSHA, the median survival time for people with VaD was 3.31 years (95% confidence preferred 2.31 to 4.31 years) *(14)*.

From: *Current Clinical Neurology,*
Alzheimer's Disease: A Physician's Guide to Practical Management
Edited by: R. W. Richter and B. Zoeller Richter © Humana Press Inc., Totowa, NJ

PATHOPHYSIOLOGY OF VCI

Recalling that the construct of VCI is heterogenous and incorporates a variety of clinical syndromes, it is to be expected that a variety of vascular mechanisms and brain changes operate. In general, VCI arises from interactions among vascular risk factors, the brain injury associated with them (for example, infarction, white matter lesions, atrophy), host factors (age, education), and premorbid cognition *(6)*. Infarction can arise from large-artery disease, embolic events, small-vessel disease and, perhaps most controversially, from hemodynamic mechanisms *(15,16)*. VCI can also rise in the setting of cerebrovascular disease (CVD) without obvious infarction *(15–19)*.

Also of note for current management is that there appears to be considerable overlap in the cognitive deficits of VaD and AD, even without pathological findings of AD. This is felt to arise from the susceptibility of cholinergic structures to ischemic damage, especially hippocampal CA1 neurons and cholinergic projection fibers found in the white matter *(18–21)*. Global ischemia is also associated experimentally with a cholinergic deficit *(22,23)*.

CLINICO-RADIOGRAPHIC CLASSIFICATION OF VCI

Given the lack of data supporting more traditional VaD criteria, there is some interest in a more recent, empirically based clinico-radiographic approach to the diagnosis of VCI *(8,24,25,29)*. This approach recognizes the three chief subtypes of VCI, which are defined clinically. Next, the clinical type can be cross-classified by one of five radiographic profiles.

Vascular Cognitive Impairment Without Dementia (Vasc CIND)

Patients diagnosed with Vasc CIND fall into one of two groups. Some patients have few cognitive deficits, no functional impairment, and are thus analogous to patients with mild cognitive impairment (MCI) in relation to AD. As such, it is not surprising that many (about half in the CSHA) *(27)* progress to dementia. A second group with Vasc CIND is represented by those patients with clinically important cognitive and functional impairment who are excluded by most dementia criteria on the grounds that they do not have prominent memory impairment. Examples are patients with ischemic frontal lobe disconnection syndromes, or those in whom functional impairment from the motoric effects of stroke make the attribution of impairment to a cognitive cause difficult.

Vascular Dementia VaD

Patients with vascular dementia have an acquired, chronic, global impairment of cognition that is sufficiently severe to interfere with social or occupational functioning, whose cause appears to be attributable to vascular disease. Features demonstrably associated with VaD are outlined in Table 1. Note that, in contrast to the Hachinski ischemia score, this does not extend to vascular risk factors alone, as are risks for all forms of late-life cognitive impairment, including so-called neurodegenerative ones *(28,29)*.

Mixed Dementia (AD With CVD)

The classification of mixed dementia has been expanded to include not just the combination of AD and VaD, but also other primary neurodegenerative disorders *(8,30)*. These patients, when diagnosed initially, present clinically with a profile suggestive of a given primary neurodegenerative dementia in the face of concomitant evident CVD injury. As noted below, however, an equally common presentation is that they have an apparently typical presentation of a pure form of a late-life dementia, but are found on neuroimaging also to have CVD *(31)*.

Radiographic Profiles

As noted, five major neuroimaging profiles are recognized. As outlined in Table 2, these consist of more than one cortical stroke, one cortical stroke (the so-called single strategic stroke), subcortical

Table 1
Clinical Clues to the Diagnosis of a Vascular Contribution to Dementia

Abrupt onset
Stepwise deterioration
Fluctuating course
Prolonged periods of plateau
History of stroke
Focal neurological symptoms
Early onset of gait disorder
Early onset of a seizure
Early onset of urinary incontinence
Patchy cognitive deficits
Focal neurological signs

Table 2
Clinical-Neuroimaging Classification of VCI

	Cortical stroke(s)	Subcortical strokes	White matter changes	No imaging used
Vascular CIND				
With mild cognitive impairment	+	+	+	–
With important cognitive and functional impairment that does not meet dementia criteria requiring memory loss or global impairment	++	++	+	–
Vascular Dementia				
With predominantly multiple cortical stroke(s)	++++	+	++	–
With predominantly subcortical ischemia	+	++++	++	+/–
Mixed neurodegenerative dementia/ cerebrovascular disease diagnosed clinically with both features	+	++	+++	+
Incidental ischemic lesions on neuroimaging in patients with otherwise typical neurodegenerative profiles (e.g., Alzheimer's disease, dementia with Lewy bodies)	+	++	+++	–

strokes, white matter changes, and combinations of the above. Taken with the clinical profiles, a clinico-neuroimaging cross-classification can provide a comprehensive account of the type of VCI profile. Note, however, that this approach is not etiologically based, so that treatments must also consider the presumed cause of the impairment.

TREATMENT OF PATIENTS WITH VCI

The treatment of patients with VCI rests on three approaches: nonspecific management, which is chiefly the treatment of vascular risk factors; specific cognitive therapy (chiefly a cholinesterase inhibitor); and treatment of behavioral and psychological symptoms.

Of the vascular risk factor treatments now available, it appears that treatment of arterial hypertension is best associated with a lower risk of dementia *(32,33)*. The agents studied include a long-acting dihydropyridine calcium channel blocker, a thiazide diuretic, and enalapril. In addition, treatment with perindopril and indapamide has been shown to lower the risk of dementia in patients treated after a first stroke who later had a second stroke *(34)*. Observational data also support the use of lipid-lowering agents in preventing all forms of late-life dementia, including VaD *(35)*.

Limited data support the use of nimodipine, another dihydropyridine calcium channel blocker, on cognitive and behavioral outcomes in patients with predominant white matter lesions with at least one subcortical stroke *(36)*. More specific cognitive effects have also been seen with memantine, an *N*-methyl-D-aspartate (NMDA) receptor antagonist. In a randomized controlled trial of patients with severe dementia of mixed etiology (51% of whom had VaD), those treated with 10 mg of memantine per day showed better function compared to those on placebo *(37)*. A second trial, in patients with mild to moderate VaD, showed that the group on 20 mg of memantine per day had improved cognition and no deterioration in global functioning and behavior *(38)*.

The use of cholinesterase inhibitors has also been investigated in VaD. At present, the most persuasive data derived from a randomized, double-blind, controlled, 6-month trial with galantamine (24 mg/day) in patients with VaD or AD, combined with CVD *(39)*. This trial showed better outcomes on all measures in the combined-groups analysis; statistically significant effects were demonstrated in the subgroup analysis only for those with mixed AD/VaD. In addition, a combined analysis of data from two trials of donepezil in patients with VaD (most of whom had an MID profile) showed significant improvements in some but not all outcome measures *(40)*.

In the management of behavioral problems in dementia patients, antipsychotics are used more widely than the available evidence suggests. Still, a meta-analysis of controlled trials showed overall improvement rates of 61% for these medications, compared with 34% for placebo *(41)*. Note, however, that adverse effects are common, including anticholinergic effects that can worsen cognition, and produce gastrointestinal and cardiac side effects. Anti-dopaminergic side effects are also common, giving rise to drug-induced or exacerbated extrapyramidal symptoms. Perhaps the most feared adverse effect of antipsychotic use is tardive dyskinesia. This potentially irreversible movement disorder is seen especially with typical neuroleptics. Though generally related to the duration of use (becoming more common with prolonged use), it can also occur early *(42)*.

The atypical antipsychotics have been available since the mid-1990s, and generally have better data to support their use, although precise data for VCI remain lacking. There is good evidence for the use of low-dose risperidone in aggression, agitation, and psychosis *(43,44)*. Street and colleagues showed that a low dose of olanzapine was effective for treatment of both aggression and psychosis *(45)*. Although data on the use of quetiapine have not yet been published, preliminary information presented at scientific meetings indicate that it too has a role *(46)*. Of particular interest with atypical antipsychotics is the relative paucity of extrapyramidal side effects when they are used at low doses. In addition, there appears to be a lack of anticholinergic effects and, as of yet, there are only few reports of tardive dyskinesia.

While many antidepressants have been used for the treatment of behavioral and psychological symptoms, much of the data come from case series and inconclusive randomized trials, as reviewed elsewhere *(47)*. Such evidence exists for trazodone, citalopram, sertraline, and fluvoxamine. The psychobehavioral metaphor of depression in VCI might be particularly useful (for example, citalopram in poststroke depression *(48)*). Unfortunately, studies too often have not made clear the baseline target symptoms that were being treated, instead proposing only that they are useful for nonspecific agitation. Many studies have found that the side effects of sedation, restlessness, and gastrointestinal distress limit the use of selective serontonine reuptake inhibitors (SSRI), while tricyclic antidepressants are associated with anticholinergic effects.

Anticonvulsants have also been used for the treatment of behavioral problems in patients with VCI, but again, definitive evidence is lacking. Thus we must rely on a survey of experts, which recommended divalproex, and, with more limited enthusiasm, carbamazepine *(49)*. Benzodiazepines also have been widely used for agitation, especially when features of anxiety and sleep disturbance are present.

Again, side effects such as falls, ataxia, sedation, and paradoxical agitation are well known, and both tolerance and withdrawal symptoms also limit their use.

Where new-onset anxiety appears in isolation, it is always worth considering depression as the cause. If this seems unlikely, then a short course of benzodiazepines can be tried, with low-dose loraza-pam or oxazepam as the drugs of choice, given their lack of active metabolites. There is also limited evidence for buspirone in these circumstances *(49)*.

SUMMARY

VCI is an important, common, and costly condition. It has distinct clinical and radiographic sub-types, with increasing evidence that both can contribute to distinct patient profiles and outcomes *(50,51)*. Treatment consists of measures directed primarily toward cardiovascular risk factors, especially hypertension.

REFERENCES

1. Torak, R.M. (ed): The pathologic physiology of dementia. With indications for diagnosis and treatment. Springer-Verlag, Berlin, Heidelberg, 1978.
2. Hackinski, V.C.; Lassen, N.A.; Marshall, J.: Multi-infarct dementia. A cause of mental deterioration in the elderly. Lancet 1974; 2: 207–210.
3. Erkinjuntti, T.; Hachinski, V.C.: Rethinking vascular dementia. Cerebrovasc Dis 1993; 3: 3–23.
4. Roman, G.C. et al.: Vascular dementia: diagnostic criteria for research studies. Report of the NINDS-AIREN International Workshop. Neurology 1993; 43: 250–260.
5. Chui, H.C. et al.: Criteria for the diagnosis of ischemic vascular dementia proposed by the State of California Alzheimer's Disease Diagnostic and Treatment Centers. Neurology 1992; 42: 473–480.
6. Erkinjuntti, T.; Rockwood, K.: Vascular dementia. Semin Clin Neuropsychiatry 2003; 8: 37–45.
7. O'Brien, J.T. et al.: Evolving concepts in vascular burden of the brain. Lancet Neurol 2003; 2: 89–98.
8. Rockwood, K. et al.: Prevalence and outcomes of vascular cognitive impairment. Neurology 2000; 54: 447–451.
9. Rockwood, K. et al.: Societal costs of vascular cognitive impairment in older adults. Stroke 2002; 33: 1605–1609.
10. Lobo, A. et al.: Prevalence of dementia and major subtypes in Europe: a collaborative study of population-based cohorts. Neurology 2000; 54: S4–S9.
11. Fratiglioni, L. et al.: Incidence of dementia and major subtypes in Europe: a collaborative study of population-based cohorts. Neurology 2000; 54: S10–S15.
12. Hébert, R. et al.: Vascular dementia. Incidence and risk factors in the Canadian Study of Health and Aging. Stroke 2000; 31: 1487–1493.
13. Desmond, D.W.: Vascular dementia: a construct in evolution. Cerebrovasc Brain Metab Rev 1996; 8: 296–325.
14. Wolfson, C. et al.: A re-evaluation of the duration of survival from the onset of dementia. N Engl J Med 2001; 344: 1111–1116.
15. Erkinjuntti, T. et al.: Accuracy of the clinical diagnosis of vascular dementia: a prospective clinical and post-mortem neuropathological study. J Neurol Neurosurg Psychiatry 1988; 51: 1037–1044.
16. Mielke, R. et al.: Severity of vascular dementia is related to volume of metabolically impaired tissue. Arch Neurol 1992; 49: 909–913.
17. Olsson, Y.; Brun, A.; Englund, E.: Fundamental pathological lesions in vascular dementia. Acta Neurol Scand Suppl 1996; 168: 31–38.
18. Vinters, H.V. et al.: Neuropathologic substrates of ischemic vascular dementia. J Neuropathol Exp Neurol 2000; 59: 931–945.
19. Pohjasvaara, T. et al.: MRI correlates of dementia after first clinical ischemic stroke. J Neurol Sci 2000; 181: 111–117.
20. Roessmann, U.; Friede, R.L.: Changes in butyryl cholinesterase activity in reactive glia. Neurology 1966; 16: 123–129.
21. Selden, N.R. et al.: Trajectories of cholinergic pathways within the cerebral hemispheres of the human brain. Brain 1998; 121 (Pt12): 2249–2257.
22. Zhou, J.; Zhang, H.Y.; Tang, X.C.: Huperzine A attenuates cognitive deficits and hippocampal neuronal damage after transient global ischemia in gerbils. Neurosci Lett 2001; 313: 137–140.
23. Block, F.: Global ischemia and behavioural deficits. Prog Neurobiol 1999; 58: 279–295.
24. Rockwood, K. et al.: Prevalence and outcomes of vascular cognitive impairment. Neurology 2000; 55: 66–73.
25. Rockwood, K. et al.: Spectrum of disease in vascular cognitive impairment. Neuroepidemiology 1999; 18: 248–254.
26. Wentzel, C. et al.: Inter-rater reliability of the diagnosis of vascular cognitive impairment at a memory clinic. Neuroepidemiology 2000; 19: 186–193.

27. Wentzel, C. et al.: Progression of impairment in patients with vascular cognitive impairment without dementia. Neurology 2001; 57: 714–716.

28. Hachinski, V.C. et al.: Cerebral blood flow in dementia. Arch Neurol 1975; 32: 632–637.

29. Rockwood, K.: Vascular risk factors in dementia. J Geriatr Care 2002; 1: 141–146.

30. Ballard, C. et al.: Neuropathological substrates of dementia and depression in vascular dementia, with a particular focus on cases with small infarct volumes. Dementia Geriatr Cogn Disord 2000; 11: 59–65.

31. Rockwood, K. et al.: The diagnosis of "mixed" dementia in the Consortium for the Investigation of Vascular Impairment of Cognition (CIVIC). Ann N Y Acad Sci 2000; 903: 522–528.

32. Forette, F. et al.: Prevention of dementia in randomized double-blind placebo-controlled systolic hypertension in Europe (Syst-Eur) trial. Lancet 1998; 352: 1347–1351.

33. Birkenhager, W.H. et al.: Blood pressure, cognitive functions, and prevention of dementias in older patients with hypertension. Arch Intern Med 2001; 161: 152–156.

34. Progress investigators. Randomized trial of a perindopril-based blood-pressure-lowering regimen among 6105 individuals with previous stroke or transient ischaemic attack. Lancet 2001; 358: 1033–1041.

35. Tuokko, H. et al.: Five-year follow-up of cognitive impairment with no dementia. Arch Neurol 2003; 60: 577–582.

36. Pantoni, L. et al.: A preliminary open trial with nimodipine in patients with cognitive impairment and leukoaraiosis. Clin Neuropharmacol 1996; 19: 497–506.

37. Winblad, B.; Poritis, N.: Memantine in severe dementia. Results of the 9M-Best Study (Benefit and efficacy in severely demented patients during treatment with memantine). Int J Geriatr Psychiatry 1999; 14: 135–146.

38. Orgogozo, J.-M. et al.: Efficacy and safety of memantine in patients with mild to moderate vascular dementia. Stroke 2002; 33: 1843–1839.

39. Erkinjuntti, T. et al.: Efficacy of galantamine in probable vascular dementia and Alzheimer's disease combined with cerebrovascular disease: a randomized trial. Lancet 2002; 359: 1283–1290.

40. Pratt, R.D.: Patient populations in clinical trials of the efficacy and tolerability of donepezil in patients with vascular dementia. J Neurol Sci 2002; 203–204: 57–65.

41. Lanctot, K.L. et al.: Efficacy and safety of neuroleptics in behavioural disorders associated with dementia. J Clin Psychiatry 1998; 59: 550–561.

42. Jeste, D.V. et al.: Low incidence of persistent tardive dyskinesia in elderly patients with dementia treated with risperidone. Am J Psychiatry 2000; 157: 1150–1155.

43. De Deyn, P.P. et al.: A randomized trial of risperidone, placebo, and haloperidol for behavioural symptoms of dementia. Neurology 1999; 53: 946–955.

44. Katz, I.R. et al.: Comparison of risperidone and placebo for psychosis and behavioural symptoms associated with dementia: a randomized, double-blind trial. J Clin Psychiatry 1999; 60: 107–115.

45. Street, J.; Clark, S.; Gannon, K.S.: Olanzepine treatment of psychotic and behavioral symptoms in patients with Alzheimer's disease in nursing care facilities: a double-blind, randomized, placebo-controlled trial. Arch Gen Psychiatry 2000; 57: 968–977.

46. Tariot, P.N.; Ismail, M.S.: Use of quetiapine in elderly patients. J Clin Psychiatry 2002; 63 (Suppl 13): 21–26.

47. Rockwood, K.; Shea, C.: Behavioural and psychological symptoms in vascular cognitive impairment. In: Bowler, J.V.; Hachinski, V.: The vascular dementias: a review and critical appraisal. Oxford University Press, Oxford, UK, 2002.

48. Gottfries, C.G.; Karlsson, I.; Nyth, A.I.: Treatment of depression in elderly patients with and without dementia disorders. Int Clin Psychopharm 1992; 6; 55–64.

49. Alexopoulos, G.S. et al.: Treatment of agitation in older persons with dementia: the Expert Consensus Guideline. Postgraduate Medicine Special Report, April 1998.

50. Ingles, J.L. et al.: Neuropsychological predictors of incident dementia in patients with vascular cognitive impairment without dementia. Stroke 2002; 33: 1999–2002.

51. Bennett, H.P. et al.: Subcortical vascular disease and functional decline: a 6-year predicator study. J Am Geriatr Soc 2002; 50: 1969–1977.

13

Lewy Body Disease

Robert Barber, Jane Newby, and Ian G. McKeith

INTRODUCTION

Our understanding of the clinical and pathological features of dementia in late life is changing. Indeed, the way we conceptualize, investigate, and manage dementia has altered radically over recent times. An increasing public awareness, coupled with greater expectations, changing demography, and an ever more productive research alliance among specialist clinicians, the scientific community, and the pharmacological industry are all influencing clinical practice. This is particularly true for dementia with Lewy bodies (DLB).

Clinically, DLB is set apart from other causes of dementia by its distinct pattern of cognitive, psychiatric, and motor symptoms, as discussed in more detail below. It is now recognized to be the second most common cause of degenerative dementia in late life, after Alzheimer's disease (AD). DLB accounts for up to 20% of all hospital-assessed elderly cases of dementia reaching autopsy, although its community prevalence is probably lower.

Pathologically, Lewy bodies (LB) have been recognized for many years but only associated with dementia in recent times. They were first detected in the brainstem by Friederich Lewy (1885–1950), a one-time pupil of Aloys Alzheimer, in 1912, and subsequently linked to the motor symptoms of Parkinson's disease (PD). However, from the 1980s, new immunocytochemical staining techniques were developed, which improved the detection and characterization of LB occurring in other brain areas, particularly the cortex and limbic system. The clinical significance of this more diffuse distribution of LB has subsequently been the focus of much research and debate. In 1996 consensus clinical criteria were introduced under the rubric of "dementia with Lewy bodies" to capture the growing recognition of a link between the LB in the cortex and limbic areas and the characteristic cognitive and neuropsychiatric symptoms of DLB, without necessarily implying a direct causal relationship (1).

This chapter summarizes the principal clinical and pathological features of dementia with Lewy bodies and outlines a step-by-step practical guide to the assessment and management of this disease from primary care to specialist involvement.

CLINICAL IMPORTANCE OF DLB

DLB has significant implications for patients, their families, and clinicians. It can present in many guises. The distinct pattern of cognitive, psychiatric, and motor symptoms that lie at the heart of the disorder can be relevant to clinicians across a range of specialties, including primary care, psychiatry, neurology, and elderly/geriatric medicine. Invariably, patients will need a great deal of support and care, and in a proportion of them the illness progresses at a distressingly rapid pace and leads to early institutionalization.

Despite being the second most common cause of degenerative dementia in late life, DLB often remains underdetected and therefore under-treated. When DLB is diagnosed, the management of any

From: *Current Clinical Neurology,*
Alzheimer's Disease: A Physician's Guide to Practical Management
Edited by: R. W. Richter and B. Zoeller Richter © Humana Press Inc., Totowa, NJ

associated psychiatric disturbance and parkinsonism that feature so prominently can be challenging and at times unpredictable. There is a high risk of adverse events to medication, and patients with DLB can be exquisitely sensitive to antipsychotic (neuroleptic) medication. Indeed, the use of antipsychotic agents has been associated with increased mortality and will often exacerbate motor deficits. Conversely, drugs used to treat parkinsonism can exacerbate psychosis. To complicate matters further, there is a limited evidence base to inform treatment decisions, though emerging reports that cholinergic enhancers, such as rivastigmine and donepezil, are particularly effective in DLB are a source of optimism. Because of these difficulties and the frequent need for multidisciplinary involvement, whenever DLB is suspected, patients should be referred to a specialist for further assessment and management.

CLINICAL FEATURES OF DLB

In contrast to AD, which stereotypically presents with memory impairments, the presentation of DLB is more heterogeneous. It may present either individually or in combination with cognitive, neuropsychiatric, and/or motor symptoms, including parkinsonism, autonomic dysfunction, and falls. DLB primarily affects people over the age of 70 years and is slightly more common in men. On average the illness lasts 6 years or so, but there is a considerable spread, from 1 to 20 years, with some individuals deteriorating rapidly (2,3). The clinical features of DLB are divided into central, core, and supportive symptoms.

Central Features

Central to its diagnosis is the presence of a progressive, irreversible form of cognitive decline or dementia sufficient to undermine normal functioning. In broad terms this is similar to AD, but initial memory deficits can be relatively mild. Patients with DLB usually have significant problems focusing, maintaining, and switching their attention, and performing visuospatial tasks. Their thinking can be slow and effortful.

Core Features

The core features of this disorder are the triad of fluctuating cognitive impairment, persistent visual hallucinations, and spontaneous parkinsonism (1). Fluctuations in cognitive performance occur in 50–75% of patients. The frequency, duration, and severity of these fluctuations are variable. They can be observed over minutes, hours, or days and are associated with reduced attention and alertness. Short-lived fluctuations can be difficult to detect, but they may be witnessed during conversation as a glazed expression, loss of alertness or attention, or muteness. More dramatically, fluctuations can mimic delirium-like episodes, with patients switching from periods of relative lucidity to an acute confusional state. This level of confusion not only affects a person's alertness and cognitive performance but also his or her level of day-to-day functioning and communication. Changes can be so marked that the patient can have difficulty standing, dressing, talking, washing, and feeding. It has been hypothesized that fluctuations result from unstable activity in the ascending cholinergic projections that regulate attention.

Visual hallucinations occur in the majority of patients. In contrast to patients with AD, in which hallucinations are rare with Mini-Mental State Examination (MMSE) scores above 20, visual hallucinations in DLB tend to present much earlier and are often associated with other psychiatric symptoms, such as delusions and depression. Understandably, they can be distressing for both the patients and their family. Typically they are vivid, rich in detail and color, and often involve animals or people. They are usually present for weeks or months at a time and occur on most days. Retrospective insight is often present.

Parkinsonian symptoms are a core but not an inevitable feature of DLB. Approximately half of subjects with DLB have parkinsonism at presentation, but around a quarter remain symptom-free throughout the course of their illness. Typically, bradykinesis and symmetrical body rigidity as opposed to tremor characterize the parkinsonian syndrome, though consensus is lacking. Not surprisingly, these symptoms can have a detrimental impact on self-confidence, functioning, quality of life, and caregiver burden.

Supportive Features

In addition to the core features, DLB can be accompanied by changes that have been classified as "supportive" features. These include increased sensitivity to antipsychotic (neuroleptic) medication (up to 50%), recurrent falls (30%), depression (up to 50%), auditory hallucinations (20%), secondary delusions (65%), and, less commonly syncope and transient loss of consciousness.

Differential Diagnosis

The differential diagnosis of DLB includes other subtypes of dementia, particularly AD and vascular dementia (VaD), co-morbid medical disorders that can cause visual hallucinations and/or delirium, certain neurological disorders, such as PD, and psychiatric disorders with psychotic features. Table 1 summarizes the key clinical features of AD, DLB, and VaD for comparison.

Accuracy of Clinical Diagnosis

Specialists diagnose DLB using consensus clinical criteria introduced in 1996 *(1)*. This sets two levels of diagnostic confidence, probable and possible, depending on the weight of clinical evidence. Two of three core symptoms, mentioned above, need to be present to make a diagnosis of probable DLB; if only one is present, a diagnosis of possible DLB is made. These criteria enable DLB to be diagnosed to the same level of accuracy (80–90% specificity) as AD, PD, and VaD. However, the criteria are less sensitive, and clinico-pathological studies indicate that DLB is more likely to be under- rather than overdiagnosed. In primary care, possible DLB should be suspected in a patient presenting with cognitive decline/dementia and any one of the three core features.

PATHOLOGY OF DLB

DLB shares a number of pathological changes with AD, including cortical beta-amyloid deposition and senile plaque formation, but there are also distinct important differences. In AD, intracellular neurofibrillary tangles (NFT) are found in abundance, and in conjunction with amyloid plaques they represent the pathological hallmarks of this condition. At the molecular level NFT result from errors in the metabolism of a protein called tau. In DLB, tangle formation is minimal and LBs are associated with dysregulation of another key protein called α-synuclein. This protein probably has a crucial role in the regulation of synaptic function *(4)*, and its dysregulation is relatively specific to DLB (and PD). To reflect these molecular differences, DLB has been classified as an α-synucleinopathy and AD as a tauopathy. It remains to be seen whether this classification has implications for further treatment interventions.

Like Alzheimer-type pathology in AD, LB are not randomly distributed in DLB. They appear to have predilection for certain areas of the brain, namely the neocortex, limbic cortex, subcortical nuclei, and brainstem. The precise pathological significance of LB-type pathology is not known. However, it is probable that a spectrum of LB disorders exist, with the clinical features reflecting the distribution and type of pathology *(5)*. In Parkinson's disease, LBs in the brainstem (e.g., substantia nigra) are prominent and associated with the prevalent motor symptoms. In DLB, LBs are more widely distributed. LBs in the limbic and neocortical regions are probably implicated in the cognitive and neuropsychiatric symptoms of DLB. In addition, LBs can occur in the spinal cord sympathetic neurons and dorsal vagal nuclei, leading to autonomic failure and dysphagia, respectively. Although "pure" presentations are documented, heterogenous combinations of parkinsonism, cognitive impairment, neuropsychiatric symptoms, and signs of autonomic failure reflecting multisite (diffuse) pathology are most frequent, especially in the elderly.

Table 1
Main Clinical Features of DLB, AD, and VaD[a]

	DLB	AD	VaD
Key features in clinical history	Fluctuations Visual hallucinations Parkinsonism Plus signs of autonomic instability, falls, depression, or other psychotic symptoms	Gradual onset of amnesia Later emergence of apraxia, agnosia, aphasia, agraphia, alexia, acalculia, and visuospatial impairment	Varied symptoms and progression (e.g., depending on location and severity of vascular disease Evidence of vascular risk factors
Key findings physical exam	Bradykinesia Rigidity Automatic instability	No specific finding until moderately to severely advanced	Focal neurological signs Evidence of vascular disease/risk factors for stroke disease
Key findings on mental state exam	Hallucinations +/– secondary delusions Cognitive impairment, especially visuospatial deficits Impaired attention	Impaired recall, language, and praxis Preserved personality in early stages	Patchy/variable cognitive impairment (e.g., reflecting location and extent of ischemia) Slow thinking and evidence of impaired executive functioning
Neuroimaging	CT/MRI: generalized ventricular enlargement and relative preservation of medial temporal lobe structures SPECT: parietal deficits similar to AD but more marked occipital deficits IDAT scan: reduced D2 receptor density and dopamine transporter	CT/MRI: generalized cerebral atrophy and ventricular enlargemnt and reduced medial temporal lobe width; similar white matter changes to DLB but less extensive than VaD SPECT: bilateral tempo-parietal hypoperfusion	CT/MRI: Significant white matter lesions and/or infarcts; generalized atrophy and ventricular enlargement SPECT: patchy deficits
Response to AChEI	+++	++	(?)+
Special comment	Sensitivity to neuroleptic medication	Most common form of dementia	Treat/modify vascular risk factors

[a]DLB, dementia with Lewy bodies; AD, Alzheimer's disease; VaD, vascular dementia; CT, computed tomography; MRI, magnetic resonance imaging; SPECT, single photon emission computed tomography; DaTscan, dopamine transporter scan; D2, dopamine receptor subtype 2; and AChEI, acetylcholinesterase inhibitors.

Neurochemical changes also feature prominently in the pathophysiology of DLB, particularly deficits in acetylcholinergic (ACh) and dopaminergic pathways. In comparison to AD, subjects with DLB have greater preservation of postsynaptic cholinergic mechanisms, but a more pronounced reduction in ACh neurotransmission *(6)*. These changes may explain why patients with DLB respond to drug treatments that enhance ACh neurotransmission. In addition, deficits in ACh are thought to contribute to cognitive impairment and fluctuations in attention. It has also been hypothesized that the underactivity in ACh function relative to monoaminergic function could generate visual hallucinations—especially when coupled with impaired arousal *(6)*.

Defects in the nigrostriatal dopamine pathway in DLB have also been observed using functional neuroimaging *(7,8)*. These neurons undergo degeneration in patients with PD and DLB but remain unaffected in AD. These techniques can be useful in the differential diagnosis of neurologic disease.

PRACTICAL GUIDE TO THE ASSESSMENT AND MANAGEMENT OF DLB

When diagnosing dementia, it is important to remember that this is a syndromal diagnosis analogous to chronic brain failure, which can be associated with altered cognition, behavior, personality, neurology, and functioning. It results from a myriad of pathologies. The clinician is tasked with the responsibility to determine, where possible and appropriate, the underlying disease(s) and plan interventions accordingly. Key steps in the assessment and management of DLB include the following.

Step 1. Initial medical detection and early diagnosis of the illness
Step 2. Providing information
Step 3. Establishing the key issues to target interventions and planning multidisciplinary assessment
Step 4. Introducing additional supports focusing on nonpharmacological, multiprofessional interventions
Step 5. Referring to a specialist for further advice on diagnosis and pharmacological therapies and involvement of specialist services

Step 1. Initial Detection and Benefits of Early Diagnosis

The diagnosis of DLB is, like that of nearly all cases of dementia, clinically based. There are no biological diagnostic markers, although certain investigations can be helpful in providing information that may make a diagnosis of DLB more or less likely. Ultimately, an accurate and timely diagnosis will rely on piecing together findings from the medical history, mental and physical examinations, and relevant investigations. The clinician should remain mindful of changes that can help confirm DLB but also factors that make a diagnosis of DLB less likely, such as stroke disease. Indeed, it is important to exclude any other physical illness or brain disorder sufficient to account for the clinical picture.

In terms of the medical history, vigilance to the varied presentations of DLB will also be necessary. This is particularly the case when an older person presents with cognitive decline colored by the core features of DLB, namely, unexplained fluctuations, recurring vivid visual hallucinations, or parkinsonism. Additional warning signs are unexplained falls and autonomic instability, low tolerance to neuroleptic medication, and recurrent unexplained episodes of delirium. In common with other subtypes of dementia, family members or caregivers will have a crucial role in helping to establish an accurate clinical history and in reality are likely to initiate the first contact with a family physician.

Initial physical and mental state examination should be completed. The physical examination should at least include the cardiovascular as well as neurological system. Inevitably, the examination will need to be tailored to the specific situation and differential diagnosis in question.

Mental state examination should gauge the presence and severity of any psychiatric and cognitive features (hallucinations, delusions, depression). A standardized screening tool such as the MMSE is a useful way to detect deficits (and areas of preserved functioning). The clock drawing test can quickly and usefully reveal signs of dyspraxia. Indeed, patients with DLB may be disproportionately impaired on this task compared with recall.

Initial routine examinations should include a standard dementia screen, e.g., full blood count, erythrocyte sedimentation rate (ESR), urea and electrolytes, liver function, thyroid function, vitamin B_{12}/folate, and cholesterol. Appropriate consideration should be given to further investigations as relevant, e.g., electrocardiogram (ECG), chest X-ray, and urine analysis.

The aim of any examination and investigation is at least twofold. First, it should help clarify the specific diagnosis and exclude other potential causes. Second, when DLB is present, it is important to detect any co-morbid factors that could influence treatment options (e.g., presence of cardiac arrhythmias, impaired renal or liver function), and/or exacerbate symptoms of the illness (such as anemia, infections, cardiac failure).

The benefits of early detection can be significant, although families and individuals vary in how they adjust to a diagnosis of dementia and the amount of information and external support they feel ready to accept or require. As a general rule, early diagnosis allows for early intervention and a more managed approach to planning for future change. This in turn should help to reduce caregiver burden and unforeseen crises. It also allows more time to be spent at home and less time in institutional care. Information can be imparted in a more sensitive way, and it creates greater scope to undertake any financial and legal planning. Importantly, early detection should reduce the risk of inadvertently using neuroleptic medication, with its associated hazards. Finally, it also unlocks opportunities for using cholinergic enhancers at an earlier stage of disease progression, with possible benefits on cognition, behavior, and functioning, as discussed below.

Step 2. Providing Information

Not surprisingly, patients and their families are often alarmed and anxious about the changes that are taking place. Explaining the diagnosis and providing information to individuals and their families is an important but potentially difficult area. For the clinician, the boundaries between AD, DLB, and PD can be difficult to describe, and there are underlying uncertainties about the precise osological status of DLB. There is also a general lack information about the condition in the public domain for caregivers, patients, and professionals to access. The Alzheimer Society in the UK (www.alzheimers.org.uk) and the U.S.-based Alzheimer Association (www.alz.org) have some useful information as well as links to other websites providing information about DLB.

Step 3. Establishing the Key Issues to Target Interventions and Planning Further Assessments

Invariably, given the chronic, changing, and often complex issues involved in the assessment and management of DLB, the clinician will need to work with other professionals and agencies hand-in-hand with the patient and his or her family. In order to plan and target interventions, key concerns need to be identified. Consideration needs to be given to a range of issues including level of functioning, safety, risks, mobility, as well as environmental, social, personal, and nutritional needs. Expectations and wishes of the patient and the family need to be clarified, as do the strains and strengths of the care network.

Input may be sought in the form of occupational therapy, environmental adaptations and mobility aids, social workers, home care, day care, respite care, financial and legal advice, physiotherapy, community psychiatric nurses, and other specialist nurses, such as a PD nurse.

Step 4. Initial Management: The Importance of Nonpharmacological Approaches

There has been no systematic appraisal of psychosocial interventions in DLB. Nevertheless, until safe and effective medications are developed, the provision of educational, practical, and emotional support for patients and caregivers will form the backbone of clinical management.

Interventions can be targeted for each of the three core symptoms; strategies for cognitive symptoms include orientation and memory prompts and attentional cues.

For psychiatric symptoms, options include explanation, education, reassurance, and targeted behavioral interventions. Anecdotally, visual hallucinations and reduced alertness may be exacerbated by an understimulating environment and improve in response to increased stimulation and novelty.

Motor impairments may benefit from physiotherapy, mobility aids, and the involvement of a PD nurse.

Step 5. Referral to a Specialist: Further Investigations and Pharmacological Management

Referral to a specialist is usually advisable and often necessary to complete further diagnostic assessments and management, particularly pharmacological treatments and involvement of specialist services. If necessary, the specialist is likely to request further structural and functional neuroimaging. The main neuroimaging changes in DLB are summarized in Table 1.

Table 2
Main Drug Treatments for Symptoms in DLB*[a]*

	Medication Options	Comments
Motor symptoms—parkinsonism	Levodopa (with either carbidopa or benserazide), dopamine agonists, and COMT inhibitors	Treatment is best achieved under specialist guidance. Risk of exacerbating psychosis. If necessary, low-dose levodopa is probably best first choice.
Depression	Selective serotonin reuptake inhibitors (SSRI: e.g., fluoxetine, citalopram, sertraline, paroxetine)	Depressive symptoms may resolve with support, advice, and monitoring. SSRI are likely to be safer and better tolerated than older tricyclics.
Rapid-eye-movement (REM) sleep behavior disorder (RBD)	Low-dose clonazepam (0.5–1 mg)	Disorder characterized by acting out of dreams during REM sleep
Psychosis	Cholinesterase inhibitors (ChEI); atypical neuroleptics used with *caution* and low starting doses, e.g., 0.25–0.5 mg risperidone; 2.5–5 mg olanzapine; and 12.5–25 mg quetiapine	Minimize exacerbating factors first. AChEI are safer and better tolerated than neuroleptics. Neuroleptics should only be used under specialist advice.
Cognitive impairment	Cholinesterase inhibitors (AChEI), e.g., rivastigmine, donepezil, and galantamine	AChEI have a broad therapeutic effect and can improve cognition, attention, psychosis, anxiety, and apathy.

*[a]*DLB, dementia with Lewy bodies; AChEI, acetylcholinesterase inhibitors; COMT, catechol-o-methyltransferase.

Currently, no disease-modifying therapies are available. Symptomatic treatment exists for neuropsychiatric (psychosis, depression, sleeping disturbance), cognitive, and motor symptoms. As summarized in Table 2, the treatment options are antipsychotics, antiparkinsonian medication, benzodiazepines, antidepressants, and cholinesterase inhibitors.

Managing Depression

Depressive symptoms are relatively common in DLB. In a proportion of patients they will resolve spontaneously, without the need for medication. Advice, support, and monitoring will be sufficient. If the symptoms persist and cause distress and impairment, then treatment with an antidepressant needs to be considered. There is insufficient published data to provide specific guidance, but extrapolating from general principles, selective serotonin reuptake inhibitors (SSRIs: e.g., fluoxetine, citalopram, sertraline, paroxetine) are preferable to tricyclic antidepressants (TCAs). Overall, they are safer and better tolerated, and they avoid the risk of anticholinergic side effects. The starting dose of SSRIs is close to the treatment and maintenance dose. Compliance is eased by once-a-day dosing, and as a rule they are a sensible first-line choice in the absence of more definitive evidence.

Managing Sleep Disturbance

Rapid-eye-movement (REM) sleep behavior disorder (RBD) is a recognized early feature of DLB. Due to a failure of normal muscle atonia, patients act out their dreams during REM sleep, and may kick, hit, or carry out actions such as swimming. Treatment with low-dose clonazepam (0.5–1 mg) can be effective. Occasionally, brief treatment with a hypnotic, such as a short-acting benzodiazepine or chlormethiazole, is necessary to help reestablish a sleep pattern.

Managing Motor Symptoms

The treatment of parkinsonism can be complex and fraught with difficulties. Specialist advice should be sought. The clinician is often walking a therapeutic tightrope between improving parkinsonism and worsening psychosis. Options include levodopa (with either carbidopa or benserazide), dopamine agonists, and COMT (catechol-O-methyltransferase) inhibitors. Again, definitive evidence and consensus is lacking regarding which drug or combination to use, and the likely responsiveness to dopaminergic treatments, with reported response rates varying from 40% to 100%.

The clinician must ascertain which symptoms are most troublesome for the sufferer and explain the risks and benefits associated with changes in medication. The patient and his or her caregiver may only be able to decide the best compromise after a trial treatment. If indicated, then treatment with levodopa monotherapy is a reasonable starting point, using the lowest effective dose. Dopamine agonists may be more prone to induce hallucinations and sedation.

Treating Psychosis

To treat psychosis, there are two main options: neuroleptics and acetylcholinesterase inhibitors (AChEI). The use of neuroleptics in DLB can be hazardous. They should be used cautiously and only when careful supervision and monitoring can be guaranteed—usually under specialist advice. Treatment can exacerbate parkinsonian symptoms, as well as precipitate a life-threatening reaction called neuroleptic sensitivity (2). This reaction is recognized by the onset of sedation, immobility, rigidity, postural instability, falls, and increased confusion. Its outcome is poor, with a two- to threefold increased mortality.

In the absence of published clinical trials of antipsychotics for DLB, specific guidance is limited. Overall, however, it is likely that newer atypical antipsychotics are safer than traditional agents, although neuroleptic sensitivity reactions may still occur. Slow titration—start low, go slow—is probably more significant than the use of any specific drug, as side effects are likely to emerge at higher doses even with atypical neuroleptics (9). Examples of starting dosages are 0.25–0.5 mg risperidone, 2.5–5 mg olanzapine, or 12.5–25 mg quetiapine.

Whenever possible, before using antipsychotic medication, factors that may exacerbate psychosis should be addressed. If indicated clinically, dose reduction or even withdrawal of antiparkinsonian drugs should be carefully thought about, at least on a trial basis. Empirically, drugs for PD can be reduced/withdrawn in order of anticholinergics, amantadine, l-deprenyl (selegeline), dopamine agonists, and levodopa preparations.

AChEI have been shown in open-label studies and one randomized placebo-controlled trial to be well tolerated and effective in treating cognitive and psychiatric symptoms in DLB. Indeed, subjects with DLB have a similar if not greater therapeutic response to AChEI than those with AD (10–15).

Interestingly, symptoms that respond best to treatment with AChEI are apathy, anxiety, delusions, hallucinations, and attention. Dose titration and adverse effects are similar to those experienced with AD. Parkinsonian symptoms tend not to worsen on treatment, although emergent tremor has been noted in a small number of patients.

Although further studies are needed, drugs enhancing central cholinergic function, such as rivastigmine, donepezil, and galantamine, therefore appear to offer a new treatment strategy in DLB. AChEI have broader therapeutic benefits than antipsychotics and are better tolerated. They can be effective in treating cognitive impairment and attention as well as hallucinations, delusions, and apathy, and may become first-line therapy.

SUMMARY

DLB is the second most common form of degenerative dementia and is characterized by fluctuating cognitive impairment, spontaneous parkinsonism, and recurrent visual hallucinations. Pathologically, further research is required, but it is probable that a spectrum of Lewy body disorders exists, with the clinical features reflecting the distribution and severity of pathology. In practice, DLB is underdiagnosed but clinically important, as the management of the cognitive, neuropsychiatric, and motor symptoms can be complex and at time hazardous. Specialist referral is often necessary, but a broad-based, multiprofessional approach to management is essential throughout the course of the illness. Optimistically, acetylcholinesterase inhibitors have recently been shown to be well tolerated and effective in treating cognitive and psychiatric symptoms in DLB. They may become first-line therapies.

REFERENCES

1. McKeith, I.G. et al.: Consensus guidelines for the clinical and pathologic diagnosis of dementia with Lewy bodies (DLB): report of the Consortium on DLB International Workshop. Neurology 1996; 47: 1113–1124.
2. McKeith, I.G. et al.: Neuroleptic sensitivity in patients with senile dementia of Lewy body type. Br Med J 1992; 305: 673–678.
3. Armstrong, T.P. et al.: Rapidly progressive dementia in a patient with the Lewy body variant of Alzheimer's disease. Neurology 1991; 41: 1178–1180.
4. Spillantini, M.G. et al.: Alpha-synuclein in Lewy bodies. Nature 1997; 388: 839–848.
5. Lowe, J.S. et al.: Pathological significance of Lewy bodies in dementia. In: Perry, R.; McKeith, I.G.; Perry, E. (eds.): Dementia with Lewy bodies: clinical, pathological, and treatment issues. Cambridge University Press, New York, 1996: 195–203.
6. Perry, E.K.; Perry, R.H.: Altered consciousness and transmitter signalling in Lewy body dementia. In: Perry, R.; McKeith, I.G.; Perry, E. (eds.): Dementia with Lewy bodies: clinical, pathological, and treatment issues. Cambridge University Press, New York, 1996: 397–413.
7. Donnemiller, E. et al.: Brain perfusion scintigraphy with 99mTc-HMPAO or 99mTc-ECD and 123I-beta-CIT single-photon emission tomography in dementia of the Alzheimer-type and diffuse Lewy body disease. Eur J Nuclear Med 1997; 24: 320–325.
8. Walker, Z. et al.: Dementia with Lewy bodies: a study of post-synaptic dopaminergic receptors with iodine-123 iodobenzamide single-photon emission tomography. Eur J Nuclear Med 1997; 24: 609–614.
9. McKeith, I.G. et al.: Neuroleptic sensitivity to risperidone in Lewy body dementia. Lancet 1995; 346: 699.
10. Levy, R. et al.: Lewy bodies and response to tacrine in Alzheimer's disease. Lancet 1994; 343: 176.
11. Wilcock, G.K.; Scott, M.I.: Tacrine for senile dementia of Alzheimer's or Lewy body type. Lancet 1994; 344: 544.
12. Liberini, P. et al.: Lewy-body dementia and responsiveness to cholinesterase inhibitors: a paradigm for heterogeneity of Alzheimer's disease? Trends Pharmacol Sci 1996; 17: 155–160.
13. Shea, C. et al.: Donepezil for treatment of dementia with Lewy bodies: a case series of nine patients. Int Psychogeriatr 1998; 10: 229–239.
14. McKeith, I. et al.: Efficacy of rivastigmine in dementia with Lewy bodies: a randomized, double-blind, placebo-controlled international study. Lancet 2000; 356: 2031–2036.
15. Samuel, W. et al.: Better cognitive and psychopathologic response to donepezil in patients prospectively diagnosed as dementia with Lewy bodies: a preliminary study. Int J Geriatr Psychiatry 2000; 15: 794–802.

14

Frontotemporal Lobe Dementia

Malgorzata Franczak, Diana Kerwin, and Piero Antuono

INTRODUCTION

Frontotemporal lobe degeneration (FTLD) is the term currently used for what was formerly called Pick's disease—a condition in which behavioral symptoms (of the frontal and/or temporal lobe syndrome) precede memory loss *(1)*. Since Pick's bodies are found in only 25% of patients with frontotemporal dementia, the diagnosis of Pick's disease should be reserved for pathologically confirmed cases. From a clinical perspective these cases should be referred to as frontotemporal lobe degeneration (FTLD) or frontotemporal dementia (FTD). The diagnosis of FTLD is based mainly on the clinical presentation and can be confirmed by postmortem examination *(1,2)*. The clinical diagnosis can be supported by the performance of structural as well as functional brain imaging.

The prevalence of FTLD varies among studies. In a large series, 8–10% of all patients with presenile dementia showed this syndrome *(3)*; other series suggest that 15–20% of all cases of degenerative dementia represent FTLD *(4,5)*. FTLD occurs in people between 35 and 75 years of age, and affects both sexes equally. The disease has an insidious onset, and its progression is slow. In the early stage, behavioral, personality, and language changes occur, whereas the memory may be preserved. Death usually occurs within 2 to 15 years of onset.

Four clinical types of dementia can be identified as a result of changes in the frontal lobes:

1. Frontotemporal lobe dementia (FTD)
2. Primary progressive aphasia (PPA)
3. Semantic dementia (SD) *(6)*
4. Corticobasal ganglionic degeneration (CBGD)

CBGD has also been defined as a frontal lobe dementia with pathological changes in the frontal as well as parietal lobes.

FRONTOTEMPORAL DEMENTIA

Twenty to forty percent of FTD cases are familial, with autosomal dominant inheritance, whereas the majority of cases occur sporadically. The most characteristic and distinguishing clinical feature of FTD is an early change in personality and behavior, which can vary from apathy and indifference to inappropriate social behavior, and disinhibition, with relative preservation of memory. Emotional blunting, anhedonia, and loss of insight occur early in the disease. The patients frequently become self-centered and often are described by family members as being cold, lacking motivation, or uninterested.

Other symptoms of FTD, such as hyperorality, jocularity, hypersexuality, perseveration, or utilization behavior, are often grouped under the term "Kluever-Bucy syndrome," as the pathology is thought to be related to dysfunction of the amygdala and hippocampus. Hyperorality frequently is man-

From: *Current Clinical Neurology,*
Alzheimer's Disease: A Physician's Guide to Practical Management
Edited by: R. W. Richter and B. Zoeller Richter © Humana Press Inc., Totowa, NJ

ifested by overeating of certain foods, often leading to weight gain. Changes in oral/dietary behavior, such as excessive drinking, smoking, or overeating, were observed in about 30% of FTD cases. Utilization behavior refers to the patient as grasping and repeatedly using objects lying in his or her visual field (for instance, if given a pair of glasses, the patient may repeatedly put them on and take them off). Dyscalculia (impairment of arithmetic skills) is often present as an early symptom. Other changes consistent with FTD are a decline in personal hygiene and grooming, perseverative and stereotyped behavior (hand clapping or rubbing, dancing), as well as mental rigidity and inflexibility. Because of these unpredictable behavioral features, a patient may be rejected by his or her family or community, and may even run into trouble with the law.

Despite many (for his environment) obvious changes, the patient shows little insight into his deficit. Emotional and affective changes are common in the early stages of FTD, but cognitive decline becomes evident later as the disease progresses. Emotional changes, such as elated mood, may be mistaken for manic episodes. Some patients may demonstrate obsessive/compulsive traits, such as preoccupation with certain activities, or obsession about their daily routines. Distractibility and impersistence are other features commonly seen in FTD patients. Primitive reflexes (such as the palmomental, snout, or glabellar) can be present early in the disease. Urinary incontinence may also be present as a sign of frontal lobe disinhibition. Early onset of these abnormal behaviors, while short-term memory may still be preserved, distinguishes this type of dementia from that seen in Alzheimer's disease (AD).

Structural imaging techniques, such as magnetic resonance imaging (MRI) or computed tomography (CT), may show atrophy of the frontal and anterior temporal lobes. Functional brain imaging, such as positron emission tomography (PET), or single photon emission computed tomography (SPECT), typically demonstrates decreased perfusion of the frontal and temporal lobes (Fig. 1). These changes differ from those seen in AD, in which decreased perfusion and atrophy occur typically in the temporoparietal areas in the early disease stages.

Neuropsychological testing may demonstrate typical changes indicating frontal lobe dysfunction. Also, patients may have difficulty with abstract thinking, generating words, as well as defects in executive function. They may also demonstrate a poor performance on tests of mental flexibility. Visuospatial skills are usually preserved for a longer period. These patients are often able to copy geometric figures long after their language and behavior are impaired, which is in contrast to AD patients, who typically demonstrate early impairment of spatial and verbal memory.

Neuropsychological testing early in the disease may help differentiate FTD from nonorganic mental illness and AD.

PRIMARY PROGRESSIVE APHASIA

Primary progressive aphasia (PPA) was first described by Mesulam in six patients with language disturbance and focal atrophy involving the left perisylvian region *(7)*. Clinically, the patient presents with a slowly progressive difficulty in expressive language as well as a presenile age of onset.

Core features of PPA are nonfluent spontaneous speech, with at least one of the following impairments:

> Difficulty with naming objects (anomia)
> Sound-based errors, e.g., "gat" for "rat" (phonemic paraphasia)
> Agrammatism (incorrect use of common grammatical terms)

The first complaint by the patient is the difficulty in finding words (not memory loss). Initially a patient with PPA looks more like someone who has had a stroke, rather than a demented person. PPA patients initially may have preserved memory. AD patients, in contrast, in addition to anomia, show impairment of memory, visuospatial skills, and in other cognitive domains. PPA patients sometimes progress to nonfluent aphasia and subsequently to mutism. Despite the patients being mute, their visuospatial skills and memory may still be relatively preserved and they may function well in the com-

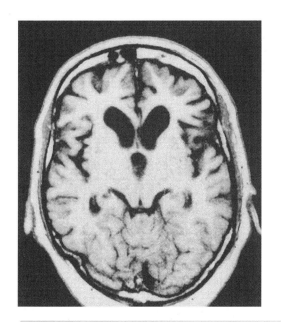
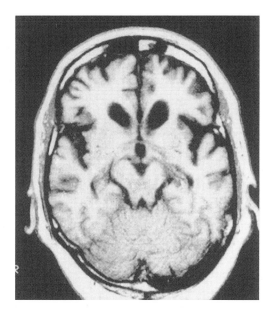
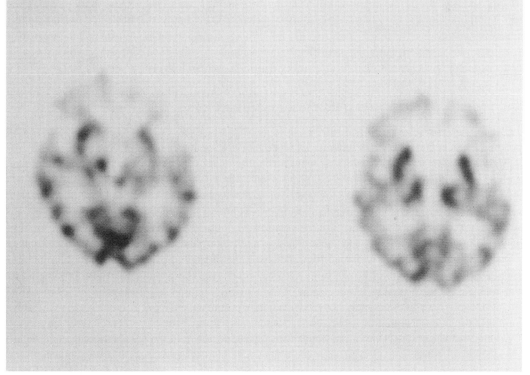

Fig. 1. Frontotemporal lobe degeneration (FTLD). *(Top)* MRI scan of the case of FTLD showing predominantly frontal gyral atrophy and widening of the sulci. *(Bottom)* SPECT scan of the same patient showing the typical pattern of cortical hypometabolism involving frontal lobes.

munity. Although mute, they may maintain some of their activities of daily living intact. Difficulty with reading and writing is frequently observed.

PPA patients may also develop ideomotor apraxia and thus signal "no" when they mean "yes," creating difficulties in interpreting test results. The understanding of the meaning of words is usually well preserved, but their expression is impaired. Behavioral changes involving frontal lobes may occur later in the disease. Some patients with PPA may develop a variant, associated with motor neuron disease like amyotrophic lateral sclerosis (ALS), usually with bulbar symptoms.

Neuroimaging studies, such as CT or MRI, reveal left perisylvian atrophy. SPECT demonstrates hypometabolism involving frontal and/or temporal lobes (Fig. 2).

SEMANTIC DEMENTIA

Semantic dementia (SD) was first described by Snowden et al. *(8,9)*. SD patients often present with difficulty in naming and comprehension. Core features include fluent aphasia, characterized by effortless, spontaneous speech, but with empty content and inability to convey information pertinent to the conversation. The ability to read aloud and to write is preserved. Associative agnosia (loss of the ability to recognize previously known objects or their function) may also be present. These patients may be classified as having transcortical sensory aphasia, since they retain fluency and repetition but lose comprehension. Articulation, syntax, and phonology (intonation) remain intact. In contrast to AD patients, those with SD show preservation of episodic memory and visuospatial skills. SD patients often become nonfluent later in the disease. Behavioral problems may also be seen at a later stage.

Neuropsychological testing reveals impairment of language function, manifested as an impairment of word comprehension, naming, identification of famous faces, or impairment of object identity. Performance on visuospatial skills and memory testing may be relatively preserved.

CORTICOBASAL GANGLIONIC DEGENERATION

CBGD was first described by Rebeiz et al. in 1968 *(10)*. Often, the presenting symptom is limb apraxia, or rigidity involving the upper and, less commonly, the lower limbs. Upper limb apraxia may manifest itself as clumsiness or difficulty with fine finger movements. If the lower extremities are involved, the patient may have problems picking up or dragging the feet, or tripping. Sometimes, a patient may not be able to initiate walking. As the disease progresses, the limb becomes flexed, clenched, and a dystonic postures may develop. True weakness is not an initial feature, but as the limb eventually becomes useless (secondary to rigidity, or apraxia), motor weakness may appear. Other parkinsonian features, such as bradykinesia, gait disorder, and tremor, may also be present at an early stage.

Ocular symptoms may be seen early in the disease, manifested as difficulty with initiating voluntary saccades to commands, although spontaneous saccades may be present. Saccadic hypometria for both horizontal and vertical gaze may occur. Early vertical supranuclear gaze palsy raises the suspicion of progressive supranuclear palsy (PSP), another progressive degenerative disease with prominent frontal lobe involvement.

Another feature of CBGD is "alien limb" phenomena, a slow, semipurposeful movement typically seen in the hand. It was first described clinically as involvement of the corpus callosum, and later found in patients with medial frontal cortex lesions. In a minority of patients, stimulus-sensitive myoclonus may appear early in the disease, raising the suspicion of CBGD. Dysarthria, dysphagia, pseudobulbar palsy with emotional lability, as well as sensory symptoms are usually not present in the early disease stages, but may occur as the disease progresses. Other frontal lobe motor abnormalities, such as primitive frontal release signs (grasp, or snout), reflex may also appear at later stages. Cognitive changes often do not occur early in the disease.

The disease usually affects people after age 50, and affects both sexes equally. There is no clear genetic linkage, although advances in the molecular genetics of non-Alzheimer dementias will ulti-

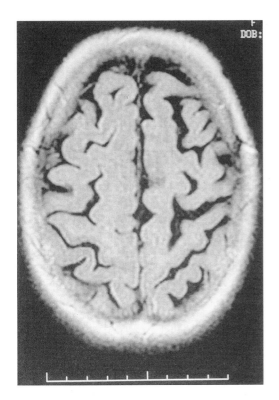 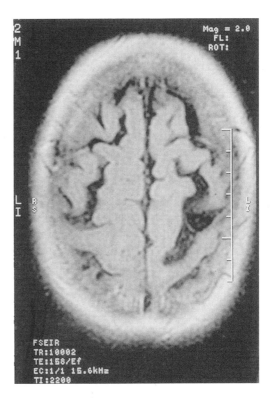

Fig. 2. Progressive aphasia. Axial MRI images of a woman with primary progressive aphasia representing asymmetric widening of the superior frontal and pre-central sulci on the left.

mately offer a better basis for classifying these disorders. Death usually occurs within 5–10 years after onset, due to generalized immobility.

DIFFERENTIAL DIAGNOSIS

Currently, FTLD and CBGD can only be diagnosed with certainty through neuropathological examination. The clinical diagnosis is now based on clinical and neuropsychological criteria, and supported by neuroimaging. There are, however, many other causes of behavioral, language, and cognitive changes. The primary differential diagnosis is AD. Patients with FTLD initially present with behavioral or language problems, unlike AD patients, who initially present with memory deficits; behavioral symptoms are unusual at this stage. Patients with FTLD usually present with presenile dementia, unlike AD patients, in whom disease prevalence increases with age. In FTLD, visuospatial skills are well preserved, whereas in AD these skills are impaired early in the disease. Language dysfunction can be present early in FTD and PPA. In AD patients, language problems may not occur until later in the disease.

Lewy body dementia (LBD) may be very difficult to differentiate from FTLD. Parkinsonian features such as gait disturbance and rigidity have been seen in patients with FTD as well as in patients with LBD. Behavioral abnormalities are usually seen early in FTD but can also be seen in some cases of LBD. Behavioral changes in LBD may fluctuate considerably in early stages.

CBGD should be differentiated from Parkinson's disease (PD). The early onset of apraxia, alien hand phenomena, myoclonus, and lack of response to levodopa therapy is suggestive of CBGD. The diagnosis of progressive supranuclear palsy (PSP) may be very difficult, and in some cases may only be confirmed pathologically. Both diseases may present in similar ways. If myoclonus occurs, CBGD should be more highly suspected.

Other conditions that can cause behavioral and cognitive changes, such as frontal white matter infarctions and Huntington's disease, also need to be differentiated.

NEUROPATHOLOGY

In frontotemporal dementia (FTD), there is prominent bilateral and symmetrical atrophy involving the frontal lobes. In primary progressive aphasia (PPA), the atrophy is often asymmetric, and involves the left frontal lobe to a greater extent. In semantic dementia (SD), atrophy is often bilateral and mostly involves the anterior temporal neocortex. These localized atrophies can be identified on MRI. Functional imaging techniques (SPECT, PET) may help identify these changes at earlier stages. Histopathological changes in FTD can vary.

Pathognomonic Pick bodies are found in about 25% of patients with FTD. Pick bodies are not seen in normal aging but may occasionally be seen in other conditions, such as Binswanger's disease, glioma, encephalitis, or lead poisoning. Immunohistochemical testing for ubiquitin is also very important, as some of the characteristic lesions in FTLD are negative for tau protein yet positive for ubiquitin. Pick cells are enlarged ballooned neurons with displaced nuclei and silver-staining cytoplasm. Electron microscopy reveals cytoplasm filled with neurofilaments and neurotubules similar to those found in Pick bodies. In the remaining 75% of FTD, nonspecific changes, such as gliosis, neuronal loss, and superficial linear spongiosis, are found.

Cases lacking these features have also been described, and are often called "dementia lacking distinctive pathology" (DLDH). Some of the cases previously called DLDH have tau-negative, ubiquitin-positive inclusions.

Pathologically, CBGD is characterized by asymmetric cortical atrophy involving the frontal and parietal cortex. The substantia nigra may become depigmented. Neuronal loss and gliosis with basophilic inclusions predominantly involves the substantia nigra and pallidum, but other subcortical structures such as the putamen, subthalamic nucleus, dentate nucleus, or brainstem nuclei may be involved. Ballooned neurons are a characteristic feature of CBGD and are present in the cortical regions as well as in the brainstem and subcortical areas.

GENETIC BACKGROUND

A positive family history of dementia is present in 20–40% of FTD cases (3–5). Of those, a mutation in tau protein on chromosome 17 constitutes about 10–14% of all familial FTLD cases (11,12). Patients with this mutation are known as chromosome 17-linked frontotemporal dementia with parkinsonism (FTDP-17). Another locus has been found on chromosome 9. These are cases of familial FTLD with motor neuron disease (MND). Recently an additional locus was found on chromosome 3 (13). The disease may also be inherited through an autosomal dominant trait with high penetrance.

The clinical spectrum of chromosome 3-linked dementia is similar to typical frontal dementia. In these patients the dementia usually starts with subtle personality and behavioral changes. Dyscalculia and hyperorality are frequently present, suggesting involvement not only of the frontal lobes but also of the parietal and temporal lobes. Some patients may present with parkinsonian features. On postmortem analysis, global atrophy, with predominance of frontal lobe involvement, may be seen. Microscopic examination may also reveal gliosis and neuronal loss. FTD-3 is known as dementia lacking distinctive histology (DLDH).

TREATMENT

There is no therapy available to prevent or slow the progression of FTLD, and treatment is symptomatic. Patients with FTLD have marked decrease in serotonin (14). Selective serotonin reuptake inhibitors (SSRI) have been administered to patients with FTLD with resultant improvement in some of the behavioral symptoms. Acetylcholinesterase inhibitors (AChEI) have not shown significant benefit. Trazadone has been used for treatment of agitation and compulsive behavior with some benefit.

Antipsychotics may be indicated for aggressive and sexually disinhibited behavior. Because these medications can cause extrapyramidal symptoms, the drug selected must be monitored very carefully. Estrogen therapy has been advocated to reduce hypersexual behavior.

The evaluation by a speech pathologist is very important, not only for the diagnosis of PPA, but for counseling and teaching the patients alternative speech strategies. Emotional support for caregivers and other family members is also needed. Support groups are an excellent resource for family members, but the typical Alzheimer support group may not fully address the particular needs of FTLD caregivers. Advances in understanding the underlying pathology and genetics of FTLD will allow for better counseling of patients and their families.

Treatment for CBGD is symptomatic and often ineffective. Levodopa and dopamine agonists may have little effect. Clonazepam may be useful for treating the symptoms of associated myoclonus.

SUMMARY

Frontotemporal lobe degeneration (FTLD) represents a heterogenous group of progressive neurodegenerative disorders involving frontal and temporal lobe dysfunction. The disease accounts for 10–20% of all dementia cases. The disease has an insidious onset and slow progression. Unlike AD, the presenting symptoms include personality changes with disinhibition or apathy, as well as language dysfunction. Memory loss becomes apparent as the disease progresses. The different clinical types of FTLD can be identified as a result of change in the frontal and temporal lobes: frontotemporal lobe dementia (FTD), primary progressive aphasia (PPA), and semantic dementia (SD). Corticobasal ganglionic degeneration (CBGD) has also been included in this group, because of the clinical and pathological relationship to the frontal lobes. The diagnosis is based on clinical presentation and can be supported by structural and functional brain imaging consistent with atrophy of the frontal and temporal lobes or decreased perfusion of the frontal and temporal lobes. The pathological profile of FTLD can vary greatly. The most common findings are neuronal loss, superficial linear spongiosis, and gliosis. In a minority of cases, Pick cells are found in affected cortical areas. Treatment of FTLD is predominantly symptomatic, addressing the behavioral problems.

REFERENCES

1. The Lund and Manchester Groups: Clinical and neuropathological criteria for frontotemporal dementia. J Neurol Neurosurg Psychiatry 1994; 57: 416–418.
2. McKhann, G.M. et al.: Clinical and pathological diagnosis of frontotemporal dementia. Arch Neurol 2001; 58: 1803–1809.
3. Gustafson, L.; Brun, A.; Passant, U.: Frontal lobe degeneration of non-Alzheimer Type. In: Rossor, M.N. (ed.): Unusual dementias. Balliere Tindall, London, 1992: 559–582.
4. Knopman, D.S. et al.: Dementia lacking distinctive histologic features: a common non-Alzheimer degenerative dementia. Neurology 1990; 40: 251–256.
5. Neary, D.: Non Alzheimer's disease forms of cerebral atrophy. J Neurol Neurosurg Psychiatry 1990; 53: 929–931.
6. Neary, D. et al.: Frontotemporal lobar degeneration. A consensus on clinical diagnostic criteria. Neurology 1998; 51: 1546–1554.
7. Mesulam, M.-M.: Slowly progressive aphasia without generalized dementia. Ann Neurol 1982; 11: 592–598.
8. Snowden, J.S.; Goulding, P.J.; Neary, D.: Semantic dementia; a form of circumscribed cerebral atrophy. Behav Neurol 1989; 2: 167–182.
9. Snowden, J.S.; Neary, D.; Mann, D.M.A.: Fronto-temporal lobar degeneration: fronto-temporal dementia, progressive aphasia, semantic dementia. Churchill Livingstone, London, 1996.
10. Rebeiz, J.J.; Kolodny, E.H.; Richardson, E.P. Jr: Corticodentatonigral degeneration with neuronal achromasia. Arch Neurol 1968; 18: 20–33.
11. Houlden, H. et al. Frequency of tau mutations in three series of non-Alzheimer degenerative dementias. Ann Neurol 1999; 46: 243–248.
12. Poorkaj, P. et al.: Frequency of tau gene mutations in familial and sporadic cases of non-Alzheimer dementia. Arch Neurol 2001; 58: 383–387.
13. Gydesen, S. et al.: Chromosome 3 linked frontotemporal dementia (FTD-3). Neurology 2002; 59: 1585–1594.
14. Swartz, J.R. et al.: Frontotemporal dementia: treatment response to serotonin reuptake inhibitors. J Clin Psychiatry 1997; 58: 212–216.

IV The Transitional Stage

15

Mild Forgetfulness
Distinguishing Early AD from Normal Aging

Scott A. Small

INTRODUCTION

Localizing a lesion is a time-honored tenet in clinical neuroscience. Pinpointing the brain region most affected by a disease process aids in diagnosing and, ultimately, treating neurological disorders. Historically, this localizing process has relied on visualizing structural changes in the brain, either under the microscope or more recently with imaging techniques. The last decade of careful investigation has established that aging has no clear histological marker *(1)*. The absence of neuronal damage in the face of obvious behavioral deficits suggests that age-related memory decline is caused by biochemical changes in intact cells, changes that alter normal physiological functions, which somehow interfere with mechanisms of brain plasticity. Indeed, animal studies have shown that age-related memory decline is associated with changes in the electrophysiological properties of structurally intact hippocampal neurons *(2)*. Even early neurodegenerative processes, such as AD, appear to cause electrophysiological changes before histological lesions, as demonstrated in transgenic mouse models *(3)*. Thus, aging is by and large invisible to the microscope, and isolating the neurons most affected by aging cannot rely on histological analysis of postmortem tissue. Rather, "functional techniques"—techniques whose measures reflect the physiology of living tissue—are nowadays required to explore the aging brain.

In our own experiments we used a newly developed, high-resolution magnetic resonance imaging (MRI) approach, designed to detect functional changes in various hippocampal subregions. With this approach we have tried to distinguish changes that occur in hippocampal function as a result of normal aging, from changes that reflect the earliest stages of Alzheimer's disease (AD).

THE GROSS ANATOMY OF THE AGING BRAIN

Isolating neuronal populations requires a stepwise analysis, moving from techniques with lower to higher magnifications. For this reason the search should begin with neuropsychological testing. The first question that can be addressed by neuropsychological analysis is whether aging affects cognition diffusely, or whether aging targets a select cognitive domain.

One reason this question remained open throughout decades of investigation was because—if not adequately addressed—neuropsychological test results suffer from two confounding effects. The cohort effect is the more common confound, and this effect beleaguers cross-sectional studies. For example, although a group of 80-year-olds may be found to have lower test scores than a group of 20-year-olds, the possibility always exists that the older cohort never scored better even when they were younger. The plausibility of this interpretation rests on clear evidence that younger generations increas-

From: *Current Clinical Neurology,*
Alzheimer's Disease: A Physician's Guide to Practical Management
Edited by: R. W. Richter and B. Zoeller Richter © Humana Press Inc., Totowa, NJ

ingly perform better on standardized tests because of their exposure to school curricula modified for this very purpose.

Although studies with a longitudinal design address the cohort effect, they in turn suffer from the "learning" effect—administering cognitive tests to the same cohort repeatedly over time will artificially boost test scores, thereby masking an underlying cognitive decline. A few recent studies, including our own work *(4)*, have attempted to address these confounds by designing studies with a mixed cross-sectional/longitudinal design, where an old and a younger cohort are recruited. Both cohorts are followed in parallel over time.

> **Memory is the cognitive domain most sensitive to aging.** Using this approach we have found that memory is the cognitive domain most sensitive to the effects of aging. Other cognitive domains, in contrast, such as language ability or abstract reasoning, are relatively insensitive to the passage of time.
>
> **Memory decline localizes to the hippocampal formation.** Furthermore, within the memory domain we found that aging affects the acquisition of declarative memories more than memory retrieval *(4)*. Since the ability to acquire new declarative memories requires an intact hippocampal formation, our results suggest that age-related memory decline resides somewhere within the hippocampus.

THE MICROANATOMY OF THE AGING BRAIN

The hippocampal formation is made up of anatomically separate subregions: the entorhinal cortex, the dentate gyrus, the CA (cornu ammonis) subfields, and the subiculum. Recent gene expression studies have confirmed what early neuroanatomists suspected: that each hippocampal subregion is comprised of distinct neuronal populations, each with its own molecular profile *(5)*. Unique molecular profiling accounts for why the separate subregions of the hippocampus are differentially sensitive to mechanisms of dysfunction *(6)*.

For example, the high expression of NMDA (N-methyl-D-aspartate) receptors in CA1 neurons can account for why this subregion is most sensitive to hypoperfusion. The high expression of steroid receptors can account for why CA3 neurons are most sensitive to corticosteroid elevation. The high expression of aldosterone receptors can account for why the dentate gyrus neurons are most sensitive to a decline in adrenal hormones.

Properties of the Hippocampal Formation

Although causes of memory dysfunction typically target select subregions, the one most affected by aging has until recently remained unknown. One reason for this persistent state of ignorance is that hippocampal subregions are interconnected, so that the hippocampus functions as a circuit. Dysfunction in any hippocampal subregion will equivalently interrupt the hippocampal circuit and produce overlapping memory deficits. Neuropsychological tests, therefore, are designed to assess global hippocampal function. In their current form, however, these tests are ill-equipped to isolate the ultimate circuit-breaking subregion.

High Resolution Techniques Are Required to Visualize Hippocampal Subregions

What is required, therefore, is a technique that can assess the functional integrity of the hippocampal subregions—independently and simultaneously. Since MRI is the imaging technique with the highest spatial resolution, we first explored conventional functional magnetic resonance imaging (fMRI). fMRI can map acute changes in metabolism elicited by a behavioral task. In order to reliably visualize the hippocampal subregions, however, a technique needs to possess submillimeter or microscopic resolution, which cannot be achieved by conventional fMRI.

Mapping Chronic Brain Metabolism With MRI

In our attempt to isolate dysfunctional subregions, we have moved away from mapping acute metabolic changes and instead have focused on mapping the chronic changes in brain metabolism caused by disease or aging. There are a number of reasons for this departure. First, measures of acute metabolism reflect a region's bioelectrical state, while measures of chronic metabolism are more sensitive to the cell's biochemistry. Aging, like most causes of brain dysfunction, appears to alter neuronal plasticity by targeting the biochemistry of neuronal function—for example, signal transduction, covalent modification of existing proteins, and *de novo* protein synthesis—and so measures of chronic metabolism are simply a more direct measure of brain dysfunction. Second, by relying on measures of chronic metabolism, we can acquire images with much higher spatial resolution, easily achieving the microscopic levels required to visualize hippocampal subregions. Third, a growing number of studies are showing that fMRI measures of acute metabolism are dependent on the brain's chronic "resting" state. Since the chronic state varies with age and disease, uncalibrated maps of acute metabolism are difficult to interpret.

IS MEMORY DECLINE NORMAL?

In a recent study *(7)* we have used an MRI approach designed to map the chronic state of the hippocampus in order to address the simplest but most intractable question asked by older individuals: Is memory decline normal? Prior findings allowed us to postulate that the hippocampal formation is susceptible both to the affects of normal aging as well as by the earliest stages of AD pathology. Each process would target separate hippocampal subregions. Although we had shown previously that our MRI approach detects dysfunction in isolated hippocampal subregions *(8)*, the problem was how to establish which subregion reflected early AD and which normal aging.

We imaged healthy individuals across the life span—from 20 to 88 years of age—and applied formal parametric criteria of normal aging in assessing patterns of decline in each subregion. A key assumption underlying these criteria is that if an age-related change in bodily function occurs normally, the change should occur stochastically within a given population of older individuals. In contrast, if the change in bodily function reflects a disease process, it should systematically target a subpopulation of elders. These different patterns of decline—normal vs pathological—should be reflected in the parametric distribution of functional measures. Although, specifically, the average of the distribution of function in a young and in an old group of subjects is expected to be different, the distribution variance should be the same in the case of normal aging. The variance, however, should be significantly larger in the older group in the case of pathological aging.

Anatomical Patterns of Hippocampal Dysfunction Distinguishes Early AD from Normal Aging

Using these parametric criteria, we found that age-related decline in the entorhinal cortex and the CA subfields reflects a pathological process, which we assume represents the earliest phases of AD. In contrast, we found that age-related decline in the dentate gyrus and to a lesser extent in the subiculum represents normal aging *(7)*.

CLINICAL IMPLICATIONS

With these results we can begin to formulate answers to basic diagnostic questions. First, these results show that age-related hippocampal dysfunction can occur as part of the normal trajectory of the aging process, but may also be the first symptom of disease. Second, and more important, these results suggest that we can rely on the microanatomy of the hippocampus to disambiguate two fundamentally distinct causes of memory decline—early AD and normal aging.

Of course, this dichotomy does not fully capture the heterogeneity of age-related memory decline. Age-related hippocampal dysfunction has multiple potential causes. The ultimate goal, therefore, is to investigate a large group of older individuals and to segregate them into four or five subgroups, based on the hippocampal subregion with the greatest dysfunction.

Beyond diagnostics, segregating patients with memory decline into separate anatomical subgroups will allow us to pursue the ultimate goal—the treatment of memory decline. If future studies establish, for example, that patients with CA1 dysfunction are more likely to have cardiovascular disease, or that patients with dentate gyrus dysfunction are more likely to suffer from oxidative stress, this would allow us to target more aggressive diagnostic tests and to tailor appropriate therapy.

FUTURE DIRECTIONS

A number of outstanding questions and issues need to be highlighted. First, although our focus has been on the hippocampal formation, there is no question that the prefrontal cortex is another brain area targeted by aging. Similar questions, as well as similar analytic approaches, can be applied to the aging prefrontal cortex. For example, like the hippocampus, the prefrontal cortex is targeted both by normal aging as well as by early neurodegenerative processes; like the hippocampus, the prefrontal cortex is a complex circuit made up by interconnected neuronal populations that are differentially sensitive to causes of dysfunction.

Second, we need to continue improving imaging techniques. In our original study, we relied on a MRI signal sensitive to resting deoxyhemoglobin content—an indirect correlate of chronic metabolism. Nevertheless, the signal is also sensitive to tissue constituents that are independent of metabolism, which constitute a main source of noise. Noise needs to be minimized as much as possible, particularly for diagnostic purposes. Toward this goal, we are working on MRI approaches that generate purer measures of chronic metabolism.

Third, we need to continue our search by using techniques that can zoom in on the hippocampal subregion itself, keeping in mind that a subregion contains neurons as well as interneurons and glial cells that mediate and support neuronal function. Although memory decline is a readout of neuronal dysfunction, *a priori*, we do not know which cell type within a subregion expresses the primary biochemical defect.

SUMMARY

Clinicians are increasingly confronted with elderly patients who are quite healthy—independently living individuals leading full and demanding lives—whose chief complaint is mild forgetfulness. Examination is typically nonfocal, and even cognitive testing might be within normal limits, or perhaps suggestive of mild memory decline. These patients pose an assortment of questions that all circle around the same diagnostic dilemma: is forgetfulness in later-life normal? Is this the first stage of Alzheimer's disease? If not AD, what else can cause forgetfulness? Are there any treatment options? All good questions—as simple to ask as they are difficult to answer. The anatomy and mechanisms of brain dysfunction associated with age-related memory decline are reviewed in this chapter, accounting for why this entity continues to confuse. With this as a background, recent findings that rely on functional techniques (fMRI) to investigate age-related memory decline will be discussed, as well as their clinical implications. Main result of these "zooming-on-the-brain" MRI studies: Memory decline can be caused by different mechanisms. Hippocampal dysfunction in specific subregions seems to be the major contributor to pathological and age-related memory decline in elderly subjects.

ACKNOWLEDGMENT

This work was funded in part by federal grants AG08702, AG00949; the Beeson Faculty Scholar Award from the American Federation of Aging; and the Institute for the Study of Aging.

REFERENCES

1. Rapp, P.R.; Gallagher, M.: Preserved neuron number in the hippocampus of aged rats with spatial learning deficits. Proc Natl Acad Sci USA 1996; 18: 9926–9930.

2. Barnes, C.A.; Rao, G.; Shen, J.: Age-related decrease in the N-methyl-D-aspartate-mediated excitatory postsynaptic potential in hippocampal region CA1. Neurobiol Aging 1997; 18: 445–452.
3. Mucke, L. et al.: High-level neuronal expression of Abeta1-42 in wild-type human amyloid protein precursor transgenic mice: synaptotoxicity without plaque formation. J Neurosci 2000; 20: 4050–4058.
4. Small, S.A. et al.: Selective decline in memory function among healthy elderly. Neurology 1999; 52: 1392–1396.
5. Zhao, X. et al.: Transcriptional profiling reveals strict boundaries between hippocampal subregions. J Comp Neurol 2001; 441: 187–196.
6. Small, S.A.: Age-related memory decline; current concepts and future directions. Arch Neurol 2001; 58: 360–364.
7. Small, S.A. et al.: Imaging hippocampal function across the human life span: is memory decline normal or not? Ann Neurol 2002; 51: 290–295.
8. Small, S. et al.: Imaging physiologic dysfunction of individual hippocampal subregions in humans and genetically modified mice. Neuron 2000; 28: 653–664.

16

Mild Cognitive Impairment

What the Physician Should Know

Brigitte Zoeller Richter

INTRODUCTION

Early disease recognition is a growing concern in modern medicine, particularly in areas where prevention may be of benefit. Certain neurodegenerative disorders, however, are still far from being diagnosed at an early stage or before clinical manifestations are apparent through typical symptoms. Alzheimer's disease (AD) certainly is one of these difficult-to-diagnose diseases. Not only is dementia often not detected in time, it actually is being reported to be poorly recognized and underdiagnosed in the primary-care setting *(1)*. The detection rate is even worse when individuals present with features that do not (yet) meet the diagnostic criteria for probable AD, but could be considered as suffering from mild cognitive impairment.

WHAT IS MILD COGNITIVE IMPAIRMENT?

Persons who would be classified as having mild cognitive impairment (MCI) are neither demented nor normal. They usually fulfill a set of criteria associated with or caused by a mild degree of cognitive impairment. These features today are utilized as diagnostic criteria for MCI *(2)*. The patients must present with (isolated) memory complaints/abnormal memory function, but normal general cognition. Their activities of daily living must be intact, and they are not demented.

Other cognitive domains, such as attention, language, executive function, and visuospatial skills, are usually not affected in persons with MCI. This means that individuals with MCI are otherwise normal and well functioning, and they are (still) capable of decision making and planning for the future *(2)*.

The prevalence of MCI is not well studied yet because of difficulties in diagnosis. In a recently published population-based study from Finland, 5.3% of elderly subjects (60–76 years) met the MCI criteria *(3)*. According to a study in the United States, the prevalence of MCI increases from 1% at age 60 to 42% at age 85 *(4)*. The conversion rate from nonaffected patients to MCI increased in the same study from 1% per year at age 60 to 11% at age 85.

WHAT CAUSES MCI?

There is growing evidence that vascular factors may contribute to the development of late-life dementia as well as MCI. A relationship has been suggested to elevated blood pressures as well as high serum levels of cholesterol. Long-standing hypercholesterolemia may induce thickening of the intima and alterations in endothelial function in cerebrovascular arterioles and capillaries. These changes might impair brain metabolism.

From: *Current Clinical Neurology,*
Alzheimer's Disease: A Physician's Guide to Practical Management
Edited by: R. W. Richter and B. Zoeller Richter © Humana Press Inc., Totowa, NJ

Cognitive decline in MCI and in AD patients seems to be associated not only with regional but with widespread structural brain damage, as was reported from a study using magnetization transfer imaging (MTI) *(5)*.

WHAT IS THE PROBLEM WITH MCI?

The main problem with MCI is that it is even more difficult to diagnose then AD. Since there appears to be an overlap between normal aging and MCI, this represents a real challenge for the clinician.

Neuropsychological tests appear to be useful in the recognition of patients at increased risk for cognitive impairment *(6)*. However, MCI subjects are not easily identified. Some information may be gained in the primary-care setting using the Mini-Mental State Examination (MMSE), the Global Deterioration Scale (GDS), or the Clinical Dementia Rating scale (CDR). An MMSE score greater than 24 (out of 30), mostly in the range 26–28, is typical for MCI *(6)*. A 0.5 rating on the CDR is assigned for the questionable dementia that characterizes MCI. The rating on GDS (score range 1–7) for MCI patients is typically documented as between 2 and 3.

More sophisticated are learning measures such as the free and cued selective reminding test (FCSRT) and the auditory verbal learning test (AVLT), used mainly for memory testing. They are considered possible predictors for decline in research settings.

Cognitive decline in very intelligent people is particularly difficult to diagnose. Their high cognitive reserve can mask early changes on testing for several years, and this may result in a delayed diagnosis *(7)*.

WHY SHOULD MCI BE RECOGNIZED?

MCI should be recognized by the clinician, because these patients also complain about their memory impairment. Interestingly, this subjective impression turns out to be the best predictor for the conversion of MCI to AD.

The main reason why MCI should be recognized and diagnosed is related to the natural course of the disease. Persons who meet the criteria for MCI tend to progress to clinically probable AD at a rate of 10–15% per year. That means that approximately 80% of MCI subjects will have converted to dementia in a period of 6 years *(2)*. This is in contrast to a conversion rate of 1–2% in the normal elderly population.

Though the actual prodromal or precursor phase of MCI is uncertain but probably spans many years, there appears to be a gradual progression of symptoms. With this conceptual viewpoint, MCI represents a transitional stage between normal (healthy) aging and AD. Thus it is distinct from what historically was termed age-associated memory impairment or age-associated cognitive decline *(6)*.

Dementia may also be preceded by MCI in some subtypes of vascular dementia (VaD), particularly those caused by subcortical microvascular disease (small-vessel dementia), which has similar domains of cognitive impairment *(8)*.

DOES THE PRESENCE OF MCI PREDICT AD?

Individuals characterized as being cognitively impaired but not meeting clinical criteria for dementia or AD are thus considered as having MCI and have a high risk of progressing to dementia or AD. The progression/conversion rate varies in the literature (due to different diagnostic criteria and methodological differences), from 6% and 25%.

HOW CAN MCI BE VERIFIED?

Anatomically, MCI subjects present with a reduced hippocampal volume, related to atrophy, which can be detected with the use of magnetic resonance imaging (MRI). MRI spectroscopy studies also revealed a reduced myoinositol/creatine ratio in the posterior cingulate. Postmortem data reveal the presence of characteristic AD features in approximately half of MCI subjects, including fibrillary changes and neuritic plaques as well as diffuse amyloid depositions in the neocortex *(2)*.

Volumetric magnetic resonance imaging (MRI) measurements of the medial temporal lobe regions appear to be useful in identifying patients with mild to moderate AD as well as individuals with MCI, thus separating both groups from normal elderly individuals *(9)*.

WHICH QUESTIONS SHOULD THE PHYSICIAN ASK?

Though the subjective impression of the patient regarding memory problems is a valid one, the physician should not rely only on this information. Useful observations frequently are made and reported by close relatives or partners of the patient. Separate interviews with potential informants are therefore recommended. Clinicians should ask about any apparent change in memory, problem-solving ability, and the ability to handle tasks the patient used to be able to perform well.

WHAT CAN BE DONE FOR THE PATIENT WITH MCI?

No approved or recommended treatment for MCI is available. Acetylcholinesterase inhibitors (AChEI) seem to be effective, although they are currently approved for the treatment of mild to moderate AD only. Several long-term studies with various compounds are underway, however—for example, with AChEI, memantine, anti-inflammatory drugs, and statins, as well as antioxidants and nootropics. Emerging data from AD studies suggest that initiating therapy at an early stage may help maintain function at a higher level.

On the other side there are more skeptical voices in the scientific community, such as Peter Whitehouse, who, as cited in an article in *Neurology Reviews,* cautioned that we should not necessarily jump into thinking that screening and early recognition naturally does lead automatically to benefits in patients *(10)*.

NEUROPSYCHIATRIC SYMPTOMS HIGHLY PREVALENT IN MCI

Neuropsychiatric symptoms are frequent in AD. The recently published first population-based estimates for neuropsychiatric symptoms in MCI indicate a high prevalence of such symptoms in MCI as well *(11)*. Forty-three percent of MCI participants in a cross-sectional study derived from the Cardiovascular Health Study exhibited mostly clinically significant neuropsychiatric symptoms, such as depression (20%), apathy (15%), and irritability (15%), compared to 75% of AD participants. This finding supports the status of MCI as an intermediate condition between normal cognition and dementia, and warrants special attention.

REFERENCES

1. Valcour, V.G. et al.: The detection of dementia in the primary care setting. Arch Intern Med 2000; 160: 2964–2968.
2. Petersen, R.C.: Mild cognitive impairment: transition from aging to Alzheimer's disease. In: Iqbal, K.; Sisodia, S.; Winblad, B.: (eds.): Alzheimer's disease: advances in etiology, pathogenesis and therapeutics. Wiley, New York, 2001: 141–151.
3. Hanninen, T. et al.: Prevalence of mild cognitive impairment: a population-based study in elderly subjects. Acta Neurol Scand 2002; 106: 148–154.
4. Yesavage, J.A. et al.: Modeling the prevalence and incidence of Alzheimer's disease and mild cognitive impairment. J Psychiatric Res 2002; 36: 281–286.
5. Van der Flier, W.M. et al.: Cognitive decline in AD and mild cognitive impairment is associated with global brain damage. Neurology 2002; 59: 874–879.
6. Petersen, R.C. et al.: Practice parameter: early detection of dementia: mild cognitive impairment (an evidence-based review). Report of the Quality Standards Subcommittee of the American Academy of Neurology. Neurology 2001; 56: 1133–1142.
7. Rentz, D.R. et al.: Detecting early cognitive decline in high functioning elders. J Geriatr Psychiatry 2000; 33: 27–48.

8. Meyer, J.S. et al.: Is mild cognitive impairment prodromal for vascular dementia like Alzheimer's disease? Stroke 2002; 33: 1981–1985.
9. Bottino, C.M. et al.: Volumetric MRI measurements can differentiate Alzheimer's disease, mild cognitive impairment, and normal aging. Int Psychogeriatr 2002; 14: 59–72.
10. Whitehouse, P.J.: In: Are we ready to begin screening for Alzheimer's disease? Neurol Rev 2001; 9: 1.
11. Lyketsos, C.G. et al.: Prevalence of neuropsychiatric symptoms in dementia and mild cognitive impairment. JAMA 2002; 288: 1475–1483.

17

Diagnosis of Predementia AD in a Clinical Setting

Pieter Jelle Visser

INTRODUCTION

Alzheimer's disease (AD) is a slowly progressing neurodegenerative disorder. The first symptoms include mild cognitive impairments (MCI) in activities of daily living, which are not yet severe enough to meet the criteria of dementia. The period in which these symptoms start to occur will be referred to as the predementia phase of AD. It is important to identify subjects with predementia AD in a clinical setting, because they may be candidates for trials with drugs that might improve cognition, such as acetylcholinesterase (AChE) inhibitors, and agents that might slow down the progression of AD. Furthermore, it is important to provide subjects with predementia AD with a diagnosis and a prognosis with regard to the potential progression of the cognitive impairment. This may relieve the patient from anxiety and uncertainty concerning the underlying disorder, and it will give subjects the opportunity to anticipate the future. Finally, persons who are likely to have predementia AD should remain under clinical supervision in order to be advised on how to deal with the cognitive impairment and to receive early psychosocial interventions if deterioration occurs.

The outline of this chapter is as follows. First will be described how subjects with predementia AD present in clinical practice. Second will be discussed which variables can help differentiate these subjects from those with MCI for other reasons. Then, a number of diagnostic approaches to predementia AD will be presented. Finally, a summary and recommendations for clinical practice and future research will be given.

The data that are presented here derive mainly from studies that have been performed in second- or third-line health care settings, such as memory clinics or geriatric, neurological, or psychiatric outpatient clinics. The term MCI will be used to refer to nondemented subjects who experience cognitive impairments; it does not refer to any specific set of criteria.

PRESENTATION OF PREDEMENTIA AD IN CLINICAL PRACTICE

Subjects with predementia AD may present in many different ways. The clinical presentation will be described on the basis of a study with 31 subjects with predementia AD who were identified after a 5-year follow-up of 199 subjects with mild cognitive impairments older than 40 years from the Maastricht Memory Clinic (1). The average age of the subjects with predementia AD was 70 years at baseline (range 48–81 years). Ninety percent were older than 60. The most common cognitive symptoms as measured by the Blessed Dementia Rating Scale (BDRS) were inability to remember a short list (80%) and inability to recall recent events (50%). The severity of interference of the cognitive impairment with activities of daily living (ADL) was mild [a score of 3 on the Global Deterioration Scale (GDS) (2)] in 74% of the subjects, very mild (a score of 2 on the GDS) in 23%, and moderate (a score of 4 on the GDS) in 3%. The average Mini-Mental State Examination (MMSE) score was 26.5 at baseline (range 21–30). The MMSE score was 27 or higher in 59% of the subjects.

From: *Current Clinical Neurology,*
Alzheimer's Disease: A Physician's Guide to Practical Management
Edited by: R. W. Richter and B. Zoeller Richter © Humana Press Inc., Totowa, NJ

Table 1
Examples of Causes of Mild Cognitive Impairment Other Than Predementia AD

A. *Disorders with strong relationship to mild cognitive impairment, which often can be easily recognized*
   by clinical examination and/or ancillary tests
   Parkinson's disease, Huntington's disease, severe brain trauma, brain infections, large intracerebral tumors, cerebral bleeding, large cerebral infarcts, extensive white matter pathology, severe depression, psychotic disorders, long-standing and severe alcohol intoxication, drug intoxication (i.e., prolonged use of high doses of benzodiazepines), severe thiamine or vitamin B_{12} deficiency, uncontrolled diabetes mellitus or thyroid disorders

B. *Disorders with strong relationship to mild cognitive impairment but difficult to recognize*
   by clinical assessment and/or ancillary tests
   Predementia or prodromal stage of Lewy body disease, frontotemporal dementia, vascular dementia, Parkinson's disease, multiple system atrophy, Huntington's disease

C. *Disorders with weak relationship to mild cognitive impairment*
   Mild brain trauma, transient ischemic attack, epilepsy, disorders that chronically or temporarily impair brain perfusion (hyper/hypotension, stenosis of the carotid artery, generalized artherosclerosis, cardiac surgery), mild depression, bipolar disorders, anxiety disorders, regulated diabetes mellitus or thyroid disorders, mild thiamine or vitamin deficiency, heart failure, chronic obstructed pulmonary diseases, anemia, severe liver or kidney disorders, hearing loss, "normal aging," and psychosocial problems in relation to work, relationships, life-phase change, somatic disorders, or fear of dementia

The most common noncognitive symptoms as measured by the Hamilton Depression Rating Scale and the BDRS were general somatic complaints (42%), psychological anxiety (42%), depressed mood (39%), decreased work and interests (35%), somatic anxiety (26%), sleep disturbances early in the morning (23%), impaired emotional control (43%), hobbies relinquished (23%), and diminished initiative (20%). Hallucinations, delusions, offensive behavior, or wandering were not observed. The main diagnosis at baseline was cognitive impairment not otherwise specified (77%), amnestic disorder (9%), or no cognitive impairment (3%). A co-diagnosis of an affective disorder was made in 61% of the subjects and included depression (48%) and anxiety (13%). These affective disorders were mild, as none of the subjects performed higher than 20 on the Hamilton Depression Scale.

In summary, the results of this study indicated that subjects with predementia AD generally present with mild impairments in ADL and mild affective symptoms, but that marked heterogeneity also exists. These findings are consistent with other studies *(3,4)*. It ensues that there is no single clinical profile that can characterize subjects with predementia AD. The high frequency of affective symptoms in these subjects indicates that a diagnosis of predementia AD should be considered when people present with mild cognitive impairments and mild depression. This is in contrast to the general clinical assumption that cognitive symptoms in mildly depressed patients always appear secondary to depression.

VARIABLES THAT CAN DISTINGUISH BETWEEN SUBJECTS WITH PREDEMENTIA AD AND THOSE WITH MCI FOR OTHER REASONS

Not only predementia AD but also numerous other conditions can cause MCI without dementia. Some of the symptoms of these other conditions may overlap with symptoms of predementia AD. It is therefore a major clinical question how these other conditions can be differentiated from predementia AD. Conditions other than predementia AD that can cause cognitive impairment can be divided into three groups on the basis of a number of diagnostic properties. The first group of conditions are obvious causes for MCI, which means they are sufficient cause for the impairments and can be identified by clinical examination and/or ancillary tests (such as laboratory tests or neuroimaging; *see* Table 1, part A, for examples). The second are conditions that are sufficient cause for the MCI but can presently not be diagnosed by clinical examination or ancillary tests (*see* Table 1, part B). The third group are conditions with a weak relation to MCI; that is, these subjects may have MCI on a group level, but it is not clear whether the disorder itself could be the cause for the condition in the individual patient (*see* Table 1, part C).

Studies that have investigated markers of predementia AD focused mainly on the differentiation of subjects with predementia AD from those with MCI due to causes listed in parts B and C of Table 1; they excluded subjects with obvious causes for MCI. Long-term follow-up studies indicated that, after exclusion of subjects with obvious causes for MCI, 50–80% of the those with mild cognitive impairments have predementia AD *(5,6)*.

A large number of variables have been tested as markers of predementia AD. These markers include demographic factors, clinical rating scales for functional impairment, depressive symptoms, short cognitive screening tests (such as MMSE), neuropsychological test performance, brain imaging parameters, electrophysiological measures, biochemical, and genetic variables. The diagnostic accuracy of these markers will be described shortly. If markers have been tested in at least four different studies with similar design, we will provide pooled estimates of diagnostic accuracy based on a meta-analysis *(3)*.

Demographic Variables

The meta-analysis indicated that subjects older than 75 years of age had an odds ratio (OR, global measure of diagnostic accuracy—an OR of 25 or more indicates good diagnostic accuracy) of 2 for predementia AD compared to subjects aged 60–75 years. The corresponding sensitivity (i.e., the percentage of subjects with predementia AD in which the marker is present) was low (47%), as was the positive predictive value (54%) (i.e., the percentage of subjects in which the marker is present and which have predementia AD). Sex and educational level were weak or no markers of predementia AD (OR lower than 1.5).

Clinical Rating Scales for Functional Impairment

Examples of clinical rating scales for functional impairment are the GDS *(2)* and the Clinical Dementia Rating Scale (CDRS) *(7)*. The meta-analysis indicated that the OR for predementia AD in subjects with mild functional impairment (defined as a score of 3 on GDS, or CDRS overall score of 0.5 or sum of boxes score more than 1) compared to subjects with very mild functional impairment was 6.8. The sensitivity was good (77%), but the positive predictive value was modest (51%). One study showed that the discrepancy in self-reported and informant-reported functional deficits may be a useful marker of predementia AD (OR 8, sensitivity 62%, positive predictive value 53%) *(8)*.

Depression

Although mood disorders are common in predementia AD, the meta-analysis indicated that the presence of depression had no diagnostic value for predementia AD (OR 0.9).

Short Cognitive Screening Scales

The scale that has most often been investigated as marker of predementia AD is the MMSE. The meta-analysis indicated that the OR for predementia AD was 3.8 if subjects with an MMSE score below 27 were compared with those with a higher score. Both the pooled sensitivity and positive predictive value were poor (57% and 49%, respectively).

Neuropsychological Test Performance

A large number of neuropsychological tests from different cognitive domains have been tested as markers for predementia AD. Generally, tests that assess memory impairment are the strongest marker for predementia AD. The meta-analysis indicated that the odds ratio for predementia AD was 7.6 if subjects with memory impairment were compared to those without. The corresponding sensitivity was 74%, the positive predictive value 59%. Impairment of language function (as measured by the Boston

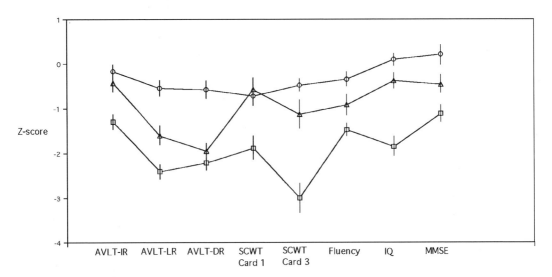

Fig. 1. Profile of cognitive test performance (mean and standard error) of subjects with predementia AD in a clinical setting (*n* = 23) (triangles, middle line). For reference purposes the cognitive performance of subjects with nonprogressive mild cognitive impairment (*n* = 44) (circles, upper line), and subjects with very mild Alzheimer-type dementia (*n* = 25) (squares, lower line) are shown. Z-score, number of standard deviations difference from expected value given age, sex, and education; AVLT-IR, immediate recall of Auditory Verbal Learning Test (AVLT); AVLT-LR, learning measure of AVLT; AVLT-DR, delayed recall of AVLT; SCWT, Stroop Colour Word Test; IQ, intelligence quotient; MMSE, Mini-Mental State Examination. (Reproduced from *International Psychogeriatrics [27]* with permission of Springer Publishing Company.)

Naming Test or verbal fluency), executive functions (as measured by the Stroop Color Word test card 3 or the Trail Making Test B), or attention (as measured by the Symbol Digit Substitution Test) were also markers for predementia AD, but the diagnostic accuracy appeared to be generally less. Several studies showed that impairments in these other domains could increase the diagnostic accuracy compared to that of memory impairment alone. One study indicated that a decreased olfaction score is strongly associated with predementia AD (OR 42, sensitivity 100%, positive predictive value 40%) *(9)*. The profile of neuropsychological test performance in subjects with predementia AD is illustrated in Fig. 1.

Neuroimaging

The most frequent finding on neuroimaging in subjects with predementia AD is atrophy of the medial temporal lobe, which includes the hippocampus, entorhinal cortex, amygdala, and parahippocampal gyrus. The meta-analysis indicated that the OR for predementia AD was 4.6 in subjects with medial temporal lobe atrophy, compared to those without atrophy. The corresponding sensitivity was 59%, and the positive predictive value 61%. Atrophy in other parts of the brain, such as the gray matter at the bank of the superior temporal sulcus, the caudal part of the cingulate gyrus, the fusiform gyrus, and dilatation of the third ventricle, the suprasellar cistern, and other cortical and ventricular cerebrospinal liquor spaces, generally had a lower diagnostic accuracy *(10,11)*. In one study, the presence of white matter was a marker with modest accuracy for predementia AD *(12)*. SPECT assessment of hypoperfusion has yielded conflicting results with respect to diagnostic accuracy. One study showed that a quantitative rating of asymmetry in parietal temporal perfusion was a marker of predementia AD *(13)*, but another showed that a qualitative rating of hypoperfusion was not *(14)*. Recently, it was demonstrated that hypoperfusion in the posterior cingulate gyrus might be a good diagnostic marker for predementia AD, with an area under the curve between 0.76 and 0.87 *(15,16)*.

The predictive accuracy of hypometabolism has been investigated in three PET studies. One study demonstrated that a decrease in glucose metabolism in the temporoparietal area was a marker for predementia AD, with an overall predictive accuracy of 75% *(17)*. Another PET study showed that hypometabolism in the entorhinal cortex was predictive of cognitive decline in subjects who had very mild functional impairment at baseline *(18)*. A third study found that an abnormal parietal index tended to be associated with predementia AD *(19)*. However, hypometabolism in the frontal, parietal, temporal, or occipital region were not markers of predementia AD in this study *(19)*.

Electrophysiological Studies

A combination of different background frequencies accurately identified subjects with predementia AD, with an overall accuracy of 82% in one small study *(20)*. Another small study showed that event-related potentials may be useful for the diagnosis of predementia AD, with an overall diagnostic accuracy of 85% *(21)*.

Biochemical Markers

Biochemical markers that have most often been investigated in predementia AD are tau protein and beta-amyloid (Aβ) ending at amino acid 42 (Aβ_{42}) in cerebrospinal fluid. An elevated concentration of total tau protein had a sensitivity of 70% for detecting subjects with predementia AD *(22)*. The sensitivity of the combination of an elevated concentration of total tau protein and decreased Abeta42 was about 90% *(23,24)*. The OR of this combination for predementia AD was 18, the positive predictive value 60% *(24)*.

Another biomarker that has been investigated is the level of F_2-isoprostane 8,12-iso-iPF$_{2\alpha}$-VI in CSF, plasma, or urine. Preliminary data indicate that an elevated level of F_2-isoprostane 8,12-iso-iPF$_{2\alpha}$-VI in CSF, plasma, or urine may be a marker of predementia AD *(25)*.

Genetic Markers

Genetic markers for AD can be divided into autosomal dominant inherited mutations and genetic risk factors. The autosomal dominant mutations may have a high diagnostic value in subjects with MCI from families with a high frequency of early-onset AD. The diagnostic accuracy of these mutations in other samples of subjects with MCI has not been investigated but is likely to be low, because these mutations are rare. The only genetic risk factor of AD that has been tested in predementia AD is the apolipoprotein E (ApoE) genotype. The meta-analysis indicated that the OR for predementia AD was 3.4 if carriers of at least one ApoE$_{e4}$ allele were compared to those without this allele. The corresponding sensitivity was 61%, the positive predictive value 45%.

In conclusion, there is no single variable that can accurately identify subjects with predementia AD from those with MCI for other reasons. The meta-analysis of variables that have been investigated in at least four studies indicated that no variable has an OR higher than 8. Several promising new markers of predementia AD have been investigated in small studies, but larger ones are needed to further assess their diagnostic accuracy.

DIAGNOSTIC APPROACH FOR PREDEMENTIA AD

Since a single-variable approach has insufficient accuracy for diagnosing subjects with predementia AD, several studies have used a multivariable approach. Two of them will be discussed here, which can be easily used in clinical practice: the concept of amnestic MCI *(6)* and the Preclinical Alzheimer's Disease Scale (PAS) *(26)*. Amnestic MCI is defined as mild functional impairment in combination with impairment on a memory test *(6)*. Longitudinal studies in subjects with amnestic MCI, who were

Table 2
Preclinical Alzheimer's Disease Scale (PAS)

	−1	0	1	2	Score
A. Age	≤59	60–64	65–74	≥75	
B. MMSE[a]	—	≥28	26, 27	≤25	
C. Functional impairment[b]					
C.1 GDS	—	GDS 1	GDS 2	GDS 3	
C.2 CDRS					
C.2.1. Total Box score	—	<0.5	0.5–1	≥1.5	
C.2.2. Final score	—	CDRS = 0	—	CDRS = 0.5	
C.3 CAMDEX	—	—	—	Min Dem	
D. Neuropsychological tests[c]	Memory ≥50 perc	Other	1 test impaired	2 tests impaired	
E. MTL atrophy[d]					
E.1 Qualitative rating					
Age < 75yr	—	0	1	2	
Age ≥ 75yr	0	1	2	3	
E.2 Volumetry	≥66 perc	33–66 perc	10–33 perc	≤10 perc	
F. ApoE genotype	—	Other	e2e4/e3e4	e4e4	_____
				Total Score	

[a]The MMSE should be corrected for age and education: if age is 75 years or older, or if the period of education was 8 years or less, 1 point should each time be added to the observed score; if the period of education was 14 years or more, 1 point should be subtracted from the observed score.

[b]One option should be used. The CDR can be scored using the Sum of Boxes score (preferred) or the final rating.

[c]At least two and maximal four tests including one memory test for delayed recall or learning. An impairment is a score below the 10th percentile (perc) or above the 90th percentile (for speed-related tasks) after correction for age, sex, and education.

[d]One option should be used. A qualitative score can be performed on a CT scan or a MRI scan *(29,30)*. Volumetry should measure the hippocampus (preferred), parahippocampal gyrus, or entorhinal cortex. The percentile score is relative to age, sex, and intracranial volume.

The table indicates which score corresponds with the test result. The total score is an indication for the risk of predementia AD. More information can be found in ref. *26* and at www.np.unimaas.nl/pas

MMSE, Mini-Mental State Examination; GDS, Global Deterioration Scale *(2)*; CDRS, Clinical Dementia Rating Scale *(7)*; MTL, medial temporal lobe; ApoE, apolipoprotein E; Min Dem, minimal dementia; Perc, percentile; and CAMDEX, Cambridge Mental Disorders of the Elderly Examination *(28)*.

Reproduced from ref. *26* with permission of Springer-Verlag.

on average 79 years old, showed that about 80% of them had predementia AD at long-term follow-up *(6)*. Data regarding the positive predictive value of amnestic-MCI in younger age samples and the sensitivity of amnestic MCI have not been published yet. Unpublished data from a 5-year follow-up study of the Maastricht Memory Clinic, however, indicated that the positive predictive value was much lower in younger compared to higher age samples: 7% of subjects with amnestic MCI in the age range 50–60 had predementia AD, 50% in the age range 60–70, and 100% in the age range 70–85 years. In the same sample, the sensitivity of amnestic MCI for predementia AD reached 33–56%, depending on the age group.

Another multivariable approach is the PAS (Table 2) *(26)*. The PAS combines six markers for predementia AD, which were selected on the basis of the above-mentioned meta-analysis. Each variable is scored on a 3- to 4-point scale, and the total sum score indicates the risk for predementia AD. A retrospective validation study of the PAS in two samples of subjects with MCI older than 55 years indicated that the best cutoff score was 6 for the full PAS and 5 for PAS without the neuroimaging variable

(26). The OR at the best cutoff score was 25, the sensitivity 82%, the positive predictive accuracy 75%. Subjects with a score of 7 or higher had a very high risk (93%) for predementia AD in both samples, those with a score lower than 4 a very low risk (7%), while those with a score between 3 and 7 had an intermediate risk for predementia AD (46%). These intermediate scores were seen in 38% of the subjects. This means that in a substantial number of subjects the diagnosis of predementia AD remains uncertain.

In summary, multivariable approaches may be useful for detecting subjects at high risk for predementia AD. The concept of amnestic MCI has the advantage of offering a high positive predictive value in samples with a high median age. The positive predictive value in younger samples, however, is low, as well as the sensitivity. The PAS may be a useful tool to identify subjects at low, intermediate, and high risk for predementia AD, but the scale needs cross-validation.

RECOMMENDATIONS FOR CLINICAL PRACTICE AND FUTURE RESEARCH

The clinical presentation of predementia AD is heterogeneous. There is no single marker of predementia AD that can accurately distinguish it from other causes of MCI. A multivariable approach, however, can reach good diagnostic accuracy. Low-risk and high-risk subjects can be accurately identified by a multivariable approach, though there remains a substantial group of subjects with an intermediate risk for predementia AD, in which the diagnosis remains uncertain. It is expected that the diagnostic accuracy for these subjects might increase with the inclusion of new markers for predementia AD in the multivariable approach, such as the concentration of tau and $A\beta_{42}$ in cerebrospinal fluid.

In clinical practice, it seems advisable to keep subjects at intermediate or high risk for predementia AD under clinical supervision. There is, however, no evidence yet that subjects at high risk for predementia AD will benefit from pharmacological treatment with, for example, AChE inhibitors.

Information concerning diagnostic markers of predementia AD is rapidly expanding. It will, however, take time to investigate the diagnostic value of new markers, as they will have to be tested in longitudinal studies of subjects with MCI. Since it may take more than 5 years before a person with MCI becomes demented, the length of any study should ideally be at least 5 years.

Diagnostic research should not be limited to subjects at high risk for predementia AD only (for example, elderly people with amnestic MCI), because many patients with predementia AD do not fulfil the inclusion criteria for high-risk predementia AD. Therefore, the overall sensitivity of tests performed in subjects at high risk will be low. New variables should preferably be investigated together with known markers of predementia AD, in a way that a potential additional diagnostic value can be recognized. In addition, this would open the opportunity to investigate the order in which diagnostic tests might best be performed. Serial testing would have the advantage that the number of diagnostic assessments could be reduced, which might reduce the burden of diagnostic testings for patients and also reduce costs. Since the number of potential diagnostic markers is high, large studies are necessary to address these issues. In order to increase the generalizability of the results, those studies should preferably be performed in multicenter settings.

SUMMARY

Many patients with AD come under clinical attention before they are demented but when they have only mild cognitive impairments. In this chapter we discussed ways to identify subjects with predementia AD among subjects with mild cognitive impairments for other reasons. It was shown that the clinical presentation of subjects with predementia AD is heterogeneous and that there is no single marker of predementia AD that could allow an accurate distinction from other causes of mild cognitive impairment. If a number of markers are combined, however, it is possible to accurately identify subjects with a low or a high risk for predementia AD.

REFERENCES

1. Visser, P.J. et al.: Characteristics of preclinical Alzheimer's disease. Int J Geriatric Psychiatry 2002; 17: 88–89.
2. Reisberg, B. et al.: The global deterioration scale for assessment of primary degenerative dementia. Am J Psychiatry 1982; 139: 1136–1139.
3. Visser, P.J. et al.: Predictors of dementia in subjects with mild cognitive impairment—a quantitative meta-analysis [abstr]. Neurobiol Aging 2002; 23: S138.
4. Tierney, M.C. et al.: Do depressive symptoms in memory-impaired elders predict probable Alzheimer's disease? Aging Mental Health 1999; 3: 88–93.
5. Morris, J.C. et al.: Mild cognitive impairment represents early-stage Alzheimer disease. Arch Neurol 2001; 58: 397–405.
6. Petersen, R.C. et al.: Current concepts in mild cognitive impairment. Arch Neurol 2001; 58: 1985–1992.
7. Morris, J.: The Clinical Dementia Rating (CDR): current version and scoring rules. Neurology 1993; 43: 2412–2414.
8. Tabert, M.H. et al.: Functional deficits in patients with mild cognitive impairment: prediction of AD. Neurology 2002; 58: 758–764.
9. Devanand, D.P. et al.: Olfactory deficits in patients with mild cognitive impairment predict Alzheimer's disease at follow-up. Am J Psychiatry 2000; 157: 1399–1405.
10. Killiany, R.J. et al.: Use of structural magnetic resonance imaging to predict who will get Alzheimer's disease. Ann Neurol 2000; 47: 430–439.
11. Convit, A. et al.: Atrophy of the medial occipitotemporal, inferior, and middle temporal gyri in non-demented elderly predicts decline to Alzheimer's disease. Neurobiol Aging 2000; 21: 19–26.
12. Wolf, H. et al.: Do white matter changes contribute to the subsequent development of dementia in patients with mild cognitive impairment? A longitudinal study. Int J Geriatric Psychiatry 2000; 15: 803–812.
13. Celsis, P. et al.: Age related cognitive decline: a clinical entity? A longitudinal study of cerebral blood flow and memory performance. J Neurol Neurosurg Psychiatry 1997; 62: 601–608.
14. McKelvey, R. et al.: Lack of prognostic significance of SPECT abnormalities in non-demented elderly subjects with memory loss. Can J Neurol Sci 1999; 26: 23–28.
15. Huang, C. et al.: Cingulate cortex hypoperfusion predicts Alzheimer's disease in mild cognitive impairment. BMC Neurol 2002; 2: 9.
16. Okamura, N. et al.: Combined analysis of CSF tau levels and [(123)I]iodoamphetamine SPECT in mild cognitive impairment: implications for a novel predictor of Alzheimer's disease. Am J Psychiatry 2002; 159: 474–476.
17. Arnaiz, E. et al.: Impaired cerebral glucose metabolism and cognitive functioning predict deterioration in mild cognitive impairment. Neuroreport 2001; 12: 851–855.
18. De Leon, M.J. et al.: Prediction of cognitive decline in normal elderly subjects with 2-[^{18}F]fluoro-2-deoxy-d-glucose/positron-emssion tomography (FDG/PET). Proc Natl Acad Sci USA 2001; 98: 10966–10971.
19. Berent, S. et al.: Neuropsychological function and cerebral glucose utilization in isolated memory impairment and Alzheimer's disease. J Psychiatric Res 1999; 33: 7–16.
20. Jelic, V. et al.: Quantitative electroencephalography in mild cognitive impairment: longitudinal changes and possible prediction of Alzheimer's disease. Neurobiol Aging 2000; 21: 533–540.
21. Olichney, J.M. et al.: Abnormal verbal event related potentials in mild cognitive impairment and incipient Alzheimer's disease. J Neurol Neurosurg Psychiatry 2002; 73: 377–384.
22. Arai, H. et al.: Elevated cerebrospinal fluid tau protein level as a predictor of dementia in memory-impaired individuals. Alzheimer's Res 1997; 3: 211–213.
23. Andreasen, N. et al.: Cerebrospinal fluid tau and A-beta-42 as predictors of development of Alzheimer's disease in patients with mild cognitive impairment. Neurosci Lett 1999; 273: 5–8.
24. Riemenschneider, M. et al.: Cerebrospinal fluid tau and beta-amyloid 42 proteins identify Alzheimer disease in subjects with mild cognitive impairment. Arch Neurol 2002; 59: 1729–1734.
25. Pratico, D. et al.: Increase of brain oxidative stress in mild cognitive impairment: a possible predictor of Alzheimer's disease. Arch Neurol 2002; 59: 972–976.
26. Visser, P.J. et al.: Diagnostic accuracy of the Preclinical AD Scale (PAS) in cognitively mildly impaired subjects. J Neurol 2002; 249: 312–319.
27. Visser, P.J. et al.: Diagnosis of preclinical Alzheimer's disease in a clinical setting. Int Psychogeriatr 2001; 13: 411–424.
28. Roth, M. et al.: A standardised instrument for the diagnoses of mental disorder in the elderly with special reference to the early detection of dementia. Br J Psychiatry 1986; 149: 698–709.
29. De Leon, M.J. et al.: The radiologic prediction of Alzheimer's disease: the atrophic hippocampal formation. Am J Neuroradiol 1993; 14: 897–906.
30. Scheltens, P. et al.: Atrophy of medial temporal lobes on MRI in "probable" Alzheimer's disease and normal ageing: diagnostic value and neuropsychological correlates. J Neurol Neurosurg Psychiatry 1992; 55: 967–972.

18

Loss of Olfactory Function in Patients With Alzheimer's Disease

Claire Murphy and Paul E. Gilbert

INTRODUCTION

Alzheimer's disease (AD) is a progressive degenerative dementia disorder that affects more than 5 million Americans. The prevalence is projected to rise substantially as the U.S. population ages. Progressive memory impairment and one or more of the following cognitive disturbances characterize AD behaviorally: aphasia, apraxia, agnosia, or deficits in executive function. Characteristic neuropathological changes in AD include cell loss, granulovacuolar degeneration, and an increased number of neuritic plaques and neurofibrillary tangles. Plaques and tangles develop first in the temporal lobe *(1–3)*, and as the disease progresses, plaques and tangles also are found in the frontal cortex and eventually in areas of association cortex *(1,2)*. As noted by Van Hoesen and Solodkin *(4)*, the neuropathological changes in AD affect the primary regions of the brain involved in olfaction but have little effect on other sensory systems.

Although diagnostic criteria have been established for AD, a definite diagnosis is possible only following autopsy or biopsy when the neuritic plaques and neurofibrillary tangles are identified in the brain *(3,5)*. The neuropathological diagnosis of AD requires sufficient senile plaques to meet National Institute on Aging (NIA) criteria *(6)* and Consortium to Establish a Registry for Alzheimer's Disease (CERAD) neuropathological criteria for AD *(7)*. Therefore, since the diagnosis of AD cannot be made until death, the diagnosis of "probable AD" is given in the living patient, which is based on neuropsychological assessment and genetic testing. The diagnosis of probable AD is given according to the criteria for primary degenerative dementia, outlined in the *Diagnostic and Statistical Manual of Mental Disorders* (DSM), 4th Edition (American Psychiatric Association, 1994), and according to the criteria developed by the National Institute on Communicative Disorders and Stroke—Alzheimer's Disease and Related Disorders Association *(5)*.

The difficulty in accurately diagnosing AD in the living patient has motivated a tremendous amount of research to determine the genetic risk factors for AD and to learn the mechanisms that underlie the neural degeneration. However, it is clear that to improve the early assessment and diagnosis of AD, it is necessary to improve the diagnostic accuracy in the living patient. Based on a substantial amount of evidence, the assessment of olfactory function in patients with AD and those at risk for the disease is of great theoretical important and may be potentially useful in the diagnosis. Inclusion of olfactory measures into test batteries for AD is important, since olfactory loss is often not reported by patients and may not be detected without special measurement *(8)*.

From: *Current Clinical Neurology,*
Alzheimer's Disease: A Physician's Guide to Practical Management
Edited by: R. W. Richter and B. Zoeller Richter © Humana Press Inc., Totowa, NJ

NEUROPATHOLOGICAL SUBSTRATE FOR OLFACTORY DYSFUNCTION

The plaques and tangles associated with AD develop first in temporal lobe structures. The neurofibrillary tangles first appear in the entorhinal and transentorhinal cortex *(1)*. Gomez-Isla demonstrated that individuals with very mild cognitive impairment showed a 32% reduction in the number of entorhinal cortex neurons, with a 60% decrease specifically in layer II *(9)*. In patients with severe dementia, a decrease of 90% was reported in layer II of the entorhinal cortex *(9)*. The lesions in layer II of the entorhinal cortex are likely to affect stellate projection cells that form the primary afferent input into the hippocampus. As the disease progresses, degeneration is then found throughout other temporal lobe structures including the hippocampus, periamygdala, and anterior olfactory nucleus *(1–3)*. The brain areas affected early in the progression of AD are primary regions involved in processing olfactory information *(4)*. Degeneration in the anterior olfactory nucleus, entorhinal cortex, and amygdala has been shown in individuals with moderate and even mild AD, therefore degeneration may occur very early in the progression of the disease *(3)*. The most severe lesions associated with AD have been reported in entorhinal cortex, the CA1/subicular subregions of the hippocampus, the amygdala, and association areas *(1)*. A proliferation of neurofibrillary tangles also has been shown in the olfactory bulb early in disease progression *(10)*.

As the disease progresses, plaques and tangles are found throughout many regions of the neocortex, including regions of the orbitofrontal cortex *(1,3,11,12)*. Morris and colleagues have shown that the brains of patients with AD show a relatively high presence of plaques in the frontal cortex *(13)*. Neuroanatomical studies have shown that the projections from the hippocampal formation, the entorhinal cortex, and the basal nuclei of the amygdala form efferent projections to the prefrontal cortex, which has reciprocal afferent inputs back to the amygdala *(11,12)*. A portion of limbic system efferents have been shown to project to the ventral striatum and then to the mediodorsal nucleus of the thalamus before terminating in the medial and orbitofrontal regions of the frontal cortex *(11,12)*. Therefore, even in the early stages of AD, plaques and tangles are found in limbic system structures that provide afferent inputs to the frontal cortex, and as the disease progresses, plaques are found in regions of the frontal cortex *(11)*.

In conclusion, the neuropathological changes associated with AD affect regions of the brain involved in processing olfactory information. Therefore, tests of olfactory function may be useful in understanding sensory and cognitive changes in AD.

IMPAIRED ODOR IDENTIFICATION IN AD

One of the most consistent findings in the literature is the association between AD and impaired odor identification. Impaired odor identification was one of the first documented olfactory deficits in patients with AD, and an impairment has been reported by multiple investigators using a variety of odor identification tests *(8,14–17)*. Tests of odor identification typically involve the presentation of an odor to the subject, and the subject is asked to name the odor, usually with the aid of a list of words or using pictures. The sensitivity and specificity for odor identification tests are very high and comparable to many of the existing neuropsychological tests used in the assessment of AD *(8,18)*. Since patients with AD show deficits in odor identification, researchers have suggested that this measure may be useful in the assessment of AD *(18)*. Using two different odor identification tests, the University of Pennsylvania Smell Identification Test (UPSIT) *(19)* and the San Diego Odor Identification Test *(20)*, Morgan et al. examined the sensitivity and specificity of odor identification *(8)*. The UPSIT is a lexically based 40 item microencapsulated scratch-and-sniff test with four written responses for each odor—for example, gasoline, pizza, peanuts, and lilac. The San Diego Odor Identification Test is a nonlexical, picture-based task, in which odors are presented in opaque jars and the subject is asked to either point to the correct picture or say the name of the odor.

Individuals who were diagnosed with either questionable AD or who were determined to be at risk for the disease were tested on both odor identification tests. The sensitivity and specificity were high for both in persons with questionable AD and those at risk for AD. Since subjects were impaired on both the lexical and the nonlexical odor identification tests, the results suggest that deficits on the tests were not due to lexical difficulty in interpreting the words. Furthermore, AD patients score in the normal range on the Picture Identification Test (PIT), which is identical to the UPSIT except that line-drawn pictures are used rather than odors *(8)*.

This finding demonstrates that AD patients have the cognitive ability to perform an odor identification task, indicating that AD patients are cognitively able to perform an identification task. Therefore, these findings suggest that tests of odor identification are sensitive to dementia in individuals in the early stages of AD as well as those at risk for the disease.

It has been have suggested that the lesions in the entorhinal cortex, which is the primary input into the hippocampus, disconnect the hippocampus from the isocortex, thus preventing the transfer of information essential to memory function *(21)*. Therefore, in addition to memory problems resulting from direct damage to the hippocampus in patients with AD, damage to the entorhinal cortex may also contribute to deficits in memory, particularly for olfactory stimuli. Furthermore, the flow of information to the orbital frontal cortex also may be disrupted in AD and could contribute to impaired performance in higher-order olfactory memory tasks, such as odor identification. As a result, memory for olfactory stimuli may be particularly impaired in AD patients and those at risk for the disease and would be particularly sensitive in the early stages of disease progression. Therefore, the pattern of neuropathological changes in brain regions involved in olfaction associated with AD are consistent with impairments in odor identification.

A number of tests have been developed to assess odor identification. A commercially available version of the UPSIT is known as the Smell Identification Test™ (SIT) *(19)*. However, the expense of the commercially available tests has motivated the development of tests such as the San Diego Odor Identification Test, which can be assembled quickly and easily from common household odors. Furthermore, each test can be administered to large numbers of subjects with minimal maintenance. The San Diego Odor Identification Test also uses pictures rather than written words, so that the test can be administered to individuals for whom reading might be a problem.

IMPAIRED ODOR DETECTION IN AD

Since AD affects regions of the brain critical to olfaction, it seems likely that AD also may be associated with impaired odor detection, as well as impaired odor identification. A number of tests have been developed to measure odor threshold. Most tests rely on a two-alternative or forced-choice procedure involving a concentration series of an odorant dissolved in a dilutent. Each dilution step represents an increased concentration of the odorant. On each trial, a subject is presented with a bottle containing water (blank) and a bottle containing a sample of an odor. The subject is instructed to indicate which of the two bottles contains the odorant. This procedure is used to reduce a response bias or the tendency of a subject to report smelling an odor because he or she believes the experimenter expects this response. Beginning with the lowest concentration, an incorrect choice (selecting the blank) leads to the presentation of a dilution with a one-step increase in concentration. A correct choice (selecting the odorant) leads to the presentation of the same concentration to a criterion of a set number of consecutive correct choices. A predetermined criterion is used to avoid the selection of the correct odor simply by chance. A 45-second intertrial interval is typically implemented to avoid adaptation *(22)*.

Although deficits in odor identification have been consistently noted in the literature, early investigations have reported inconsistent findings for an association between AD and impaired odor detection. Some studies have documented deficits in odor detection associated with AD *(23)*, whereas others have not *(15)*. Murphy et al. reported that the patients with moderate AD showed impaired odor threshold, but taste threshold was not impaired *(24)*. Impaired odor threshold but not taste threshold in AD patients suggests that the patients are cognitively able to perform a threshold task.

Furthermore, the data illustrate that the neuropathological changes associated with AD affect olfactory processing specifically and are not only affecting the basic cognitive processing required to perform a threshold test. In addition, Murphy et al. demonstrated that olfactory threshold impairment in AD was related to the level of dementia assessed by performance of neuropsychological tests *(24)*. In a subsequent study Nordin and Murphy showed that individuals with questionable AD also showed impaired odor threshold; however, subjects with moderate AD showed greater impairments in odor threshold *(25)*. Furthermore, the study revealed a relationship between the progression of olfactory impairment and cognitive decline. Patients who showed more rapid olfactory impairment over time also showed increased progression of dementia *(25)*.

Therefore, the data suggest that an association may exist between olfactory function and severity of dementia. These findings may account for some of the inconsistent findings from early studies of odor detection in AD. Impairments in odor threshold may have been related to the severity of the dementia of the subjects and likely varied across the samples used in each study.

Since AD is associated with impaired odor threshold, one may question whether the olfactory loss in AD is due to changes in neuropathology or whether it is due simply to nasal disease. However, Feldman and colleagues have reported that impairments in olfactory threshold in AD are not associated with peripheral nasal disease *(26)*. Odor threshold was recorded in a sample of mild to moderately demented AD and normal control subjects. Patients with AD showed poorer odor thresholds than controls; however, endoscopic examinations of the olfactory epithelium showed no abnormalities in either group of patients. These data suggest that impairments in odor threshold in AD patients are likely centrally based and not due to peripheral nasal disease.

A number of odor threshold tests have been used in previous experiments *(24,27)*. In addition, there are a number of commercially available tests, such as the Smell Threshold Test™ (Sensonics, Haddon Heights, NJ) and the "Sniffin' Sticks" test *(28)*. The test kits for odor threshold are often quite cumbersome due to the large number of different concentrations needed for the odorant. However, the Alcohol Sniff Test (AST) is a simple odor detection test that was developed for use by a physician or his/her staff for rapid screening of anosmia *(29)*. The test involves the use of a 70% isopropyl alcohol pad and measuring tape. The distance from the nose to where the subject detects the odor is used as the metric, rather than concentration of an odorant.

IMPAIRED ODOR MEMORY IN AD

AD leads to deterioration within the hippocampus, which has been shown to play a critical role in the formation of episodic and declarative memories. It has been suggested that the lesions in the entorhinal cortex, which is the primary input into the hippocampus, disconnect the hippocampus from the isocortex, thus preventing the transfer of information essential to memory function *(21)*. Therefore, in addition to memory problems resulting from direct damage to the hippocampus in AD patients, damage to the entorhinal cortex may also contribute to deficits in memory, particularly for olfactory stimuli. As a result, memory for olfactory stimuli may be more impaired in AD patients than memory for other types of stimuli.

Impairments in odor identification associated with AD offer support for this hypothesis, since odor identification requires a memory component *(8,14–16)*. As a result, multiple studies have been designed to examine odor memory in individuals with AD. Kesslack et al. demonstrated that patients with AD were significantly impaired on a delayed-match-to-sample discrimination task involving novel olfactory stimuli *(30)*, a task that involves a short-term or working-memory component. On the sample phase, subjects were presented with an odor. Then, following a delay, the subject was presented with three odors. One of the odors was the same as the sample odor and the other two were distractors. The subject was asked to report which of the three odors was the same as the odor presented during the sample phase. Impaired remote memory for odors also has been shown in AD patients as well as in patients with questionable AD *(25,31)*. Remote memory was measured by familiarity ratings for odors and visual stimuli. Patients with AD rated odors, but not visual stimuli, as less familiar than did controls.

Multiple studies have shown that AD is associated with deficits in recognition memory for olfactory stimuli *(23,25,32)*. Nordin and Murphy showed that recognition memory for odors was significantly impaired in subjects with questionable AD *(25)*. Furthermore, subjects with AD committed significantly more false-positive errors for olfactory stimuli than did controls. Another group of researchers demonstrated that although there were detectable differences in odor discrimination between AD patients and elderly controls, the latter outperformed AD patients on a recognition memory test for odors *(33)*. Furthermore, feedback was shown to enhance the memory performance in the control group but did not benefit patients with AD *(33)*.

Impaired odor fluency has also been reported to be associated with AD *(34)*. Subjects were presented with an odor and then asked to report all of the odors associated with the odor stimulus. When they were able to identify an odor, more exemplars were generated than when a subject was unable to identify it. This finding is consistent with the hypothesis that a semantic network for olfactory information is damaged in AD.

Based on the aforementioned data, it has been suggested that recognition memory and identification of odors may be more affected than memory for visual stimuli even very early in the progression of AD and therefore may contribute to an early diagnosis of this disease *(35)*.

OLFACTORY PROCESSING IN INDIVIDUALS AT RISK FOR AD

Multiple risk factors have been identified for AD, including positive family history, age, Down's syndrome, mutations of the presenilin-1 and -2 genes found on chromosomes 14 and 1, respectively, and the e4 allele of the apolipoprotein E (ApoE) gene. The gene for ApoE is localized on the proximal long arm of chromosome 19q in a region that has previously been shown to be linked to late-onset familial AD. ApoE is a lipoprotein involved in lipid transport and is found throughout the brain and cerebral spinal fluid. ApoE has been shown to bind to soluble and insoluble forms of Aβ, which is the principal component of neuritic plaques found in the brains of patients with AD. Three different isoforms of ApoE have been identified, including the e2, e3, and e4 allele. The presence of at least one e4 allele has been associated with both familial and sporadic AD. The identification of the e4 allele provided one genetic risk factor for sporadic AD. The e4 allele has been shown to be more common in subjects with AD compared to the general population.

A number of studies have examined olfactory function in individuals at risk for AD. A study conducted by Devanand et al. showed that patients with mild cognitive impairment (MCI), who demonstrated low scores on the UPSIT odor identification test, were more likely to develop AD at a 2-year follow-up than patients with higher scores *(36)*. Patients with low olfactory scores, who did not report an awareness of olfactory loss, were particularly at risk *(36)*. Schiffman et al. have shown that individuals at risk for AD, based on multigenerational evidence of family history (multiplex families), were impaired relative to controls in odor detection and odor memory *(37)*. However, the study did not find a difference in olfactory function based on ApoE status in individuals with a family history of AD. Other studies have shown that the e4 allele may be linked to deficits in olfactory functioning. A recent study examined odor threshold the year preceding a change in diagnosis from normal control to AD *(38)*. The results indicated that individuals with the e4 allele showed greater impairments in odor threshold compared to e4-negative individuals.

A recent study assessed odor identification in nondemented individuals who were at risk for AD by virtue of the e4 allele *(39)*. The results indicated that odor identification was impaired in individuals with the e4 allele compared to e4-negative controls. This finding suggests that impairments in odor identification may be present during the preclinical, silent stage of AD.

The early deficits on odor identification tests may be due to early neuropathological changes in the entorhinal cortex. A recent study also demonstrated that the e4 allele was associated with deficits in odor identification in individuals with MCI *(40)*. Therefore, odor identification tests may be of clinical utility in early assessment and diagnosis of AD. Additional studies also have shown that the presence of the e4 allele may be associated with impaired olfactory processing in nondemented elderly individuals at risk for AD. A longitudinal study conducted by Graves et al. also demonstrated relationships among the e4 allele, cognitive decline, and olfactory dysfunction *(41)*. Individuals who were anosmic when first examined were documented to be twice as likely to show cognitive decline over a 2-year period than normosmics. However, e4-positive anosmics showed a 5 times greater risk of cognitive decline compared to that of e4-negative normosmics *(41)*. The results demonstrate that the presence of the e4 allele both in AD patients and in individuals at risk for AD may be associated with impaired olfactory processing. The results also suggest that impairments in olfactory processing may be associated with future cognitive decline, particularly in individuals with the e4 allele. Furthermore, the finding that nondemented, elderly e4-positive individuals at risk for AD show impaired odor identification, a measure of remote memory for odors, suggests that memory tasks involving olfactory stimuli may be useful in the early detection of AD.

OLFACTORY EVENT-RELATED BRAIN POTENTIALS IN AD

Event-related potentials (ERP) directly measure the ongoing electrical activity of the brain. Early components of the ERP (e.g., N1) are considered to be more exogenous measures that reflect the processing of the stimulus by auditory cortex *(42)*. The P300 (P3) component is more endogenous and cognitive in nature. The later P3 component is considered to reflect the ability to attend to and evaluate a stimulus *(43,44)* and its latency is considered to be a measure of stimulus classification speed *(42,45)*. The P3 is typically elicited during the "oddball" paradigm, in which a standard stimulus with a high probability of occurrence is presented along with a target stimulus with a low probability of occurrence. The processing of the target stimulus (the "oddball") elicits the P3. Early studies suggested abnormal P3 activity in an auditory "oddball" paradigm in patients with AD and that the latency and amplitude of the P3 might be associated with the degree of dementia *(46–48)*. Because AD disrupts brain connectivity and communication, the ERP might be expected to reflect the neuropathology of the disease. Findings from the auditory ERP have been mixed, with some suggestion of delayed latency and smaller amplitude of the P3 component in AD patients, although the magnitude of the reported effects has been variable *(49–53)* and the sensitivity and specificity of the measures for clinical diagnosis has been debated *(52,54,55)*.

Because the effects of the disease on the olfactory system are profound, Morgan and Murphy investigated the possibility that olfactory ERPs may show greater disruption in patients with AD *(56)*. Techniques for recording the olfactory ERP (OERP) recently have been developed *(57–61)*. Olfactory stimuli elicit the same waveform components (N1, P2, N2, and P3) as auditory and visual stimuli in ERP paradigms. Morgan and Murphy reported significantly longer OERP latencies in AD patients than in age- and gender-matched normal controls *(56)*. These latencies were associated with dementia status, and correctly classified up to 92% of participants. The olfactory ERP proved to be more sensitive at correctly classifying AD patients and controls than the auditory ERP. When results of AD patients and controls on an odor identification test (the San Diego Odor Identification Test) and the OERP P3 latency were combined, the combination resulted in a correct classification rate of 100%. The consonance of these findings with the psychophysical results discussed above suggests that the OERP and psychophysical measures of olfactory function in AD are particularly sensitive to the neuropathology in brain regions vulnerable to the disease.

CONCLUSION

The vulnerability of the olfactory system to the neuropathological changes associated with AD is profound. Patients with AD show marked impairment in odor threshold, odor identification, odor memory, and olfactory event-related potentials. The association of olfactory impairment with

AD suggests the potential clinical utility of including olfactory tasks in the assessment battery for detection of AD.

SUMMARY

The earliest neuropathological changes associated with Alzheimer's disease (AD) are observed in the areas of the brain central to olfactory processing. As a result, the assessment of olfactory function in AD patients and those at risk for the disease is of great theoretical importance and may be potentially useful in the diagnosis. AD has been shown to be associated with impairments in odor threshold, odor identification, odor memory, and odor fluency. Individuals genetically at risk for AD and those with a positive family history of the disease also show impaired olfactory function. In this chapter we reviewed studies conducted to assess olfactory function in patients with AD and those at risk for the disease. Some measures of olfactory function may detect impairments earlier than others. Furthermore, impairments on some measures have been shown to increase as a function of increasing age and may be related to the onset of dementia. The results suggest the use of olfactory measures in test batteries designed for the early detection of AD.

ACKNOWLEDGMENTS

We gratefully acknowledge Drs. Robert Katzman, Leon Thal, and David Salmon for access to patients, and we thank the patients and staff of the UCSD Alzheimer's Disease Research Center and the participants and staff of the SDSU Lifespan Human Senses Laboratory for their participation. Supported by National Institutes of Health grants AG04085 and DC02064 to CM and training grant DC00032 to T. M. Davidson (PG).

REFERENCES

1. Braak, H.; Braak, E.: Frequency of stages of Alzheimer's-related lesion in different age categories. Neurobiol Aging 1997; 18: 351–357.
2. Esiri, M.M.; Wilcox, G.K.: The olfactory bulbs in Alzheimer's disease. J Neurol Neurosurg Psychiatry 1984; 47: 56–60.
3. Price, J.L. et al.: The distribution of tangles, plaques and related immunohistochemical markers in early aging and Alzheimer's disease. NeurobiolAging 1991; 12: 295–312.
4. Van Hoesen, G.W.; Solodkin, A.: Cellular and systems neuroanatomical changes in Alzheimer's Disease. Ann NY Acad Sci 1994; 747: 12–35.
5. McKhann, G. et al.: Clinical diagnosis of Alzheimer's disease: report of the NINCDS-ADRDA Work Group under the auspices of Department of Health and Human Services Task Force on Alzheimer's Disease. Neurology 1984; 34: 939–944.
6. Khachaturian, Z.S.: Diagnosis of Alzheimer's disease. Arch Neurol 1985; 42: 1097–1105.
7. Mirra, S.S. et al.: The Consortium to Establish a Registry for Alzheimer's Disease (CERAD). Part II. Standardization of the neuropathologic assessment of Alzheimer's disease. Neurology 1991; 41: 479–486.
8. Morgan, C.D.; Nordin, S.; Murphy, C.: Odor identification as an early marker for Alzheimer's disease: impact of lexical functioning and detection sensitivity. J Clin Exp Neuropsychol 1995; 17: 793–803.
9. Gomez-Isla, T.: Profound loss of layer II entorhinal cortex neurons occurs in very mild Alzheimer's disease. J Neurosci 1996; 16: 4491–4500.
10. Hyman, B.T.: The neuropathological diagnosis of Alzheimer's disease: clinical-pathological studies. Neurobiol Aging 1997; 18: S27–S32.
11. Braak, H.; Braak, E.: Neuropathological stageing of Alzheimer-related changes. Acta Neuropathol 1991; 82: 239–259.
12. Braak, H. et al.: Pattern of brain destruction in Parkinson's and Alzheimer's diseases. J Neural Transmission 1996; 103: 455–490.
13. Morris, J.C. et al.: Cerebral amyloid deposition and diffuse plaques in "normal" aging: evidence for presymptomatic and very mild Alzheimer's disease. Neurology 1996; 46: 707–719.
14. Doty, R.L.: Olfactory dysfunction in neurodegenerative disorders. In: Getchell, T.V. et al. (eds.): Smell and taste in health and disease. Raven Press, New York: 1991: 735–751.
15. Koss, E. et al.: Olfactory detection and recognition in Alzheimer's disease. Lancet 1987; 1: 622.
16. Serby, M. et al.: Olfaction in dementia. J Neurol Neurosurg Psychiatry 1985; 48: 848–849.
17. Rezek, D.L.: Olfactory deficits as neurological sign in dementia of the Alzheimer's type. Arch Neurol 1987; 44: 1030–1032.
18. Murphy, C.: Loss of olfactory function in dementing disease. Physiol Behav 1999; 66: 177–182.

19. Doty, R.L. et al.: Development of the University of Pennsylvania Smell Identification Test: a standardized microencapsulated test of olfactory function. Physiol Behav 1984; 32: 489–502.

20. Murphy, C. et al.: Psychophysical assessment of chemosensory disorders in clinical populations. In: Kurihara K. (ed.): ISOT XI. Springer-Verlag, Berlin, 609–613.

21. Braak, H.; Braak, E.: The human entorhinal cortex: normal morphology and lamina-specific pathology in various diseases. Neurosci Res 1992; 15: 6–31.

22. Ekman, G.et al.: Perceived intensity of odor as a function of time of adaptation. Scand J Psychol 1967; 8: 177–186.

23. Knupfer, L.; Spiegel, R.: Differences in olfactory test performance between normal aged, Alzheimer, and vascular type dementia individuals. Int J Geriatr Psychiatry 1986; 1: 3–14.

24. Murphy, C. et al.: Olfactory thresholds are associated with degree of dementia in Alzheimer's disease. Neurobiol Aging 1990; 11: 465–469.

25. Nordin, S.; Murphy, C.: Impaired sensory and cognitive olfactory function in questionable Alzheimer's disease. Neuropsychology 1996; 10: 113–119.

26. Feldman, J.I. et al.: The rhinologic evaluation of Alzheimer's disease. Laryngoscope 1991; 101: 1198–1202.

27. Cain, W.S. et al.: Evaluation of olfactory dysfunction in the Connecticut Chemosensory Clinical Research Center. Laryngoscope 1984; 98: 83–88.

28. Hummel, T. et al.: "Sniffin' sticks": olfactory performance assessed by the combined testing of odor identification, odor discrimination and olfactory threshold. Chem Senses 1997; 22: 39–52.

29. Davidson, T.M.; Murphy, C.: Rapid clinical evaluation of anosmia. Arch Otolaryngol Head Neck Surg 1996; 123: 591–594.

30. Kesslack, J.P. et al.: Olfactory tests as possible probes for detecting and monitoring Alzheimer's disease. Neurobiol Aging 1988; 9: 399–403.

31. Niccoli-Waller, C.A. et al.: Remote odor memory in Alzheimer's disease: deficits as measured by familiarity. J Adult Development 1999; 6: 131–136.

32. Moberg, P.J. et al.: Olfactory recognition: differential impairments in early and late Huntington's and Alzheimer's disease. J Clin Exp Neuropsychol 1987; 9: 650–664.

33. Hughes, L.F. et al.: Olfaction in elderly and patients with Alzheimer's disease: differing feedback conditions. J Alzheimer's Dis 2001; 3: 367–375.

34. Bacon-Moore, A.S.; Paulsen, J.S.; Murphy, C.: A test of odor fluency in patients with Alzheimer's and Huntington's disease. J Clin Exp Neuropsychol 1999; 21: 341–351.

35. Nordin, S.; Murphy, C.: Odor memory in normal aging and Alzheimer's disease. Ann N Y Acad Sci 1998; 855: 686–693.

36. Devanand, D.P. et al.: Olfactory deficits in patients with mild cognitive impairment predict Alzheimer's disease at follow-up. Am J Psychiatry 2000; 157: 1399–1405.

37. Schiffman, S.S. et al.: Taste, smell and neuropsychological performance of individuals at familial risk for Alzheimer's disease. Neurobiol Aging 2002; 23: 397–404.

38. Bacon, A.W. et al.: Very early changes in olfactory functioning due to Alzheimer's disease and the role of apolipoprotein E in olfaction. Ann N Y Acad Sci 1998; 855: 723–731.

39. Murphy, C. et al.: Apolipoprotein E status is associated with odor identification deficits in non-demented older persons. Ann N Y Acad Sci 1998; 855: 744–750.

40. Wang, Q. et al.: (2002). Olfactory identification and apolipoprotein E e4 allele in mild cognitive impairment. Brain Res 2002; 951: 77–81.

41. Graves, A.B. et al.: Impaired olfaction as a marker for cognitive decline. Neurology 1999; 53: 1480–1487.

42. Polich, J.: Cognitive brain potentials. Am Psychol Soc 1993; 2: 175–179.

43. Kramer, A.F.; Strayer, D.L.: Assessing the development of automatic processing: an application of dual-task and event-related brain potential methodologies. Biol Psychol 1988; 26: 231–267.

44. Wickens, C. et al.: Performance of concurrent tasks: a psychophysiological analysis of the reciprocity of information-processing resources. Science 1983; 221: 1080–1082.

45. Donchin, E.; Coles, M.G.: Is the P300 component a manifestation of context updating? Behav Brain Sci 1988; 11: 357–427.

46. Goodin, D.S.; Squires, K.C.; Starr, A.: Long latency event-related components of the auditory evoked potential in dementia. Brain 1978; 101: 635–648.

47. Squires, K.C. et al.: Electrophysiological assessment of mental function in aging and dementia. In: Poon, L.W. (ed.): Aging in the 1980s: selected contemporary issues in the psychology of aging. American Psychological Association, Washington, DC, 1980: 125–134.

48. Pfefferbaum, A. et al.: Clinical application of the P3 component of event-related potentials. Electroencephalogr Clin Neurophysiol 1984; 59: 85–103.

49. Filipovic, S. et al.: Auditory event-related potentials in different types of dementia. Eur Neurol 1990; 30: 189–193.

50. Verleger, R.; Koempf, D.; Neukaeter, W.: Event-related EEG potentials in mild dementia of Alzheimer type. Electroencephalogr Clin Neurophysiol 1992; 84: 332–343.

51. O'Mahony, D. et al.: Primary auditory pathway and reticular activating system dysfunction in Alzheimer's disease. Neurology 1994; 44: 2089–2094.

52. Cohen, R.A. et al.: ERP indices and neuropsychological preformance as predictors of functional outcome in dementia. J Geriatr Psychol Neurol 1995; 8: 217–225.
53. Yamaguchi, S. et al.: Event-related brain potentials in response to novel sounds in dementia. Clin Neurophysiol 2000; 111: 195–203.
54. Goodin, D.S.: Clinical utility of long latency "cognitive" event-related potentials (P3): the pros. Electroencephalogr Clin Neurophysiol 1990; 76: 2–5.
55. Pfefferbaum, A.; Ford, J.M.; Kraemer, H.C.: Clinical utility of long latency "cognitive" event-related potentials (P3): the cons. Electroencephalogr Clin Neurophysiol 1990; 76: 6–12.
56. Morgan, C.D.; Murphy, C.: Olfactory event-related potentials in Alzheimer's disease. J Int Neuropsychol Soc 2002; 8: 753–763.
57. Kobal, G.; Hummel, T.; Van Troller, S.: Differences in human chemosensory evoked potentials to olfactory and somatosensory chemical stimuli presented to left and right nostrils. Chem Senses 1992; 17: 233–244.
58. Murphy, C. et al.: Olfactory-evoked potentials: assessment of young and elderly, and comparison to psychophysical threshold. Chem Senses 1994; 19: 47–56.
59. Pause, B.M. et al.: The nature of the late positive complex within the olfactory event-related potential (OERP). Psychophysiology 1996; 33: 376–384.
60. Morgan, C.D. et al.: The olfactory P3 in young and older adults. Psychophysiology 1999; 36: 281–187.
61. Murphy, C. et al.: Olfactory event-related potentials and aging: normative data. Int J Psychophysiology 2000; 36: 133–145.

V Treatment Options

19

Treatment of Alzheimer's Disease
Basic Considerations

Brigitte Zoeller Richter and Ralph W. Richter

INTRODUCTION

Alzheimer's disease (AD) is a slow progressive disease, starting with mild memory disturbances and ending with severe destruction of certain brain areas. The course of the disease varies individually. AD patients may live from 4 years and in rare cases as many as 20 years. The main problems that evolve in later stages of AD include difficult-to-treat behavioral changes, which frequently require the patient to be placed in a nursing home.

HOW TO TREAT AD

AD is not yet curable; no pharmacological treatment can now stop the degenerative process. Certain drugs, however, are available now that are assumed (from controlled clinical trials) to delay deterioration for a maximum of 24 months. These drugs have mostly been tested in mild to moderately affected patients, that is, in the earlier and middle stages of AD. Most effective to date, according to the results of clinical trials, are acetylcholinesterase inhibitors (AChEI). Four such agents currently are approved: tacrine (Cognex[R], not used any longer because of severe side effects), donepezil (Aricept[R]), rivastigmine (Exelon[R]), and galantamine (Reminyl[R]). Clinical trials with these established medications are ongoing.

Some patient in the earlier stages of AD might receive benefit in the areas of cognition from additional ginkgo medication, others from vitamin E administration. Data to support their efficacy, however, are relatively weak.

Many other compounds and therapeutic strategies are currently under investigation, either in animal models or in clinical trials. There is also extensive testing of preventative strategies. Drugs that are thought to be of benefit in AD from observational studies include nonsteroidal anti-inflammatory drugs (NSAIDs), lipid-lowering agents (so-called statins), estrogen, nootropics, neuroprotective compounds, vitamins, herbal/plant medicines, and nutrients/nutraceuticals. For these potential medications, however, there is yet no evidence for significant beneficial effects in randomized controlled trials in AD patients. Other promising clinical trials are underway. The results are being awaited impatiently by the research community as well as by AD patients and their caregivers.

It is important in the treatment of AD not to forget to include complementary options, such as mental training, physical exercise, or sensory stimulation and regular leisure activity. These measures often appear to be beneficial for managing behavioral problems. Aromatherapy and bright light therapy are alternative interventions currently under investigation for the management of behavioral and psychological symptoms *(1)*.

From: *Current Clinical Neurology,*
Alzheimer's Disease: A Physician's Guide to Practical Management
Edited by: R. W. Richter and B. Zoeller Richter © Humana Press Inc., Totowa, NJ

TREATMENT PLAN

Once the clinical diagnosis of AD has been made, it is useful to develop a treatment plan—which is done in close communication with the patient, the caregiver, and other family members. Future perspectives should be discussed and treatment goals defined. According to the overall medical status, the stage of the disease, and the neuropsychiatric behavioral changes, the most adequate medications are then chosen.

The pharmacological and nonpharmacological treatment should address cognitive deficits, psychiatric and mood disorders, as well as co-morbid illnesses. Guidelines for the management of AD patients in the primary-care setting are now available *(2)*.

REFERENCES

1. Burns, A. et al.: Sensory stimulation in dementia (editorial). Br Med J 2002; 325: 1312–1313.
2. Cummings, J.L. et al.: Guidelines for managing Alzheimer's disease. Part II. Treatment. Am Fam Physician 2002; 65: 2525–2534.

20

Donepezil in Treatment of AD

Ging-Yuek Robin Hsiung and Howard Feldman

INTRODUCTION

Donepezil is the second cholinesterase inhibitor to have become commercially available. It is considered a "second-generation" acetylcholinesterase inhibitor (AChEI) because of its safety profile with clear advantages over the acridine-based cholinesterase inhibitor tacrine, the first AChEI approved for symptomatic treatment of Alzheimer's disease (AD). Because of considerable toxicity, tacrine is no longer used since the advent of the second generation of AChEIs.

Donepezil is a piperidine derivative and acts as a noncompetitive reversible AChEI. The compound is highly selective for acetylcholinesterase (AChE), which is the predominant cholinesterase in the brain *(1)*.

PHARMACOKINETICS

After oral administration, peak plasma donepezil concentration is achieved within 3–5 hours. Absorption is not affected by food. Under clinical trials condition, mean trough plasma drug concentration are 25.9 ± 0.7 µg/L with therapeutic doses of 5 mg/day, and 50.6 ± 1.9 µg/L at 10 mg/d *(2)*. A plateau effect of acetylcholinesterase inhibition (80–90%) in red blood cells is reached at concentrations higher than 50 µg/L. Donepezil is highly protein bound in plasma (total 96%; 75% to albumin and 21% to α-glycoprotein) *(3)*. Steady-state pharmacokinetics are achieved in about 2–3 weeks after daily administration *(4)*.

Donepezil is predominantly metabolized in the liver by CYP2D6, CYP3A4, and UDP-glucuronosyl transferase, and undergoes extensive first-pass metabolism. It does not significantly affect the metabolism of other drugs metabolized by the cytochrome P450 system, such as cimetidine, digoxin, furosemide, theophylline, and warfarin. However, donepezil metabolism is inhibited by ketoconazole and quinidine, and caution is warranted when concurrent use of these drugs is considered *(5)*.

It is noteworthy that the half-life of donepezil is significantly longer (104 vs 60 hours) in the elderly (over 65 years of age) compared to young adults (20–27 years), but the area under the curve and clearance do not differ significantly between the two age groups *(5)*. In turn, no dosage adjustments are necessary in the elderly population.

Donepezil elimination is not affected by renal or hepatic impairment, but the peak concentration is 37.5% higher in patients with impaired liver function. Thus, close monitoring for adverse effects is needed for hepatic patients.

EFFICACY

To date, the efficacy of donepezil on symptomatic management of AD has been demonstrated in 10 randomized double-blind placebo-controlled clinical trials (Level 1 evidence) *(2,6–14)*. However,

From: *Current Clinical Neurology,*
Alzheimer's Disease: A Physician's Guide to Practical Management
Edited by: R. W. Richter and B. Zoeller Richter © Humana Press Inc., Totowa, NJ

the primary outcome measure is not uniform across these studies. Eight trials have focused on mild to moderate-severity AD patients *(2,6,8–12,14)*, whereas two trials have aimed at moderate to severe patients *(7,13)*. The main characteristics and findings of each trial are summarized in Table 1.

Short-Term (12–24 Weeks) Studies of Mild to Moderate AD Patients (MMSE 10–26)

In the initial safety and efficacy study, donepezil at doses of 1, 3, and 5 mg was compared with placebo over a 12-week double-blind phase followed by a 2-week single-blind placebo washout phase *(8)*. A total of 161 patients entered the study, and 141 completed treatment. The improvements in cognition as measured on the Alzheimer Disease Assessment Scale—cognitive subscale (ADAS-cog) were significantly greater in subjects treated with 5 mg/d than in those given placebo *(15)*. There was also a significant correlation between plasma concentration of donepezil and AChE inhibition. The incidence of adverse effects with all three dosages of donepezil (66–68%) was comparable to that observed with placebo (65%).

Subsequently, four placebo-controlled, multicenter clinical trials were conducted using a double-blind, parallel-group design to examine the effect of 5–10 mg/d of donepezil in mild to moderate (MMSE 10–26) AD patients *(2,6,9,10)*. Two studies were conducted in the United States, another international study was conducted in European countries, Canada, and New Zealand, and one was conducted in Japan.

In the 12-week U.S. study, 468 patients were randomized to three groups receiving placebo, 5 mg or 10 mg of donepezil per day *(2)*. Ninety-seven percent of the patients were included in the intention-to-treat analysis of all randomized subjects. The mean drug–placebo improvements for the 5-mg/day and 10-mg/day groups, respectively, were 2.5 and 3.1 units ($p < 0.001$) on the ADAS-cog, and 1.0 and 1.3 units on the MMSE ($p < 0.008$). On assessment of global functioning by the Clinician's Interview Based Impression of Change-plus scale (CIBIC+) *(16)*, 32% and 38% of patients, treated with 5 and 10 mg/day of donepezil, respectively, demonstrated clinical improvement at the approved study endpoint at 12 weeks compared with placebo (18%).

In the 24-week U.S. study, 473 subjects were randomized to treatment with placebo ($n = 162$), 5 mg/day donepezil ($n = 154$), or 10 mg/day donepezil ($n = 157$) *(9)*. Cognition and global function both significantly benefited from 5- and 10-mg/day donepezil treatment compared to placebo at weeks 12, 18, and 24. The mean drug–placebo differences on the ADAS-cog were 2.49 and 2.88 for the 5- and 10-mg/day groups, respectively ($p < 0.00001$). Significant improvements were also noted in both the 5- and 10-mg/day donepezil treatments on the CIBIC+ scale, first evident at week 12 and persistent to the end of treatment at week 24 ($p < 0.005$).

In the international study of 818 patients with the same study design, similarly consistent results were found *(6)*. At endpoint, the donepezil vs placebo differences in ADAS-cog scores in least-square (LS) means were 1.5 and 2.9 points for the 5- and 10-mg/day donepezil groups, respectively. There were statistically significant greater numbers of donepezil-treated patients judged clinically improved on the CIBIC+ scale as compared to placebo. In this study, the Clinical Dementia Rating Scale (CDR) *(17)* sum of the boxes score was also used as a secondary outcome to measure a composite of cognitive and functional performance rating. There was significant benefit with donepezil treatment at week 12, 18, 24, and study endpoint ($p < 0.05$).

In the study performed in Japan, 268 patients were randomized to placebo and 5 mg/day of donepezil *(10)*. Using an intention-to-treat analysis, there was a 2.32-point improvement ($p < 0.001$) on the Japanese version of ADAS-cog (ADAS-J-cog) in the donepezil group compared to placebo. The improvement rates (percentage of slightly improved or better) as measured with the Japanese version of the Clinical Global Impression of Change (J-CGIC) *(18)* were 52% and 22% ($p < 0.001$, U-test) in the donepezil and placebo groups, respectively.

In a study by Greenberg and colleagues, a randomized, placebo-controlled, double-blind crossover design was used *(12)*. Sixty subjects with probable AD and scores of 20 or less on the information-memory-concentration subscale of the Blessed Dementia Scale (BDS) *(19)* received placebo wash-in, followed in randomized sequence by (1) 5 mg/day donepezil therapy for 6 weeks, followed by placebo wash-out for 6 weeks, and (2) placebo treatment for 6 weeks. During donepezil therapy, ADAS-cog score improved by 2.17 units ($p = 0.04$) relative to placebo. However, there was no associated change in caregiver-rated global impression or on specific tests of explicit memory or verbal fluency. In this study, the presence of ApoEe4-allele did not predict treatment response.

Medium-Term Studies (1 Year) of Donepezil in Mild to Moderate AD

Two studies have been performed to examine the medium-term effects of donepezil compared with placebo over the course of 1 year. The study by Mohs and colleagues used a survival design in a double-blind, prospective, placebo-controlled, parallel group trial to evaluate the primary outcome measure of "time to clinically evident decline in function" *(11)*. The criteria for clinically evident decline in function was defined as any one of the following: (1) a clinically evident decline in the ability to perform one or more basic activities of daily living (ADL) from the AD functional assessment and change scale (ADFACS) *(20,21)* present at baseline, excluding a decline from 0 (no impairment) to 1 (mild impairment), which was not considered clinically significant; (2) a clinically evident decline in ability to perform 20% or more of the instrumental ADL in the ADFACS present at baseline, excluding a decline from 0 (no impairment) to 1 (mild impairment), which was not considered clinically significant; (3) an increase in global CDR (clinical dementia rating) *(22)* score of 1 point or more compared with baseline. The median time to clinically evident functional decline was 208 days (95% CI: 165, 252) for the placebo group, and 357 days (95% CI: lower limit 280) for donepezil-treated patients. The Kaplan-Meier survival curves were significantly different, favoring donepezil, by log-rank ($p = 0.0019$) and Wilcoxon ($p = 0.0051$) test results. The probability of survival with no clinically evident functional decline for donepezil-treated patients at 48 weeks was 51% (95% CI: 43, 58) compared with 35% (95% CI: 27, 42) in the placebo group. The hazard ratio for reaching endpoint (donepezil/placebo) was 0.62.

In the study by Winblad and colleagues, 286 subjects from five Northern European countries with possible or probable AD were randomized to receive either donepezil or placebo for 1 year *(14)*. The primary outcome measure was the Gottfries-Bråne-Steen scale (GBS) *(23,24)*, a global assessment for rating dementia symptoms. Significant differences in favor of donepezil over placebo were demonstrated at weeks 24, 36, and 52 by mean change from baseline on the GBS total score. As a secondary outcome measure, the mean change from baseline MMSE total scores was significantly different at weeks 24, 36, and 52, favoring the donepezil-treated group. Treatment response was not predicted by ApoE genotype or sex in this population.

Studies Including Moderate to Severe AD Patients

Two clinical trials have investigated the efficacy of donepezil in more advanced AD. In the study reported by Feldman and colleagues, 290 patients with moderate to severe AD (MMSE scores 5–17) were randomized to receive donepezil (5 mg/day for the first 28 days and 10 mg/day thereafter as per the clinician's judgment) or placebo *(7)*. The primary outcome measure was the CIBIC+. Significant clinical improvements were noted in the donepezil-treated group compared with placebo at week 4 ($p < 0.008$) and persisted at week 8, 12, 18, and 24. With last observation carried forward analysis at week 24, 63% of donepezil- and 42% of placebo-treated patients were rated as improved or no change ($p < 0.0001$). Significant differences favoring donepezil were also seen in a number of secondary measures, with mean difference of 1.79 ($p < 0.0001$) on MMSE, 5.62 ($p < 0.0001$) on the Severe Impairment Battery (SIB) *(25)*, 8.23 ($p < 0.0001$) on the Disability Assessment for Dementia scale (DAD) *(26)*, and 5.64 ($p = 0.005$) in the Neuropsychiatric Inventory total score (NPI) *(27)*.

In a study by Tariot and colleagues in nursing-home patients with possible or probable AD or AD with cerebrovascular disease (MMSE range 5–26), 208 patients were randomized to receive donepezil

Table 1
Summary of Randomized Controlled Trials of Donepezil on Alzheimer's Disease

Study	Location	Design	Duration (wk)	Dosing (mg/day)	Inclusion MMSE	Subjects	Primary outcome measure(s)	Main findings Donepezil vs placebo difference
Rogers et al., 1996 (8)	Multicenter U.S.	Double-blind, placebo-controlled, parallel-group	12	1, 3, 5	10–26	161	ADAS-cog	1 mg/day 1.6, NS; 3 mg/day 2.1, $p < 0.05$; 5 mg/day 3.2, $p < 0.01$
							CGIC	Donepezil 5 mg/day/d vs placebo, $p < 0.05$
Rogers et al., 1998 (2)	Multicenter U.S.	Double-blind, placebo-controlled, parallel-group	12	5, 10	10–26	468	ADAS-cog	5 mg/day 2.5, 95% CI 3.59–1.29; 10 mg/day 3.1, 95% CI 4.22–1.92
							CIBIC+	Combine donepezil groups vs placebo, $p < 0.05$; NS between 5 and 10 mg/day of donepezil
Rogers et al. 1998 (9)	Multicenter U.S.	Double-blind, placebo-controlled, parallel-group	24	5, 10	10–26	473	ADAS-cog	5 mg/day 2.49, $p < 0.0001$; 10 mg/day 2.88, $p < 0.0001$
							CIBIC+	Combinedonepezil groups vs placebo, $p < 0.05$
Burns et al., 1999 (6)	Multicenter Europe, Canada, and New Zealand	Double-blind, placebo-controlled, parallel-group	24	5, 10	10–26	818	ADAS-cog	5 mg/day 1.5, $p = 0.002$; 10 mg/day 2.9, $p < 0.001$
							CIBIC+	Combine donepezil groups vs placebo, $p < 0.05$; NS between 5 and 10 mg/day of donepezil
Grenberg et al., 2000 (12)	Two-center U.S.	Double-blind, placebo-controlled, crossover	6 + 6	5	21.8 ± 13.7	60	ADAS-cog	2.17 (SE 0.98)

Homma et al., 2000 (10)	Multicenter Japan	Double-blind, placebo-controlled, parallel-group	24	5	10–26	268	ADAS-J-cog	Protocol compatible 2.44, $p = 0.003$ ITT analysis 2.32, $p < 0.001$ Donepezil 5 mg/day vs placebo, $p < 0.05$; no difference betwen PC and ITT analyses
Mohs et al., 2001 (11)	Multicenter U.S.	Double-blind, placebo-controlled, parallel-group	54	5–10	12–20	431	Survival from functional decline at 48 wks	Probability of no clinically evident functional loss = 51% in donepezil vs 35% placebo, $p = 0.002$
Winblad et al., 2001 (14)	Multicenter Scandinavia and Netherlands	Double-blind, placebo-controlled, parallel-group	52	5–10	10–26	286	Gottfries-Bråne-Steen scale	Favor donepezil at 24, 36, and 52 wks $p < 0.05$
Feldman et al., 2001 (7)	Multicenter Canada, France, and Australia	Double-blind, placebo-controlled, parallel-group	24	5–10	5–17	290	CIBIC+	Favor donepezil up to 24 wks $p < 0.001$, and at 24 wks last observation carried forward, $p < 0.0001$
Tariot et al., 2001 (13)	Multicenter U.S. nursing home patients	Double-blind, placebo-controlled parallel-group	24	5–10	5–26	208	NPI-NH	NS

NS, not significant.

or placebo *(13)*. The primary outcome measure was the NPI-NH 12-item total score, a modified version of the Neuropsychiatric Inventory for use with nursing-home residents *(28)*. Both groups improved relative to baseline, with no significant differences observed between the groups at any assessment. In some planned secondary outcome analyses, the mean change from baseline CDR-SB improved significantly with donepezil compared with placebo at week 24 ($p < 0.05$), and differences in mean change from baseline on MMSE favored donepezil over placebo at weeks 8, 16, and 20 ($p < 0.05$).

Longer-Term Efficacy

At the moment, there have been no randomized placebo-controlled clinical trials of donepezil in AD longer than 1 year yet published. Most of the available longer-term data derive from comparisons of open-label treatment with observational cohort or modeled data. A study by Doody and colleagues showed a slower rate of symptomatic decline in subjects treated continuously with donepezil for up to 2.8 years *(29)*. Recent data suggest that there is a delay to nursing-home placement for individuals treated with donepezil continuously over periods of up to 70 months *(30)*. There have not yet been any randomized studies addressing mortality rates and long-term treatment with donepezil. However, an observational study by López and colleagues did not find any differences in AChEI vs non-AChEI subjects in mortality rates *(31)*.

SAFETY PROFILE OF DONEPEZIL

In general, donepezil was quite well tolerated across all of the clinical trials, with adverse events usually transient and of mild to moderate severity. The highest frequency of adverse events were reported by Feldman and colleagues, with 83% of the donepezil group and 80% of the placebo group experiencing adverse events *(7)*. However, the majority of them were rated mild in severity. Eight percent of donepezil and 6% of placebo-treated patients discontinued because of adverse events. In the study by Burns and colleagues, higher incidences of nausea, vomiting, diarrhea, and central nervous disturbances (such as dizziness, confusion, insomnia) were noted in patients receiving 10 mg/d donepezil compared with those receiving 5 mg/d donepezil or placebo *(6)*. These adverse effects were not unexpected for a cholinomimetic drug, and most resolved without the need for change of treatment or withdrawal.

CONCLUSION

There is convincing and quite consistent data demonstrating the efficacy of donepezil in delaying cognitive decline and improving global functioning in patients with mild to moderate AD for at least 1 year. From uncontrolled data it is suggested that benefits may extend for a number of years and with a possible delay in the time to nursing-home placement. There is some emerging evidence also for the utility of donepezil in the more advanced stages of AD. Further confirmatory studies will be required by the regulatory authorities before the current labeled indication can be expanded beyond the score range of 10–26 on the MMSE.

Looking forward, the potential utility of donepezil in the symptomatic management of patients with mild cognitive impairment (MCI) has been considered. Currently, a large multicenter clinical trial by the Alzheimer Disease Study Cooperative Group is being undertaken to examine this option. In addition, some encouraging preliminary data have been presented from clinical trials with donepezil in the treatment of vascular dementia, Lewy body dementia, and AD associated with Down's syndrome. Forthcoming publications of these studies are anticipated. There have also been some publications reporting the pharmacoeconomic benefit of donepezil treatment in AD *(32,33)*. The acceptance of donepezil into clinical practice has been quite promising in allowing improved symptomatic management of AD patients.

SUMMARY

Donepezil, a piperidine derivative, is the second acetylcholinesterase inhibitor (AChEI) to become commercially available for treatment of AD. To date, 10 randomized clinical trials have been conducted on donepezil. Its efficacy in mild to moderate AD has been consistently demonstrated, and its utility in moderate to severe AD has also been suggested. Its benefit may last up to one year or longer. It has a long half-life and requires only once-a-day dosing. Although side effects are common, which include nausea, vomiting, diarrhea, dizziness, and sleep disturbances, they are generally mild and most resolve without need for change of treatment or withdrawal. Donepezil represents an important clinical advance in the symptomatic management of patients with AD.

REFERENCES

1. Dooley, M.; Lamb, H.M.: Donepezil: a review of its use in Alzheimer's disease. Drugs Aging 2000; 16: 199–226.
2. Rogers, S.L. et al.: Donepezil improves cognition and global function in Alzheimer disease: a 15-week, double-blind, placebo-controlled study. Donepezil Study Group. Arch Intern Med 1998; 158: 1021–1031.
3. Barner, E.L.; Gray, S.L.: Donepezil use in Alzheimer disease. Ann Pharmacother 1998; 32: 70–77.
4. Rogers, S.L. et al.: Pharmacokinetics and pharmacodynamic profile of donepezil HCl following multiple oral dose. Br J Clin Pharmacol 1998; 46: 7–12.
5. Jann, M.W.; Shirley, K.L.; Small, G.W: Clinical pharmacokinetics and pharmacodynamics of cholinesterase inhibitors. Clin Pharmacokinet 2002; 41: 719–739.
6. Burns, A. et al.: The effects of donepezil in Alzheimer's disease—results from a multinational trial. Dement Geriatr Cogn Disord 1999; 10: 237–244.
7. Feldman, H. et al.: A 24-week, randomized, double-blind study of donepezil in moderate to severe Alzheimer's disease. Neurology 2001; 57: 613–620.
8. Rogers, S.L.; Friedhoff, L.T.: The efficacy and safety of donepezil in patients with Alzheimer's disease: results of a US multicentre, randomized, double-blind, placebo-controlled trial. The Donepezil Study Group. Dementia 1996; 7: 293–303.
9. Rogers, S.L. et al.: A 24-week, double-blind, placebo-controlled trial of donepezil in patients with Alzheimer's disease. Donepezil Study Group. Neurology 1998; 50: 136–145.
10. Homma, A. et al.: Clinical efficacy and safety of donepezil on cognitive and global function in patients with Alzheimer's disease. A 24-week, multicenter, double-blind, placebo-controlled study in Japan. E2020 Study Group. Dement Geriatr Cogn Disord 2000; 11: 299–313.
11. Mohs, R.C. et al.: A 1-year, placebo-controlled preservation of function survival study of donepezil in AD patients. Neurology 2001; 57: 481–488.
12. Greenberg, S.M. et al.: Donepezil therapy in clinical practice: a randomized crossover study. Arch Neurol 2000; 57: 94–99.
13. Tariot, P.N et al.: A randomized, double-blind, placebo-controlled study of the efficacy and safety of donepezil in patients with Alzheimer's disease in the nursing home setting. J Am Geriatr Soc 2001; 49: 1590–1599.
14. Winblad, B. et al.: A 1-year, randomized, placebo-controlled study of donepezil in patients with mild to moderate AD. Neurology 2001; 57: 489–495.
15. Rosen, W.G.; Mohs, R.C.; Davis, K.L.: A new rating scale for Alzheimer's disease. Am J Psychiatry 1984; 141: 1356–1364.
16. Schneider, L.S. et al.: Validity and reliability of the Alzheimer's Disease Cooperative Study-Clinical Global Impression of Change. The Alzheimer's Disease Cooperative Study. Alzheimer's Dis Assoc Disord 1997; 11: S22–S32.
17. Berg, L. et al.: Mild senile dementia of the Alzheimer type. 4. Evaluation of intervention. Ann Neurol 1992; 31: 242–249.
18. Guy, W.: Clinical global impressions (CGI). In Guy, W. (ed.), ECDEU assessment manual for psychopharmacology, revised. Alcohol Drug Abuse and Mental Health Administration, NIMH Psychopharmacology Research Branch, Division of Extramural Research Programs, Rockville, MD, 1976.
19. Blessed, G.; Tomlinson, B.E.; Roth, M.: The association between quantitative measures of dementia and of senile change in the cerebral grey matter of elderly subjects. Br J Psychiatry 1968; 114: 797–811.
20. Lawton, M.P.; Brody, E.M.: Assessment of older people: self-maintaining and instrumental activities of daily living. Gerontologist 1969; 9: 179–186.
21. Schmeidler, J.; Mohs, R.C.; Aryan, M.: Relationship of disease severity to decline on specific cognitive and functional measures in Alzheimer's disease. Alzheimer's Dis Assoc Disord 1998; 12: 146–151.
22. Morris, J.C.: The Clinical Dementia Rating (CDR): current version and scoring rules. Neurology 1993; 43: 2412–2414.
23. Gottfries, C.G. et al.: A new rating scale for dementia syndromes. Arch Gerontol Geriatr 1982; 1: 311–330.
24. Bråne, G.; Gottfries, C.G.; Winblad, B.: The Gottfries-Bråne-Steen scale: validity, reliability and application in anti-dementia drug trials. Dement Geriatr Cogn Disord 2001; 12: 1–14.

25. Panisset, M. et al.: Severe impairment battery. A neuropsychological test for severely demented patients. Arch Neurol 1994; 51: 41–45.
26. Gélinas, I. et al.: Development of a functional measure for persons with Alzheimer's disease: the disability assessment for dementia. Am J Occup Ther 1999; 53: 471–481.
27. Cummings, J.L. et al.: The Neuropsychiatric Inventory: comprehensive assessment of psychopathology in dementia. Neurology 1994; 44: 2308–2314.
28. Wood, S. et al.: The use of the neuropsychiatric inventory in nursing home residents. Characterization and measurement. Am J Geriatr Psychiatry 2000; 8: 75–83.
29. Doody, R.S. et al.: Open-label, multicenter, phase 3 extension study of the safety and efficacy of donepezil in patients with Alzheimer disease. Arch Neurol 2001; 58: 427–433.
30. McRae, T. et al.: Donepezil delays time to nursing home placement in patients with Alzheimer's disease. J Am Geriatr Soc 2001; 49: 132.
31. Lopez, O.L. et al.: Cholinesterase inhibitor treatment alters the natural history of Alzheimer's disease. J Neurol Neurosurg Psychiatry 2002; 72: 310–314.
32. Small, G.W.; Donohue, J.A.; Brooks, R.L.: An economic evaluation of donepezil in the treatment of Alzheimer's disease. Clin Ther 1998; 20: 838–850.
33. Wimo, A. et al.: An economic evaluation of donepezil in mild to moderate Alzheimer's disease: results of a 1-year, double-blind, randomized trial. Dement Geriatr Cogn Disord 2003; 15: 44–54.

21

Rivastigmine for Treatment of AD

Martin R. Farlow

INTRODUCTION

Alzheimer's disease (AD), the most common form of dementia in persons over the age of 65 years, is a progressive neurodegenerative disease of the central nervous system that is clinically characterized by memory impairment and other cognitive disturbances. The disease also causes declines in function in activities of daily living (ADL), behavior, and personality. The costs in the United States of this illness are estimated to exceed $100 billion.

Neuropathologically, AD is characterized by loss of neurons, extracellular amyloid plaques, and intracellular neurofibrillary tangles. Some regions of the brain are affected earlier and more severely than others, with the cholinergic system (basalis and septal nuclei and their projections to many areas of the cortex) being affected most prominently. The cholinergic hypothesis suggests that associated deficits in levels of the neurotransmitter acetylcholine are responsible for much of the learning and memory difficulties that are the most prominent symptoms in AD. Therapeutic approaches have focused on improving cholinergic function to potentially reverse these deficits. Drugs that block the enzyme acetylcholinesterase (AChE) have been proven in clinical trials to have significant beneficial effects in patients with AD. They have become the standard of care for the treatment of cognitive and functional deficits in patients with mild to moderate-stage AD. Rivastigmine, a cholinesterase inhibitor with unique pharmacological properties, has proven effective in the treatment of AD symptoms. The agent may delay symptomatic or biological progression of the disease.

PHARMACOLOGY

Rivastigmine is a cholinesterase inhibitor that reversibly covalently bonds to sites in the enzymatic clefts of both acetylcholinesterase and butyrylcholinesterase (1). AChE is the predominant enzyme at the synapse that breaks down acetylcholine (ACh). It is produced predominantly in neurons; levels of this enzyme decline as the illness progresses (2). Inhibition of AChE is the major mechanism by which rivastigmine and the other cholinesterase inhibitors are thought to act.

Butyrylcholinesterase (BuChE) also degrades acetylcholine, but is produced mainly by glial cells (3), though recent studies suggest that BuChE-predominant neurons are found commonly in the amygdala and hippocampus (areas known to be prominently affected by AD) (4). As AD progresses, BuChE levels increase rather than decrease, and the additional enzyme has been suggested to increase cholinergic deficits and consequent cognitive symptoms. BuChE has also been found to decorate neuritic amyloid plaques, and it has been proposed that this enzyme may play a role in the transformation of diffuse amyloid deposits to more compact, fibrillary plaques (5).

Studies in aged rats have suggested that AChE-specific and BuChE-specific inhibitors each will independently improve learning and memory in aged rats (6). Studies examining levels of AChE inhi-

From: *Current Clinical Neurology,*
Alzheimer's Disease: A Physician's Guide to Practical Management
Edited by: R. W. Richter and B. Zoeller Richter © Humana Press Inc., Totowa, NJ

bition and BuChE inhibition measured in CSF obtained by indwelling lumbar catheter at different time points have suggested that improvements in cognitive functioning after rivastigmine dosing actually correlate more closely with BuChE inhibition *(7)*.

Another differentiating pharmacological characteristic of rivastigmine is that it binds predominantly to the G1 forms of both AChE and BuChE *(8)*. In normal adults the G4 form of this enzyme is prominent in the brain. In AD, however, levels of G4 decline markedly in the cortex and basalis nucleus, such that G1 levels become equal or higher *(9)*. Interestingly, the G4 form of the enzyme remains predominant in the basal ganglia, as well as in cardiac and other peripheral organ systems. This may explain why rivastigmine has little action at these sites, giving potential advantage for fewer adverse cardiac effects and or less potential to exacerbate extrapyramidal symptoms in patients with Parkinson's dementia or diffuse Lewy body disease *(10)*.

Rivastigmine bonds covalently at the active site in a cleft in the cholinesterase enzymes, so the half-life of cholinergic inhibition is determined by the rate at which this bond breaks down (9 hours), rather than the half-life in plasma (60–90 minutes). Breaking of this covalent bond is the first and most significant step in the metabolism, as the metabolite is not processed further via cytochrome P450 enzymes in the liver (like the other cholinesterase inhibitors), but rather is excreted unchanged by the kidney. The relatively short half-life of rivastigmine in plasma and the absence of liver metabolism explain the lack of reported drug–drug interactions, with none being seen between rivastigmine and 22 other therapeutic classes of drugs *(11)*.

With a 9-hour half-life of cholinergic inhibition, rivastigmine is administered twice daily (bid). It is recommended that the drug be given after meals. Food significantly increases the time to maximum concentration while simultaneously decreasing the maximum concentration, but actually increasing the area under the curve, potentially increasing pharmacological effects while decreasing side effects *(12)*.

The starting oral dose is 1.5 mg bid for 1 month, after which the patient should be increased to 3 mg bid, which is a therapeutically effective dose. Patients may then be electively uptitrated on a monthly basis to 4.5 mg bid or to a maximum oral dose of 6 mg bid. The potential for greater efficacy as well as the risk for adverse effects increases with the total daily dosage and patients should be individually titrated to the level where clinical benefits are greatest and adverse effects are least.

CLINICAL EFFICACY

Four large, double-blind, placebo-controlled, 26-week trials with rivastigmine in more than 3000 patients with mild to moderate-stage AD have demonstrated consistent benefits in measures of cognition, global functioning, and activities of daily living *(13,14)*.

Cognition was assessed using the ADAS-cog, which measures memory, praxis, and language, and which was previously proven to be a reliable test in mild to moderate-stage patients with AD *(15)*. The magnitude of improvement in ADAS-cog scores in patients treated with 6–12 mg/day of rivastigmine vs placebo in the U.S. study (699 patients) was the largest reported in a cholinesterase inhibitor trial in AD—4.9 points. As comparison, the expected rate of deterioration in ADAS-cog would be 7–11 points per year. Interestingly, deterioration in the placebo group (reflecting natural progression rate) was somewhat greater than seen in other trials, which may have contributed to the apparent large magnitude of cognitive benefit. The ADAS-cog was given at screen before baseline in this trial, and drug dose was flexibly titrated up to the maximum tolerated dose or 12 mg/day in each patient. These differences may have increased the effect size. A consequence of this maximum-tolerated-dose approach was increased side effects, particularly during titration. The three other pivotal trials, which were conducted internationally, also showed significant benefits with rivastigmine in ADAS-cog, but of lesser magnitude.

Global function was assessed by the clinician interview-based impression of change test with caregiver input (CIBIC+), in which an experienced clinician evaluated cognition, function in ADL, and psychiatric and behavioral symptoms by interviewing the patient and the caregiver. With these data, global change from baseline was assessed using a 7-point scale *(16)*. Clinically significant therapeutic effects with rivastigmine were seen in these trials for patients in the 6–12 mg/day group *(13,14)*.

ADL in these trials were assessed by the progressive deterioration scale (PDS), an instrument filled out by the caregiver, which assesses a variety of instructional and basic ADL that are known to deteriorate during mild to moderate-stage AD *(17)*. Function in ADL for the 6–12 mg/day rivastigmine-treated groups was significantly preserved during each of these four large trials, with minimal change from baseline, while placebo groups deteriorated significantly.

It should be noted that in the three different domains of cognition, global functioning, and function in ADL, individuals showed considerable variability in their response to rivastigmine. Improvement in cognition did not always correlate with improvements in global functioning or change in ADL. Response probably should not be judged by change in a single domain such as cognition as assessed by the Mini-Mental State Examination (MMSE). In the pooled data for these studies, 30–55% of patients had stabilization or improvement in any one domain, but overall 86% had a beneficial response in one or more domains *(18)*.

Behavioral change was not one of the principal outcomes measured in the original rivastigmine trials in mild to moderate-stage AD. However, later studies have strongly suggested that this drug improves or delays onset of psychiatric symptoms and or behavioral abnormalities, with beneficial effects being demonstrated in a large open nursing-home trial of rivastigmine in patients with AD and in a double-blind, placebo-controlled trial of patients with diffuse Lewy body disease *(19,20)*.

RESPONDER ANALYSES

Patients with moderate-stage disease were more likely to show significant improvements than those with milder-stage disease as measured by change in cognition (ADAS-cog) and ADL (PDS), but not global functioning (CIBIC+) or disease stage (global deterioration scale, GDS) *(21)*.

A more rapid rate of decline in placebo patients during the initial double-blind phase, as measured by ADAS-cog and PDS in the rivastigmine trials, predicted larger response to rivastigmine therapy when the patients started the medication during the following open-label phase *(22)*. This finding suggests that patients with more rapidly progressive symptoms may be more likely to respond to rivastigmine. Patients with vascular risk factors (Hachinski score 1–4; predominantly history of hypertension) also responded significantly better to rivastigmine than patients with Hachinski ischemia score of 0 *(23)*. Demographic variables (age, gender, ethnicity) and ApoE status were not predictors of drug response (M. Mullan, ApoE and Rivastigmine Subgroup, personal communication, 2001; ref. *13*).

DURABILITY OF BENEFITS AND EFFECTS
ON LONGER-TERM DISEASE PROGRESSION

Ethical concerns about denying effective therapy probably preclude trials of longer than 26 weeks, which were not conducted during the initial development program that led to approval of this drug by the Food and Drug Administration (FDA) *(24)*. However, rivastigmine appears to have beneficial effects that persist for at least 2 years, as demonstrated by follow-up studies of over 2000 patients who participated in the original double-blind trials *(25)*.

Patients treated with 6–12 mg/day of rivastigmine showed significantly less deterioration on the ADAS-cog at 52 weeks than would be expected for projected decline for patients on placebo, with the difference increasing by 104 weeks. The U.S. 26-week, double-blind, placebo-controlled trial with its 6-month extension was also analyzed together to approximate a delayed-start trial design *(26)*. The delayed-start trial design has been suggested as a means for demonstrating whether a drug delays disease progression *(27)*. If rivastigmine delayed disease progression, treated patients should deteriorate less during the first 6 months on therapy as compared to those on placebo. Differences between these groups would not resolve in the next 6 months, when both groups of patients were taking rivastigmine. In the U.S. trial, patients originally on placebo responded well to rivastigmine, but never caught up on either cognitive or ADL measures, when compared to those taking rivastigmine from the start of the trial. These results suggest a possible effect of rivastigmine on disease progression.

Patients with AD in the U.S. trial who dropped out before the end of the trial were urged to return for cognitive assessments at the 26-week end time point, even though they had been off study medication for various periods of time. Retrieved patients who had been on rivastigmine deteriorated statistically significantly less, as measured by ADAS-cog, compared to subjects who were on placebo *(28)*. The less severe deterioration after withdrawal of treatment suggests an effect on disease progression.

The original pivotal trials of rivastigmine included only patients with mild to moderate-stage AD. Rivastigmine has recently been assessed for clinical utility in more severe-stage nursing-home patients *(19)*. Preventing psychiatric or behavioral problems at this point in the illness may be clinically more important than improving cognitive function. The neuropsychiatric inventory (NPI) is an instrument with which the caregiver rates the frequency and severity of behavioral and psychiatric symptoms along several domains during the preceding 2 weeks *(29)*. In a large open study of nursing-home patients receiving rivastigmine and repeatedly evaluated using this instrument, significant stabilization and/or improvement in behavioral symptoms were seen at both 26 and 52 weeks *(19)*. Over half of these patients achieved a 30% or greater improvement in their NPI ratings. These findings are even more remarkable because the natural history of AD is for psychiatric symptoms to increase with disease progression. Significant reductions in the use of psychotropic medications, particularly in the use of atypical antipsychotics for agitation, hallucinations, and delusions, were also documented corresponding with these improvements in behavior *(30)*.

Another retrospective subanalysis determined the rate of disease progression for up to 3 years (change in ADAS-cog scores over time) in more than 2000 AD patients who participated in the open-label trials of rivastigmine that followed the original four double-blind pivotal trials *(31)*. Patients were grouped into those taking less than 6 mg per day of rivastigmine and those taking 6 mg/day or more of the drug. Patients taking 6 mg/day or more had 50% less deterioration compared to those maintained on lower dosages, suggesting longer-term effects on the disease beyond immediate symptomatic behavior. As in any retrospective analysis, an unknown factor might create bias between the groups. Nonetheless, these data further suggest a disease progression-delaying effect for rivastigmine.

SAFETY AND TOLERABILITY

The original rivastigmine therapeutic trials in AD utilized a maximum-tolerated dosage design *(13,14)*. Patients were uptitrated on drug dose until either side effects occurred or until a dosage of 12 mg/day was achieved. Using this approach to titration, adverse effects in the 6-month pivotal trials were significantly higher for the 6–12-mg/day group vs placebo, with side effects including nausea (48%), vomiting (27%), and anorexia (20%) *(13,14)*. Most of the drug-related adverse effects occurred during titration (34%), vs a much lower rate during maintenance on stable drug dosage (13%). Adverse gastrointestinal effects generally occurred within the first one or two doses after uptitration. They were usually transient and self-limited. In these studies, 13% of rivastigmine patients discontinued due to adverse effects, compared to 4% of patients on placebo. Later studies have demonstrated a considerable reduction in side effects when uptitration is slowed to monthly and rivastigmine is taken only after full meals. Clinically significant beneficial effects are seen at dosages of 6 mg/day and higher. For patients who stop drug for 1 week or longer, it is recommended that they retitrate up to their therapeutic dose, since tolerability of immediately reinstituting high-dose therapy is unknown.

Follow-up assessments of patients, at 26 weeks, who had discontinued rivastigmine for various reasons at earlier times during the four large double-blind, placebo-controlled trials have not revealed any evidence of accelerated deterioration or support for withdrawal syndrome *(28)*.

SUMMARY

Rivastigmine is both an acetylcholinesterase and a butyrylcholinesterase inhibitor, designed to treat symptoms of AD. Four large double-blind, placebo-controlled trials of 26 weeks duration in over 3000 patients have demonstrated that it improves cognition, global functioning, and ability to perform activities of daily living relative to placebo. Rivastigmine has a half-life at the synapse of 9 hours, so dosing is twice daily. Metabolism of this drug occurs at the synapse rather than in the liver, minimizing the potential for drug–drug interactions. Therapy is initiated at 1.5 mg per os twice daily, with the drug taken after meals. The first titration at 1 month is up to 3.0 mg per os twice daily. Potential adverse effects are nausea, vomiting, and diarrhea, which are most likely to occur during the titration phase. There is the option of further dose increases, if there are no adverse symptoms, to 4.5 mg per os twice daily and/or up to 6.0 mg per o.s. twice daily, with the higher dosage providing greater benefits in some patients. The effectiveness of rivastigmine was originally demonstrated in 6-month trials in patients with mild to moderate-stage disease. Recent studies, however, suggest continued effectiveness for patients followed up to 3 years and in more severely affected nursing-home patients, where the most clinically significant effects may be reduction in new psychiatric and or behavioral symptoms.

REFERENCES

1. Weinstock, M. et al.: Pharmacological activity of novel anticholinesterase agents of potential use in the treatment of Alzheimer disease. In: Fisher, A.; Hanin, I.; Lachman, P. (eds.): Advances in behavioral biology, Vol 29. Plenum Press, New York, 1986: 539–549.
2. Perry, E.K. et al.: Changes in brain cholinesterases in senile dementia of Alzheimer type. Neuropath Appl Neurobiol 1978; 4: 273–277.
3. Guillozet, A.L. et al.: Butyrylcholinesterase in the life cycle of amyloid plaques. Ann Neurol 1997; 42: 909–918.
4. Darvesh, S.; Grantham, D.L.; Hopkins, D.: Distribution of butyrylcholinesterase in human amygdala and hippocampal formation. J Comp Neurol 1988; 393: 374–390.
5. Guillozet, A.L. et al.: Butyrylcholinesterase in the life cycle of amyloid plaques. Ann Neurol 1997; 42: 909–918.
6. Greig, G.H. (personal communication) 2003.
7. Giacobini, E. et al.: Inhibition of acetyl and butyric-cholinesterase in the cerebrospinal fluid of patients with Alzheimer's disease by rivastigmine: correlation with cognitive benefit. J Neural Transmission 2002; 109: 1053–1065.
8. Enz, A.; Chappuis, A.; Probst, A.: Different influence of inhibitors on acetylcholinesterase molecular forms G1 and G4 isolated from Alzheimer's disease and control brains. In: Shafferman, A., Velan, B. (eds.): Multidisciplinary approaches to cholinesterase functions. Plenum Press, New York, 1992: 243–249.
9. Siek, G.C. et al.: Molecular forms of acetylcholinesterase in subcortical areas of normal and Alzheimer disease brain. Biol Psychol 1990; 27: 573–580.
10. Enz, A. et al.: Brain selective inhibition of acetylcholinesterase: a novel approach to therapy for Alzheimer's disease. Prog Brain Res 1993; 98: 431–438.
11. Grossberg, G.T. et al.: Lack of adverse pharmacodynamic drug interactions with rivastigmine and twenty-two classes of medications. Int J Geriatr Pscychol 2000; 15: 242–247.
12. Farlow, M.R.: Do cholinesterase inhibitors slow progression of Alzheimer disease? Int J Clin Pract 2002; suppl 127: 1–5.
13. Schneider, L.S.; Anand, R.; Farlow, M.R.: Systematic review of the efficacy of rivastigmine for patients with Alzheimer's disease. Int J Geriatr Psychopharmacol 1998; 1: S2–S6.
14. Rosler, M. et al.: Efficacy and safety of rivastigmine in patients with Alzheimer's disease: international randomized controlled trial. Br Med J 2001; 318: 633–638. [Erratum Br Med J 2001; 322: 1456.]
15. Rosen, W.G.; Mohs, R.C.; Davis, K.L.: A new rating scale for Alzheimer's disease. Am J Psychiatry 1984; 141: 1356–1364.
16. Reisberg, B. et al.: Clinical global measures of dementia. Alzheimer's Dis Assoc Disord 1997; 11: 8–18.
17. Dejong, R.; Osterlund, O.W.; Roy, G.W.: Measurement of quality-of-life changes in patients with Alzheimer disease. Clin Therapeut 1989; 11: 545–554.
18. Farlow, M.R.; Anand, R.; Hartman, R.: Response to rivastigmine treatment in the key domains of Alzheimer's disease. Proc Am Psychiatric Assoc 2001: 208.
19. Edwards, K. et al.: Flexible titration reduces side effects of rivastigmine. Proc Am Ass Geriatr Psychiatry 2001.
20. McKeith, I. et al.: Efficacy of rivastigmine in dementia with Lewy bodies: a randomized, double blind, placebo-controlled international study. Lancet 2000; 356: 2031–2036.
21. Farlow, M.R. et al.: Moderate Alzheimer's disease is responsive to therapy with rivastigmine. Neurology 2003; in press.

22. Farlow, M.R. et al.: Response of patients with Alzheimer disease to rivastigmine treatment is predicted by the rate of disease progression. Arch Neurol 2001; 58: 417–422.

23. Kumar, V. et al.: An efficacy and safety analysis of Exelon in Alzheimer's disease with concurrent vascular risk factors. Eur J Neurol 2000; 7: 159–169.

24. Kawas, C.H. al.: Clinical trials in Alzheimer's disease: the debate on the use of placebo controls. Alzheimer's Dis Assoc Disord 1999; 13: 124–129.

25. Farlow, M.R.; Messina, J.; Anand, R.: Long-term cognitive benefits associated with the use of rivastigmine in the treatment of Alzheimer's disease: Results following two years of treatment. Proc Am Geriatric Assoc 2000; 172: 396.

26. Farlow, M.R. et al.: A 52-week study of the efficacy of rivastigmine in patients with mild to moderately severe Alzheimer's disease. Eur Neurol 2000; 44: 236–241.

27. Leber, P.: Slowing the progression of Alzheimer disease: methodologic issues. Alzheimer's Dis Assoc Disord 1997; 11 (suppl 5): 10–21.

28. Anand, R.: Analysis of outcome of patient dropouts originally treated with rivastigmine versus placebo in a 26-week, Alzheimer's disease trial. Neurology 2001; 56 (Suppl 3): A339.

29. Cummings, J.L.: The neuropsychiatric inventory: assessing psychopathology in dementia patients. Neurology 1997; 48 (5 Suppl 6): S10–S16.

30. Messina, J. et al.: Evaluation of the changes in concomitant psychotropic medications for patients with Alzheimer's disease treated with rivastigmine in a long-term care setting. Proc Third Int Meeting College Psychiatric Neurologic Pharmacists, Washington, DC, April 16–19, 2002.

31. Farlow, M. et al.: Dose dependent effect of rivastigmine on progression of cognition deterioration in Alzheimer's disease. Sixth Int Stockholm/Springfield Symp on Advances in Alzheimer Therapy, Stockholm, Sweden, 2000.

22

Galantamine in Treatment of AD

M. Saleem Ismail and Pierre N. Tariot

INTRODUCTION

The cholinergic hypothesis proposes that well-defined deficits in cholinergic neurotransmission contribute to cognitive dysfunction in Alzheimer's disease (AD), and that enhancing cholinergic transmission will lead to improved outcome *(1)*. Several acetylcholinesterase inhibitors (AChEI) have been approved during the past few years on the basis of clinical trials, demonstrating that these agents improve or maintain cognitive function in patients with possible AD. Thus far all AChEI have been shown to be efficacious as a class and are considered a mainstay of AD treatment. Galantamine is the newest member of this class of agents at present.

PHARMACOLOGY

Galantamine (Table 1) is a reversible, weakly competitive inhibitor of acetylcholinesterase (AChE), the major enzyme that degrades acetylcholine (ACh). The functional significance of this inhibition is presumed to be slowed breakdown of ACh, increased concentration within the synaptic cleft, and prolonged physiological effect. Galantamine also allosterically modulates nicotinic acetylcholine receptors (nAChR). Allosteric modulators are ligands that interact with receptor-binding sites that are different from those to which the natural agonist binds. Allosteric nicotinic receptor modulation results in increased uptake of components for synthesis of ACh, such as choline and acetic acid, increased packaging and release of ACh, and increased resynthesis of ACh. Through these mechanisms and by enhancing the sensitivity of nAChR to available ACh, galantamine enhances both pre- and postsynaptic cholinergic receptor function. Through its effects on nicotinic receptor modulation, galantamine increases release of other neurotransmitters as well, such as glutamate, serotonin, and γ-aminobutyric acid (GABA), transmitters that may in part mediate the behavioral symptoms of AD.

Nicotinic AChR play an important role in learning and memory *(2)*. A reduction in number of these receptors occurs in patients with AD, particularly in hippocampus and neocortex—regions of the brain that are known to be involved in learning and memory tasks that are fundamentally impaired in AD *(3–6)*. Furthermore, a reduction in number of these receptors in the central nervous system (CNS) is highly correlated with the severity of AD. Studies in animal models, healthy volunteers, and patients with AD have shown that nicotinic agents can improve deficits in memory and psychomotor functions *(7–9)*. These data argue for the importance of nAChR in AD, although the clinical significance of galantamine's action on nAChR is not fully established yet. Since galantamine is a weak inhibitor of AChE, it would seem logical that, at a minimum, its nicotinic effects may contribute to enhanced cholinergic neurotransmission. Both codeine and physostigmine have similar effects, whereas none of the other marketed AChEI do, to our knowledge.

From: *Current Clinical Neurology,*
Alzheimer's Disease: A Physician's Guide to Practical Management
Edited by: R. W. Richter and B. Zoeller Richter © Humana Press Inc., Totowa, NJ

Table 1
Galantamine: Clinical Pharmacology

Pharmacodynamics
    Competitive inhibition of acetylcholinesterase (AChE)
    Allosteric modulation at nicotinic acetylcholine receptors (nAChR)
Phamacokinetics
    Linear elimination kinetics
    Low plasma protein binding
    Metabolized by CY2D6 and CY3A4
    $t_{1/2}$-7-h
    Food delays the rate but not the extent of absorption in healthy individuals
    Available as tablets and oral solution
Clinical use
    Dosing: twice daily
    Starting dose: 8 mg/d
    Lowest effective dose: 16 mg/d
    Maximum: 24 mg/d
    Dose increase schedule: escalate to 16 mg/d after a minimum of 4 wk; a further increase to 24 mg/d may
    be attempted after 4 wk at previous dose
Adverse effects
    Anorexia, weight loss, nausea, syncope, bradycardia;
    exercise special caution in patients with cardiac conduction abnormality and those with a history of peptic
    ulcer disease
Potential drug interactions
    Possible with other cholinergic agents;
    may interfere with action of anticholinergic agents;
    none observed with digoxin or warfarin at therapeutic dose;
    reduce dose when co-administered with paroxetine, ketoconazole, and erythromycin
Hepatic and renal disease
    Mild: no dose adjustment needed, monitor
    Moderate: reduce dose, monitor closely
    Severe: contraindicated

It has been hypothesized that galantamine's effects on nicotinic receptors may also confer neuro-protection by directly stimulating target neurons and indirectly stimulating neighboring neurons *(10)*. There have been suggestions that AChEI and some other cholinergic agents may prevent formation of amyloid and promote normal processing of amyloid precursor protein (APP) *(11)*. It is also possible that stimulation of muscarinic and nicotinic receptors may influence tau phosphorylation, apoptosis, and cell death induced by glutamate *(12,13)*. These findings suggest—but do not prove—that cholinergic therapy, including galantamine, could alter the natural history of AD, but this optimistic view remains speculative *(14)*.

CLINICAL PHARMACOLOGY

Galantamine is absorbed rapidly, has linear pharmacokinetics, and has a half-life of about 7 hours (Table 1). It is metabolized primarily via cytochrome isoenzymes in the liver (CYP2D6 and CYP3A4). A reduction of galantamine dose should be considered when potential CYP2D6 inhibitors such as paroxetine, or CYP3A4 inhibitors such as ketoconazole, are also being administered. Caution is required in patients with hepatic and renal impairment. Galantamine is contraindicated in patients with severe hepatic or renal disease, although no metabolic monitoring is required for other patients on maintenance treatment.

The recommended starting dose is 8 mg/day, a dose not associated with statistically significant improvement in cognitive function compared to placebo, although a trend to this effect is evident in the data. Usual treatment entails an increase to 16 mg/day after 4 weeks. A further increase after another 4 weeks to 24 mg/day is possible, based on clinical assessment of response. Higher doses are usually not well tolerated.

GOALS OF TREATMENT IN AD: REDEFINING TREATMENT SUCCESS

As this class of drugs evolved, regulatory guidelines were adopted that focused primarily on cognitive outcomes but did not necessarily address the ranges of issues that would define clinical practice. The cognitive subscale of the Alzheimer Disease Assessment Scale (ADAS-cog) is the most widely used measure of cognitive function in clinical studies of dementia *(15)*. Compared to other cognitive assessment scales that are used commonly, it is more sensitive to a wider range of disease severity and has greater specificity for the key features of cognitive function in AD.

It has been estimated that after 12 months patients with mild to moderate AD treated with placebo decline by approximately 5–6 points on ADAS-cog *(16)*. For regulatory purposes, clinical trials of AChEI define a "responder" as someone who has an improvement of 4 points on ADAS-cog.

A broader definition of treatment response may provide a richer appreciation of the clinical meaningfulness of AChEI therapy. For example, the progressive nature of AD results in the continued emergence of symptoms, albeit at a slower rate than if patients were not treated. What is the evidence about the effect of treatment over the long haul? Further, behavioral and psychological signs and symptoms occur commonly and adversely affect the quality of life of both patients and caregivers. Behavioral symptoms are also a major determinant of nursing-home placement. New evidence points to a role for impaired cholinergic function in mediating some of the behavioral features of AD as well, further rationalizing efforts to address this aspect of response to therapy *(17,18)*.

Clinical trial programs have begun to address the shortcomings inherent in the initial regulatory trials that were conducted to obtain approval of antidementia therapies. Newer studies examine effects of treatment on behavioral problems, on rate of decline in performance of activities of daily living (ADL), on quality of life, and on caregiver burden. As greater social and economic burdens are imposed on society due to the increased prevalence of this chronic illness, pharmacoeconomic benefits of treatment have also become an important goal of study as well as treatment.

In general, the effectiveness, rather than simply the efficacy, of these agents approved as "cognitive enhancers" is being assessed using complex outcomes that more meaningfully address broader potential benefits for patients, caregivers, and society. With this context in mind, the evidence regarding efficacy and effectiveness of galantamine will be reviewed.

EVIDENCE FROM CLINICAL TRIALS

The galantamine clinical development program clarified its effective dose range and titration schedule, addressed international regulatory requirements for approval, and incorporated newer outcomes addressing effectiveness of treatment. The efficacy of galantamine for AD has been established in several pivotal trials of up to 6 months duration *(19–23)* (Table 2). More than 3000 patients were enrolled, and some of these trials were followed by open-label treatment up to 1 year. Important but unpublished long-term data (up to 3 years) regarding galantamine treatment in patients with AD has also been presented *(24)*. New information has recently come out about the effects of galatamine in patients with probable vascular dementia and AD plus cerebrovascular disease. These studies, summarized here, firmly established galantamine as a therapeutic option in the treatment of AD.

Effects on Cognitive Function

Findings in four pivotal clinical trials in patients with AD showed that treatment with 16–32 mg/day galantamine for 3–6 months resulted in statistically significant beneficial effects on cognition relative

Table 2
Galantamine: Efficacy in Clinical Trials

Trial	Duration (mo)	N/Dx	Dose regimen	Doses (mg/d)	Efficacy measures[a]							
					ADAS-cog	CIGIC-plus	CIBIC+	NPI	PDS	DAD	ADCS-ADL	Ref.
Wilkinson	3	285	2-wk dose	18	–0.8*	81.6			83.9			22
		AD	escalation	24	–1.9**	77.1			95.4*			
				36	–1.8**	93.1			79.3			
				P	2.3	71.6			78.4			
Rockwood	3	386	Flexible	24–32	–1.1*		80.8*	–0.3		–0.4**		23
		AD	dose	P	0.6		62.6	0.5		–5.2		
Tariot	5	978	4–8 wk	8	0.4		53	2.3			–3.2	19
		AD	escalation	16	–1.4**		66**	–0.1*			–0.7**	
				24	–1.4**		64**	0*			–1.5*	
				P	1.7		49	2			–3.8*	
Wilcock	6	653	Fixed dose	24	–0.6**		65*			–2.7		21
		AD		32	–1.3**		66.8**			–2.4*		
				P	2.2		51.8			–5.8		
Raskind	6	636	Fixed dose	24	–1.9**		73.1*					20
		AD		32	–1.4**		69*					
				P	2		56.7					
Erkinjuntti	6	592	6-wk dose	24	–1.7**		74**	–1.2*		0.2*		26
		VaD, or	escalation to	P	1		59	1		–4.4		
		AD+CVD	24 mg/d									

[a]Expressed as percent of patients showing no change or improvement; *$p < 0.05$; **$p < 0.001$ vs placebo. ADAS-cog, Alzheimer's Disease Assessment Scale—cognitive subscale; ADCS-ADL, Alzheimer's Disease Cooperative Study; AD, Activities of Daily Living; CIBIC+, Clinician's Interview-Based Impression of Change plus caregiver input; CVD, cardiovascular disease; Dx, diagnoses; DAD, Disability Assessment in Dementia; NPI, Neuropsychiatric Inventory; P, placebo; PDS, Progressive Deterioration Scale; VaD, vascular dementia.

to placebo *(19–21,23)*. A mean treatment difference of 3–4 points on the ADAS-cog was seen after treatment periods of up to 6 months, an effect size similar to that seen with other AChEI. Improvements in ADAS-cog scores were maintained above baseline with galantamine treatment of both 5 and 6 months, whereas scores fell significantly below baseline in patients randomized to placebo.

In a multicenter international pivotal trial *(23)*, 386 patients with probable AD and baseline Mini-Mental State Examination (MMSE) of 11–24 were randomized to treatment with placebo ($n = 125$) or galantamine ($n = 261$). The galantamine dose was escalated over 4 weeks to a dose of 24–32 mg/day. At the end of 3 months, treatment with galantamine produced a significantly better outcome on cognitive function—as measured by change in ADAS-cog score—compared to treatment with placebo (treatment difference of 1.9 points on ADAS-cog).

Similar cognitive benefits were seen in a 5-month randomized, placebo-controlled trial with 978 patients *(19)*. This trial employed a 4-week placebo run-in followed by a randomization phase, in which study medication dose was escalated over 4 weeks to a maintenance dose of 8, 16, or 24 mg/day galantamine. Galantamine–placebo differences in mean ADAS-cog change scores were 3.3 points for the 16-mg group and 3.6 points for the 24-mg group, respectively. The 8-mg dose group was included to address possible dose dependency of cognitive effects. Drug–placebo differences in ADAS-cog change were not significant for this dose group, although there was a trend in favor of the drug. These results helped clarify the effective dose range and titration schedule for galantamine.

The results of two randomized 6-month placebo-controlled studies *(20,21)* further reinforced these findings. Pooled efficacy data from these two pivotal trials showed that at 6 months, 24 mg/day galantamine maintained patients' cognitive function above baseline, whereas patients receiving placebo experienced a significant deterioration. These two trials had similar designs and patient populations. Overall, the difference in mean ADAS-cog scores between galantamine- and placebo-treated patients in the pooled analysis was 3.4–3.9 points.

Secondary Analyses of Cognitive Data

Galantamine's effects on cognition were independent of age or sex. In patients with mild and moderate disease, both doses of galantamine (24 and 32 mg/day) were superior to placebo on the ADAS-cog. The benefit was greater, however, for patients with moderately severe disease (baseline MMSE below 18). The presence of one or more apolipoprotein E (ApoE)e4-alleles in patients with AD did not influence treatment response to galantamine—a finding that contrasts with reports from studies of tacrine treatment *(25)*.

Pooled data from the two 6-month double-blind trials have been analyzed in order to clarify the clinical significance of the observed changes in mean ADAS-cog scores. Treatment response in this case was defined as either maintaining cognitive function at baseline or improving it from baseline during the study period. The magnitude of improvement was defined operationally as any (change in ADAS-cog from baseline > 0), moderate (improvements in ADAS-cog > 4), or marked (improvement in ADAS-cog > 7 points). The data showed that patients treated with 24 mg/day galantamine had approximately twice the response rate of placebo-treated patients. Rates of treatment response with 24 mg galantamine were 64.8%, 32.1%, and 16.7% respectively (Reminyl® Product Information). All three responder rates were highly statistically significantly different from rates with placebo treatment. Similar results have been demonstrated with high-dose donepezil treatment (10 mg/day) in patients with AD (Aricept® Product Information).

LONG-TERM COGNITIVE DATA

Given the fact that AChEI are known to be beneficial in patients with AD, prolonged placebo-controlled trials are difficult to conduct for ethical reasons. An alternative strategy to obtain long-term data has been to use open extension studies to provide an estimate of the impact of treatment relative to baseline. The absence of a placebo arm limits the ability to quantify the treatment effect, however. Sometimes other informative methods (though less robust) have been adopted, such as use of historical placebo data for comparison. Another approach is to conduct open treatment studies. These methods are valuable, although such data should be interpreted with caution.

In one study, the 6-month double blind phase was followed by a 6-month open extension period, in which all eligible patients were given 24 mg/day galantamine *(20)*. The investigators remained blinded to the original treatment assignments. By the end of 1 year, the patient group still receiving 24 mg galantamine had not experienced a decline in mean ADAS-cog performance relative to baseline (182/353 = 51.5%). On the other hand, patients who received placebo in the double-blind phase and were then crossed over to open treatment showed the expected initial decline in cognitive performance followed by the expected improvement when galantamine therapy was initiated. However, by the end of 12 months of observation, this group of patients experienced a mean decline of 2.2 points in mean ADAS-cog scores compared to baseline (86/353 = 24.3%). Thus the placebo/galantamine group did not catch up to the level reached by the galantamine/galantamine group, suggesting (but not proving) that delayed therapy might deprive some patients of an optimal long-term response. Interpretation of such data is limited by the fact that dropouts occurred continually in both groups over the 12 months and that testing in the last 6 months was not conducted in a blinded fashion.

COGNITIVE EFFECTS OF GALANTAMINE IN CEREBROVASCULAR DISEASE

In a 6-month, double-blind, placebo-controlled trial, patients with a diagnosis of probable vascular dementia or AD combined with cerebrovascular disease (CVD) were randomly assigned to treatment with 24 mg/day galantamine ($n = 396$) or placebo ($n = 196$). At 6 months, the mean difference in ADAS-cog change scores was 2.7 points ($p < 0.0001$) in patients treated with galantamine (26). The results of the open-label 6-month extension to this trial have recently been presented (27). Continuous treatment with galantamine maintained cognition in patients diagnosed with probable vascular dementia (VaD) or AD plus CVD for at least 12 months. Patients who received continuous galantamine treatment did significantly better than those who received placebo during the placebo-controlled phase, suggesting (but not proving) that early therapy may be beneficial. These data extend our understanding of the potential value of AChEI therapy, although they may not be sufficient to gain regulatory approval for a new indication.

GLOBAL RATINGS

The Clinician's Interview-Based Impression of Change-plus caregiver input (CIBIC+) has been used in AChEI trials for AD following FDA guidelines (28). This yields a global assessment of the patient's behavior, general psychopathology, cognition, and ADL. It asks simply whether the patient has improved, stayed the same, or worsened overall, and is used to validate arithmetic change seen in cognitive test scores.

In clinical trials, CIBIC+ outcomes have been consistently better in patients treated with galantamine compared with those receiving placebo. In a 3-month study, 21% of patients on galantamine deteriorated, compared with 37% of those in the placebo group (23). In the 5-month study, 64–68% of patients in the 16- and 24-mg/day galantamine groups remained stable or improved, compared with 47% of those in the placebo group (19). Similar results were seen in the two 6-month double-blind studies (20,21). In both studies, the effect of galantamine on CIBIC+ rating was significantly better than that of placebo at 6 months (Table 2).

EFFECTS ON DAILY FUNCTION

Functional disability in AD is an important determinant of patient dependence, caregiver burden, and cost of care. A treatment that preserves functional abilities would add to the meaning of successful antidementia therapy. Both short and long-term data point toward a significant benefit on daily function in AD patients treated with galantamine. Historical 12-month placebo data from previous studies in patients with mild to moderate AD indicate that the annual decrease on the disability assessment in dementia (DAD) scale in untreated patients is 11–13 points (29). During 3 months of treatment with galantamine (24–32 mg/day), there was a significant galantamine/placebo difference of 4.3 points in mean change in DAD scores from baseline (23). The 5-month galantamine trial using a different ADL assessment scale (ADCS-ADL) also showed that patients on 16 and 24 mg galantamine had better functional outcomes than those on placebo. Their functional ability was not only preserved (16 mg) over the study period of 5 months, patients treated with both 16 and 24 mg showed a significantly smaller decrease in their mean ADCS-ADL score (indicating benefit) than those treated with placebo (19).

The long-term data suggest sustained functional benefit. Two 6-month placebo-controlled studies followed by 6-month open extension phases have been completed; both had a similar design and patient population. One study has been published and showed that, in contrast to patients who received placebo for the initial 6 months, those who received galantamine continuously for 12 months maintained functional abilities as measured by the DAD (20). Pooled data from both studies have been presented in abstract form (30). Galantamine produced highly statistically significant reductions in functional decline as assessed by the DAD over 12 months compared with a pooled historical placebo group.

In addition to the cognitive benefits described above, patients treated with galantamine also had significant functional benefit compared to those treated with placebo in a 6-month study involving patients with VaD and mixed AD and CVD (26). These data underscore the potential benefit of galantamine in patients with AD who may also have significant vascular disease.

BEHAVIORAL EFFECTS

It is estimated that about 90% of patients with AD develop psychopathological features during the course of illness *(31)*. The emergence of behavioral symptoms has a major impact on caregiver burden and is often the primary reason for nursing-home placement. It is only recently that studies of anti-dementia agents have incorporated behavioral outcomes as efficacy measures.

It has been suggested that galantamine postponed the emergence of behavioral symptoms during the 5-month dose-ranging study *(19)*. Most of the patients enrolled in this study lacked significant psychopathology at baseline. Patients who received 16 and 24 mg/day galantamine maintained baseline levels of behavioral symptoms; that is, they had a reduced likelihood of emergent psychopathology over the trial in comparison to those receiving placebo. This was assessed with the neuropsychiatric inventory (NPI). Among the NPI items, the galantamine effect was greatest for symptoms of aberrant motor behavior, anxiety, disinhibition, and hallucinations. An earlier 3-month efficacy study did not show any change in the mean NPI scores from baseline for both the galantamine and placebo groups *(23)*. A secondary analysis of patients with VaD or those with AD and CVD showed that galantamine treatment was associated with significantly better outcome on the NPI than treatment with placebo (2.2 points, $p < 0.018$) *(32)*.

It is not clear to what extent there is clinically meaningful behavioral benefit in patients using AChEI *(33)*. Favorable effects appear to fit two basic patterns: delay of emergent psychopathology in patients who lack behavioral problems to begin with, as described above, or a reduction of some behavioral symptoms when present *(34)*. The data available are encouraging, and are consistent with what we see in clinical practice. More long-term peer-reviewed studies, however, are needed before definitive conclusions are possible.

CAREGIVER-RELATED BENEFITS

The amount of time spent by caregivers assisting patients with AD and the amount of time caregivers spent supervising patients was evaluated in a clinical trial using a caregiver time questionnaire *(21)*. The average daily time spent by caregivers increased steadily over time for placebo-treated patients, reaching an additional 23 minutes by month 6, while the average time caregivers spent each day assisting patients with AD decreased relative to baseline by 15–38 minutes for patients treated with galantamine. Similarly, the time caregivers spent supervising patients increased gradually relative to baseline with placebo, reaching an additional 2 hours by month 6. However, there was no significant change in supervision time from baseline with galantamine (24 and 32 mg/day) *(35)*. These encouraging preliminary findings bear more detailed examination as well as replication. *(36)*.

EFFECTS ON RESOURCE UTILIZATION

Public health models of clinical research emphasize inclusion of resource utilization outcomes to assess direct and indirect savings from treatment. One of these models adapted to Canada compared treatment with galantamine vs no pharmacological intervention. Galantamine treatment has been shown to reduce the period full-time care (FTC) was required by 10% in patients with mild to moderate AD. This study predicted a cost saving ranging from $US528 per patient with mild to moderate AD to $US2533 per patient for moderate AD *(37)*. There is further evidence that cognitive enhancement treatment in AD results in substantial economic benefits *(38)*. Such findings predict that AD patients treated with pharmacological agents will remain at home longer or will require briefer periods of full-time care while at home. This view is also supported by observational data from an open-label trial of tacrine treatment in AD that suggested a delay to nursing-home placement *(14,39)*.

SAFETY AND TOLERABILITY

In clinical trials of galantamine, higher rates of treatment discontinuation were seen with more rapid titration (for example, 1–2 weeks) compared to slower schedules (4–6 weeks). Similarly, adverse events occurred at higher frequencies during the dose-escalation phase compared to fixed dose-maintenance phase (42% vs 16%) *(20)*. As expected in studies of cholinergic treatments, most common adverse events of galantamine therapy included gastrointestinal side effects. These events were generally described as mild to moderate, although significantly more patients discontinued due to nausea and vomiting than due to other adverse events. Headache, dizziness, diarrhea, anorexia, and weight loss are also among the side effects seen in these studies. A mean body weight decline of 2.1 to 2.5 kg was reported in galantamine-treated patients, compared to a slight increase in weight (0.1 kg) in the placebo group *(20)*. Reports of muscle weakness on galantamine treatment were rare and no more common than on placebo. Rarer events, such as syncope, can occur with this and other AChEI, although precise frequency estimates are not available. There were no clinically relevant differences among treatment groups in vital signs other than weight, laboratory values, or EKG measures.

It appears that the tolerability of galantamine improved with duration of treatment, and no unexpected adverse events were seen in patients who continued to receive galantamine in extension phase following 6 months of double-blind treatment. During the extension phase of one of the pivotal trials of galantamine *(20)* 10.6% of patients experienced nausea, 9.2% had diarrhea, and 6.9% reported dizziness. Sixteen percent of patients in the extension phase withdrew due to adverse events, compared to 23% of those who received 24 mg of galantamine in the double-blind phase.

Available evidence favors a slower titration of galantamine over an 8-week period to therapeutic dose of 24 mg/day. Although patients in the low-dose galantamine group experienced fewer side effects than those receiving 16 or 24 mg/day, a dose lower than 16 mg is considered ineffective. Available data do not conclusively show a dose–response effect with galantamine at higher dose range, as a dose of 32 mg/day produced substantially higher rate of adverse events—without significant differences in outcome efficacy measures. Most of the adverse events seen in patients receiving galantamine are expected from cholinergic stimulation and have been reported in studies of other AChEI, albeit with some apparent differences in their frequency *(40)*.

SUMMARY

Clinical trials conducted according to regulatory guidelines for antidementia therapy have shown that galantamine is a safe and effective treatment for AD. Specifically, modest improvement in cognitive performance relative to placebo has been demonstrated in clinical trials up to 6 months in duration. The clinical relevance of this has been supported by global impressions of change. Significant reduction in rate of decline of daily functioning has been demonstrated. There is evidence of statistically significant effects on ratings of behavior, chiefly indicating delayed incidence of psychopathology in asymptomatic patients begun on treatment, supported by evidence of symptomatic benefit as well. The effective doses are 16 and 24 mg/day, with lower doses being ineffective and higher doses associated with higher side-effect rates. The major safety and tolerability concerns center on gastrointestinal distress, particularly at times of dose change. Strong evidence exists indicating efficacy for patients with AD combined with cerebrovascular disease. Galantamine is marketed in numerous countries worldwide for treatment of mild to moderate AD. It can be considered a first-line treatment for AD, along with the other approved acetylcholinesterase inhibitors (AChEI) *(41)*. Emerging evidence supports the effectiveness as well as efficacy of galantamine. We lack information about treatment in patients with advanced dementia, with very mild dementia, in nursing-home residents, and in patients receiving memantine.

REFERENCES

1. Bartus, R.T. et al.: The cholinergic hypothesis of geriatric memory dysfunction. Science 1982; 217: 408–414.
2. Levin, E.D.; Simon, B.B.: Nicotinic acetylcholine involvement in cognitive functions in animals. Psychopharmacology 1998; 138: 217–230.
3. Whitehouse, P.J. et al.: Alzheimer's disease and senile dementia: loss of neurons in the basal forebrain. Science 1982; 215: 1237–1239.

4. Schroeder, H. et al.: Nicotinic cholinoreceptive neurons of the frontal cortex are reduced in Alzheimer's disease. Neurobiol Aging 1991; 12: 259–262.
5. Nordberg, A.; Lundqvist, H.; Hartvig, P.: Kinetic analysis of regional (S) (–) 11C- nicotinic binding in normal and Alzheimer brains—in vivo assessment using positron emission tomography. Alzheimer's Dis Assoc Disord 1995; 9: 21–27.
6. Perry, E. et al.: Alteration in nicotinic binding sites in Parkinson's disease, Lewy body dementia and Alzheimer's disease: possible index of early neuropathology. Neuroscience 1995; 64: 385–395.
7. Decker, M.W.: Animal models of cognitive functions. Crit Rev Neurobiol 1995; 9: 321–343.
8. Levin, E.D.; Rezvani, A.H.: Development of nicotinic drug therapy for cognitive disorders. Eur J Pharmacol 2000; 393: 141–146.
9. Parks, R.W. et al.: Increased regional cerebral glucose metabolism and semantic memory performance in Alzheimer's disease: a pilot double-blind transdermal nicotine positron emission tomography study. Neuropsychol Rev 1996; 6: 61–79.
10. Maelicke, A.; Albuquerque, E.X.: Allosteric modulation of nicotinic acetylcholine receptors as a treatment strategy for Alzheimer's disease. Eur J Pharmacol 2000; 393: 165–170.
11. Inestrosa, N.C. et al.: Acetylcholinesterases accelerate assembly of amyloid B-peptides into Alzheimer's fibrils: possible role of the peripheral site of the enzyme. Neuron 1996; 16: 881–889.
12. Williams, M.; Arneric, S.P.: Alzheimer's disease: prospects for treatment in the next decade. In: Brioni, J.D.; Decker, M.W. (eds.): Pharmacological treatment of Alzheimer's disease. Wiley-Liss, New York, 1997: 525–542.
13. Meyer, E.M. et al.: Cytoprotective actions of nicotinic receptor stimulation (abst). Fifth Int Conf Alzheimer's Disease and Related Disorders, Osaka, Japan, 1996.
14. Lopez, O.L. et al.: Cholinesterase inhibitor treatment alters the natural history of Alzheimer's disease. J Neurol Neurosurg Psychiatry 2002; 72: 310–314.
15. Rosen, W.G.; Mohs, R.C.; Davis, K.L.: A new rating scale for Alzheimer's disease. Am J Psychiatry 1984; 141: 1356–1364.
16. Torfs, K.; Feldman, H., on behalf of the Sabeluzole Study Groups. 12-month decline in cognitive and daily function in patients with mild to-moderate Alzheimer's disease: two randomized, placebo-controlled studies (poster). World Alzheimer Congress, Washington, DC, July 9–13, 2000.
17. Bartus, R.T.: On neurodegenerative diseases, models and treatment strategies, lessons learned and lessons forgotten a generation following the cholinergic hypothesis. Exp Neurol 2000; 163: 495–529.
18. Cummings, J.L.; Kaufer, D.: Neuropsychiatric aspects of Alzheimer's disease: the cholinergic hypothesis revisited. Neurology 1996; 47: 876–883.
19. Tariot, P.N. et al.: A 5-month, randomized placebo-controlled trial of galantamine in Alzheimer's disease. Neurology 2000; 54: 2269–2276.
20. Raskind, M.A. et al. and the Galantamine USA-1 Study Group: Galantamine in AD: a 6-month randomized placebo-controlled trial with a 6-month extension. Neurology 2000; 54: 2261–2268.
21. Wilcock, G.K.; Lilienfeld, S.; Gaens, E. on behalf of the Galantamine International-1 Study Group. Efficacy and safety of galantamine in patients with mild to moderate Alzheimer's disease: multicenter randomized controlled trial. Br Med J 2000; 321: 1445–1449.
22. Wilkinson, D.; Murray, J.: Galantamine: a randomized, double-blind, dose comparison in patients with Alzheimer's disease. Int J Geriatr Psychiatry 2001; 16: 852–857.
23. Rockwood, K. et al.: Effects of flexible galantamine dose in Alzheimer's disease: a randomized, controlled trial. J Neurol Neurosurg Psychiatry 2001; 71: 589–595.
24. Raskind, M.A.; Peskind, E.; Truyen, L.: Galantamine provides long-term cognitive benefits for at least 36 months in patients with Alzheimer's disease (poster). American Psychiatric Association 155th Annual Meeting, Philadelphia, May 18–23, 2002.
25. Farlow, M.R. et al.: Treatment outcome of tacrine therapy depends on apolipoprotein genotype and gender of the subjects with Alzheimer's disease. Neurology 1998; 50: 669–677.
26. Erkinjutti, T. et al: Efficacy of galantamine in probable vascular dementia and Alzheimer's disease combined with cerebrovascular disease: a randomized trial. Lancet 2002; 1359: 1283–1290.
27. Small, G.W.; Lilenfield, S.: Galantamine demonstrates sustained cognitive benefits in patients with Alzheimer's disease, vascular dementia, or Alzheimer's disease with cerebrovascular disease (poster). American Psychiatric Association 155th Annual Meeting, Philadelphia, May 18–23, 2002.
28. Leber, P.: Guidelines for the clinical evaluation of anti-dementia drugs, 1st draft. U.S. Food and Drug Administration, Rockville, MD, 1990.
29. Feldman, H. et al.: The disability assessment for dementia scale: a 12-month study of functional ability in mild to moderate severity Alzheimer' disease. Alzheimer's Dis Assoc Disord 2001; 15: 89–95.
30. Mintzer, J.E.; Faison, W.E.: Prolonged benefits with acetylcholinesterase inhibitors are exhibited in patients with Alzheimer's disease (poster). American Association for Geriatric Psychiatry 15th Annual Meeting, Orlando, Fla, February 24–27, 2002.
31. Tariot, P.N.; Blazina, L.: The psychopathology of dementia. In: Morris, J. (ed.): Handbook of dementing illnesses. Marcel Decker, New York, 1993: 461–475.

32. Burke, E.; Lilienfeld, S.: Galantamine improves behavior and reduces caregiver distress in patients with Alzheimer's disease, vascular dementia, or Alzheimer's disease with cerebrovacular disease (poster). American Psychiatric Association 155th Annual Meeting, Philadelphia, May 18–23, 2002.

33. Tariot, P.N.: Treating non-cognitive problems: other classes of psychotropics in dementia. In: Qizilbash, N.; et al. (eds.): Evidence-based practice of dementia. Blackwell, Oxford, UK, 2002: 671–694.

34. Feldman, H. et al.: A 24-week randomized, double blind study of donepezil in moderate to severe Alzheimer's disease. Neurology 2001; 57: 613–620.

35. Wilcock, G.; Lilienfeld, S.: Galantamine alleviates caregiver burden in Alzheimer's disease: a 6- month-placebo-controlled study (poster). World Alzheimer's Congress, Washington, DC, July 9–18, 2000.

36. Lilenfeld, S.; Gaens, E.: Galantamine alleviates caregiver burden in Alzheimer's disease: a 12-month study (poster). 5th Congress European Federation of Neurological Studies, Copenhagen, October 14–18, 2000.

37. Getsios, D. et al.: The AHEAD Study Group. Assessment of Health Economics in Alzheimer's Disease (AHEAD): galantamine treatment in Canada. Neurology 2002; 57: 972–978.

38. Ernst, R.L. et al.: Cognitive function and cost of Alzheimer disease. Arch Neurol 1997; 54: 687–693.

39. Knopman, D. et al.: Long term tacrine treatment: effects on nursing home placement and mortality: tacrine study group. Neurology 1996; 47: 166–177.

40. Kaye, J.; Schneider, L.S.; Qizilbash, N.: Therapies for cognitive symptoms, disease modification and prevention. In: Qizilbash, N.; et al. (eds.): Evidence-based practice of dementia. Blackwell, Oxford, UK, 2002: 461–588.

41. Qizilbash, N.; Schneider, L.S.: Summary, practical recommendations and opinion on therapies for cognitive symptoms, disease modification and prevention. In: Qizilbash, N.; et al. (eds.): Evidence-based practice of dementia. Blackwell, Oxford, UK, 2002: 560–588.

23

Memantine in Treatment of AD

Hans Jörg Möbius

INTRODUCTION

None of the currently available treatment strategies effectively alleviates symptoms and stabilizes disease in moderate to severe Alzheimer's disease (AD). However, memantine* is a moderate-affinity, voltage-dependent, noncompetitive *N*-methyl-D-aspartate (NMDA) receptor antagonist that has both demonstrated clinical benefit in improving individual symptoms of AD and produced preclinical evidence for neuroprotection in various models *(1)*.

HOW THE NMDA RECEPTOR WORKS

It is widely acknowledged that glutamate-mediated neurotoxicity is a likely pathogenic mechanism contributing to neurodegeneration in dementia, as disruption of normal glutamate function promotes cortical and subcortical neuronal cell damage *(2)*. Additionally, glutamate-sensitive NMDA receptors regulate synaptic plasticity necessary for learning and memory processes. Under conditions of glutamate homeostasis the NMDA channel remains blocked in a use- and voltage-dependent manner by magnesium ions. After AMPA (α-amino-3-hydroxy-5-methyl-4-isoxazole propionic acid) receptor activation evoked by glutamate, during learning and memory processes, postsynaptic membranes are depolarized, drawing the magnesium ion out of the NMDA receptor channel and allowing calcium ions to enter the channel, thereby enhancing physiological signal transmission.

The long-term potentiation (LTP) model is the standard neurophysiological approach to investigate compounds that potentially affect memory formation. Various processes—for example, energy deprivation—may lead to sustained pathogenic concentrations of glutamate, partial depolarization of the postsynaptic membranes, and ultimately a chronic state of glutamatergic excitotoxity. NMDA receptors subjected to overactivation lead to reduction of LTP and finally induction of neuronal cell damage through necrosis and apoptosis *(2,3)*. Concurrently, postsynaptic calcium levels may remain too high to permit signal detection, due to increased background noise. Both processes, functional and structural in nature, are thought to represent causes of the cognitive loss characteristic of AD progression.

Because NMDA receptors mediate excitatory neurotransmission, receptor antagonists whose receptor kinetics are fast enough to allow physiological transmission but have appropriate receptor affinity to inhibit excitotoxic activity have been the focus of intense research. Memantine has been shown to effectively limit glutamate-induced neurotoxicity under conditions of overactivity of this system, while restoring LTP, and is to date the only fully developed NMDA receptor antagonist in dementia therapeutics *(3–9)*.

---

*Axura® is the registered trademark for memantine, patented by Merz Pharmaceuticals, Frankfurt, Germany.

From: *Current Clinical Neurology,*
Alzheimer's Disease: A Physician's Guide to Practical Management
Edited by: R. W. Richter and B. Zoeller Richter © Humana Press Inc., Totowa, NJ

PHARMACOLOGY OF MEMANTINE

Preclinical studies performed with whole-cell patch clamp technique with cultured and freshly dissociated neurones, retinal ganglion cells, hippocampal, and striatal slices have clearly defined the mechanism of action of memantine *(10–17)*. Memantine inhibits NMDA receptor channels in a use- and voltage-dependent manner with IC_{50} of 0.5–3 μM at –100 to –70 mV. Memantine's antagonistic properties at –70 mV were not minimized by increasing concentrations of glycine *(14,18)*.

At concentrations of 2–33 µmol/L, memantine inhibited the effects of 100 µmol/L NMDA in superior collicular and hippocampal neurons in a concentration-dependent manner (a concentration of 2.92 µmol/L produced 50% inhibition) *(18)*. Memantine induces open-channel blockade of NMDA receptors, and has been observed to be only "partially trapped" in NMDA receptor channels *(14,16)*. Experiments with NMDA receptors composed of the NR1-1a, NR2A, or NR2B subunits, produced by recombinant DNA-technology and expressed in Chinese hamster ovary cells, confirmed these results *(16)*.

Memantine produced a protective effect on cultured neurons from excitotoxic cell death *(19)*. The drug prevented glutamate-induced cell death in rat cerebellar, cortical, mesencephalic, and hippocampal neurons, and calcium ion-induced death in retinal ganglions in animal models *(19–22)*.

Memantine has produced neuroprotective benefit in a number of models of brain injury. At higher doses, it attenuated neuronal injury instigated by traumatic brain injury, ischemic stroke induced by occlusion of cerebral or carotid arteries, and cerebral focal ischemia *(23–28)*. Loss of cholinergic neurons in the central nervous system (CNS) induced by injection of NMDA in rats was markedly ameliorated at therapeutically relevant doses of memantine, as was quinolinic acid-induced damage *(29,30)*.

Human Pharmacology

Memantine is completely absorbed from the gastrointestinal tract (absolute bioavailability 100%) *(1)*. Maximum plasma concentrations (C_{max}) occur between 3 and 8 hours after oral administration (t_{max}); the dose–plasma concentration relationship is linear over the range 10–40 mg in healthy volunteers *(1)*. Food does not affect the bioavailability *(1)*.

Approximately 80% of an administered dose of memantine circulates unchanged from the parent drug composition *(1)*. Several identified metabolites are inactive; no cytochrome P450-catalyzed metabolism has been detected in vitro *(1)*. The mean terminal elimination half-life ($t_{1/2}$) of memantine is 60–100 hours *(1)*. Memantine is eliminated renally through renal tubular secretion and reabsorption via cationic transport proteins. A mean of 84% of oral-dose ^{14}C-labeled memantine was recovered within 20 days, 99% of which was recovered in urine. Marked urinary alkalinisation may reduce renal excretion of memantine. In healthy volunteers with normal renal function, total renal clearance (CL_{tot}) was 170 mL/min/1.73 m^2, whereas in elderly volunteers with different levels of renal function (creatinine clearance between 100 and 50 mL/min/1.73 m^2) significant decreases were observed in CL_{tot} of memantine with increasing degrees of renal impairment. Creatinine clearance correlated with total body clearance of memantine *(1)*.

CLINICAL TRIAL RESULTS

In a Phase I study, memantine significantly increased intracortical inhibition and reduced intracortical facilitation in 7 healthy volunteers, effects that were both negatively correlated with plasma levels of the drug (all $p < 0.05$ vs placebo) *(31)*. In this randomized, double-blind, crossover study, 10–30 mg memantine administered for 8 days also blocked cortico-cortical excitability. The drug did not affect variables of motor excitability, including motor threshold, silent period duration after transcranial magnetic stimulation, and M- and F-wave amplitudes.

Memantine did not produce significant effects on mood, attention, or immediate and delayed verbal and visuospatial memory in a separate study with 16 healthy male volunteers *(32)*. In another randomized, double-blind, placebo-controlled, study memantine improved vigilance in healthy elderly volunteers (mean age 65 years) *(33)*. Single doses of memantine (20 mg) counteracted negative time-dependent EEG changes indicative of diminished vigilance. In healthy male volunteers memantine did not affect performance on perceptual and psychomotor tasks *(34)*.

A first placebo-controlled trial in Europe included 166 (intention-to-treat, ITT) severely demented nursing-home patients with approximately equal numbers of patients with AD or vascular dementia (VaD) (overall baseline Mini-Mental State Examination, MMSE, 6.9). A subgroup analysis per etiology was predefined. The analysis of the total trial population as well as the AD group showed statistically significant superiority of memantine after 3 months of treatment on predefined endpoints assessing care dependency (subscale of BGP *[35]*, $p < 0.05$) and clinical global impression (CGI-C, $p = 0.006$) *(4)*.

To date, the safety and efficacy of memantine in AD have been shown in two large-scale state-of-the-art Phase III trials in the United States; in addition, two large-scale Phase III trials in VaD have been completed in Europe.

Evidence of the benefits of memantine treatment in patients with moderately severe to severe AD was observed in a first investigation of the efficacy and long-term tolerability of this drug *(7,8)*. This was a placebo-controlled, 28-week, double-blind, randomized, two-arm parallel, fixed-dose multi-center trial with optional 6-month open-label extension study of randomized patients receiving 20 mg/day memantine or placebo *(7)*. The three main outcome measures included the clinician's inter-view-based impression of change plus caregiver input (CIBIC+, New York University version), the Alzheimer's Disease Cooperative Study activities of daily living inventory modified for severe dementia (ADCS-ADLsev, 19 items), and the Severe Impairment Battery (SIB) as performance-based cognition test. Additional endpoints included Mini-Mental State Examination (MMSE), Functional Assessment Staging (FAST), Geriatric Depression Scale (GDS), Neuropsychiatric Inventory (NPI, 12 items), and—as pharmacoeconomic endpoint—the Resource Utilization in Dementia Scale (RUD).

A total of 252 patients, who met the protocol inclusion criteria (NINCDS-ADRDA criteria and MRI or CT scan), were randomized to the two treatment groups ($n = 126$ each) at 32 trial sites. A total of 181 patients completed the 28-week study. These included 84 patients (67%) randomized to the placebo group and 97 (77%) randomized to receive memantine tablets. The mean MMSE score at baseline was 7.9.

Results: Memantine-treated patients experienced less deterioration in functioning relative to placebo patients as measured by the ADCS-ADLsev ($p = 0.003$). Single-item analysis of ADCS-ADLsev also revealed significant advantages for memantine patients for key activities of daily living (ADL). At endpoint or week 28, changes in CIBIC+ scores demonstrated that memantine-treated patients showed less decline as compared to the placebo patients ($p = 0.025$). Memantine significantly reduced further cognitive decline relative to the placebo-treated patients, as assessed by the SIB mean change from baseline scores; the placebo patients showed substantially more worsening ($p = 0.002$). Significant single-item differences between the two groups were observed in memory and visuospatial abilities. The NPI results were inconclusive. These results are detailed in a recent publication *(7)*. Significantly positive results with the pharmacoeconomic endpoint (RUD) analysis were also observed *(36)*.

Patients completing the double-blind phase were eligible for memantine treatment in a 24-week open-label extension study *(8)*. Clinical assessors, patients, and caregivers remained blinded to the initial double-blind treatment allocation throughout the end of the full 52-week treatment period. Improvements in cognition, functioning, and global impression were maintained for patients continuing memantine therapy from the initial treatment period. Slope analysis after 52 weeks showed statistically significant differences in SIB, ADCS-ADLsev, and CIBIC+ score decline over time for placebo patients switched to memantine treatment.

The most frequent adverse events reported in the double-blind study were agitation (18% vs 32% in memantine and placebo cohorts, respectively), insomnia (10% vs 8%), diarrhea (10% vs 8%), urinary tract infection (6% vs 13%), and urinary incontinence (11% in both cohorts). The most common adverse events reported during the 24-wk extension study (agitation and urinary incontinence) were consistent with data from the double-blind period. These results support the use of memantine for long-term treatment of patients with advanced AD.

The second trial was a randomized, double-blind, placebo-controlled, parallel-group study with a 1- to 2-week single-blind placebo screening period followed by 24 weeks of double-blind treatment *(9)*. Again, memantine was given at 20 mg/day maintenance dose (10 mg twice daily, titrated over a four-week period). Male or female outpatients 50 years of age with a diagnosis of probable AD consistent with NINCDS-ADRDA criteria and MRI or CT scan consistent with diagnosis of probable AD with a MMSE of 5–14 (inclusive) at baseline were eligible. In addition, they had to have at least 6 months of ongoing daily donepezil monotherapy, at a stable dose (5 or 10 mg/day) for the immediately preceding 3 months and throughout the study period.

The primary efficacy assessments included the SIB and the ADCS-ADLsev (modified 19 items). Secondary efficacy assessments included the CIBIC+ (format adapted from the ADCS-CGIC), the NPI, and the Behavioral Rating Scale for Geriatric Patients (BGP) care dependency subscale (adapted from the Stockton Geriatric Rating Scale). A total of 404 patients were randomized with 403 patients (202 memantine, 201 placebo) treated at 37 sites. The majority of memantine/donepezil- (85%) and placebo/donepezil- (75%) treated patients completed the 6-month study.

Results: There was a statistically significant difference in cognitive performance favoring memantine/donepezil combination over placebo/donepezil, as measured by the SIB ($p < 0.001$). Patients treated with memantine/donepezil appeared to show improvement relative to baseline over the 24-week course of the study, whereas patients receiving placebo/donepezil exhibited progressive cognitive decline over the same duration. Patients treated with memantine/donepezil showed a statistically significant superiority in function, as measured by the ADCS-ADLsev ($p = 0.028$) and BGP-care dependency subscale, when compared to patients treated with placebo/donepezil. Also, patients treated with memantine/donepezil demonstrated a statistically significant global improvement over patients treated with placebo/donepezil as measured by the CIBIC+ ($p = 0.027$). In addition, statistically significant superiority in behavior, as measured by the change from baseline in the NPI total score, was observed in patients treated with memantine/donepezil compared to those treated with placebo/donepezil alone.

Summarizing this second Phase III trial in AD and examining the effects of the combination of an NMDA receptor antagonist and an AChEI in patients with AD, beneficial effects of combining memantine with a stable dosage of donepezil in patients with moderate to severe AD (mean baseline MMSE 10) were consistently observed on measures of cognition, daily functioning, clinical global status, and behavior.

Memantine, given at a dose of 20 mg/day administered concomitantly with donepezil, was safe and well tolerated in patients with moderate to severe Alzheimer's disease. In general, the incidence of treatment-emergent adverse events was similar in both groups, and the profile of adverse events was similar to what had been previously observed in other clinical trials. Patients were significantly more likely to complete the treatment trial when on combination treatment; the incidence of premature discontinuations due to adverse events was lower in the memantine/donepezil group compared to the placebo/donepezil group.

Beyond these AD trials, two large-scale, placebo-controlled Phase III trials in mild to moderate VaD have shown clinical benefits with memantine treatment *(5,6)*. Patients in both trials met diagnostic criteria for probable VaD (consistent with NINDS-AIREN). In the MMM300 study (a multicentre, 28-week trial conducted in France), 321 patients with MMSE scores between 12 and 20 received 10 mg memantine or placebo twice a day *(5)*. Primary endpoints were the ADAS-cog and CIBIC+ (New York University version). At 28 weeks, analysis of the intention-to-treat (ITT) population ($n = 288$) demonstrated that the memantine group experienced a significant benefit in cognitive performance: the ADAS-cog total score mean for treated patients showed an improvement of 0.4 point over baseline, while the placebo group mean score declined by 1.6 points. This 2.0-point difference

Table 1
Adverse Events Seen in the Memantine Trials

Preferred term (WHO ART)	Memantine ($n = 299$)	Placebo ($n = 288$)
Agitation	27 (9.0%)	50 (17.4%)
Inflicted injury	20 (6.7%)	20 (6.9%)
Urinary incontinence	17 (5.7%)	21 (7.3%)
Diarrhea	16 (5.4%)	14 (4.9%)
Insomnia	16 (5.4%)	14 (4.9%

was significant (ITT LOCF analysis, $p = 0.0016$, 95% confidence interval, 0.49–3.60). The global end-point difference favoured memantine treatment but did not reach statistical significance.

In the MMM500 study, a 28-week, double-blind, parallel-group, randomized controlled trial in the United Kingdom, 579 VaD patients were randomized to receive 20 mg/day memantine or matching placebo *(6)*. Inclusion criteria required MMSE total scores between 10 and 22. Primary efficacy parameters were the ADAS-cog and the Clinical Global Impression of change (CGI-C).The ITT LOCF analysis ($n = 548$) at endpoint established that memantine improved cognition with respect to placebo: the ADAS-cog total score mean change from baseline differed significantly ($p < 0.05$) for the memantine-treated group compared to the placebo-treated group (–0.53 and –2.28, respectively). The CGI-C was inconclusive.

In both VaD trials, subgroup analyses by baseline MMSE scores of ADAS-cog mean change revealed cognitive improvements with memantine treatment across all groups, with larger effect size as a function of baseline severity (up to 3.46 ADAS-cog points for baseline MMSE < 15) *(37)*.

In a pooled, post-hoc ITT population analysis from these two studies, patients were grouped according to baseline neuroradiological findings *(38)*. Subgroups were categorized as patients with small-vessel disease (no evidence of macrolesions) vs patients with large-vessel disease (presence of macrolesions, most frequently overt stroke). Cognitive benefits were experienced by memantine-treated patients in both subsets. In the large-vessel disease group, a descriptive advantage of 0.93 points ($p > 0.05$) in ADAS-cog mean change was observed with memantine treatment. However, in patients with small-vessel disease, the difference in ADAS-cog mean change between the memantine treatment and placebo cohorts was 2.0 points ($p = 0.002$) in favor of the memantine group. Accelerated cognitive decline was experienced by placebo patients with small-vessel disease as compared to placebo patients with large-vessel disease. These therapeutic benefits shown in VaD patients appear to fit with the hypothesized mode of action *(39)*.

SAFETY AND TOLERABILITY

To date, more than 3000 healthy volunteers and patients have been evaluated for adverse events and adverse drug reactions with memantine in Phase I through Phase IV studies. Little differences in safety and tolerability have been observed between memantine and placebo treatment cohorts and observing exclusion criteria. No drug–drug interactions have been detected in this multimorbid population. In clinical trials in moderately severe to severe dementia, overall incidence rates for adverse events did not differ from placebo treatment, and adverse events were usually mild to moderate in severity.

Table 1 gives an overview of the most frequent (more than 5% for memantine) adverse events (regardless of causal relationship) that were observed in the trial population of patients with moderately severe to severe dementia (without data from the AChEI add-on trial *[9]*). These figures obviously are subject to adjustments as additional large clinical trials are being completed.

CONCLUSION AND IMPLICATIONS

Acetylcholinesterase inhibitors (AChEIs, such as donepezil, rivastigmine, and galantamine) have been approved for treating symptoms in patients with mild to moderate AD. Current evidence, however, does not indicate a clear role for these drugs in the slowing of disease progression. Memantine is the first drug to demonstrate cognitive benefit in moderate to severe AD as well as in mild to moderate vascular dementia, with a comprehensive body of preclinical evidence showing its potential for slowing disease progression. In contrast to AChEI, treatment with memantine provides superior tolerability, and is the only treatment with demonstrated advantages for patients with advanced dementia *(1,4–9)*.

A well-established body of evidence indicates that memantine is a safe and effective treatment that provides cognitive, functional, behavioral, and global improvement for patients with AD; cognitive benefit has also been shown for VaD. To date, memantine has been approved in the European Union for the treatment of patients with moderately severe to severe AD and an approval file has been submitted in the United States for the treatment of moderate to severe AD. This drug may be one of the long-awaited answers for dementia patients, their families, and clinicians in urgent need of safe and effective treatments for all stages of dementia.

REFERENCES

1. Committee for Proprietary Medicinal Products (CPMP): European Public Assessment Reports (EPAR) for Axura (CPMP/982/02 and CPMP/1604/02). London, 2002.
2. Cacabelos, R.; Takeda, M.; Winblad, B.: The glutamatergic system and neurodegeneration in dementia: preventive strategies in Alzheimer's disease. Int J Geriatr Psychiatry 1999; 14: 3–47.
3. Danysz, W. et al.: Neuroprotection and symptomatological action of memantine relevant for Alzheimer's disease—a unified hypothesis on the mechanism of action. Neurotox Res 2000; 2: 85–98.
4. Winblad, B.; Poritis, N.: Memantine in severe dementia. Int J Geriatr Psychiatry 1999; 14: 135–146.
5. Orgogozo, J.M. et al.: Efficacy and safety of memantine in patients with mild to moderate vascular dementia: a randomized, placebo-controlled trial (MMM 300). Stroke 2002; 33: 1834–1839.
6. Wilcock, G.; Möbius, H.J.; Stöffler, A.: A double-blind, placebo-controlled multicentre study of memantine in mild to moderate vascular dementia (MMM500). Int Clin Psychopharmacol 2002; 17: 297–305.
7. Reisberg, B. et al.: Memantine, an uncompetitive NMDA antagonist, in patients with moderate to severe Alzheimer's disease. N Engl J Med 2003; 348: 1333–1341.
8. Reisberg, B. et al.: Long-term treatment with the NMDA antagonist memantine: results of a 24-week, open-label extension study in moderately severe to severe Alzheimer's disease. Neurobiol Aging 2002; 23: S555, abstr 2039.
9. Internal communication, Forest Labs, New York, NY, 2002.
10. Chen, H.S.; Lipton, S.A.: Mechanism of memantine block of NMDA-activated channels in rat retinal ganglion cells: uncompetitive antagonism. J Physiol 1997; 499: 27–46.
11. Rohrbacher, J.; Bijak, M.; Misgeld, U.: Suppression by memantine and amantadine of synaptic excitation intrastriatally evoked in rat neostriatal slices. Neurosci Lett 1994; 182: 95–98.
12. Parsons, C.G. et al.: Comparative patch-clamp studies with freshly dissociated rat hippocampal and striatal neurons on the NMDA receptor antagonistic effects of amantadine and memantine. Eur J Neurosci 1996; 8: 446–454.
13. Frankiewicz, T. et al.: Effects of memantine and MK-801 on NMDA-induced currents in cultured neurones and on synaptic transmission and LTP in area CA1 of rat hippocampal slices. Br J Pharmacol 1996; 117: 689–697.
14. Sobolevsky, A.I.; Koshelev, S.G.; Khodorov, B.I.: Interaction of memantine and amantadine with agonist-unbound NMDA-receptor channels in acutely isolated rat hippocampal neurons. J Physiol 1998; 512: 47–60.
15. Frankiewicz, T.; Parsons, C.G.: Memantine restores long term potentiation impaired by tonic N-methyl-D-aspartate (NMDA) receptor activation following reduction of Mg^{2+} in hippocampal slices. Neuropharmacology 1999; 38: 1253–1259.
16. Blanpied, T.A. et al.: Trapping channel block of NMDA-activated responses by amantadine and memantine. J Neurophysiol 1997; 77: 309–323.
17. Bormann, J.: Memantine is a potent blocker of N-methyl-D-aspartate (NMDA) receptor channels. Eur J Pharmacol 1989; 166: 591–592.
18. Parsons, C.G. et al.: Patch clamp studies on the kinetics and selectivity of N-methyl-D-aspartate receptor antagonism by memantine (1-amino-3,5-dimethyladamantan). Neuropharmacology 1993; 32: 1337–1350.
19. Krieglstein, J.; Lippert, K.; Poch, G.: Apparent independent action of nimodipine and glutamate antagonists to protect cultured neurons against glutamate-induced damage. Neuropharmacology 1996; 35: 1737–1742.

20. Erdo, S.L.; Schafer, M.: Memantine is highly potent in protecting cortical cultures against excitotoxic cell death evoked by glutamate and N-methyl-D-aspartate. Eur J Pharmacol 1991; 198: 215–217.

21. Weller, M.; Finiels-Marlier, F.; Paul, S.M.: NMDA receptor-mediated glutamate toxicity of cultured cerebellar, cortical and mesencephalic neurons: neuroprotective properties of amantadine and memantine. Brain Res 1993; 613: 143–148.

22. Pellegrini, J.W.; Lipton, S.A.: Delayed administration of memantine prevents N-methyl-D-aspartate receptor-mediated neurotoxicity. Ann Neurol 1993; 33: 403–407.

23. Rao, V.L. et al.: Neuroprotection by memantine, a non-competitive NMDA receptor antagonist after traumatic brain injury in rats. Brain Res 2001; 911: 96–100.

24. Gorgulu, A. et al.: Reduction of edema and infarction by memantine and MK-801 after focal cerebral ischaemia and reperfusion in rat. Acta Neurochir (Wien) 2000; 142: 1287–1292.

25. Dogan, A. et al.: Protective effects of memantine against ischemia reperfusion injury in spontaneously hypertensive rats. Acta Neurochir (Wien) 1999; 141: 1107–1113.

26. Seif el Nasr, M. et al.: Neuroprotective effect of memantine demonstrated in vivo and in vitro. Eur J Pharmacol 1990; 185: 19–24.

27. Heim, C.; Sontag, K.H.: Memantine prevents progressive functional neurodegeneration in rats. J Neural Transm Suppl 1995; 46: 117–130.

28. Stieg, P.E. et al.: Neuroprotection by the NMDA receptor-associated open channel blocker memantine in a photothrombotic model of cerebral focal ischemia in neonatal rat. Eur J Pharmacol 1999; 375: 115–120.

29. Misztal, M. et al.: Learning deficits induced by chronic intraventricular infusion of quinolinic acid—protection by MK-801 and memantine. Eur J Pharmacol 1996; 296: 1–8.

30. Wenk, G.L.; Danysz, W.; Mobley, S.L.: MK-801, memantine and amantadine show neuroprotective activity in the nucleus basalis magnocellularis. Eur J Pharmacol 1995; 293: 267–270.

31. Schwenkreis, P. et al.: Influence of the N-methyl-D-aspartate antagonist memantine on human motor cortex excitability. Neurosci Lett 1999; 270: 137–140.

32. Schugens, M.M. et al.: The NMDA antagonist memantine impairs classical eyeblink conditioning in humans. Neurosci Lett 1997; 224: 57–60.

33. Schulz, H. et al.: The use of diurnal vigilance changes in the EEG to verify vigilance-enhancing effects of memantine in a clinical pharmacological study. Neuropsychobiology 1996; 33: 32–40.

34. Rammsayer, T.H.: Effects of pharmacologically induced changes in NMDA-receptor activity on long-term memory in humans. Learn Mem 2001, 28; 8: 20–25.

35. Van der Kam, P.; Mol, F.; Wimmers, M.F.H.C.: Beoordelingsschaal voor oudere Patienten (BOP). Van Loghum Slaterus, Deuenter, The Netherlands, 1971.

36. Wimo, A. et al.: Resource utilisation and cost analysis of memantine in patients with moderate to severe Alzheimer's Disease. Pharmacoeconomics, 2003; 21: 327–340.

37. Möbius, H.J. and Stöffler, A.: Memantine in vascular dementia. Int Psychogeriatrics 2003; 15 (suppl. 1): 207–213.

38. Wilcock, G. et al.: Neuro-radiolgical findings and the magnitude of cognitive benefit by memantine treatment. A subgroup analysis of two placebo-controlled clinical trials in vascular dementia. Eur J Neuropsychopharm 2001; 10 (suppl 3): S360.

39. Möbius, H.J.: Pharmacologic rationale for memantine in chronic cerebral hypoperfusion, especially vascular dementia. Alzheimer's Dis Assoc Disord 1999; 13 (suppl 3): 172–178.

24

Alternative Treatment Options

Brigitte Zoeller Richter

INTRODUCTION

Alzheimer's disease (AD) is one of the most dreaded degenerative disorders in the population. As AD is not yet curable the market for alternative treatments is huge and the use of unproven therapies therefore very common. Although this behavior is understandable, it exposes vulnerable individuals to potential side effects and involves the risk of possible exploitation and creating false hope *(1)*.

Many of the products made available and advertised in magazines are so-called natural and often of herbal nature, which of course does not necessarily guarantee that they are safe and lack the potential for drug-interactions. Consulting physicians therefore have to be aware of possible side effects and potentially dangerous incompatibilities with prescribed medications.

How Often Are Alternative Treatments Used?

In a descriptive survey of primary caregivers of persons with AD 55% of caregivers reported that they had tried at least one alternative therapy in order to improve the patient's memory; 20% of caregivers tried three or more unproven therapies *(1)*. Vitamins were most frequently used (84%), followed by health foods (27%), herbal medicines (11%), and "smart pills" (9%) *(1)*. Alternative treatments are mostly tried in the early stage of the disease. Most caregivers however reported they did not notice significant improvement *(1)*.

HERBAL PRODUCTS, PHYTOCHEMICALS, AND NUTRIENTS FOR THE TREATMENT OF AD

The use of complementary medicines such as plant extracts for the treatment of dementia and AD varies according to different cultural traditions. While not widely used in Western countries, medicinal plants in China and the Far East since ancient times have not only been widely utilized but also thoroughly investigated (though not by modern analytical means). As important parts of the traditional medicine their pharmacological properties usually were known from critical observation. Particular well studied were plants such as ginseng (for a long life) and ginkgo (for memory enhancement).

A certain therapeutic efficacy of an extract of *Ginkgo biloba* on cognition in AD was suggested with the results of a placebo-controlled trial *(2)*. A more recent controlled study using Ginkoba®, however, suggests that ginkgo provides no measurable benefit on memory or related cognitive function to adults with healthy cognitive function *(3)*. The study was designed to investigate a claimed memory enhancing effect in elderly (60 years and older) individuals.

Old European reference books document a variety of other plants such as sage *(Salvia officinalis)* and balm *(Melissa officinalis)* with cholinergic activity and memory improving and additional properties *(4)*. These effects, however, though they may in fact exist, have not been investigated to date by modern scientific methods.

From: *Current Clinical Neurology,*
Alzheimer's Disease: A Physician's Guide to Practical Management
Edited by: R. W. Richter and B. Zoeller Richter © Humana Press Inc., Totowa, NJ

Several other nutrients and botanicals are made available for the integrative management of cognitive dysfunction *(5)*: phosphatidylserine (PS), acetyl-L-carnitine (ALCAR), vinpocetine, and *Bacopa monniera*.

PS represents a phospholipid that is essential to all cells in the human body enriched in the brain. It has been studied in AD about a decade ago, but showed no long-term efficacy in improving cognitive abilities in humans *(6)*. The short-term benefit on different measures of brain function was overcome by the progressive pathological changes at the end of the treatment period in a 6-month study conducted in Germany *(7)*. In a more recent study the oral administration of soybean lecithin transphosphatidylated phosphatidylserine (SB-tPS) showed some nootropic action in aged rats *(8)*.

ALCAR is regarded as an energizer and metabolic cofactor, which also is supposed to benefit various cognitive functions. No controlled trials to confirm this claim are available. It contains carnitine and acetyl moieties, both of which have neurobiological properties *(9)*. In a 1-year placebo-controlled and prospectively performed trial with 229 patients with early-onset AD ALCAR failed to slow decline (cognitively and clinically) *(10)*.

The *Vinca minor* alkaloid vinpocetine is thought to increase cerebral (hypo-) perfusion and with this improve cerebral vascular dysfunction or cerebrovascular insufficiency. It could have a role in vascular cognitive dysfunction as "cerebral metabolic enhancer" *(5)*. Controlled studies in AD are not available.

Bacopa monniera is an Ayurvedic botanical that has been shown to exert cognitive enhancing effects in animals. The active principle in this plant seems to be the glycosidic fraction. Three new phenylethanoid glycosides along with the known analog plantainoside B have been isolated recently *(11)*. A small placebo-controlled study in 38 healthy subjects did not reveal any acute effects of *Bacopa* (300 mg) on cognitive functioning *(12)*.

Among the new compounds that are under investigation for the prevention, treatment or delay of AD and other age-related neurological changes are certain dietary components. Increased attention is focused particularly on phytochemicals found in fruits and vegetables *(13)*.

A group of researchers in Los Angeles tested curcumin, a well-known curry spice and alternative NSAID, in transgenic mice with Alzheimer-like pathology. Low and high doses of curcumin significantly reduced inflammatory markers in the brains of the animals *(14)*. Beta-amyloid (Aβ) and plaque-burden were significantly decreased by nearly 50%. The authors conclude that this Indian spice component in view of its efficacy and low toxicity shows promise for the prevention of AD *(14)*.

One problem that has to be considered and physicians have to be aware of is the potential of interactions of herbal remedies and drug therapy. Older people with dementia particularly are often prescribed numerous medications. A systematic review to identify all studies that examined interactions between herbal and conventional drug therapies revealed 28 published articles between 1980 and 2000 that describe such interaction *(15)*. Of these articles, 11 examined St. John's Wort, 4, Ginkgo biloba, 5, Kava kava, 7, ginseng, and 1, valerian.

Coenzyme Q10

Coenzyme Q (CoQ) or ubiquinone, a lipophilic substituted benzoquinone, occurs naturally in all animal or plant cells. CoQ is an obligatory component of the respiratory chain in the inner mitochondrial membrane coupled to the synthesis of ATP (adenosine triphosphate). Its additional localization in different subcellular fractions is probably associated with its multiple functions in the cell (as a part of extramitochondrial electron transport chains, a powerful antioxidant agent or a membrane stabilizer) *(16)*. CoQ-deficiency is associated with mitochondrial diseases and encephalopathies. The natural compound has not been tested in AD. A synthetic CoQ-analog however—low molecular weight benzoquinone or idebenone—has been investigated in the treatment of AD. The global results probably were not favorable enough to further develop this drug, although sustained efficacy on cognition was reported in a controlled long-term multicenter-study in AD patients *(17)*.

Interestingly the serum levels of CoQ seem not to differ in subjects with or without AD or VaD and therefore cannot be considered as indicators for dementia risk *(18)*.

BRIGHT LIGHT THERAPY IN AD

Bright light therapy (BLT) is becoming increasingly popular in the treatment of circadian rhythm disturbances in demented patients. Evidence suggests that patients may experience benefit from BLT. BLT (2500 lux) usually is administered 2 hours/day for a period of 2 weeks or more. Preliminary study data show beneficial effects also on cognitive performance in dementia patients (AD and VaD), as documented by a significant increase in the MMSE score *(19)*.

REFERENCES

1. Coleman, L.M. et al.: Use of unproven therapies by people with Alzheimer's disease. J Am Geriatr Soc 1995; 43: 747–750.
2. Le Bars, P.L. et al.: A 26-week analysis of a double-blind, placebo-controlled trial of the ginkgo biloba extract EGb 761 in dementia. Dement Geriatr Cogn Disord 2000; 11: 230–237.
3. Solomon, Paul R. et al.: Ginkgo for memory enhancement. A randomized controlled trial. JAMA 2002; 288: 835–840.
4. Perry, E.K. et al.: Medicinal plants and Alzheimer's disease: Integrating ethnobotanical and comtemporary scientific evidence. J Altern Complement Med 1998; 4: 419–428.
5. Kidd, P.M.: A review of nutrients and botanicals in the integrative management of cognitive dysfunction. Altern Med Rev 1999; 4: 144–161.
6. Alzheimer's Association: Alternative treatments. In: Alzheimer's disease and related disorders, 2001.
7. Heiss, W.D. et al.: Long-term effects of phosphatidylserine, pyritinol, and cognitive training in Alzheimer's disease. A neuropsychological, EEG, and PET investigation. Dementia 1994; 5: 88–98.
8. Suzuki, S. et al.: Oral administration of soybean lecithin transphosphatidylated phosphatidylserine improves memory impairment in aged rats. J Nutr 2001; 131: 2951–2956.
9. Pettegrew, J.W. et al.: Acetyl-L-carnitine physical-chemical, metabolic, and therapeutic properties: relevance for its mode of action in Alzheimer's disease and geriatric depression. Mol Psychiatry 2000; 5: 616–632.
10. Thal, L.J. et al.: A 1-year controlled trial of acetyl-L-carnitine in early-onset AD. Neurology 2000; 55: 805–810.
11. Chakravarty, A.K. et al.: New phenylethanoid glycosides from *Bacopa monniera*. Chem Pharm Bull (Tokyo) 2002; 50: 1616–1618.
12. Nathan, P.J. et al.: The acute effects of an extract of *Bacopa monniera* (Brahmi) on cognitive function in healthy normal subjects. Hum Psychopharmacol 2001; 16: 345–351.
13. Youdim, K.A.; Joseph, J.A.: A possible emerging role of phytochemicals in improving age-related neurological dysfunctions: a multiplicity of effects. Free Radic Biol Med 2001; 30: 583–594.
14. Lim, G.P. et al.: The curry spice curcumin reduces oxidative damage and amyloid pathology in an Alzheimer transgenic mouse. J Neurosci 2001; 21: 8370–8377.
15. Gold, J.L. et al.: Herbal-drug therapy interactions: a focus on dementia. Curr Opin Clin Nutr Metab Care 2001; 4: 29–34.
16. Rauchova, H.; Lenaz, G.: Coenzyme Q and its therapeutic use. Ceska Slov Farm 2001; 50: 78–82.
17. Gutzmann, H.; Hadler, D.: Sustained efficacy and safety of idebenone in the treatment of Alzheimer's disease: update on a 2-year double-blind multicentre study. J Neural Transm 1998; 54 (suppl): 301–310.
18. De Bustos, F. et al.: Serum levels of coenzyme Q10 in patients with Alzheimer's disease. J Neural Transm 2000; 107: 233–239.
19. Graf, A. et al.: The effects of light therapy on mini-mental state examination scores in demented patients. Biol Psychiatry 2001; 50: 725–727.

VI Late-Stage Therapy

25

Pain and Palliative Care in Late-Stage Dementia Patients

Sophie Pautex, Dina Zekry, Gilbert Zulian,
Gabriel Gold, and Jean-Pierre Michel

INTRODUCTION

Dementia is certainly one of the most dramatic medical and economic challenges that our society will face in the coming years (1). If the specificity of care appears incontestable at the early stages of the disease (959,000 new cases of dementia per year in the United States in 1994—ninth most frequent disease in incidence) (2), the care at the end of life of the 7,082,000 existing demented patients (eighth most prevalent disease in the United States) has to be better considered, provided, and studied (2). Geriatricians and palliative care specialists are particularly concerned, because for each decade after the sixth, the number of affected people doubles, so that an estimated 30% of the population older than 85 years of age is affected by Alzheimer's disease (AD) (3,4). The end-of-life care of demented patients needs to reach the best possible quality. Its intensity has to be appropriated, timely, and ethically adapted, considering the multiple circumstances, family concerns, and the different environmental conditions (living at home or in an institution).

To highlight the importance of end-of-life care of demented patients, we will consider the survival of demented vs nondemented patients and the causes of death of patients with or without dementia, before examining specific ethical issues of end of life involved in the care of cognitively disturbed patients. A discussion of the suffering of family members and caregivers will conclude this literature review.

SURVIVAL OF DEMENTED PATIENTS

A 5-year follow-up of Canadians over 65 years living in the community (2923 with and 7340 without dementia) showed that elderly with dementia have clearly increased mortality rates compared to elderly without cognitive impairment in all age/gender categories (5). The 3-year and 5-year mortality risks of demented patients living in the community reached 45–48% (6,7) and 70%, respectively (8). Median length of life from diagnosis was reported to be 5.3 years (9), 5.4 years (10), and 8.5 years (11) in three prospective studies. However, the median survival after onset of dementia (and not time of study entry) appears to be shorter, after adjustment for length bias, than previously stressed: 3.3 years (95% confidence interval 2.7–4) (12). In the Baltimore Longitudinal Study of Aging, median length of life for both genders, following the diagnosis of AD was 8.3 years for persons diagnosed at 65 years and 3.4 years for persons diagnosed at 90 years (13). A 3-year follow-up of 5362 community-dwelling Italians, aged between 65 and 84 years, confirmed that the relative risk of dying (Cox proportional hazards model) for demented patients was higher (RR = 3.61; CI = 2.55–5.11) than for patients with cancer (RR = 2.01; CI = 1.20–3.38), heart failure (RR = 1.87; CI = 1.27–2.76), or dia-

From: *Current Clinical Neurology,*
Alzheimer's Disease: A Physician's Guide to Practical Management
Edited by: R. W. Richter and B. Zoeller Richter © Humana Press Inc., Totowa, NJ

betes (RR = 1.62; CI = 1.12–2.34) *(13)*. In the same study, institutionalization appeared to be more dangerous (RR = 4.17; CI = 2.20–7.94) than any pathological process considered separately (including dementia). That is, demented patients, who are frequently institutionalized at advanced stage of the disease, are really at the highest risk of death *(14)*. This relative risk is twice as high for men compared to women *(8,14)* and increases with age, severity of dementia, and its disability consequences *(7,15)*.

The dementia etiology is also important to consider. Vascular dementia (VaD) has a higher 5-year risk of mortality than Alzheimer's disease *(8)*, while Lewy body disease has the same 3-year mortality risk as Alzheimer's disease, considering the age at onset and the age at death *(16)*. The number and importance of associated diseases were not known in this study and they could have explained these findings, particularly the worst survival prognosis of patients with VaD.

Moreover, independent of the medical conditions, the types of social care seem to affect the survival of demented patients. Participation at a day center as well as the active support of family members appear to decrease the mortality risk significantly, while the benefit of Meals on Wheels on survival is not at all proved *(6)*. This raises the question of whether individual affective support of demented patients is more important than the type and the quantity of care.

Another interesting debate relates to the impact of the new cholinesterase inhibitors on the survival of demented patients. The safety of this category of drugs has been demonstrated on a total of 208 demented patients treated with tacrine *(17)*. Treatment with tacrine, at least at doses of more than 80 mg/d, appeared to be associated with a reduced likelihood of nursing-home placement *(18)*. This tendency is supported by the results of a cost analysis based on a decision-analytic model constructed on the milestones in the progression of Alzheimer's disease *(19)*. These various analyses suggested a trend toward lower mortality for patients receiving more than 120 mg/d of tacrine *(18,19)*. This tendency was confirmed by a recent retrospective cohort study of 1449 users of tacrine compared with 6119 nonusers matched on facility, date of tacrine use, level of cognitive function, and dementia diagnosis *(20)*. The survival hazard rate ratio (HRR) was 0.76 (95% CI = 0.70–0.83) for the users of tacrine, and those who used higher doses (more than 80 mg/d) experienced the greatest survival advantage (HRR = 0.74; 95% CI = 0.56–1.0) *(20)*. These data on increased survival of AD patients treated with tacrine require us to reconsider the negative impact of institutionalization *(14)* and to raise the same debate with the other cholinesterase inhibitor drugs *(21)*. Moreover, the economic impact of such treatments needs to be reevaluated.

CAUSES OF DEATH OF DEMENTED AND NONDEMENTED PATIENTS

At the end stage of the disease, persons with dementia are often bedridden and vulnerable to developing other medical conditions and dying earlier than if they were not demented *(22)*. This is consistent with several studies reporting that the main causes of death of demented patients are pneumonia and cardiovascular disease *(23–26)*. Bronchopneumonia occurred in severely impaired patients, more often with AD (70.9%) than with vascular dementia (VaD) *(26)*. Heart disease and stroke predominated in the less cognitively impaired patients with VaD *(25)*. However, the above data were based almost exclusively on death certificate reports, which may not be sufficiently reliable. Morbidity and mortality statistics arising from death certificates are seriously flawed, because of the omission of important information *(27)*.

In practice, deciding which disorders should be included on death certificates reflects the opinion of the physician completing the form, and very often underlying causes of death are not mentioned *(28)*. This can explain why comparison of data from death certificates completed by either attending physicians or by doctor-coroners and necropsy reports show large deviations in causes of death, ranging from –91.6% to +74.8% *(29)*. The Canadian Study of Health and Aging proves that the sensitivity of the death certificate and the question regarding diagnosis of dementia is low (33% and 44%), although their specificity is very high (93%) *(30)*. A prospective, 11-year, longitudinal study of behavioral and psychological changes in dementia, with autopsy follow-up, showed that the immediate cause of death recorded at autopsy agreed with the cause of death on 53% of death certificates *(12)*.

Similar discrepancies have also been reported by others, resulting in an increased interest in geriatric autopsy studies *(31,32)*. Pathological series are rare in the literature. An autopsy series based on 72 cases showed that pneumonia was the immediate cause of death in 72% of clinically demented patients, while cardiovascular diseases represented only 24% of the causes of death *(33)*. Another complete autopsy study performed in 120 hospitalized demented with VaD ($n = 34$), mixed dementia (MD, $n = 65$), and AD ($n = 21$) neuropathologically confirmed and 222 nondemented elderly (mean age 84.9 ± 6.9 years) showed that the number of reported causes of death per patient was 1.7 in both groups *(34)*. Among the reported causes of death in each group, bronchopneumonia was identified as the main immediate cause of death in 40.8% of demented and in 34.2% of nondemented patients. Infections of various origins, including pulmonary tract infections, represented 53.3% and 48.6% of the causes of death in demented and nondemented patients, respectively. The combination of cardiac and cerebrovascular diseases (cardiac failure plus pulmonary embolism plus myocardial infarction plus central nervous system hemorrhage) corresponded to 68.2% and 73.7% of the identified immediate causes of death in demented and nondemented patients, respectively. No difference in infectious causes was observed among the various dementia types, although the combined cardio- and cerebrovascular causes of death were significantly more frequent in VaD (91.0%) than in MD (61.3%) and in AD (52.1%) cases ($p = 0.001$). The major differences in these various pathological cases occurred in the rate of cardiac failure: VaD (44.1%), AD (19%), and MD (15.3%) *(34)*.

In opposition with current opinion *(35,36)*, this study *(34)*, like many others *(31,37–39)* strongly suggests that dementia can only be considered as an underlying cause of death. Moreover, demented patients died from the same causes as nondemented hospitalized subjects, when quality of care was not influenced by cognitive status.

ETHICAL CONSIDERATIONS IN END-OF-LIFE ISSUES

Dementia is associated with a wide variety of underlying conditions: poor nutrition resulting from diminishing intake of fluids and nutrients, urinary incontinence, skin breakdown, and various types of infections that accelerate the progression of common age-associated diseases (diabetes, chronic heart failure, hip fracture) and precipitate the demented patient into functional dependency *(13,40)*. Although the end-of-life issues are similar in demented and nondemented patients, the intensity and types of care are really different in these two patient groups. A 13-month retrospective study compared the hospital charts of two kinds of end-of-life patients: demented ($n = 80$) and metastatic cancer patients ($n = 84$) *(41)*. Complex invasive or noninvasive diagnostic tests were used significantly more frequently in cancer patients than in demented patients (respectively 41% vs 13%, $p < 0.002$, and 49% vs 23%, $p < 0.02$), while enteral tube feeding and use of antibiotics for an identifiable infection were significantly less in cancer than in demented patients (respectively 9% vs 26%, $p < 0.02$, and 45% vs 65%, $p < 0.004$) *(41)*. Cardiopulmonary resuscitation was practiced with the same frequency in the two different groups of patients *(41)*. These disturbing findings raise the difficult issues of appropriate quality of care during terminal stages of dementia.

Some of the most troublesome complications of advanced dementia, and particularly during the terminal phase of dementia, are the behavioral symptoms: physical aggression and delusions, wandering, agitation, sleep problems, and anxiety are among the most important (42). Behavioral and psychological symptoms of dementia (BPSD) is a recently coined term to describe this heterogeneous range of noncognitive symptoms occurring in people with dementia of any etiology *(43)*. They result in emotional suffering for patients and caregivers, excess disability and mortality, premature institutionalization, and increased financial cost *(43)*. Antipsychotic neuroleptics are the most commonly used medications for the treatment of psychotic symptoms in AD. Although a number of antipsychotics and antidepressants are available to treat behavioral symptoms in AD, none of these drugs has been approved specifically for this purpose. Nonetheless, physicians prescribe such medications without proper labeling and despite a dearth of published controlled studies supporting their use. A meta-analysis of the available placebo-controlled trials by Schneider et al. *(44)* found that the use of these drugs produced only modest effect and that no single antipsychotic medication had greater efficacy than another. However, more recent data have shown a significant effect of atypical antipsychotics in reducing behavioral disturbances *(45,46)*. Side-effect profiles and co-morbidities must also be considered when prescribing these drugs. Several studies have shown that acetylcholinesterase inhibitors also may reduce behavioral and psychological symptoms, including agitation, apathy, anxiety, pacing, and visual hallucinations *(9,10)*.

Nonpharmacological intervention is also an important part of dementia care. Few controlled trials have been published on the effectiveness of various nonpharmacological strategies *(47–49)*.

Frequently BPSD is the atypical clinical presentation of pain and suffering *(50)*. Assessment of discomfort in 104 late-stage demented patients (mean age 85 years) with the "Assessment of Discomfort in Dementia" scales showed that the most frequent displayed behaviors were tense body language, sad facial expression, persevering verbalizations, and verbal outbursts *(50)*. These nonverbal cues and subjective states are very difficult to identify. In a study of severely disabled nursing-home residents, aggressive behaviors were significantly more frequent in subjects with two or more pain-related diagnoses *(51)*. This point was not supported, however, by a recent retrospective study of 154 patients with dementia *(52)*. This study did not demonstrate that a single point-in-time measurement of pain in demented patients was associated with an increase of behavioral problems.

Cognitive impairment is a major barrier to proper pain assessment. A number of studies have confirmed that it is possible to assess pain in cognitively impaired patients and that their reports of pain should be taken seriously *(52,53)*. A French study compared the estimation of pain recognition and adequate treatment in hospitalized late-stage demented patients: physicians thought they recognized pain in 96% of the cases, assistant nurses estimated that it was true only in 68%, and nurses were more severe, thinking that pain is not recognized and not adequately treated in 44% of the cases *(54)*. Moreover, the same study shows that physicians estimated that the care decision was really the result of an interdisciplinary consensus in 87% of the cases, while assistant nurses and nurses, respectively, thought that this was the case in only 55% and 51% of the cases *(54)*. These differences attest to the inability of the caregivers to identify pain and suffering in advanced dementia patients. The main consequence is the tendency to undermedicate pain in these patients *(55–58)*. This has led to the recognition of pain as the fifth vital sign, with the hope that this will increase the awareness of inadequately treated pain in older persons *(59)*.

Unfortunately, instead of providing pain control and spiritual support during the dying process, there is a tendency of the medical system to concentrate on life-prolonging interventions *(60)*. Four main medical interventions are considered as life-prolonging and are indeed raising ethical debates: cardiopulmonary resuscitation, renal dialysis, tube feeding, and antibiotic administration. At the advanced stage of dementia, only enteral nutrition and antibiotic use raise an ethical debate.

A review of evidence of the usefulness of tube feeding in patients with advanced dementia (including all Medline peer-reviewed papers published between 1996 and 1999) found that tube feeding does not clinically improve important outcomes, such as survival, functioning, risk of pressure sores, risk of infection, or risk of aspiration *(61)*. However, it must be recognized that malnutrition and vitamin deficiencies may worsen dementia *(62)*.

Infectious complications are very common causes of death in the demented *(34)*. The atypical clinical presentation of infections is frequent. When an infection is recognized, antibiotic use needs to be discussed and integrated into the comprehensive care assessment (physiological reserves of the patient, severity of dementia). Sometimes, the patient's discomfort is linked to an evident clinical infection, particularly of the pulmonary tract. In this case, antibiotic usage is beneficial, whatever the dementia stage, but the antibiotic choice has to be accurate, adequate, and timely *(63,64)*. A prospective cohort study conducted in 61 nursing homes in the Netherlands assessed the suffering (with the Discomfort Scale—Dementia of Alzheimer Type) in demented patients (*n* = 662) with pneumonia, treated with (77%) or without (23%) antibiotics at baseline and 3 months later *(65)*. Breathing problems were the most prominent. A peak in discomfort was observed at baseline. Compared with surviving patients treated with antibiotics, the level of discomfort was generally higher in patients in whom antibiotic treatment was withheld and in nonsurvivors. Some 39% of patients treated with antibiotics and 93% of patients treated without antibiotics died within 3 months.

The anguish of end-of-life patients seen in all cases exists particularly in the severely demented. The quality of terminal care depends largely on the patient's awareness, which often fluctuates. Sometimes the patient is confused and unaware of his or her condition; at other times the patient knows that she or he is dying and attempts to communicate these fears *(66)*. What is the significance of this attempt? Are there any nonverbal hidden messages; is there any expression of a wish to die? Too often these questions remain without recognizable responses. Important and difficult ethical debates arise among the caregiver staff and family members, who are frequently disappointed by the patients' fluctuating mental status.

The ethical concern about palliative drug treatment of these demented patients can be reduced but never completely resolved. Advanced health directive planning is probably the best way to respect demented patients' prior self-determination *(67,68)*. The role of euthanasia as legally practiced in the Netherlands and in the U.S. state of Oregon is beyond the scope of this review.

SUFFERING OF FAMILY MEMBERS AND CAREGIVERS

Confronted with the terminal stage of life of a demented patient, family members and health care professionals face two important features: the fear of death and the fear of dementia *(69)*. The mourning process itself is influenced by various factors, such as the symbolic role of the dying person, his or her unfulfilled requests, the death circumstances, and the quality of the last moments of life *(70)*. In the case of death of a demented patient, the mourning process is different. The loss, the separation from a loved one, who has been demented for several years, is even more difficult. The anticipation of the death, preceded by the social death, does not help to ease the mourning process *(70)*.

Thus, in the terminal phase of life of demented patients, it is important to improve communication skills with the patient and to facilitate the interdisciplinary exchange. Family members must be helped to clarify the inescapable fatal outcome of their loved one and to cope better with the mourning process. It is really fundamental to support the family during the mourning process, which always is difficult. Frequently, mourning leads to severe depression in family members and caregivers *(70)*.

REFERENCES

1. Souètre, E.J.; et al.: Economic analysis of Alzheimer's disease in outpatients: impact of symptom severity. In: Giacobini, E.; Becker, R. (eds.): Alzheimer's disease: therapeutic strategies. Birkhaeuser, Boston, 1994: 470–480.
2. Murray, C.J.; Lorez, A.D.: The global burden of disease. Harvard University Press, Cambridge, MA, 1997.
3. Katchaturian, Z.S.; Radebaugh, T.S.: AD: Where are we now? Where are we going? Alzheimer's Dis Assoc Disord 1998; 12 (suppl 3): 24–28.
4. Ritchie, K.; Kildea, D.: Is senile dementia "age related" or "aging related"? Evidence from a meta-analysis of dementia prevalence in the oldest old. Lancet 1995; 346: 931–934.
5. Ostbye, T.; Hill, G.; Steenhuis, R.: Mortality in elderly Canadians with and without dementia: a 5-year follow-up. Neurology 1999; 53: 521–526.
6. Orrell, M.; Butler, R.; Bebbington, P.: Social factors and the outcome of dementia. Int J Geriatr Psychiatry 2000; 15: 515–520.
7. Schaufele, M.; Bickel, H.; Weyerer, S.: Predictors of mortality among demented elderly in primary care. Int J Geriatr Psychiatry 1999; 14: 946–956.
8. Auero-Torres, H. et al.: Mortality from dementia in advanced age: a 5-year follow-up study of incident dementia cases. J Clin Epidemiol 1999; 52: 737–743.

9. Welch, H.G.; Waslsh, J.S.; Larson, E.B.: The cost of institutional care in Alzheimer's disease: nursing home and hospital use in a prospective cohort. J Am Geriatr Soc 1992; 40: 221–224.

10. Severson, M.A. et al.: Patterns and predictors of institutionalization in community-based dementia patients. J Am Geriatr Soc 1994; 42: 181–185.

11. Keene, J. et al.: Death and dementia. Int J Geriatr Psychiatry 2001; 16: 969–974.

12. Wolfson, C. et al.: A reevaluation of the duration of survival after the onset of dementia. N Engl J Med 2001; 344: 1111–1116.

13. Brookmeyer, R. et al.: Survival following a diagnosis of Alzheimer's disease. Arch Neurol 2002; 59: 1764–1767.

14. Baldereschi, M. et al.: Dementia as a major predictor of death among Italian elderly. ILSA Working Group. Italian Longitudinal Study on Aging. Neurology 1999; 52: 709–713; comments: Neurology 2000; 54: 1014.

15. Broersma, F. et al.: Survival in a population-based cohort of dementia patients: predictors and causes of mortality. Int J Geriatr Psychiatry 1999; 14: 748–753.

16. Walker, Z. et al.: Three years survival in patients with a clinical diagnosis of dementia with Lewy bodies. Int J Geriatr Psychiatry 2000; 15: 267–273.

17. Gracon, S.I. et al.: Safety of tacrine: clinical trials, treatment IND and postmarketing experience. Alzheimer's Dis Assoc Dis 1998; 12: 93–101.

18. Knopman, D. et al.: Long-term tacrine (Cognex) treatment: effects on nursing home placement and mortality. Neurology 1996; 47: 166–177.

19. Henke, C.J.; Burchmore, M.J.: The economic impact of tacrine in the treatment of Azheimer's disease. Clin Therapeut 1997; 19: 1–6.

20. Ott, B.R.; Lapane, K.L.: Tacrine therapy is associated with reduced mortality in nursing home residents with dementia. J Am Geriatr Soc 2002; 50: 35–40.

21. Lopez, O.L. et al.: Cholinesterase inhibitor treatment alters the natural history of Alzheimer's disease. J Neurol Neurosurg Psychiatry 2002; 72: 310–314.

22. National Institute of Aging (USA): Progress report on Alzheimer's disease 1998. National Institutes of Health, Bethesda, MD, 1998.

23. Hewer, W. et al.: Mortality of patients with organ-induced psychiatric disorders during inpatient psychiatric treatment. Nervenarzt 1991; 62, 170–176.

24. Inagaki, T. et al.: Five year follow-up study on dementia in institutions for the elderly. Nippon Ronen Igakkai Zasshi 1992; 29: 729–734.

25. Kukull, W.A.: Causes of death associated with Alzheimer's disease: variation by level of cognitive impairment before death. J Am Geriatr Soc 1994; 42: 723–726.

26. Olichney, J.M. et al: Death certificate reporting of dementia and mortality in an Alzheimer's disease research center cohort. J Am Geriatr Soc 1995; 43: 890.

27. Thomas, B.M.; Starr, J.M.; Whalley, L.J.: Death certification in treated cases of presenile Alzheimer's disease and vascular dementia in Scotland. Age Ageing 1997; 26, 401–406.

28. Salib, E.: Autopsy in psychiatric geriatry. Int J Geriatr Psychiatry 1998, 13: 747–748.

29. Karolyi, G.; Karolyi, P.: Value of mortality data and necropsy records in monitoring morbidity in a population. J Epidemiol Community Health 1991; 45, 238–243.

30. Stewart, M. et al: Estimating antemortem cognitive status of deceased subjects in a longitudinal study of dementia. Int Psychogeriatrics 2001; 13 (suppl) 1: 99–106.

31. Klima, M.P. et al.: Causes of death in geriatric patients: a cross cultural study. J Gerontol A Biol Sci Med Sci 1997; 52, M247–M253.

32. Blumenthal, H.T.: The autopsy in gerontological research: a retrospective. J Gerontol A Biol Sci Med Sci 2002; 57 A: M433–M437.

33. Burns, A. et al.: Cause of death in Alzheimer's disease. Age Ageing 1990; 19: 341–344.

34. Kammoun, S. et al.: Immediate causes of death of demented and non-demented elderly: clinical and pathological comparisons. Acta Neurol Scand 2000; 176 (suppl): 96–99.

35. Hoyert, D.L.; Rosenberg, H.M.: Mortality from Alzheimer's disease: an update. Natl Vital Stat Rep 1999; 47: 1–5.

36. Anderson, R.N.: Leading causes for 2000. Natl Vital Stat Rep 2002; 50: 1–85.

37. Molsa, P.K. et al.: Survival and cause of death in Alzheimer's disease and multi-infarct dementia. Acta Neurol Scand 1986; 74: 103–107.

38. Chandra, V. et al.: Patterns of mortality from types of dementia in the United States, 1971 and 1973–1978. Neurology 1986; 36: 204–208.

39. Hwang, J.P. et alL.: Mortality in geriatric psychiatric inpatients. Int J Psychiatry Med 1998; 28: 327–331.

40. Shuster, J.L.: Palliative care for advanced dementia. Clin Geriatr Med 2000; 16: 373–386.

41. Abronheim, J.C. et al.: Treatment of the dying in the acute care hospital: advanced dementia and metastatic cancer. Arch Intern Med 1996; 156: 2094–2100.

42. Michel, J.P.; Gold, G.: Behavioural symptoms in Alzheimers'disease: validity of targets and present treatments. Age Ageing 2001; 30: 105–106.

43. Finkel, S.I.; Burns, A.: Behavioural and psychological symptoms of dementia (BPSD): a clinical and research update. Intern Psychogeriatrics 2000; 12: 9–12.
44. Schneider, L. et al.: A meta-analysis of controlled trials of neuroleptic treatment in dementia. J Am Geriatr Soc 1990; 38: 553–563.
45. Lane, H.Y. et al.: Shifting from haloperidol to risperidone for behavioral disturbances in dementia: safety, response predictors and mood effects. J Clin Psychopharmacol 2002; 22: 4–10.
46. Davidson, M. et al.: A long-term, multicenter, open-label study of risperidone in elderly patients with psychosis. Int J Geriatr Psychiatry 2000; 15: 506–514.
47. Teri, L. et al.: Behavioural management of depression in demented patients: a controlled trial. J Gerontol 1997; 52B: 159–166.
48. Procter, R. et al.: Behavioural management in nursing and residential homes: a randomized controlled trial. Lancet 1999; 354: 26–29.
49. Gormley, N. et al.: Behavioural management of aggression in dementia: a randomized controlled trial. Age Ageing 2001; 30: 141–145.
50. Kovach, C.R. et al: Assessment and treatment of discomfort for people with late-stage dementia. J Pain Sympt Manage 1999; 18: 412–419.
51. Feldt, K.S. et al.: Examining pain in aggressive cognitively impaired older adults. J Gerontol Nurs 1998; 24: 14–22.
52. Brummel-Smith, K. et al.: Outcomes of pain in frail older adults with dementia. J Am Geriatr Soc 2002; 50: 1847–1851.
53. Pautex, S. et al.: Pain assessment in elderly hospitalized demented patients. Abstract, Congress International Association Study of Pain, San Diego, CA, 2002.
54. Gonthier, R. et al: Séméiologie et évaluation de la douleur chez le dément ou non-communicant. Info Kara 1998; 53: 12–23.
55. Farrell, M.J. et al.: The impact of dementia on the pain experience. Pain 1996; 67: 7–15.
56. Weissman, D.E.; Matson, S.: Pain assessment and management in the long-term care setting. Theor Med Bioethics 1999; 20: 31–43.
57. Feldt, S.; Ryden, M.; Myles, S.: Treatment of pain in cognitively impaired compared to cognitively intact older patients with hip fracture. J Am Geriatr Soc. 1998; 46: 1079–1085.
58. Morrison, R.S.; Siu A.L.: A comparison of pain and its treatment in advanced dementia and cognitively intact patients with hip fracture. J Pain Sympt Manage 2000; 19: 240–248.
59. Flaherty, J.H.: Who is taking about the 5th vital sign? J Gerontol Med Sci 2001; 56A: M397–M399.
60. Volicer, L. et al.: Scales for evaluation of end of life care in dementia. Alzheimer's Dis Assoc Dis 2001; 15: 194–200.
61. Finucane, T.E. et al.: Tube feeding in patients with advanced dementia: a review of the evidence. JAMA 1999; 282: 1365–1370; comments: JAMA 1999; 282: 1380–1381, JAMA 2000; 283: 1563, 1564.
62. Reynisch, W. et al.: Nutritional factors and Alzheimer's disease. J Gerontol Med Sci 2001; 56A: M675–M680.
63. Michel, J.P. et al.: Ethique de l'antibiothérapie en médecine de l'âge avancé. Schweiz Med Wochenschr 1994; 124: 2220–2225.
64. Van Nes, M.C. et al.: Considérations sur l'utilisation des antibiotiques chez les malades très âgés. Gériatrie Pratique 1998; 4: 39–42.
65. Van Der Steen, J.T. et al.: Pneumonia: the demented patient's best friend? Discomfort after starting or withholding antibiotic treatment. J Am Geriatr Soc. 2002; 50: 1681–1688.
66. Benbow, S.M.: Dementia, grief and dying. Palliative Med 1990, 4: 87–92.
67. Hurley, A.C.; Volicer, L.: Alzheimer's disease: it's okay mama, if you want to go, it's okay. JAMA 2002; 288: 2324–2331.
68. Hurley, A.C. et al.: Nursing role in advance proxy planning for Alzheimer patients. Caring 1994; 13: 72–76.
69. Franken, E. et al.: La mort du vieillard dément. Thanatologie 1997; 31: 143–146.
70. Dell'Accio, E.: Le vécu de deuil des familles ayant accompagné un parent âgé dément. JALMALV 2000; 60: 35–39.

26

Cardiological Issues in Late-Stage Alzheimer's Disease

A Clinician's Approach

José R. Medina

INTRODUCTION

Practicing clinicians face an ever-aging population afflicted by severe cardiovascular and cognitive disorders, which pose clinical dilemmas and are a challenge for families and caregivers. Cardiovascular diseases are the leading cause of hospital admissions and of morbidity and mortality in the elderly *(1,2)*. Proper allocation of resources, increasing costs, and consumer pressures are a daily experience. Ethical decisions for patients afflicted by terminal diseases are difficult and require the participation of specialized teams.

Medical societies have published Practice Guidelines based on clinical evidence to help practitioners in the decision-making process. They are implemented in hospitals across the country and enforced by quality assurance committees. The application of these guidelines to special populations, i.e., the elderly, demented, or patients at the end of life, is difficult. Advanced medical directives are critical in the implementation of these recommendations.

THE HEART AND THE BRAIN: A CONNECTION OF UTMOST IMPORTANCE

Although the brain comprises only 2% of total body weight, it utilizes 20% of cardiac output and 20% of total body oxygen uptake. Brain cell function and survival are related directly to the cerebral blood flow, the perfusion pressure, and the availability of metabolic substrates of oxygen and glucose. The loss of cortical neurons begins after 4 minutes of a cardiac arrest with the associated cessation of flow of oxygen and nutrients to the brain *(3)*.

The integrity of the extracranial and intracranial circulation is of vital importance for the adequate delivery of oxygen and glucose to the brain. Of equal importance are normal glucose levels (plasma), hemoglobin concentration, blood viscosity, and arterial oxygen saturation, as well as arterial perfusion pressure.

Disorders that affect cardiac output, oxygen transport, blood pressure, and cerebral blood flow can create acute and chronic dysfunction of the brain or of certain brain areas. Vascular dementia (VaD) is secondary to cardiovascular conditions that decrease the cerebral perfusion and lead to multiple infarcts, and hypoperfusion of watershed brain areas. Clinical syndromes of dementia therefore are not only related to cerebrovascular diseases but also and frequently to cardiovascular conditions *(4)*.

AGE-RELATED CARDIOVASCULAR CHANGES

Life expectancy in the United States rose from 47 years in 1900 to 76 years in 1996, and is expected to be 82 years of age by the year 2026. Despite a decrease in the incidence of coronary artery disease,

From: *Current Clinical Neurology,*
Alzheimer's Disease: A Physician's Guide to Practical Management
Edited by: R. W. Richter and B. Zoeller Richter © Humana Press Inc., Totowa, NJ

the number of deaths has increased in individuals older than 65 years. The aged population consumes one-third of the drugs and spends one-third of all health-care dollars.

Congestive heart failure (CHF) is the most common cause of hospitalization in the elderly, with an incidence of 550,000 new cases per year and a mortality rate ranging between 10% and 40%, depending on the severity of the illness. Myocardial infarction accounts for about 1.5% of cases in the population over 65, with a male preponderance that equalizes after the age of 80 *(5)*.

Hypertension and hypercholesterolemia aggravate atherosclerosis. Adequate treatment of these conditions can lead to a reduction in cardiovascular mortality and cardiovascular events. Systolic hypertension increases with age due to a decrease in aortic compliance. An increase in pulse pressure of 10 mmHg is associated with a 12% increase in coronary artery disease (CAD), a 14% increase in heart failure risk, and a 6% increase in mortality *(6)*.

Age-related changes in the cardiac skeleton promote calcification of the aortic valve, the mitral annulus, and the interventricular septum. Aging affects the conduction system of the heart with prolongation of the QT interval in women with the appearance of significant arrhythmias. Sick sinus syndrome, atrial fibrillation, bilateral bundle branch blocks, and complete AV block are common and may cause sudden death *(7)*.

Significant vascular changes—both structural and functional—affect vascular compliance. These changes may decrease the cerebral blood flow and increase the risk of ischemic cerebral damage, leading to conditions such as Alzheimer's disease (AD). The concept that AD is a vascular disorder has recently been proposed. De la Torre and colleagues present evidence that AD represents a vascular disease with a decreased cerebral perfusion and microvascular changes, which precede the neurodegenerative changes and the cognitive decline *(8)*.

Newer studies suggest that lipid-lowering agents (such as statins) can help prevent the development of dementia. These findings support the importance of vascular changes in the development of AD.

CARDIOVASCULAR DISEASE PRACTICE GUIDELINES

The American College of Cardiology and the American Heart Association in association with other medical societies have published recommendations for the evaluation and treatment of cardiovascular diseases.

Congestive Heart Failure

The Congestive Heart Failure Practice Guidelines have been recently updated, and a new classification of CHF was presented *(9–12)*. The emphasis lies on the prevention of organ damage, and emphasizes the need of recognizing and treating hypertension, diabetes, and hypercholesterolemia, as well as alcohol or drug overuse.

CHF is a disease that affects a significant percentage (5–10%) of individuals older than 65 years of age. It has been reported that nearly 5 million people in the United Sates suffer from CHF, and approximately 900,000 hospital admissions show a primary diagnosis of this disease, with substantial economical implications for the Medicare budget. CHF derives from improper emptying of the left ventricle (systolic dysfunction) or is secondary to a difficulty in its filling (diastolic dysfunction). These abnormalities lead to pulmonary vascular congestion, pulmonary hypertension, hepatic congestion, and peripheral edema.

Poorly managed hypertension and degenerative valvular as well as ischemic diseases are the most common causes of CHF. Infiltrative diseases such as amyloidosis may also be present in the myocardium of elderly patients. Dyspnea, progressive fatigue, and inability to cope with daily physical activities are frequent symptoms. The presence of pulmonary rales, neck vein distention and abnormal heart sounds (S4, S3 gallops and murmurs), enlargement of the liver, and peripheral edema are frequent findings. The chest X-ray usually confirms the presence of pulmonary edema.

Laboratory findings, including the determination of cardiac enzymes, serum electrolytes, and the newly developed brain natriuretic peptide (BNP), help diagnose CHF. Increased concentrations of BNP have been found to be a marker in patients with elevated left atrial pressure. BNP decreases with a decrease in left atrial pressure and has become a useful marker for separating cardiac from pulmonary dyspnea.

The echocardiogram helps with the determination of the systolic vs diastolic dysfunction. A decrease in ejection fraction is associated with systolic dysfunction. An abnormal transmitral flow (measured by Doppler) is the hallmark of diastolic dysfunction. Echocardiography also helps in the diagnosis of valvular structural changes and function. The determination of correctable causes of heart failure by means of invasive and noninvasive diagnostic procedures is recommended.

Treatment modalities, which include ACE inhibitors, β-blockers, and diuretics, have been shown not only to relieve CHF symptoms, but also to improve survival. Digitalis is useful to control the cardiac rate in patients with atrial fibrillation and has been shown to decrease the number of readmissions in patients with systolic dysfunction. Correction of lipid abnormalities is important in patients with ischemic heart disease and heart failure. Correction of valvular disease, revascularization procedures, and in some cases plastic procedures to modify the left ventricular dimensions are to be considered in the management of patients with CHF.

Recently, a new therapeutic modality using biventricular pacing has been found to be of help in modifying the contractility of the two ventricles and to ease CHF symptoms *(13)*.

Coronary Artery Disease and Myocardial Infarction in the Elderly

CAD is prevalent in patients over 65 years; by the age of 80, 70% of patients have pathological evidence of CAD.

The clinical manifestations can be atypical in the elderly. Patients may complain more frequently of dyspnea or fatigue rather than angina. Silent myocardial infarctions are common in the elderly, and the first manifestation is the presence of CHF. Patients with clinically evident myocardial infarction (MI) usually present to the emergency room with considerable delay.

Patients with a suspected MI need to have an immediate electrocardiographic evaluation to establish the presence of ST-segment elevation, -depression, and of Q-wave abnormalities. The treatment of Q-wave infarction may vary from that of non-Q-wave infarctions. Patients with Q-wave infarct usually have a total occlusion of the coronary artery due to a fibrin-enriched thrombus. Patients with non-Q-wave infarct are usually found to have a platelet-rich thrombus, which responds to antithrombotic agents *(14,15)*.

MI patients with ST-segment elevation need to receive either thrombolysis or primary percutaneous coronary intervention (PCI). Older individuals are at risk for intracranial bleeding, as they frequently have an elevated blood pressure. In patients with ST-segment elevation, our primary approach consists of coronary angiography and immediate percutaneous coronary intervention, namely, angioplasty and stenting, if indicated.

Patients with non-Q-wave infarcts are usually treated with low-molecular heparin and GPIIb/IIIA inhibitors, and elective angiography, if clinical or imaging manifestations of residual ischemia are present.

The complications of thrombolytic therapy include a slight increase in the incidence of hemorrhagic stroke. Old age, prior history of stroke, and severe hypertension are predisposing causes of intracranial bleeding after thrombolytic therapy.

Myocardial damage may lead to intracavitary thrombosis, which predisposes to cerebral embolization and may provoke vascular dementia. The proper use of warfarin and antiplatelet agents may prevent recurrent embolic problems.

Atrial Fibrillation

Atrial fibrillation (AF) is a common form of arrhythmia, either as a complication of myocardial infarction or secondary to left ventricular disease with left atrial enlargement. It is also present with sick sinus syndrome. Atrial arrhythmias are common in the postoperative state.

Table 1
Major Risk Factors for Cardiogenic Embolism

Atrial fibrillation
Mitral stenosis, mitral calcification
Prosthetic cardiac valves
Recent myocardial infarction
Left ventricular thrombus, left ventricular wall motion abnormalities
Atrial myxoma
Endocarditis
Cardiomyopathy (dilated)
Atrial septal aneurysm
Aortic arch atherosclerotic plaques

AF also is the most important predisposing cardiac condition for cerebral embolism. Cerebral manifestations of cardiogenic embolism may include monocular visual loss, focal visual field cuts, transient ischemic attacks (TIAs) with focal or nonfocal findings, speech disturbances, strokes, and later multi-infarct dementia. Cardiac risk factors for cerebral embolism are outlined in Table 1. It has to be noted that essential hypertension is a recognized risk factor for AF.

The prevalence of AF increases with age. By the age of 80, 6% of all adults are affected. The evaluation of AF requires a good history for the determination of its onset, the frequency of the attacks or chronicity, and the associated symptoms. The physical examination is helpful in the determination of valvular heart disease, associated CHF, or thyroid or hypertensive cardiovascular disease.

The echocardiogram aids in the identification of valvular disease, the left atrial and left ventricular size and contractility, as well as the presence of pulmonary hypertension or pericardial disease. Transesophageal echocardiogram is frequently used to identify the presence of thrombus in the left atrial appendage and is used prior to electrical or chemical cardioversion.

A recently published practice guideline for AF outlines the treatment approach *(16)*. Paroxysmal AF may require no treatment after conversion to sinus rhythm. The management of persistent AF includes two modalities: rate control or attempts to reverse to sinus rhythm. Both modalities need anticoagulation with warfarin *(17)*.

The results of a randomized controlled study comparing these two treatment modalities suggest no difference in mortality with either measure. From this report, it appears reasonable that in older individuals one could attempt to control the ventricular response and prevent peripheral embolization with adequate anticoagulation. Warfarin prevents 62% of strokes in patients with AF, compared to aspirin, which prevents only 22%.

Older individuals are at risk for intracranial or gastrointestinal bleeding. Older people are also susceptible to falls. The fear of complications prevents many clinicians in the proper use of anticoagulation. Clinical evidence indicates that warfarin should be used in all patients with AF. The INR should be maintained between 2 and 3. It is well established that the benefit of anticoagulation is greater than the risk. Frequent monitoring of the prothrombin time helps in the prevention of significant hemorrhage. The use of gastric acid inhibiting agents (proton-pump inhibitors, H_2-receptor blocker) may prevent bleeding complications *(18,19)*.

Valvular Heart Disease

Aortic valvular disease, sclerosis, and stenosis in association with aortic regurgitation are common the elderly. Wear-and-tear phenomena of the aortic leaflets cause sclerotic, calcific, and degenerative changes, leading to stenosis and malfunction of the valve. It appears that lipid abnormalities aggravate this process.

The aortic valve becomes stenotic and insufficient as the valve becomes calcified. A systolic pressure gradient develops between the left ventricle and the aorta. The degree of gradient depends on the severity of the stenosis. Valvular stenosis of less than 0.7 cm^2 causes significant compromise in the left ventricular function and is the cause of symptoms manifested by dyspnea, CHF, angina-like discomfort, and sudden death. Valvular replacement is the treatment of choice in the symptomatic patient. Statins are being used to decrease the progression of aortic stenoses in the elderly. Valvuloplasty has been plagued by a significant number of restenoses and sudden death *(20–22)*.

Elderly patients tolerate valve replacement well. Usually tissue valves are used in the elderly, although mechanical valves should be preferred in physiologically young patients to prevent reoperation after the expected degeneration in biological valves. The risks of anticoagulation have to be taken into account in patients who receive mechanical prostheses. Newer pericardial valves appear to offer an advantage in longevity and durability.

In addition to the physical examination, echocardiography and Doppler determination of the gradient across the valve are the best measures to determine the progression of the disease.

Complications of aortic stenosis include the development of AF. Patients with this condition usually do not tolerate increases in the cardiac rate. The loss of the atrial contribution for ventricular filling may precipitate heart failure in patients with hyperthrophic ventricles and impaired diastolic function. Aggressive management of AF contributes to the patient's comfort and improves the hemodynamic malfunction.

Mitral Insufficiency

Mitral insufficiency in the elderly frequently is the consequence of ischemic heart disease with left ventricular dilatation. Acute papillary muscle dysfunction is secondary to acute ischemia. Chronic mitral insufficiency is due to myocardial fibrosis or papillary muscle infarction.

Hemodynamic consequences are those related to left ventricular (LV) dilatation, elevation of left atrial pressure, and fibrosis that ensues as the left atrium dilates. Left atrial pressure elevation leads to pulmonary edema, especially in cases of mitral regurgitation that follows acute myocardial infarction or ruptured cordae tendini. Annular dilatation secondary to LV dilatation is frequently seen in patients with CHF. Chronic mitral insufficiency leads to marked dilatation of the left atrium, which in turn predisposes to AF and left atrial thrombosis with the complications of peripheral embolization.

Mitral valve repair is the treatment of choice. This can be accomplished in association with coronary bypass surgery if indicated. Medical management includes agents to unload the left ventricle and prevent the recurrence of myocardial infarction. ACE inhibitors and β-blockers are used with this purpose.

Cardiovascular surgery using extracorporeal circulation may predispose to loss of memory and dementia. Present techniques, however, avoid the use of extracorporeal circulation in bypass operations.

Carotid Disease

Cerebrovascular accidents, either thromboembolic or hemorrhagic, are the third leading cause of death in the United States. The incidence of strokes is increasing with the increasing age of the population. The mortality from the acute episode is about 20%, with a late mortality of about 50% in 5 years *(23)*.

Cardiovascular causes of strokes include systemic hypertension, embolization from the left atrium, especially left atrial appendage in patients with mitral disease or AF, mural thrombus after myocardial infarction or cardiomyopathy, and carotid disease. Diabetic patients may develop small-vessel brain disease in addition to carotid disease. Paradoxical emboli through a patent foramen ovale have also been recognized as a potential cause of cerebrovascular accidents.

Significant improvements in the evaluation and treatment of strokes have been achieved over the years. The use of Doppler duplex technology and ultrasound imaging have helped in the identification of carotid stenosis. Radiological techniques such as magnetic resonance imaging (MRI and MRA), and computer tomography (CT scanning) are common practice in the evaluation of stroke patients. Transesophageal echocardiography to visualize the left atrial appendage, the presence of valvular vegetations, and right-to-left shunts, are considered routine procedures today. The use of tissue plasminogen activator (tPA) in the treatment of ischemic strokes is being incorporated with increasing frequency *(24)*.

The surgical technique of carotid endarterectomy in experienced hands has proven to be of value in symptomatic patients. Controversy still remains regarding the surgical treatment of asymptomatic carotid disease. Carotid stenting is becoming a new alternative for the management of these patients, although no large comparative studies are yet available. Clinicians should be aware of the local experience prior to surgical decisions, especially in asymptomatic patients with stenosis greater than 65%. The operative risk of stroke should be less than the incidence of strokes in asymptomatic individuals *(25)*.

The prevention of the progression of atherosclerosis with antiplatelet agents and lipid-lowering agents (such as statins) should be initiated once the diagnosis of carotid or vascular disease is established. The management of systolic and diastolic hypertension also is of paramount importance.

CARDIOVASCULAR MEDICATIONS CAN AFFECT CEREBRAL FUNCTIONS

Cardiovascular drugs have distinct, often complex effects on various brain functions, particularly pertaining to alertness and cognition. Patients suffering from dementia in addition to cardiovascular disease often take a variety of medications simultaneously. Adverse reaction should be considered, especially when mental symptoms worsen suddenly.

Antiarrhythmic agents are known to exert complex effects on the myocardium, but they also can affect the cerebrum adversely. Adverse CNS symptoms include ataxia, tremor, confusion, and delerium.

Antihypertensive agents, particularly vasodilators, can affect the brain negatively. Potentially harmful is the combination of cerebrovascular dilatation and low blood pressure, which may result in localized brain ischemia. If vasodilation is sufficient, cerebral autoregulation may be lost, and blood flow can become pressure-passive.

Ischemic brain damage and death have occurred in some cases. Reduction in cerebral blood flow has been observed in patients using calcium channel and β-blockers.

PERMANENT PACEMAKER IN OLDER INDIVIDUALS

Permanent pacemakers are indicated in the treatment of third-degree as well as advanced second-degree AV block, associated with symptomatic bradycardia, documented periods of asystole greater than 3 seconds, after catheter ablation of the AV node, and in arrhythmias and other medical conditions, which require drugs that result in symptomatic bradycardia. Newer recommendations emphasize the need of pacing in patients with cardiomegaly, left ventricular dysfunction, and asymptomatic third-degree AV block with rates greater than 40 *(26,27)*.

Permanent pacemakers are beneficial devices in older individuals. Their use is associated with low morbidity and low complication rate, and appears to be extremely helpful in the control of syncope due to bradyarrhythmias, especially in patients with prolonged QT interval and polymorphic ventricular tachycardia.

TERMINATION OF DEVICES IN THE DEMENTED PATIENT

The terminally ill patient with dementia and cardiovascular disease poses a difficult ethical problem for physicians and caregivers. Frequently, patients have not given advance directives or may no longer be mentally or cognitively competent to vocalize their wishes *(28)*. Caregivers may have optimistic or false expectations, and conflict may develop in families in the presence of the terminal illness. It is the obligation of the attending physician to establish a conversation regarding the need for advance directives and the determination of a legal guardian.

Cardiovascular consultants should be aware of the natural history of the disease in the older patient, and recommendations have to be based on the local experience in reference to specialized procedures and surgery.

Hospitals have assigned trained personnel to establish advanced directives, including cardiac resuscitation wishes. Determinations of quality of life according to age, the ability of care, and cultural factors are important aspects within the decisions. Cardiovascular surveillance committees, which evaluate the results of surgical and interventional procedures in local hospitals, can be extremely helpful to determine the local experience and outcome for anticipated procedures in the elderly.

In hospitalized patients, the participation of pastoral care services and liaison nurses between intensive care providers and the family have been helpful in the decision regarding the termination of support devices, respirators, intra-aortic balloon devices, as well as the cessation of activity of defibrillators and pacemakers. Decisions are to be made based on the patients wishes, the surrogate member of the family who has been given instructions by the patient, the family conference, by the caring team of physicians and nurses, and with the help of religious personnel. Frequently, these decisions have to be done in a step-down fashion to alleviate family emotional conflict *(28)*.

The change of attitudes from the traditional intensive rescue care to intensive palliative care demands a team approach, which respects the patient's desires, the sensitivity of the family, and the legal and ethical principles that govern the practice of medicine. Extensive knowledge of the natural history of a disease and good family communication may help to avoid the implementation of futile care *(29,30)*.

In general, the decision to stop devices, especially defibrillators and pacemakers, is based on the above considerations and the physician's insight, which recognizes that there is no hope for a meaningful life ahead.

CASE REPORTS

Late-Stage Dementia and CHF

The patient was a 79-year-old male, active until 2 years ago, when he developed progressive dementia and Parkinson's disease. His past history included a coronary bypass operation 10 years ago after an acute myocardial infarction and disabling angina. Following his surgery he was active, but as his neurological disease progressed he became bed-ridden.

He was admitted with acute pulmonary edema, markedly hypoxic, and required intubation. The laboratory tests confirmed a new myocardial infarction and markedly depressed left ventricular function.

The patient had not signed an advance directive but had expressed to his family his desire to avoid heroic measures to prolong his life. The family requested removal of the respirator and only comfort measures.

Conflict arose with the attending physician on call, who felt the patient needed respiratory support. The family requested a change of attending physician and decided to take the patient home as per his expressed wishes. Hospice Services were advised and the patient was released with morphine and comfort measures, and he expired peacefully at home 5 days later.

This case report illustrates a sensible decision of honoring the patient's request in a bed-ridden, markedly demented individual with little hope for meaningful survival.

Termination of Defibrillator-Pacemaker

The patient was a 75-year-old, white male with a history of a myocardial infarction and severe left ventricular dysfunction and signs of congestive heart failure (CHF), who developed ventricular tachycardia requiring the insertion of a pacemaker defibrillator. The patient developed small strokes leading to vascular dementia. His CHF symptoms worsened as his medication compliance diminished. He became bed-ridden, oxygen-dependent, and suffered multiple discharges of his defibrillator despite amiodarone therapy. As his condition deteriorated, the family requested no resuscitation efforts. The defibrillator-pacer was disconnected and the patient expired peacefully.

This case illustrates the need to recognize terminal illness and the need to interrupt the function of devices that may prolong the inevitable death.

REFERENCES

1. Duncan, A.K. et al.: Cardiovascular disease in elderly patients. Mayo Clin Proc 1996; 71: 184–196.
2. Braunwald, E.: The aging heart: structure, function and disease. Saunders, Philadelphia, 1998.
3. Davis, M. et al.: Cardiovascular disease and dementia. In: Alzheimer's disease. Mosby, St. Louis, MO, 1994.
4. De la Torre, J.C.: Vascular basis of Alzheimer's pathogenesis. Ann N Y Acad Sci 2002; 977: 196–215.
5. Kelly, D.T.: Our future society: a global challenge. Circulation 1997; 95: 2459–2472.
6. Wissler, R.W. et al.: Aging and cardiovascular disease. Circulation 1996; 1608–1612.
7. Yusuf, S. et al.: Global burden of cardiovascular diseases. Circulation 2001; 104: 2746–2753, 2855–2864.
8. De la Torre, J.C.: Alzheimer disease as a vascular disorder. Stroke 2002; 33: 1152.
9. Hunt, S.A. et al.: ACC/AHA guidelines for the evaluation and management of chronic heart failure in the adult. J Am Coll Cardiol 2001; 38: 2101–2113.
10. Levy, D. et al.: Long term trends in the incidence of and survival with heart failure. N Engl J Med 2002; 347: 1397–1402.
11. Redfield, M.M.: Heart failure—an epidemic of uncertain proportions. N Engl J Med 2002; 347: 1442–1444.
12. Packer, M. et al.: Consensus recommendations for the management of chronic congestive heart failure. Am J Cardiol 1999; 83: 1A–79A.
13. Abraham, W.T. et al.: Cardiac resynchronization in chronic heart failure. N Engl J Med 2002; 346: 1845–1853.
14. Braunwald, E. et al.: ACC/AHA guideline update for the management of patients with unstable angina and non ST segment elevation myocardial infarction. Circulation 2002; 106: 1893–1900.
15. Ryan, T.J. et al: 1999 update: ACC/AHA guidelines for the management of patients with acute myocardial infarction. J Am Coll Cardiol 1999; 34: 890–911.
16. Fuster, V. et al.: ACC/AHA/ESC guidelines for the management of patients with atrial fibrillation. Circulation 2001; 104: 2118–2150.
17. Wyse, D.G. et al. (AFFIRM) Investigators: A comparison of rate control in patients with atrial fibrillation. N Engl J Med 2002; 347: 1825–1833.
18. Gage, B.F. et al.: Warfarin therapy for an octogenarian who has atrial fibrillation. Ann Intern Med 2001; 134: 465–474.
19. Monette, J. et al.: Physician attitudes concerning warfarin for stroke prevention in atrial fibrillation: results of a survey of long term care practicioners. J Am Geriatr Soc 1997; 45: 1060–1065.
20. Bonow, R.O. et al.: Management of patients with valvular heart disease. J Am Coll Cardiol 1998; 32: 1486–1588.
21. Carabello, B.A.: Aortic stenosis. N Engl J Med 2002; 346: 677–682.
22. Otto, C.: Evaluation and management of chronic mitral regurgitation. N Engl J Med 2001; 345: 740–746.
23. Sacco, R.L.: Extracranial carotid stenosis. N Engl J Med 2001; 345: 1113–1118.
24. Inzitari, D. et al.: The causes and risk of stroke in patients with asymptomatic internal carotid stenosis. N Engl J Med 2000; 342: 1693–1701.
25. Brott, T. et al.: Treatment of acute ischemic stroke. N Engl J Med 2000; 343: 710–722.
26. Abrams, G.G. et al: ACC/AHA/NASPE guideline update for implantation of cardiac pacemakers and antiarrhythmic devices. J Am Coll Cardiol 2002; 40: 1703–1719.
27. Gregoratos, G.: Permanent pacemakers in older individuals. J Am Geriatr Soc 1999; 47: 1125–1135.
28. Hamel, M.B. et al.: Patient age and decisions to withhold life-sustaining treatment from seriously ill, hospitalized adults. Ann Intern Med 1999; 130: 116–125.
29. Faber-Langendoen, K. et al.: Dying patients in the intensive care unit: forgoing treatment, maintaining care. Ann Intern Med 2000; 133: 886–893.
30. Jason, H.T. et al.: A consensus-based approach to providing palliative care to patients who lack decision making capacity. Ann Intern Med 1999; 130: 835–840.

VII Prevention Strategies

27

Neuroprotection and Neurodegenerative Disease

Frank John Emery Vajda

INTRODUCTION

Genetic factors play a crucial role in the causation of Alzheimer's disease (AD), with mutations in at least three genes responsible for early-onset familial AD. A common polymorphism in the apolipoprotein E (ApoE) gene is the major determinant of risk for families with late-onset AD, as well as the general population *(1)*. Advanced age is another major risk factor, and environmental factors may influence disease expression. Some pathogenic factors include oxidative damage and mutations in messenger RNA (mRNA). Neuroprotective and multimodal therapies have not been explored yet.

Five hypotheses are currently proposed for the mechanism of AD. Hyperproduction of β-amyloid (Aβ) causes formation of amyloid deposits, which in turn induce dendrite and axon retraction and death. Hyperphosphorylation of axonal tau protein could lead to accumulation of polymerized tau in neurons, causing disturbance of intracellular communications and neuronal death. Oxidative stress and inflammation are marked by complement proteins, cytokines, and proteases—suggesting a stress response by the central nervous system (CNS). Deficits in neurotransmitters have also been proposed. Genetic hypotheses to explain the origin of the process suggest a heterogeneous disorder caused by combination of genetic and environmental factors *(2)*.

Neurodegenerative diseases are characterized by a progressive dysfunction and the death of neurons. Disorders with specific known causes are by convention excluded. There may be a commonality in pathways of degeneration. Genetic factors may interact with excitotoxic insults, involving calcium handling and mitochondrial derangements *(3)*. On a molecular level, disturbances in cellular signaling may be influenced by antiepileptic drugs (AEDs), such as valproic acid (VPA), affecting genetic expression of cytoprotective proteins, as indicated by Manji and colleagues *(4)*.

Neuroprotection may be defined as a chemically induced means of preventing neuronal damage, whose manifestations comprise clinical, cognitive, behavioral, structural, morphometric, electrical, biochemical, and molecular biological changes, correlated by clinical and laboratory measurements, supported by animal models *(5)*. The selective vulnerability of neurons, affecting nerve cells at specific sites, may involve different populations of neurons over a period. Nervous system plasticity allows for significant compensation until clinical signs appear or catastrophic failure develops *(6)*.

MODULATORS OF CNS DAMAGE

Neurochemical modulators of nervous system damage, excessive glutamate-mediated neurotransmission, impaired voltage-sensitive ion-channel functioning, impaired γ-aminobutyric acid (GABA)-mediated inhibition, and alterations in acid–base balance may trigger a cascade of events. CNS damage in response to an insult may lead to acute or delayed neuronal death *(7)*. In general, glutamate receptor-mediated excitotoxic injury results in neurodegeneration along an apopto-

From: *Current Clinical Neurology,*
Alzheimer's Disease: A Physician's Guide to Practical Management
Edited by: R. W. Richter and B. Zoeller Richter © Humana Press Inc., Totowa, NJ

sis–necrosis continuum. Effects of injury depend on the degree of brain maturity or site of lesion. Neuroprotection may be an achievable target using drugs already approved for other indications. Trials of these drugs in AD may save decades of new drug development.

NEURODEGENERATION AND THE SITE OF LESION

Degenerative disorders manifest predominantly as disorders of movement, of cognition, or a mixture. Dementia includes cortical degeneration with memory disturbance, apathy, disinhibition, and depression. Multifocal degeneration features variable cortical and subcortical deficits. The classification is syndromic. Features are related to sites of neurons, but provide no etiological insight (8). Clinical manifestations are varied, as individual sections of the CNS are geared to perform different functions (for example, extrapyramidal defects cause movement disorders, cortical insults lead to cognitive impairment or seizures) (9).

If genetic causes are augmented by comparable excitotoxicity, then similar treatment modalities may conceivably address similar processes, preventing neurons reaching a final common pathway, involving mitochondrial dysfunction (10). Environmental factors can be physical, toxic, and infection related. Trauma may be epidemiologically related to AD, toxic causes (for example, metals) may be related, but none have been proven causative. Dietary excitotoxic amino acids, bacterial infections, or viral agents may be linked to AD, but none have been proven (3).

EXCITOTOXICITY

Excitotoxicity and cerebral ischemia result in varying contributions to cell damage and causal mechanisms that may overlap (11). Increased glutamate binding to postsynaptic receptors causes channels to open, with sodium and calcium entering postsynaptic cells and causing depolarization, initiating cascades that lead to neuronal death (12). Other conditions of cerebral energy deprivation—hypoxia or hypoglycemia, for example—suggest a role for excitotoxicity. Additional factors may be peroxynitrite and oxygen free radicals (7,13,14).

The chain of events may comprise an initiating factor—excitotoxicity, oxidative stress, growth factor withdrawal, cytokines, or toxins (3). Damage may be inflicted by excessive stimulation of multiple types of glutamate receptors, ionotropic or metabotropic. A metabolic imbalance in a neuron leads to expression of immediate early genes such as c-fos, c-jun, jun-a, or jun-b. Cytoskeletal and membrane damage initially occurs in dendrites, where swelling is followed by neuronal death. In some systems this occurs by apoptosis, a process of cell destruction and shrinkage, chromatin aggregation, extensive genomic fragmentation, and nuclear pyknosis or necrosis, common to many conditions (9). It is characterized by swelling, rapid energy loss, disruption of ionic and internal homeostasis, membrane lysis, release of intracellular constituents, inflammatory reactive edema, and injury to surrounding tissue.

Indirect excitotoxicity occurs as a result of interruption of chemical synthesis, performed by aerobic generation of energy. There is altered mitochondrial energy production, a fall in membrane potential, opening of N-methyl-D-aspartate (NMDA) receptor subtypes, further ion entry, increased calcium load, and cell death (15). Neurotoxicity thus initiated and mediated by glutamate is thought to play a role in cerebral ischemia, progressive neurodegenerative diseases, and AD (16).

MITOCHONDRIAL FUNCTION

A central role for defective mitochondrial energy production resulting in increased levels of free radicals is gaining recognition (17). Energy defects in neurodegenerative disease bear similarities to known mitochondrial disorders, in which most patients present neuronal loss, gliosis, and degeneration. There is an overlap, but the nature and types of CNS lesions often allow a specific diagnosis. Different defects of cerebral energy metabolism are associated with common patterns in neuropathology. Excessive calcium is accumulated by intracellular mitochondria, affecting mitochondrial membrane potential and ATP (adenosine triphosphate) synthesis, glycolysis, and reactive oxygen species generation, resulting in failure of homeostasis *(18)*. Neuronal death, related to calcium entry, can be delayed by inhibitors of mitochondrial permeability transition pores *(19)*.

WHAT CONTRIBUTES TO THE DEVELOPMENT OF AD?

The role of genetic contribution in AD has been studied extensively *(20)*. The variety of chromosomes known to be involved in the pathogenesis of AD include chromosome 21, manifesting from birth in Down's syndrome, presenilin 1 (associated with chromosome 14), presenilin 2 (associated with chromosome 1), amyloid precursor protein (APP, associated with chromosome 21), and chromosome 19 (associated with apolipoprotein E and stability of amyloid protein deposits).

The immune system may play a role in AD. Induction of neurotoxic microglia by senile plaques may be a focus for immunosuppressive drugs. Similarities exist between neuronal injury in age-related dementia and focal cerebral ischemia. After stroke, excitotoxins may cause neuronal death and also apoptosis *(21–23)*.

Human immunodefiency virus (HIV) 1-related dementia is associated with abnormalities caused by immune-related toxins *(24)*. Tau proteins may have a role in AD, although not necessarily pivotal. Normal tau proteins are microtubular binding proteins, predominantly axonal, which stabilize the neuronal cytoskeleton. Several lines of evidence point to the primary role of amyloid in the pathogenesis of AD. Some mutations in the APP gene have been linked with rare familial forms of AD. The amyloid cascade proposes a central role for Aβ in AD pathogenesis, but links between Aβ protein generation and formation of neurofibrillary tangles (NFTs) are not known. Cognitively normal individuals can have numerous neocortical plaques, of predominantly diffuse type. Mutations in presenilin genes, causally linked to cases of early-onset inherited AD, may increase the vulnerability of cholinergic neurons to apotosis. The mechanism may involve calcium regulatory and mitochondrial dysfunction *(21,22)*.

AIMS OF TREATMENT NEED TO BE RECONSIDERED

The aims of treatment in AD need redefinition. Traditionally the focus has been on cognitive abilities, but functional abilities, behavior, caregiver burden, quality of life, and resource utilization need evaluation *(25)*.

Animal models in development of drug therapies should replicate closely key defects observed in patients. Accumulation of amyloid plaques, NFTs, loss of synapses, neurons, and markers of the cholinergic system should be observed in appropriate brain regions. Structural and functional abnormalities should worsen with age. Transgenic mice will probably provide the best model of changes and should undergo the same mutations as those found in patients with hereditary AD, such as mutations of the genes coding for APP, ApoE, or presenilin. Data for two existing models indicate that several key features of AD, including tau-containing paired helical filaments (PHF), activation of the complement pathway, and loss of synapses and neurons, do not occur in APP transgenic mice, nor does degeneration of cholinergic cells of basal forebrain. Reports of drugs modifying the process in animals must be viewed with caution. Models reflect only crude approximations of human disease *(26)*.

THERAPIES BASED ON NEUROTOXIC TRAFFIC OF AMYLOID PRODUCTION

There are excellent reviews on strategies for treatment of AD based on genetic and pathological abnormalities related to amyloid production, animal models of AD, presenilins as therapeutic targets, and plaque buster strategies to inhibit amyloid formation *(27–30)*. These will not be discussed, the focus being on neuroprotection, and possibilities of multimodal therapies employing drugs showing evidence of neuroprotection in animals or other fields of medicine *(31)*.

Evidence-Based Pharmacological Treatment of AD

Acetylcholineesterase inhibitors (AChEI) represent the only category of drugs with consistently demonstrable efficacy in well-designed clinical trials in AD, although their effect is not large. There is a lack of prospective studies for so-called nootropics. Epidemiological evidence suggests effects for estrogens and nonsteroidal antiinflammatory drugs (NSAIDs), and some benefits for selegiline. Reports exist on the effectiveness on noncognitive symptoms by narcoleptics, antidepressants, and antiepileptics, but the evidence is not robust *(32)*.

NEUROPROTECTION IN AD

Individual agents proposed for clinical evaluation in multimodal therapy include antiepileptic drugs, selegiline, NSAIDs, and estrogens.

Antiepileptic Drugs

Postulated mechanisms for antiepileptic drugs (AEDs) comprise actions on ion channels, GABA and glutamate systems, and second messengers. At a cellular level, mitochondrial mechanisms may have a role in stabilizing neurons and protection from excess calcium influx-related insults.

Topiramate (TPM) has multiple mechanisms of action and a neuroprotective potential against acquisition of kindled hippocampal seizures, prevention of prenatal hypoxia in animal models, and enhancing nerve regeneration *(33–36)*.

Clonazepam has a specific action on mitochondrial membranes *(37)*.

Lamotrigine may inhibit kainic acid neurotoxicity by affecting glutamate release *(38,39)*.

Valproate (VPA) has numerous actions on GABA, ion channels, and neurotransmitters *(40)*. Its effects on a molecular biological level has been studied extensively in psychopharmacology, indicating significant neuroprotective potential *(5)*. Similarities exist between the molecular effects of lithium and VPA, both showing benefits in manic depression *(4,41)*.

Valproate: Molecular Biological Indicators of Neuroprotective Effects

Both lithium and VPA upregulate brain concentrations of cytoreactive proteins, which exhibit neurotrophic effects, including the regeneration of CNS axons. An increase in gray matter volume on high-resolution three-dimensional magnetic resonance imaging and an increase in brain N-acetyl aspartate, a marker of neuronal viability, have been reported *(42)*. Studies have focused on the effects of VPA on intracellular signal transduction. Effects on glutamate release, decrease in inositol uptake, increase in levels of B-cell lymphoma protein-2 (bcl-2), and inhibition of glycogen synthetase-3 (GSK-3) are possible mechanisms shared between lithium and VPA *(43)*, which produce similar clinical effects, time lags on administration and cessation, and detection of the same molecular markers along signal transduction pathways (for experimental details, *see* refs. *4,41,44–46*).

G proteins are transducers of information across membranes; the phosphoinositide cycle is an intracellular messenger system. Protein kinase C (PKC) plays a role in intracellular neurotransmission of signals generated by many receptor subtypes. Activator protein 1 (AP-1) activates gene transcription. The bcl-2 may be involved in subcellular homeostasis and includes a family of proapoptotic and antiapoptotic members. Brain-derived neurotrophic factor (BDNF) is claimed to function in cell survival and plasticity. Endoplasmic reticulum (ER) cell stress proteins, which bind calcium to the ER, may play a role in clearing mal-folded proteins. All the mechanisms appear to be influenced by VPA. The implications for Alzheimer's disease are clear.

VPA elicits a neuritogenic effect in cultured neurons. Neuritogenesis has been shown to occur in the adult brain, in restricted regions, and may be related to learning and memory *(47,48)*. VPA may well have neuroprotective potential in AD.

Selegiline

Parkinson's disease (PD) is inherited as an autosomal dominant trait in some families. Environmental toxins, oxidative stress, and mitochondrial dysfunction may contribute to degeneration of substantia nigra *(49,50)*. PD is the most common Lewy body disease. Lewy bodies may be a means of removing damaged cytoskeletal proteins, including tubulin and microtubular associated proteins, APP, and synaptic protein. Selegiline is a selective, irreversible, monoamine oxidase-B (MAO-B) inhibitor, present as a glial enzyme in brain. It enhances superoxide dismutase and catalase activity in the striatum, and facilitates catecholaminergic activity. Selegiline protects nigrostriatal neurons against 6OH-dopamine, 1-methyl-4-phenyl-1,2,3,6-tetrahydropyridine (MPTP), *N*-[2-chloroethyl)-*N*-ethyl-2-bromobenzylamine (DSP-4; a noradrenergic neurotoxin), all toxic to the brain *(51–53)*. In rats, selegiline delays decline in learning and memory. In humans, selegiline may have a neuroprotective effect, which is difficult to dissect from symptomatic effects *(54)*. Selegiline may be combined with agents acting via glutamate receptors, ion channels, or GABAergic effects (valproate or topiramate).

Reports of selegiline trials in AD were examined in the Cochrane Database. Of 15 double-blind trials, 8 suggested some beneficial effects on cognition and 3 on behavior as well as mood. Although promising, the evidence is not robust enough to recommend selegiline for routine therapy in AD *(55)*.

Inflammation and AD, NSAIDs, and COX Inhibition

Neuroimmune mechanisms play a role in pathogenesis of AD *(56,57)*. Extracellular Aβ and intracellular phosphorylated tau protein form major components of senile plaques and NFT and may be factors in the neurodestructive process. Microglial cells in the region of these deposits express surface receptors for major histocompatibility complex (MHC) class 1 and 11 glycoproteins, produce complement, generate free oxygen radicals, and inflammatory cytokines, IL-1, IL-6, and tumor necrosis factor (TNF).

Classical complement pathway proteins are activated by Aβ. Stimulation of the immune system may lead to autodestruction of neurons, hence the hypothesis that NSAIDSs, which inhibit some of these processes, may protect against AD. NSAIDs reduce tissue prostaglandin levels and inflammation by cyclooxygenase (COX) inhibition.

AD has been shown to be negatively associated with arthritis *(58–60)*. Epidemiological studies have shown an inverse relationship between NSAID use and AD *(61–63)*. NSAID users have been shown to have a better performance on a range of cognitive tests and less decline over 12 months compared with nonusers *(64,65)*. Gastrointestinal toxicity is the greatest limitation in using NSAIDs. Selective COX-2 inhibitors have reduced this risk, compared to nonselective NSAIDs.

COX-1 is expressed constitutively in a number of organs and tissues, and is thought to mediate diverse homeostatic functions. COX-2 plays a role in mediating functional neuronal maturation and responses to stimuli in the brain. COX-2 expression is associated with the key pathophysiological event in AD—the deposition of Aβ and neuritic plaques within the hippocampus and cortex. This relationship, as well as the theory that neural degeneration in AD may have an inflammatory component, suggest a potential therapeutic role for COX-2 specific inhibition *(66)*.

Application for COX-2 inhibitors for the treatment of AD rests on animal data. A clinical trial of the COX-2 inhibitor celecoxib in AD showed it to be ineffective *(67)*. The appropriate target for NSAID trials in AD appears to be COX-1 rather than COX-2. There is no need for hesitation in using traditional NSAIDs with mixed COX-1/COX-2-inhibiting activity in AD *(68)*. Only two small clinical trials have been published involving NSAIDs in AD patients *(69)*. A 6-month double-blind trial with indomethacin reported arrest of the disease in the active treatment group *(70)*. In a trial of diclofenac the dropout rate was high because of gastrointestinal intolerance, despite the addition of misoprostol *(71)*.

Estrogens

The brain upregulates estrogen synthesis and estrogen receptor expression at sites of injury. Estrogen exposure may delay onset and progression of AD and enhance recovery from neurological injury, such as stroke. Mechanisms include alterations in cell survival, axonal sprouting, regenerative responses enhancing synaptic transmission and neurogenesis, action on unidentified membrane receptors, modulation of neurotransmitter function, and modification of phosphorylation cascades through direct interaction with protein kinases or signaling through trophic molecules to influence apoptotic cascades *(72)*. These mechanisms are similar to those invoked for actions of other putative neuroprotectors.

The major cholinergic projections to the frontal cortex originate from the nucleus basalis of Meynert. This is remarkably acetylcholine-deficient in AD. Cholinergic neurons appear to be sensitive to estrogens. Estrogen increases cholineacetyl-transferase (ChAT) activity in the basal forebrain of ovariectomized rats, while estrogen deprivation reduces high-affinity choline uptake in rat hippocampus, reversible with short-term estradiol replacement. Long-term estradiol replacement seems to prevent the time-independent decline in ChAT in the frontal cortex, attenuates its decline in the hippocampus, and enhances neurite growth by influencing tau protein levels and stabilizing microtubules *(73)*.

Estrogens have a secondary effect on increasing cerebral blood flow, which is reduced in AD, and antioxidant activity. Estrogen may influence learning and memory involving NMDA receptors. Evidence for the use of estrogen replacement therapy for prevention of AD at present lacks long-term prospective data. These studies are required to settle the question of possible neuroprotection by estrogens *(74–77)*.

A pilot as well as a prospective study showed protection by estrogen against AD and stabilization of cognition in people already diagnosed *(75,76)*. Subsequent case control studies confirmed some protection on postmenopausal women. However, the relative contribution to dementia by these processes remains undetermined *(78)*. There is a greater decline in glucose transport in brains of women than in men, especially affecting the hippocampus and parietal lobes. Low glucose levels may be detrimental. Estrogens may attenuate neuronal injury by affecting metabolism of APP and Apo-E polymorphism, which influence risk for AD *(79)*.

THE FUTURE: ACETYLCHOLINESTERASE INHIBITION WITH MULTIMODALITY TREATMENT

An approved AChEI in combination with a potentially neuroprotective antiepilectic drug, such as valproate, an NSAID, or estrogen could be compared against AChEI plus placebo in AD patients prospectively *(80)*.

SUMMARY

A common pathway of cell destruction in a variety of neurological diseases may involve glutamate-triggered excitotoxicity, calcium influx, and generation of free radicals leading to neuronal damage via existing mitochondrial mechanisms. In addition to amyloid-related therapeutic approaches, neuroprotection may be attempted using older drugs approved for indications other than AD, which have shown neuroprotective potential experimentally or clinically. These should be studied in randomized controlled trials in patients with AD. Applying results of basic scientists to clinical problems is scientifically justified, but is not a commercial priority. Emerging ideas from etiology and pathology, which may lead to improved therapeutics involving multimodality and neuroprotection, are presented.

REFERENCES

1. Munoz, D.G.; Feldman, H.: Causes of Alzheimers disease. J Can Med Assoc 2000; 162: 65–76.
2. Torreiles, F.; Touchon, J.: Pathogenic theories and intrathecal analysis of the sporadic form of Alzheimer's disease. Prog Neurobiol 2002; 66: 191–203.

3. Ellison, D.; Love, S.: Neurodegenerative disorders. In: Ellison, D.; Love, S. (eds.): Neuropathology, a reference text of CNS pathology. Harcourt, London, 2000: 26.1–33.11.

4. Manji, H.K. et al.: Signaling pathways in the brain: cellular transduction of mood stabilization in the treatment of manic-depressive illness. ANZ J Psych 1999; 33: S65–S83.

5. Vajda, F.J.E.: Valproate and neuroprotection. J Clin Neurosci 2002; 9: 508–514.

6. Hardy, J.; Gwinn-Hardy, K.: Genetic classification of primary neurodegenerative diseases. Science 1998; 282: 1075–1078.

7. Leist, M.; Nicotera, P.: Apoptosis, excitotoxicity and neuropathology. Exp Cell Res 1998; 239: 183–201.

8. Ellison, D.; Love, S.: Dementias. In: Ellison, D.; Love, S. (eds.): Neuropathology, a reference text of CNS pathology. Harcourt, London, 2000: 31.1–31.34.

9. Nicotera, P.; Lipton, S.A.: Excitotoxins in neuronal apoptosis and necrosis. J Cerebral Blood Flow Metab 1999; 19: 583–591.

10. Montal, M.: Mitochondria, glutamate neurotoxicity and the death cascade. Biochim Biophys Acta 1998; 1366: 113–126.

11. Martin, L.J. et al.: Neurodegeneration in excitotoxicity, global cerebral ischemia, and target deprivation: a perspective on the contributions of apoptosis and necrosis. Brain Res Bull 1998; 46: 281–309.

12. Olney, J.W.: Glutamate induced retinal degeneration in neonatal mice. Electron microscopy of the acutely evolving lesion. J Neuropathol Exp Neurol 1969; 28: 455–474.

13. Brown, G.K.; Squire, M.V.: Neuropathology and pathogenesis of mitochondrial diseases. J Inher Metab Dis 1996; 19: 553–572.

14. Lipton, S.A. et al.: Neuroprotective versus neurodestructive effects of NO-related species. Biofactors 1998; 8: 33–40.

15. Ludolph, A.C.; Meyer, T.; Riepe, M.W.: The role of excitotoxicity in ALS—what is the evidence? J Neurol 2000; 247 (suppl 1): 17–16.

16. Arias, C.; Becerra-Garcia, F.; Tapia, R.: Glutamic acid and Alzheimer's disease. Neurobiology 1998; 6: 33–43.

17. Beal, M.F.: Mitochondria, free radicals and neurodegeneration. Curr Opin Neurobiol 1996; 6: 661–666.

18. Nichols, D.G.; Budd, S.L.: Neuronal excitotoxicity: the role of mitochondria. Biofactors 1998; 8: 287–299.

19. Simpson, P.B.; Russell, J.T.: Role of mitochondrial Ca^{2+} regulation in neuronal and glial cell signaling. Brain Res Rev 1998; 26: 72–81.

20. Ellison, D.; Love, S.: Alzheimers disease. In: Ellison, D.; Love, S. (eds.): Neuropathology, a reference text of CNS pathology. Harcourt, London, 2000: 31.1–31.34.

21. Mattson, M.P.; Pedersen, W.A.: Effects of amyloid precursor protein derivatives and oxidative stress on basal forebrain cholinergic systems in Alzheimers disease. Int J Dev Neurosci 1998; 16: 737–753.

22. Blass, J.; Poirier, J.: Pathophysiology of the Alzheimer syndrome. In: Gauthier, S. (ed.): Clinical diagnosis and management of Alzheimer's disease. Martin Dunitz, London, 1996: 17–31.

23. Mark, R.J. et al.: Anticonvulsants attenuate amyloid beta peptide neurotoxicity, Ca^{2+} deregulation and cytoskeletal pathology. Neurobiol Aging 1995; 16: 187–198.

24. Lipton, S.A.: Similarity of neuronal cell injury and death in AIDS dementia and focal cerebral ischemia: potential treatment with NMDA open-channel blockers and nitric oxide-related species. Brain Pathol 1996; 6: 507–517.

25. Winblad, B. et al.: Pharmacotheapy of Alzheimer's disease: is there a need to redefine treatment success? Intern J Geriatr Psychiatry 2001; 16: 653–666.

26. Riekkinnen, P. Jr. et al.: Animal models in the development of symptomatic and preventive drug therapies for Alzheimer's disease. Ann Med Finnish Med Soc 1998; 3: 566–576.

27. Huse, J.T.; Doms, R.W.: Neurotoxic traffic: uncovering the mechanics of amyloid production in Alzheimer's disease. Traffic 2001; 2: 75–81.

28. Chapman. P. et al.: Genes, models and Alzheimer's disease. Trends Genet 2001; 17: 254–261.

29. Golde, T.E.; Younkin, S.G.: Presenilins as therapeutic targets for the treatment of Alzheimer's disease. Trends Molec Med 2001; 7: 264–269.

30. Solo, C.: Plaque busters strategies to inhibit amyloid formation in Alzheimer's disease. Molec Med Today 1999; 9: 343–359.

31. Vajda, F.J.E.: Neuroprotection and neurodegenerative disease. J Clin Neurosci 2002; 9: 4–8.

32. Emre, M., Hanagasi, A.: Evidence based pharmacological treatment of dementia. Eur J Neurol 2000; 7: 247–253.

33. White, H.S.: Basic research update: evidence for neuroprotection with topiramate. Proc 3rd Ann Topamax Symposium, Satellite Meeting of Epilepsy Society of Australia, Annual Scientific Meeting, Adelaide, 1999.

34. Perucca, E.: A pharmacological and clinical review on topiramate, a new antiepileptic drug. Pharmacol Res 1997; 35: 241–256.

35. Hanaya, R. et al.: Suppression by topiramate of epileptiform burst discharges in hippocampal CA3 neurons of spontaneously epileptic rat in vitro. Brain Res 1998; 789: 274–282.

36. Yang, Y. et al.: Neuroprotection by delayed administration of topiramate in a rat model of middle cerebral artery embolization. Brain Res 1998; 804: 169–176.

37. Macdonald, R.L.: Cellular actions of antiepileptic drugs. In: Eadie, M.J.; Vajda, F.J.E. (eds.): Antiepileptic drugs: pharmacology and therapeutics. Springer, Heidelberg/Berlin, Germany, 1999: 123–150.

38. Meldrum, R.S.: Pharmacology and mechanism of action of lamotrigine. In: Reynolds, E.H. (ed.): Lamotrigine—a new advance in the treatment of epilepsy. Royal Society of Medicine Services, London, 1993: 5–10.

39. Walker, M.C.; Sander, J.W.A.S.: Lamotrigine. In: Eadie, M.J.; Vajda, F.J.E. (eds.): Antiepileptic drugs: pharmacology and therapeutics. Springer, Heidelberg/Berlin, Germany, 1999: 331–358.

40. Loscher, W.: Valproate: a reappraisal of its pharmacodynamic properties and mechanism of action. Prog Neurobiol 1999; 58: 31–59.

41. Manji, H.K.; Moore, G.J.; Chen, G.: Clinical and preclinical evidence for the neurotrophic effects of mood stabilizers: implications for the pathophysiology and treatment of manic-depressive disorders. Biol Psychiatry 2000; 48: 740–754.

42. Moore, G.J. et al.: Lithium-induced increase in human brain grey matter. Lancet 2000; 356: 1241–1242.

43. Motohashi, N.: Valproate for the treatment of psychiatric disorders. Jpn J Neuropsychopharmacol 2001; 72: 879–882.

44. Manji, H.K. et al.: Neuroplasticity and cellular resilience in mood disorders. Molec Psychiatry 2000; 5: 578–593.

45. Manji, H.K.; Moore, G.J.; Chen, G.: Bipolar disorder: leads from the molecular and cellular mechanisms of action of mood stabilizers. Br J Psychiatry 2001; 178 (suppl 41): 107–119.

46. Chen, G. et al.: The mood-stabilizing agents lithium and valproate robustly increase the levels of the neuroprotective protein bcl-2 in the CNS. J Neurochem 1999; 72: 879–882.

47. Eriksson, P.S. et al.: Neurogenesis in the adult hippocampus. Nat Med 1998; 4: 1313–1317.

48. Kempermann, G.; Gage, F.H.: Experience-dependent regulation of adult hippocampal neurogenesis: effects of long term stimulation and stimulus withdrawal. Hippocampus 1999; 9: 321–332.

49. Ellison, D.; Love, S.: Parkinson's disease. In: Ellison, D.; Love, S. (eds.): Neuropathology, a reference text of CNS pathology. Harcourt, London, 2000: 28.1–28.16.

50. Jenner, P.; Olanow, C.W.T.: Oxidative stress and the pathogenesis of Parkinson's disease. Neurology 1996; 47 (suppl 3): S161–S170.

51. Langston, J.W.: The etiology of Parkinson's disease with emphasis on the MPTP story. Neurology 1996; 47 (suppl 3): S153–S160.

52. Gerlach, M.; Youdim, M.B.H.; Reiderer, P.: Pharmacology of selegiline. Neurology 1996; 47 (suppl 3): S137–S145.

53. Tatton, W.G.; Chalmers-Redman, R.M.: Modulation of gene expression rather than monoamine oxidase inhibition: (–)-deprenyl-related compounds in controlling neurodegeneration. Neurology 1996; 47 (suppl 3): S171–S183.

54. Olanow, C.W.: Selegiline: current perspectives on issues related to neuroprotection and mortality. Neurology 1996; 47 (suppl 3): S210–S216.

55. Birks, J.; Flicker, L.: Selegiline for Alzheimer's disease. The Cochrane Database of Systematic Reviews 1 (2001).

56. McGeer, P.L.; Rogers, J.; McGeer, E.G.: Neuroimmune mechanisms in Alzheimer disease pathogenesis. Alz Dis Assoc Disord 1994; 8: 149–158.

57. Eikelenboom, P. et al.: Inflammatory mechanisms in Alzheimer's disease. Trends Pharmacol Sci 1994; 15: 447–450.

58. Jenkinson, M.L. et al.: Rheumatoid arthritis and senile dementia of the Alzheimer's type. Br J Rheumatol 1989; 28: 86–88.

59. Broe, G.A. et al.: A case-control study of Alzheimer's disease in Australia. Neurology 1990; 40: 1698–1707.

60. McGeer, P.L. et al.: Anti-inflammatory drugs and Alzheimer disease. Lancet 1990; 335: 1037.

61. Breitner, J.C. et al.: Inverse association of anti-inflammatory treatments and Alzheimer's disease: initial results of a co-twin control study. Neurology 1994; 44: 227–232.

62. The Canadian Study of Health and Aging. Risk factors from Alzheimer's disease in Canada. Neurology 1994; 44: 2073–2080.

63. Andersen, K. et al.: Do non steroidal anti-inflammatory drugs decrease the risk for Alzheimer's disease. The Rotterdam Study. Neurology 1995; 45: 1441–1445.

64. Rich, J.B. et al.: Non-steroidal anti-inflammatory drugs in Alzheimer's disease. Neurology 1995; 45: 51–55.

65. Breitner, J.C.S. et al.: Alzheimer's disease in the NAS-NRC Registry of aging twin veterans. II. Longitudinal findings in a pilot series. National Academy of Sciences/National Research Council Registry. Dementia 1994; 5: 99–105.

66. Lipsky, P.E.: Clinical potential of cyclooxygenase-2 specific inhibitors. Am J Med 1999; 106: S51–S57.

67. Sainali, S.M. et al.: Results of a double-blind placebo controlled trial of celecoxib in the treatment of the progression of Alzheimer's disease. 6th Stockholm Springfield Symposium of Advances in Alzheimer Therapy, April 2000.

68. Dannhardt, G.; Kiefer, W.: Cyclooxygenase inhibitors—current status and future prospects. Eur J Med Chem 2001; 36: 109–126.

69. McGeer, P.: Cyclo-oxygenase-2-inhibitors. Drugs Aging 2000; 17: 1–11.

70. Rogers, J. et al.: Clinical trial of indomethacin in Alzheimer's disease. Neurology 1993; 43: 1609–1611.

71. Scharf, S. et al.: A double-blind placebo-controlled trial of diclofenac/misoprostol in Alzheimer's disease. Neurology 1999; 53: 197–201.

72. Garcia-Seguar, L.M.; Azcoitia, I.; Don Carlos, L.L.: Neuroprotection by estradiol. Prog Neurobiol 2001; 63: 29–60.

73. Monk, D.; Brodaty, H.: Use of estrogens for the prevention and treatment of Alzheimer's disease. Dement Geriatr Cognit Disord 2000; 11: 1–10.

74. Fillit, H. et al.: Observations in a preliminary open trial of estradiol therapy for senile dementia—Alzheimer type. Psychoneuroendocrinology 1986; 11: 337–345.

75. Henderson, V.W. et al.: Estrogen replacement therapy in older women. Comparison between Alzheimer's disease cases and non-demented control subjects. Arch Neurol 1994; 51: 896–900.
76. Costa, M.M. et al.: Estrogen replacement therapy and cognitive decline in memory-impaired post-menopausal women. Biol Psychiatry 1999; 46: 182–188.
77. Van Amelsvooert, T.; Compton, J.; Murphy, D.: In vivo assessment of the effects of estrogen on the human brain. Trends Endocrinol Metab 2001; 12: 273–275.
78. Panidis, K.D. et al.: The role of estrogen replacement therapy in Alzheimer's disease. Eur J Obstet Gyn Reprod Biol 2001; 95: 86–91.
79. Wiltfang, J. et al.: Molecular biology of Alzheimer's dementia and its clinical relevance to early diagnosis and new therapeutic strategies. Gerontology 2001; 47: 65–71.
80. Giulian, D.: A strategy for identifying immunosuppressive therapies for Alzheimer disease. Alz Dis Assoc Disord 1998; 12 (suppl 2): S7–S14.

28

Neurotrophic Factors for Prevention of Alzheimer's Disease

Mark H. Tuszynski

INTRODUCTION

Synapse loss and cell death are the final common pathways of cognitive decline in Alzheimer's disease. Neurotrophic factors are substances naturally produced in the nervous system that support neuronal survival during development and support neuronal function throughout adulthood. Notably, in animal models, including primates, neurotrophic factors can also prevent neuronal death after injury and can reverse spontaneous neuronal atrophy in aging. Thus, neurotrophic factor therapy has substantial potential as a means of preventing cell loss in disorders such as AD. The main challenge in clinical testing of these growth factors has been their delivery to the brain in sufficient doses to affect cell function. In this chapter the therapeutic potential of growth factors has been reviewed, as well as a clinical trial of growth factor gene therapy in AD, which currently is in progress.

Nervous system growth factors were discovered more than 50 years ago. Examining a sarcoma cell line in vitro, Rita Levi-Montalcini and Viktor Hamburger serendipitously discovered that sarcoma cells secreted a factor that promoted vigorous neurite outgrowth from sympathetic and sensory neurons *(1)*. Giving the unknown substance the name "nerve growth factor" (NGF), it was isolated and purified over several subsequent years *(2)*. The structure and biological properties of the NGF protein have subsequently been studied extensively. The rodent and human genes were identified and cloned in the mid-1980s, and their receptor complexes and signaling properties have been the subject of intense research *(3–5)*.

The effects of NGF were originally believed to be restricted to promoting neuronal survival and axon extension during development of the nervous system; no known effects of growth factors in the adult nervous system were known. This perception changed dramatically in the 1980s with the discovery that NGF was produced in the adult hippocampus and cortex, and that infusions of NGF into the injured adult brain could completely prevent the death of basal forebrain cholinergic neurons after injury (Fig. 1) *(6,7)*. It was subsequently reported that NGF reversed atrophy of basal forebrain cholinergic neurons in the aged rat brain, and that NGF improved age-related impairments in learning and memory *(8)*.

These studies delivered NGF to the adult brain by infusing it into the lateral ventricles of the cerebrospinal fluid system, because NGF is a medium-sized polar molecule and does not cross the blood–brain barrier. We and others extended the biological effects of growth factors to the primate brain, finding that NGF infusions into the lateral ventricles also prevented lesion-induced degeneration of basal forebrain cholinergic neurons *(9,10)*.

Given the evidence that NGF could prevent the death and reverse the atrophy of cholinergic neurons in rats and primates, its potential application to Alzheimer's disease (AD) was immediately evident. Extensive degeneration of cholinergic neurons occurs in AD, and this degeneration is likely to

From: *Current Clinical Neurology,*
Alzheimer's Disease: A Physician's Guide to Practical Management
Edited by: R. W. Richter and B. Zoeller Richter © Humana Press Inc., Totowa, NJ

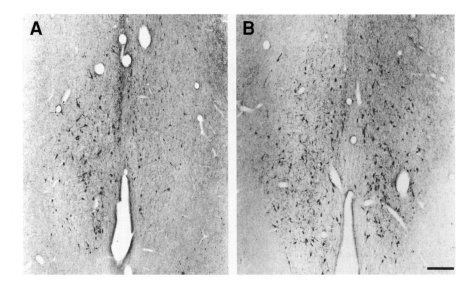

Fig. 1. NGF prevents the degeneration of basal forebrain cholinergic neurons. (**A**) Lesions of projections from the medial septal nucleus to the hippocampus cause retrograde degeneration of cholinergic neurons in the primate brain, shown on the right side of the adult primate brain with choline acetyl transferase immunolabeling. The left side of the brain is intact. (**B**) Gene delivery of human NGF to the injured, right side of the adult primate brain significantly reduces cholinergic neuronal degeneration. Scale bar = 150 μm.

contribute to cognitive dysfunction. Indeed, the only approved drugs (in the United States) for the treatment of AD target the cholinergic system, and despite only partial blockade of central cholinergic degradation, acetylcholinesterase inhibitors (AChEI) exert modestly beneficial effects on cognition *(11)*. NGF therapy, unlike other available therapies, offers the potential to prevent cholinergic cell loss before it occurs, rather than compensating for cell loss after it has taken place. Further, NGF also stimulates the production and release of acetylcholine from remaining neurons *(12)*. In the brain of AD patients, levels of NGF are diminished in cholinergic neurons *(13–15)*.

To treat human disease, NGF would require central administration to circumvent limitations of the blood–brain barrier. As preparations moved forward for clinical trials of NGF in AD in the early 1990s, however, significant toxicity resulting from intracerebroventricular delivery of NGF administration became clear. These adverse effects included pain, weight loss, and migration/proliferation of Schwann cells into the subpial space surrounding the brainstem and spinal cord *(16–18)*. The origin of these adverse effects was clear. By infusing NGF intracerebroventricularly, it was broadly distributed throughout the nervous system and reached a number of other cell populations that are NGF-sensitive, including nociceptive axons of the spinal cord dorsal horn, hypothalamic neurons, and Schwann cells of the peripheral nerve/dorsal root entry zone. Thus, whereas NGF continued to exhibit an intriguing potential to prevent cholinergic cell loss in the AD brain, the ability to deliver it safely and exclusively to cholinergic neurons of the basal forebrain was lacking. Despite these concerns, a group of investigators infused NGF into three patients with AD *(19)*. Not surprisingly, pain and weight loss forced a discontinuation of the trial. Clearly, an alternative method for delivering NGF to the brain was needed to test the possibility that this growth factor could ameliorate cholinergic neuronal atrophy in human disease.

GENE DELIVERY OF GROWTH FACTORS TO THE BRAIN

In the late 1980s, the first efforts to deliver therapeutic genes to the nervous system were reported. Indeed, the first successful application of gene therapy in the brain reported that NGF gene delivery to the brains of adult rats could prevent the loss of basal forebrain cholinergic neurons after lesions *(20)*. Subsequently it was reported that NGF gene delivery reversed age-related cognitive decline in rats, and that NGF gene therapy in the brains of adult primates prevented lesion-induced cholinergic neuron death *(21–23)*. Finally, recently it was reported that NGF gene delivery to the aged primate brain reversed age-related atrophy of cholinergic neurons, and restored cholinergic innervation to the cortex to levels equivalent to those of young monkeys *(24,25)*. These findings raised the possibility that gene therapy might represent a practical approach for preventing cholinergic decline in AD.

The potential advantages of gene therapy as a delivery system for growth factors to the brain are threefold. First, gene delivery can be directed to a specific site in the brain, thereby providing high concentrations of a growth factor to a specific brain target, while restricting delivery of the growth factor to that single site. Unlike intracerebroventricular NGF infusions, which broadly circulate a growth factor through the CNS, site-directed gene therapy restricts delivery of the growth factor to a relatively specific population of neurons, thereby potentially enhancing the safety profile of growth factor therapy. Second, gene delivery can sustain growth factor treatment for extended time periods, potentially lasting years. Unlike mechanical infusion devices that may require refilling, recharging, or removal due to infection, gene therapy can be rendered in a single session and sustain substance delivery long-term. Third, gene therapy has the advantage of simplicity: a single treatment, delivering a single natural gene, may render long-term and stable neuroprotection.

On the other hand, the preeminent disadvantage of gene therapy, at this stage of its development, is its near permanence: one gene therapy session is undertaken in the brain, and there is currently no effective and safe system for turning "off" the delivered gene product. Hence, the implementation of gene therapy in clinical trials would require a substantial body of safety and efficacy data, and evidence that the continued delivery of the gene product would not cause significant adverse effects. Such a program of experiments was therefore undertaken, as described below.

PRECLINICAL EFFICACY AND SAFETY STUDIES OF GENE THERAPY

There are two general forms of gene therapy: ex vivo and in vivo gene delivery. In ex vivo gene therapy, cells from a host are obtained from biopsy, cultured in vitro, then genetically modified (using gene therapy "vectors" that transfer a gene of interest into the host cells) *(26)*. The host cells then produce and secrete a gene product of interest (e.g., NGF). To undergo the ex vivo gene therapy process, the host cells must be sustainable in vitro; such readily available cells include fibroblasts (obtained by skin biopsy), bone marrow stromal cells (obtained by bone marrow aspiration), Schwann cells (obtained by nerve biopsy), endothelial cells, or even adult stem cells. Most early animal experiments using gene delivery to the nervous system used primary fibroblasts as vehicles of ex vivo gene delivery, due to the simplicity with which these cells can be obtained, maintained in vitro, and genetically modified.

Once the host cells are genetically modified in vitro, they are transplanted into the host region in which therapeutic gene delivery is desired. There, the genetically modified cells act as biological pumps in the host for the sustained local secretion and delivery of a therapeutic protein. Because the cells are derived from the same host, they are nonimmunogenic and are hypothetically available in limitless numbers.

In vivo gene therapy is easier to perform than ex vivo gene therapy. A vector that can directly transfer a therapeutic gene into a host cell is injected into a brain region of interest, such as the cholinergic basal forebrain of the CNS, and genetically modifies the cell in the injected region directly *(27,28)*. The most promising vectors for in vivo gene therapy to emerge in the last several years include adeno-associated virus (AAV) and retroviral-based (e.g., HIV) vectors. Unlike earlier-generation gene therapy vectors, which were immunogenic and expressed their genes of interest for limited time periods, AAV and retroviral vectors are made by removing all, or nearly all, of the virus's wild-type genes responsible for replication and disease, and replacing them with therapeutic genes of interest that can enter host cells. When injected into a host, both AAV and retroviral vectors penetrate cells and are transported to the nucleus. AAV vectors appear to persist in host cells primarily as extrachromosomal elements that do not integrate into the host genome. Retroviral vectors, however, do integrate into the host genome, and—depending on the specific site of integration—have the potential to induce host gene mutations and/or to induce malignant transformation of cells. Indeed, a clinical trial that used retroviral vectors to genetically modify bone marrow cells in severe combined immunodeficiency (SCID) has reported the development of leukemia in two patients, indicating that integrating gene therapy vectors require further study. Thus, for the present, AAV vectors may emerge as leading candidates for in vivo gene therapy.

The potential disadvantage of in vivo gene therapy relative to ex vivo gene therapy for the delivery of growth factors to the nervous system is, at this point, hypothetical. Neurons normally derive growth factor support from extracellular sources; hence, might there be disadvantages to overexpressing growth factors intrinsically in cells, which normally do not access support in this fashion? Such risks could include overstimulation of the genetically modified cells, and—paradoxically—accelerating neuronal degeneration.

Animal Models Proved Safety and Efficacy

Given the potential ability of either ex vivo or in vivo gene therapy to deliver growth factors locally to the CNS, we further investigated their potential in animal models to serve as a practical tool for safely and effectively delivering NGF in clinical trials in AD. Initial efforts focused on ex vivo rather than in vivo gene delivery, due to the superior level of development of ex vivo gene delivery techniques at the time that these studies were initiated in the early 1990s. Current development efforts are underway with in vivo gene therapy as well. In rodent and primate studies we could demonstrate that ex vivo delivery of autologous, primary primate fibroblasts, genetically modified to produce and secrete human NGF, promoted the survival of injured basal forebrain cholinergic neurons, reversed the atrophy of these neurons in aged primates, and restored cortical cholinergic inputs to levels equal to those of young monkeys *(23–25)*.

We then performed an additional set of studies to determine whether ex vivo NGF gene delivery in the primate brain could effectively restrict NGF delivery to the basal forebrain, thereby establishing the safety profile of this approach. Adult rhesus monkeys were subjected to escalating doses of gene therapy delivered to the cholinergic basal forebrain by administering progressively greater volumes of autologous fibroblasts genetically modified to secrete human NGF. Over a 50-fold variation in cell volume, from the minimally effective to the highest dose, no toxicity was observed. Primates exhibited no weight loss, no general indices of pain, and no pathological responses of Schwann cells.

Thus, unlike intracerebroventricular NGF infusions, ex vivo NGF gene delivery to the primate basal forebrain could be administered safely and effectively. In addition, persistent expression of NGF protein by the genetically modified cell implants was documented over a time period of at least 1 year—the longest time frame examined. Finally, in no case did gene delivery result in tumor formation from the genetically modified cells, and hemorrhages did not occur with introduction of the needle into the brain. Thus, the preponderance of evidence indicated that ex vivo gene delivery could effectively and safely, in the primate brain, protect cholinergic neurons.

Based on the preceding evidence, a Phase I clinical trial of NGF gene delivery for AD has been initiated at the University of California, San Diego. This ex vivo gene therapy clinical trial in patients with early-stage AD has genetically modified the subjects' fibroblasts to produce and secrete human NGF. These NGF-secreting cells have been implanted in the region of the nucleus basalis of Meynert, to determine whether cholinergic neuronal loss can be reduced and the function of remaining neurons stimulated in the AD brain.

PHASE I CLINICAL SAFETY TRIAL
OF GROWTH FACTOR GENE DELIVERY

The clinical trial, in progress, will therefore address two key questions. First, will cholinergic neurons of the AD brain respond to NGF? Because the mechanism of cholinergic neuronal death in AD is not explained yet, it is not known whether that mechanism of cell death will be prevented by NGF delivery. In animal models, NGF has been shown to prevent neuronal degeneration from several different causes, including injury-induced cell death, excitotoxicity-induced cell death, and spontaneous neuronal degeneration with aging. Thus, NGF is able to protect cholinergic neurons that are declining as a result of several distinct mechanisms, including both apoptotic (programmed) and nonapoptotic (necrotic) cell death. Whether the mechanism of cholinergic cell loss that occurs in AD will also be NGF-responsive remains to be determined in patients with the disease, because humans are the only species known to develop the pathological characteristics of AD.

Second, will preventing the cholinergic component of cell loss in AD be sufficient to significantly affect clinical progression of the disease? Many neuronal systems undergo degeneration in AD, including cortical neurons and some subsets of subcortical neurons. Of these populations, only cholinergic neurons are NGF-sensitive. However, among all neuronal systems that undergo degeneration in AD, cholinergic cell loss has been most clearly correlated with overall synapse loss in the brain *(29–31)*. Further, blockade of cholinergic function causes memory dysfunction in normal rats and humans, and restoration of this blockage improves memory *(29)*. The normal role of the cholinergic system is to modulate neuronal activity in the hippocampus and cortex, and disruption of this function would be predicted to affect learning and the efficiency of cognitive processing *(29,30,32)*. Lesions of the cholinergic system in primates also impair attention *(33)*.

Finally, the only drugs approved (in the United States) for the treatment of AD target the cholinergic system and demonstrate modest efficacy, despite the relatively modest effects of these drugs in influencing central activity of cholinergic systems. For these reasons, the delivery of a growth factor that can prevent the loss of cholinergic neurons, and augment the function of remaining neurons, could have a significant effect on clinical progression in AD. The current clinical program of NGF gene delivery will test this possibility.

Whereas the current Phase I clinical safety trial of growth factor gene delivery in AD uses ex vivo gene delivery, future clinical trials are likely to use in vivo gene delivery, due to the greater simplicity of the in vivo approach. Preclinical studies in rodents indicate that in vivo NGF gene delivery promotes a degree of cholinergic neuronal protection equal to that of ex vivo gene delivery, and efficacy and safety studies are now in progress *(34)*. Should this program continue to demonstrate efficacy and safety, then clinical trials of in vivo NGF gene delivery in AD will be initiated.

In addition, the development of a means of controlling the amount of gene product delivered to the brain will optimize the safety of gene therapy in the future. Several "regulatable" systems are under development, and have shown the ability to turn "on" or "off" the delivery of NGF to cholinergic neurons in the rodent brain (Fig. 2). Such regulatable systems require further development, however, before entering clinical trials.

ALTERNATIVE METHODS OF GROWTH FACTOR DELIVERY
TO THE BRAIN: INTRAPARENCHYMAL PROTEIN INFUSIONS

An alternative way to achieve restricted delivery of growth factors to the brain is the localized infusion of a growth factor directly into the brain parenchyma using an infusion device. This approach would allow controlled delivery of a growth factor in concentrations that would hypothetically be sufficient to rescue host neurons, while restricting diffusion of the factor from targeted regions (to avoid

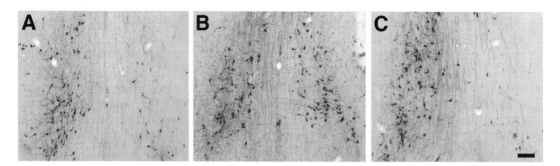

Fig. 2. Regulating gene delivery. The survival of basal forebrain cholinergic neurons can be controlled in the rat brain using regulatable gene therapy vectors. **(A)** After right-sided fimbria-fornix lesions in adult rats, basal forebrain cholinergic neurons degenerate. **(B)** Cholinergic neuronal degeneration can be prevented using regulatable gene therapy vectors, when the gene of interest (NGF in this case) is turned "on." **(C)** If a rat is treated with a regulatable NGF gene therapy vector, and the vector is turned "off" by administering doxycycline to the animal, then NGF gene expression is discontinued and cholinergic neurons are no longer rescued after fimbria-fornix lesions, as in untreated rats. These regulatable gene therapy vectors will enhance the safety and the ability to control gene delivery in future clinical trials. Scale bar = 70 μm. (From ref. *39*.)

adverse effects). The drawbacks of this approach are the need for chronic instrumentation, with the coincident risk of mechanical failure, infection, and the need for periodic pump refilling. Further, the effects of chronic hydrostatic pressure application on the brain resulting from these infusions are unknown.

Intraparenchymal growth factor infusions are currently the subject of clinical trials delivering another growth factor—glial cell line-derived neurotrophic factor (GDNF)—in Parkinson's disease. The rationale for delivering GDNF to the brain in Parkinson's disease is analogous to that of NGF delivery in AD: to rescue degenerating neurons and stimulate the function of remaining cells. Like the NGF trial in AD, this GDNF clinical trial in Parkinson's disease will be important in defining the therapeutic potential of growth factors for the treatment of neurodegenerative disorders. Growth factor infusions have been previously attempted in Parkinson's disease and amyotrophic lateral sclerosis, but using nontargeted delivery methods that caused adverse effects.

ALTERNATIVES TO GROWTH FACTOR DELIVERY: SMALL MOLECULES MIMICKING GROWTH FACTOR ACTIONS

Small peptide mimetics of the growth factors have been under development for some time. By reducing the size of the peptide, the hope is that these molecules would penetrate the CNS after peripheral administration, eliminating the need for the introduction of needles into the brain. Typically, however, these mimetics have exhibited marginal effects when tested in vivo. Perhaps of greater concern, their delivery to CNS and extra-CNS sites would be nontargeted—raising the risk of the full spectrum of adverse effects observed with nontargeted growth factor infusions. Hence, additional discovery experiments are required to determine whether small peptide mimetics of growth factors will be practical alternatives to the delivery of full-length molecules.

OTHER GROWTH FACTORS FOR AD

Approximately 100 nervous system growth factors have been discovered since the initial work of Levi-Montalcini and colleagues. The various growth factors influence a diversity of neuronal populations. For example, cortical neurons, which are vulnerable in AD, exhibit sensitivity to the growth factors brain-derived neurotrophic factor (BDNF) and fibroblast growth factor-2 (FGF-2) *(35–38)*. Thus, the possibility exists that targeted delivery of growth factors to brain regions particularly vulnerable to the neurodegeneration of AD—such as the entorhinal cortex—could rescue cells. Preclinical experiments are in progress to address these possibilities.

Growth factor delivery to the cortex presents practical challenges, however, in that the brain region targeted for growth factor treatment might be relatively large and therefore difficult to target by gene therapy or direct protein infusions. This is not the case with the delivery of NGF to the basal forebrain cholinergic system of the human, because cell groups constituting this nucleus extend over a linear distance of only 1 cm, which can be practically targeted by gene delivery.

KEY MESSAGES

Growth factor therapy offers the unique prospect of preventing cell loss early in the course of neurodegenerative disorders such as AD. Recent advances in molecular medicine also offer, for the first time, potentially practical means of delivering growth factors to the CNS by gene therapy that can provide sufficient concentrations of NGF to prevent cell loss while avoiding adverse effects of nontargeted growth factor delivery. The next decade will reveal whether these approaches will yield new possibilities for the effective treatment of what are currently essentially untreatable neurodegenerative diseases.

REFERENCES

1. Levi-Montalcini, R.; Hamburger, V.: Selective growth stimulating effects of mouse sarcoma on the sensory and sympathetic nervous system of the chick embryo. J Exp Zool 1951; 116: 321–362.
2. Levi-Montalcini, R.: The nerve growth factor 35 years later. Science 1987; 237: 1154–1162.
3. Francke, U. et al.: The human gene for the beta subunit of nerve growth factor is located on the short arm of chromosone 1. Science 1983; 222: 1248.
4. Ullrich, A. et al.: Human beta-nerve growth factor gene sequence highly homologous to that of mouse. Nature 1983; 303: 821–825.
5. Kaplan, D.R.; Miller, F.D.: Neurotrophin signal transduction in the nervous system. Curr Opin Neurobiol 2000; 10: 381–391.
6. Korsching, S.; Thoenen, H.: Quantitative demonstration of the retrograde axonal transport of endogenous nerve growth factor. Neurosci Lett 1983; 39: 1–4.
7. Hefti, F.: Nerve growth factor (NGF) promotes survival of septal cholinergic neurons after fimbrial transection. J Neurosci 1986; 6: 2155–2162.
8. Fischer, W. et al.: Amelioration of cholinergic neuron atrophy and spatial memory impairment in aged rats by nerve growth factor. Nature 1987; 329: 65–68.
9. Tuszynski, M.H. et al.: Nerve growth factor infusion in primate brain reduces lesion-induced cholinergic neuronal degeneration. J Neurosci 1990; 10: 3604–3614.
10. Koliatsos, V.E. et al.: Mouse nerve growth factor prevents degeneration of axotomized basal forebrain cholinergic neurons in the monkey. J Neurosci 1990; 10: 3801–3813.
11. Davis, K.L. et al.: A double-blind, placebo-controlled multicenter study of tacrine for Alzheimer's disease. The Tacrine Collaborative Study Group. N Engl J Med 1992; 327: 1253–1259.
12. Dekker, A.J. et al.: NGF increases cortical acetylcholine release in rats with lesions of the nucleus basalis. Neuroreport 1991; 2: 577–580.
13. Mufson, E.J.: Conner, J.M.; Kordower, J.H.: Nerve growth factor in Alzheimer's disease: defective retrograde transport to nucleus basalis. Neuroreport 1995; 6: 1063–1066.
14. Scott, S.A. et al.: Nerve growth factor in Alzheimer's disease: increased levels throughout the brain coupled with declines in nucleus basalis. J Neurosci 1995; 15: 6213–6221.
15. Crutcher, K.A. et al.: Detection of NGF-like activity in human brain tissue: increased levels in Alzheimer's disease. J Neurosci 1993; 13: 2540–2550.
16. Williams, L.R.: Hypophagia is induced by intracerebroventricular administration of nerve growth factor. Exp Neurol 1991; 113: 31–37.
17. Crutcher, K.A.: Sympathetic sprouting in the central nervous system: a model for studies of axonal growth in the mature mammalian brain. Brain Res Rev 1987; 12: 203–233.
18. Winkler, J. et al.: Reversible Schwann cell hyperplasia and sprouting of sensory and sympathetic neurites after intraventricular administration of nerve growth factor. Ann Neurol 1997; 41: 82–93.

19. Eriksdotter Jonhagen, M. et al.: Intracerebroventricular infusion of nerve growth factor in three patients with Alzheimer's disease. Dement Geriatr Cogn Disord 1998; 9: 246–257.

20. Rosenberg, M.B. et al.: Grafting genetically modified cells to the damaged brain: restorative effects of NGF expression. Science 1988; 242: 1575–1578.

21. Chen, K.; Gage, F.H.: Recovery of mnemonic function in cognitively impaired, aged rats by grafts of fibroblasts genetically modified to produce nerve growth factor. Soc Neurosci Abstr 1993.

22. Kordower, J.H. et al.: The aged monkey basal forebrain: rescue and sprouting of axotomized basal forebrain neurons after grafts of encapsulated cells secreting human nerve growth factor. Proc Natl Acad Sci USA 1994; 91: 10898–10902.

23. Tuszynski, M.H. et al.: Gene therapy in the adult primate brain: intraparenchymal grafts of cells genetically modified to produce nerve growth factor prevent cholinergic neuronal degeneration. Gene Therapy 1996; 3: 305–314.

24. Smith, D.E. et al.: Age-associated neuronal atrophy occurs in the primate brain and is reversible by growth factor gene therapy. Proc Natl Acad Sci USA 1999; 96: 10893–10898.

25. Conner, J.M. et al.: Non-tropic actions of neurotrophins: subcortical NGF gene delivery reverses age-related degeneration of primate cortical cholinergic innervation. Proc Natl Acad Sci USA 2001; 98: 1941–1946.

26. Miller, D.A.: Retrovirus packaging cells. Hum Gene Ther 1990; 1: 5–14.

27. Naldini, L. et al.: In vivo gene delivery and stable transduction of non-dividing cells by a lentiviral vector. Science 1996; 272: 263–267.

28. Rabinowitz, J.E.; Samulski, R.J.: Building a better vector: the manipulation of AAV virions. Virology 2000; 278: 301–308.

29. Bartus, R. et al.: The cholinergic hypothesis of geriatric memory dysfunction. Science 1982; 217: 408–417.

30. Coyle, J.T.; Price, P.H.; Delong, M.R.: Alzheimer's disease: a disorder of cortical cholinergic innervation. Science 1983; 219: 1184–1189.

31. Terry, R.D. et al.: Physical basis of cognitive alterations in Alzheimer's disease: synapse loss is the major correlate of cognitive impairment. Ann Neurol 1991; 30: 572–580.

32. Everitt, B.J.; Robbins, T.W.: Central cholinergic systems and cognition. Ann Rev Psychol 1997; 48: 649–684.

33. Voytko, M.L. et al.: Basal forebrain lesions in monkeys disrupt attention but not learning and memory. J Neurosci 1994; 14: 167–186.

34. Mandel, R.J. et al.: Nerve growth factor expressed in the medial septum following in vivo gene delivery using a recombinant adeno-associated viral vector protects cholinergic neurons from fimbria-fornix lesion-induced degeneration. Exp Neurol 1999; 155: 59–64.

35. Tetzlaff, W. et al.: Response of rubrospinal and corticospinal neurons to injury and neurotrophins. Prog Brain Res 1994; 103: 271–286.

36. Lu, P.; Blesch, A.; Tuszynski, M.H.: Neurotrophism without neurotropism: BDNF promotes survival but not growth of lesioned corticospinal neurons. J Comp Neurol 2001; 436: 456–470.

37. Gomez-Pinilla, F.; Lee, J.W.; Cotman, C.W.: Basic fibroblast growth factor in adult rat brain: cell distribution and response to entorhinal lesion and fimbria-fornix transection. J Neurosci 1992; 12: 345–355.

38. Peterson, D.A. et al.: Fibroblast growth factor-2 protects entorhinal layer II glutamatergic neurons from axotomy-induced death. J Neurosci 1996; 16: 886–898.

39. Blesch, A.; Conner, J.M.; Tuszynski, M.H.: Modulation of neuronal survival and axonal growth in vivo by tetracycline-regulated neurotrophin expression. Gene Ther 2001; 8: 954–960.

29

Statins in Prevention and Treatment of Alzheimer's Disease

David A. Drachman

INTRODUCTION

There are a variety of strategies by which drugs to prevent or treat Alzheimer's disease (AD) can be developed. These include:

1. Understanding the fundamental etiology of the disease, and developing drugs that interfere with this initiating process
2. Recognizing a particular step in the degenerative cascade, which is the mechanism, or immediate cause, by which neurons and other brain tissue are damaged, and interrupting this intermediate step
3. Observing serendipitous associations between AD and other disorders or their treatments, and pursuing therapeutic strategies based on these observations

The use of statins—3-hydroxy-3-methyl-glutaryl-coenzyme A reductase inhibitors—to prevent and/or treat AD has been suggested by each of these three strategic approaches. In this chapter we will briefly review the pharmacological functions of these drugs, the rationale for the use of statins in AD and other dementias, as well as the evidence so far available regarding their effectiveness in preventing and/or treating dementia.

PHARMACOLOGICAL FUNCTIONS OF STATINS

Statins competitively inhibit the key rate-limiting enzyme in the mevalonate pathway, by which cholesterol is synthesized from acetyl coenzyme A *(1)*. Introduced initially for the treatment of hypercholesterolemia, statins effectively reduce total serum cholesterol, upregulate hepatic LDL receptors (thereby lowering LDL-cholesterol), reduce serum triglycerides, increase HDL-cholesterol, and reduce atherosclerotic vascular lesions *(2)*.

Statins have a number of other important biological effects, however, which may be critical in preventing both cardiovascular disease and AD *(2,3)*. By intefering with the mevalonate pathway, statins reduce the formation of isoprenoid intermediates—geranyl pyrophosphate and farnesyl pyrophosphate *(4–6)*. These intermediates are necessary for the isoprenylation and "anchoring" to cell membranes of certain G proteins, which are responsible for signal transduction. Interference with the geranylgeranylation of rho-GTPase downregulates this signaling molecule *(4)*, with important consequences: endothelial nitric oxide synthase (eNOS) is increased in cerebral microvessels, augmenting endothelial nitric oxide; and endothelin-1 is reduced. As a consequence of these seemingly complex interactions, cerebral blood vessels are dilated, blood flow is increased, and endothelial function is improved *(7)*.

From: *Current Clinical Neurology,*
Alzheimer's Disease: A Physician's Guide to Practical Management
Edited by: R. W. Richter and B. Zoeller Richter © Humana Press Inc., Totowa, NJ

Statins also reduce inflammatory changes, by decreasing the production of inflammatory cytokines in the brain, including inducible nitric oxide synthase (iNOS), interleukin-1 (IL-1), and tumor necrosis factor-α (TNF-α) *(1)*. They also inhibit endothelial formation of free oxygen radicals *(8)*.

RATIONALE FOR THE USE OF STATINS IN AD

As noted above, statins have important effects both on cholesterol metabolism and on vascular function. AD has been associated with both cholesterol and vascular disease.

Relation Between Lipids and AD

Individuals known to have an apolipoprotein E e4 (ApoEε4) gene have approximately twice the lifetime risk of developing AD, while those with an ApoEε2 gene have half the lifetime risk *(9,10)*. The precise mechanism by which ApoEε4 favors the development of AD, and ApoEε2 reduces the risk, is uncertain *(11,12)*. Apolipoproteins are carriers of lipid moieties, however, and ApoEε4 is associated with an increased risk of systemic vascular disorders, such as myocardial infarction and stroke *(13)*.

Another mechanism by which cholesterol may favor the development of AD is through its documented effects on β-amyloid (Aβ) synthesis *(14)*. In human cell culture, for example, high cholesterol levels have been shown to increase beta-amyloid production. Using cells transfected with the amyloid precursor protein (APP) gene, cholesterol increased the β-secretase (BACE) degradation of APP, a step in the pathway that leads to the production of Aβ *(15)*. Addition of a statin to the cell culture markedly reduced both cholesterol levels and Aβ production. In a transgenic mouse model of AD, high dietary cholesterol increased the production of Aβ and both the number and the size of amyloid deposits, while cholesterol-lowering drugs reduced the Aβ deposits *(16,17)*. It is widely accepted that either accumulation of amyloid may be the underlying etiology of AD, or Aβ-toxicity may be an important mechanism of neuronal damage. In either case, cholesterol metabolism may be related to AD via this effect on the production of Aβ.

Relation Between Vascular Disorders and AD

In epidemiological studies, vascular disease and vascular risk factors have been associated with the increased occurrence of AD *(18–20)*. Myocardial infarction, diabetes, hypertension, atrial fibrillation, coronary artery disease, increased carotid wall thickness, and consumption of diets high in saturated fats have all been related to increased risks of developing AD *(21–25)*.

In affected areas of brains from patients with AD, the capillaries have been shown to be narrow and tortuous *(26)*. Microvascular endothelial cells appear abnormal on histochemical staining and on electron microscopy *(27)*. Recent studies have shown that endothelial mitochondria in regions of brain affected by the pathological features of AD appear abnormal, and mitochondrial DNA deletions are present *(28)*.

These and other observations illustrate the rationale for the use of statins in the prevention and/or treatment of AD. Although the fundamental etiology of AD remains uncertain, age-related changes (ARCs), Aβ accumulation, and microvascular impairment are potential primary causes of the sporadic form of AD *(20,29–31)*. Both the accumulation of Aβ and microvascular impairment are involved in the subsequent mechanism producing neuronal loss. Serendipitous observations demonstrate the relation of vascular risk factors and disease to the occurrence of AD. Since statins modify Aβ accumulation, improve endothelial function and cerebral blood flow, and reduce diffuse vascular disease, they are drugs with a cogent rationale for the prevention and treatment of AD.

EVIDENCE REGARDING THE USE OF STATINS
TO PREVENT OR TREAT AD

In the year 2000, two observational studies were published reporting highly significant decreases in AD or dementia in individuals taking statins for dyslipidemia. Wolozin and colleagues reported a cross-sectional study of the prevalence of AD among more than 57,000 individuals over the age of 60 in three medical centers—two Veterans' Administration centers and one University Hospital *(32)*. More than 16,500 of them were taking statins. Among the total population studied, the prevalence of AD in patients taking lovastatin or pravastatin was 69.6% lower than in the total population; patients taking simvastatin showed no decrease in prevalence of AD. To examine the data for a possible treatment bias, patients taking lovastatin or pravastatin were compared with others taking a variety of medications for the treatment of hypertension. Those patients taking lovastatin or pravastatin showed the same relative decrease in prevalence of AD as they had when compared with the entire population. The explanation for the lack of efficacy of simvastatin was not clear, since it is similar to pravastatin with regard both to efficacy in inhibiting liver HMG-CoA reductase and to blood–brain barrier penetration.

Jick and colleagues studied the incidence and relative risk of developing AD or dementia among patients taking statins, using the United Kingdom General Practice Research Database (GPRD) *(33)*. Employing a nested case control design, the authors studied a base population of about 60,000 individuals, between 50 and 89 years of age, in three groups. The first group included approximately 24,500 individuals on lipid-lowering agents (LLAs), including both statins and other drugs (such as fibrates, niacin). The second group included more than 11,000 people with hyperlipidemia and no drug treatment, the third 25,000 people with normal lipids. From these three groups, followed for more than 5 years, 284 individuals were diagnosed as developing AD or dementia. For each of these 284 cases, four nondemented controls were randomly selected from the entire base population, matched for age, sex, physician practice, years of recorded history, and multiple other risk factors and diseases. The relative risk of developing AD or dementia was reduced by 70% among those individuals on statins compared with subjects with normal lipids. The odds ratio was 0.29 (0.13 to 0.63), indicating a highly significant reduction in incidence ($p < 0.002$). The use of nonstatin LLAs produced no reduction in relative risk of AD or dementia.

These observations suggested that lowering of cholesterol may not be the primary mechanism by which statins apparently reduced the risk of developing AD. It might be, rather, another effect of statins, such as the beneficial effect on endothelial cells of the brain microvasculature (increased eNOS, decreased endothelin-1), as described above, or an anti-inflammatory effect, producing the risk reduction.

In both of these observational studies—despite the highly significant results, the efforts to match patients and controls carefully, and the statistical control for all identifiable risk factors—the question of unidentified bias producing a type 1 (false positive) error could not be completely dismissed. While misdiagnosis bias would likely reduce the probability of finding a real difference due to statin treatment, indication bias—nontreatment of individuals with early, mild cognitive impairment—could produce a spuriously positive outcome.

Rockwood and colleagues examined the issue of indication bias for statin use in the Canadian Study of Health and Aging (CSHA)—a population-based study of 2305 subjects *(34)*. In this group the authors were unable to find evidence for decreased use of statins either in subjects who considered their health to be poorer, or in those considered to have had mild cognitive impairment (MCI) but not dementia. The authors found a reduction in the odds ratio for developing incident AD or dementia among statin users of 0.21 (0.08 to 0.88), supporting the studies cited above. Other observational studies have also found a reduced prevalence of dementia among statin users *(35)*.

Two recent prospective studies have failed to find a reduction in cognitive impairment among elderly individuals at risk for vascular disease. In the PROSPER study, 5,804 individuals were treated with pravastatin or placebo for a mean of 3.2 years, with a primary outcome measure of myocardial infarction, stroke, or coronary death *(36)*. Although cardiac disease was reduced in this study, stroke was not. A secondary observation of cognitive function, measured by Mini-Mental State Examination, Stroop, and several other tests, failed to show any group differences between those treated with statins vs placebo. The authors did not report the risk of developing dementia. In the MRC/BHF Heart Protection Study, 20,536 individuals with vascular disease and/or risk factors were treated with simvastatin or placebo for 5 years *(37)*. Using a telephone cognitive screening procedure, no difference in the occurrence of dementia was found between individuals on a statin and those on placebo.

SUMMARY AND CONCLUSIONS

Many clues point to an intriguing association among vascular factors, cholesterol, and dementing disorders. There are suggestions that vascular changes may contribute to—or possibly even cause— AD, which is clearly a disorder of multiple age-related etiologies, both genetic and sporadic. Statins are known to reduce several known cardiovascular risk factors, improving dyslipidemia, reducing heart disease and stroke, and increasing dilatation of cerebral microvessels by their effects on the vascular endothelium. As of this writing, the potential efficacy of statin drugs in the prevention of dementing disorders remains suggestive, tantalizing, but as yet unresolved. No randomized studies of treatment of dementia have been published as yet. Some trials with statins in AD are ongoing. The future role of statins—and indeed, other drugs that affect the function of cerebral microvascular endothelium, reduce cholesterol, and improve general vascular health—in the prevention and treatment of dementia remains to be determined.

REFERENCES

1. Hess, D. et al.: HMG-CoA reductase inhibitors (statins); a promising approach to stroke prevention. Neurology 2000; 54: 790–796.
2. Knopp, R.: Drug treatment of lipid disorders. N Engl J Med 1999; 341: 498–511.
3. Werner, N.; Nickenig, G.; Laufs, U.: Pleiotropic effects of HMG-CoA reductase inhibitors. Basic Res Cardiol 2002; 97: 105–116.
4. Laufs, U. et al.: Neuroprotection mediated by changes in the endothelial actin cytoskeleton. J Clin Invest 2000; 106: 15–24.
5. Yamada, M. et al.: Endothelial nitric oxide synthase-dependent cerebral blood flow augmentation by L-arginine after chronic statin treatment. J Cereb Blood Flow Metab 2000; 20: 709–717.
6. Endres, M. et al.: Stroke protection by 3-hydroxy-3-methylglutaryl (HMG)-CoA reductase inhibitors mediated by endothelial nitric oxide synthase. Proc Natl Acad Sci USA 1998; 95: 8880–8885.
7. Bellosta, S. et al.: Non-lipid-related effects of statins. Ann Med 2000; 32: 164–176.
8. Wagner, A. et al.: Improvement of nitric oxide-dependent vasodilatation by HMG-CoA reductase inhibitors through attenuation of endothelial superoxide anion formation. Arterioscler Thromb Vasc Biol 2000; 20: 61–69.
9. Seshadri, S.; Drachman, D.; Lippa, C.: Apolipoprotein E e4 allele and the lifetime risk of Alzheimer's disease: what physicians know, and what they should know. Arch Neurol 1995; 52: 1074–1080.
10. Saunders, A. et al.: Association of apolipoprotein E type 4 allele epsilon 4 with late-onset familial and sporadic Alzheimer's disease. Neurology 1993; 43: 1467–1472.
11. Roses, A. et al.: Morphological, biochemical, and genetic support for an apolipoprotein E effect on microtubular metabolism. In: Wurtman, R.; Corkin, S.; Growdon, J.; Nitsch, R. (eds):. The Neurobiology of Alzheimer's Disease. New York Academy of Sciences, New York, 1996: 146–165.
12. Strittmatter, W. et al.: Apolipoprotein E: high-avidity binding to B-amyloid and increased frequency of type 4 allele in late-onset familial Alzheimer disease. Proc Natl Acad Sci USA 1993; 90: 1977–1981.
13. Contois, J.H.; Anamani, D.E.; Tsongalis, G.J.: The underlying molecular mechanism of apolipoprotein E polymorphism: relationships to lipid disorders, cardiovascular disease, and Alzheimer's disease. Clin Lab Med 1996; 16: 105–123.
14. Wood, W.G. et al.: Brain membrane cholesterol domains, aging and amyloid beta-peptides. Neurobiol Aging 2002; 23: 685–694.
15. Frears, E. et al.: The role of cholesterol in the biosynthesis of beta-amyloid. Neuroreport 1999; 10: 1699–1705.
16. Refolo, L.M. et al.: Hypercholesterolemia accelerates the Alzheimer's amyloid pathology in a transgenic mouse model. Neurobiol Dis 2000; 7: 321–331.
17. Refolo, L.M. et al.: A cholesterol-lowering drug reduces beta-amyloid pathology in a transgenic mouse model of Alzheimer's disease. Neurobiol Dis 2001; 8: 890–899.
18. Breteler, M.M.: Vascular risk factors for Alzheimer's disease: an epidemiologic perspective. Neurobiol Aging 2000; 21: 153–160.
19. Breteler, M.M. et al.: Risk factors for vascular disease and dementia. Haemostasis 1998; 28: 167–173.
20. De la Torre, J.C.: Vascular basis of Alzheimer's pathogenesis. Ann N Y Acad Sci 2002; 977: 196–215.
21. Ott, A. et al.: Diabetes mellitus and the risk of dementia: The Rotterdam Study. Neurology 1999; 53: 1937–1942.
22. Skoog. I.; Gustafson, D.: Hypertension and related factors in the etiology of Alzheimer's disease. Ann N Y Acad Sci 2002; 977: 29–36.

23. Forette, F. et al.: The prevention of dementia with antihypertensive treatment: new evidence from the Systolic Hypertension in Europe (Syst-Eur) study. Arch Intern Med 2002; 162: 2046–2052.

24. Ott, A. et al.: Atrial fibrillation and dementia in a population-based study. The Rotterdam Study. Stroke 1997; 28: 316–321.

25. Sparks, D.L.: Coronary artery disease, hypertension, ApoE, and cholesterol: a link to Alzheimer's disease? Ann N Y Acad Sci 1997; 826: 128–146.

26. Buee, L. et al.: Pathological alterations of the cerebral microvasculature in Alzheimer's disease and related dementing disorders. Acta Neuropathol 1994; 87: 469–480.

27. Drachman, D.; Smith, T.: The role of declining angiogenesis in brain aging and Alzheimer's disease; preliminary observations. In: Growdon, J. (ed.): Massachusetts Alzheimer's Disease Research Center; Twelfth Annual Scientific Poster Session, 1999, Boston, 1999.

28. Aliev, G. et al.: Atherosclerotic lesions and mitochondria DNA deletions in brain microvessels as a central target for the development of human AD and AD-like pathology in aged transgenic mice. Ann N Y Acad Sci 2002; 977: 45–64.

29. Drachman, D.: Aging and the brain: a new frontier. Ann Neurol 1997; 42: 819–828.

30. Hardy, J.; Selkoe, D.J.: The amyloid hypothesis of Alzheimer's disease: progress and problems on the road to therapeutics. Science 2002; 297: 353–356.

31. Selkoe, D.J.: The genetics and molecular pathology of Alzheimer's disease: roles of amyloid and the presenilins. Neurol Clin 2000; 18: 903–922.

32. Wolozin, B. et al.: Decreased prevalence of Alzheimer disease associated with 3-hydroxy-3-methyglutaryl coenzyme A reductase inhibitors. Arch Neurol 2000; 57: 1439–1443.

33. Jick, H. et al.: Statins and the risk of dementia. Lancet 2000; 356: 1627–1631.

34. Rockwood, K. et al.: Use of lipid-lowering agents, indication bias, and the risk of dementia in community-dwelling elderly people. Arch Neurol 2002; 59: 223–227.

35. Hajjar, I. et al.: The impact of the use of statins on the prevalence of dementia and the progression of cognitive impairment. J Gerontol A Biol Sci Med Sci 2002; 57: M414–M418.

36. Shepherd. J. et al.: Pravastatin in elderly individuals at risk of vascular disease (PROSPER): a randomized controlled trial. Lancet 2002; 360: 1623–1630.

37. MRC/BHF Heart Protection Study of antioxidant vitamin supplementation in 20,536 high-risk individuals: a randomized placebo-controlled trial. Lancet 2002; 360: 23–33.

30

Potential Role of Androgens
and Androgen Receptors in Alzheimer's Disease

Jacob Raber

INTRODUCTION

Increasing evidence indicates reductions in estrogen levels in aged women and in androgen levels in aged men and women *(1–5)*. These reductions might be risk factors for cognitive impairments and the development of Alzheimer's disease (AD). While aged people show reduced levels of sex steroid production, sex steroid receptors, and aromatase activity required to convert the androgen testosterone to the estrogen 17-β estradiol, they show improved aspects of cognition after treatment with sex steroids. Therefore, ongoing clinical trials are designed to evaluate the potential benefit of estrogen in women and of testosterone in men with AD *(1)*. In this chapter, we will review the potential roles of androgens and androgen receptors (ARs) in cognition, cognitive aging, and AD, and highlight the potential interactions of androgens with AD-related factors.

THE ROLE OF SEX STEROIDS IN THE BRAIN

Sex steroids cause sex differences in brain organization (organizational effect) *(6)* and, to a lesser degree, in behaviors in adulthood (activational effect) *(7)*. In the brain, sex steroids have effects on cell death, neuronal growth and morphology, neurotransmitter release and synaptogenesis, $GABA_A$ receptors, and the mobilization of calcium across cell membranes. Sex steroids mediate these effects by nuclear receptor pathways (genomic effects) and by mechanisms that do not involve nuclear receptors (nongenomic effects) *(8–11)*.

Androgens are steroids secreted primarily from the testes and the adrenal gland. They increase the growth of neuronal cell bodies and extensions, plasticity, and induce neuronal differentation *(12–16)*. Aromatase converts the androgen testosterone to the estrogen 17-β estradiol *(17)*, which can mediate effects of testosterone—for example, by signaling through the estrogen receptors (ER) ER-α and ER-β in the nucleus or on the plasma membrane *(18)*.

WHY FOCUS ON ANDROGENS?

Many studies focus on the effects of estrogens on cognition in women. In this chapter, we focus on androgens. The focus of androgens in women may be very relevant. In most studies, estrogen treatment was unable to slow the progression of AD *(19)*. In addition, recent clinical data indicate that estrogen has a beneficial effect on aspects of cognitive function only in healthy elderly women who do not carry the ApoE ε4 allele; no such effect is seen either in healthy elderly women who carry ε4 *(20)* nor in women with AD. Furthermore, testosterone, but not estrogen levels in serum, correlated positively with aspects of cognitive performance in older women *(21)*. Also, testosterone therapy improved

From: *Current Clinical Neurology,*
Alzheimer's Disease: A Physician's Guide to Practical Management
Edited by: R. W. Richter and B. Zoeller Richter © Humana Press Inc., Totowa, NJ

aspects of cognition in surgically menopausal women *(22)*. Finally, estrogen treatment reduces testosterone levels through feedback suppression of testosterone production.

The effects of testosterone on aspects of cognition may be mediated by ARs and/or ERs. Further research is needed to determine whether aromatization of testosterone to estrogen is required for the effects of testosterone on cognition. Aromatase inhibitors could be used to answer this important question.

AR STRUCTURE AND FUNCTION

The human AR gene contains eight exons and encodes a 110-kDa member of the nuclear receptor superfamily (Fig. 1A) *(23)*. The first exon encodes the N-terminal domain containing the major transactivation function (AF-1). This exon shows polymorphisms resulting from variable numbers of glutamine (11–35, with 21 as average in normal population) and glycine repeats (10–31, with 24 as average in normal population). Shortening of the polyglutamine or polyglycine stretch is associated with predisposition to prostatic neoplasia *(24)*. In contrast, expansion of the glutamine repeat can sequester co-activators such as the cAMP response element (CREB)-binding protein (CBP), resulting in age-dependent spinal and bulbar muscular atrophy *(25,26)*. AF-1 interacts with the glutamine-rich region of steroid receptor co-activator-1 (SRC-1) *(27)*. SRC-1 can interact with the global activator CBP/p300, and together they show synergy in inducing AR transactivation *(28)*. CBP/p300 can also interact directly with ARs.

The second and third exons encode the DNA-binding domain (DBD). This domain contains two zinc fingers, which enable ARs to bind the regulatory part of target genes. The N-terminal zinc finger is involved in sequence specificity and the C-terminal one in stabilization of the AR–DNA complex *(29)*. Interestingly, ARs and receptors for certain steroids—glucocorticoids, mineralocorticoids, and progesterone—can recognize the same DNA response element and the ligand-binding domain (LBD) folding patterns of the family members, which contain 12 α-helices, is very similar.

Exons 4–8 encode the LBD and a minor transactivation function (AF-2). AF-1 and AF-2 interact with the leucine-rich SRC-1 *(27)*. The activity of SRC-1 is regulated by phosphorylation by mitogen-activated protein kinase (MAPK), which is stimulated by androgens. In the absence of hormone, the ligand-binding domain of AR prevents the transactivation of AF-1 and the required three-dimensional structures for SRC-1 interaction at AF-2; LBD deletion results in a constitutively active receptor. Hormone binding enables AF-1 and AF-2 to associate with a multisubunit complex of co-activator proteins, which is proposed to associate additional proteins required for interaction of AR to RNA polymerase II. The relative importance of AF-1 and AF-2 for AR activity may depend on the gene and the ligand involved.

The ARs and other steroid hormone receptors can also be activated in a ligand-independent fashion. For example, the estrogen receptor in human and the progesterone receptor in chick, rat, and rabbit can be activated by dopamine, growth factors, and drugs modulating protein kinase pathways. Similarly, growth factors and interleukin-6 (IL-6) activate ARs in the absence of androgen. Such a mechanism has been suggested to underlie androgen-independent prostate cancer associated with elevated levels of SRC-1 and MAPK activity in tumor cells and of IL-6 in blood. Point mutations at different sites in exons 2–8 have been reported for partial and complete forms of androgen insensitivity. In human prostate cancer cells, the ligand-independent activation of ARs by IL-6 involves phosphorylation of SRC-1 by MAPK *(30)*. However, it should be emphasized that SRC-1 phosphorylation by itself is not sufficient for ligand-independent transactivation of ARs, as it requires the presence of IL-6 *(30)*.

Nuclear Translocation

AR not bound to hormone is localized in the cytoplasm as a complex with heat-shock proteins and immunophilins. When the endogenous androgens testosterone or 5-α-dihydrotestosterone (DHT)

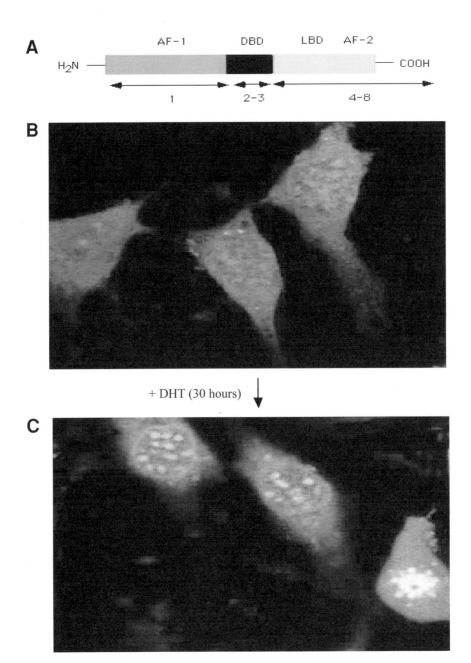

Fig. 1. (A) The AR structure (*see* text). **(B/C)** AR nuclear translocation. Mouse MC3T3 bone cells were maintained in minimum essential medium (MEM), containing 10% fetal bovine serum (FBS) and 1% penicillin-streptomycin at 37°C in 5% CO_2. Cells were treated with vehicle (95% ethanol) **(A)** or 10 nM 5-α-dihydrotestosterone (DHT) **(B)** in media containing 10% charcoal-stripped serum and 1% antibiotics for 30 hours. Following treatment with DHT or ethanol, cells were rinsed with cold phosphate-buffered saline (PBS) and incubated in 4% paraformaldehyde for 10 minutes. Cells were then rinsed in PBS twice, incubated in rabbit anti-androgen receptor antibody (Chemicon), diluted 1:250 in PBT (= PBS containing 0.2% Triton X-100 and 0.2% bovine serum albumin), and kept overnight at 4°C. Cells were washed twice in PBS, then incubated for 1 hour with the secondary antibody, Texas red-coupled donkey anti-rabbit (Jackson Immunoresearch), and diluted 1:100 in PBT. Cells were washed twice in PBS and cover slips were mounted onto slides using Vectashield (Vector Laboratories). Cells were analyzed with a Bio-Rad laser scanning confocal microscope, mounted on a (Zeiss) microscope and running Lasersharp software. Primary antibody binding was imaged and analyzed.

Four scans were averaged (Kalman filter) to obtain each final image. A 63× oil objective was used. Settings were for both images: zoom was set at 2.2, iris at 2.2, gain at 1500, and bi-level at –7. Digitized images were transferred to a PC computer and analyzed using NIH Java Image.

Images from Curley, Robertson, and Raber, Oregon Health & Science University.

bind, AR changes its confirmation, dissociates from the complex by releasing associated proteins, forms homodimers, and unmasks its nuclear localization signal. Once unmasked, this signal binds importins, which transport the hormone-bound AR into the nucleus (Fig. 1B,C). In the nucleus, active hormone-bound ARs enter nuclear foci, while antagonist-bound ARs enter the nucleus but not the nuclear foci.

Selective androgen receptor modulators (SARMs) modulate AR function by either failing to translocate ARs to the nucleus (e.g., chlozolinate or procymidone) or translocating ARs to the nucleus but not into the nuclear foci (e.g., vinclozolin or DDT or its metabolites).

ARs can modulate gene transcription by binding to specific androgen response elements (AREs) in the DNA, but are also able to *trans*-activate and *trans*-repress without interacting directly with specific DNA elements. The calcium-binding protein calreticulin is able to dissociate AR from the DNA by competing for the DBD of the AR and may export AR back to the cytoplasm, as it exports the glucocorticoid receptor from the nucleus back to cytoplasm. Hormone-dissociated AR moves back to the cytoplasm ready for another nuclear translocation.

SEX STEROIDS, THE HIPPOCAMPUS, AND SPATIAL LEARNING AND MEMORY

Studies suggest that many nonreproductive behaviors, including learning and memory *(31,32)*, are sexually dimorphic in both humans *(33)* and rodents *(6,34)*. In general, studies of spatial learning and memory in rodents have shown that males learn more quickly and exhibit superior performance compared with females *(35–43)*. Females may be more susceptible to spatial memory impairments than males. Studies of rodents with medial frontal cortical lesions showed that males were less impaired than females in mazes requiring the use of multiple visual-spatial cues for a successful solution *(44)* and by the higher susceptibility of female rodents to the cholinergic neurotoxin AF64A *(45)*. It must be noted that some studies did not show such differences between the sexes *(36)*.

Many behavioral dimorphisms are influenced by sex steroids in the perinatal environment that cause sex differences in the organization of the brain (organizational effect) *(6)*. Most behaviors remain flexible, and to a lesser degree, sex hormones also influence sexually dimorphic behaviors in adulthood (activational effect) *(7)*. Activational effects include the effects of androgens on performance on spatial tasks and of estrogens on verbal fluency, verbal memory tests, and fine motor skills and coordination of movement. It should be pointed out that it is important to distinguish potential effects of sex steroids on task performance (skills), which can affect learning and memory, from potential direct effects on learning and memory performance.

Spatial learning and memory have been attributed to the hippocampus *(46,47)*. Sex differences in hippocampal structure may contribute to sexual dimorphism in spatial cognition, including the different strategies used by males and females to solve spatial tasks *(48)*. Females tend to rely more on local cues and landmarks, whereas males rely more on the spatial relationship between fixed points.

Estrogen is associated with an increase in markers of cholinergic neurons. Cholinergic neurons in the basal forebrain and their target regions, including the hippocampus, might play a role in sex differences in spatial learning *(39)*. Importantly, fluctuations in hippocampal morphology *(49)* and in markers for cholinergic neurons *(50)* that coincide with the estrous cycle or ovariectomy do not alter spatial learning in most studies *(51)*.

These data indicate that the hippocampus is protected against the decrease in estrogen during the estrous cycle and suggest that altered estrogen levels have little effect on cognitive function during normal cycling. However, this situation might be completely different in the absence of normal cycling and/or in the presence of chronic inflammation, which have been suggested to play important roles in AD. Although ovariectomized rats showed no impairments in spatial learning and memory, they became impaired after estrogen replacement therapy or chronic inflammation *(52)*. Importantly, the combination of estrogen replacement therapy and chronic inflammation exacerbated these deficits.

The presence of ovaries or fluctuating estrogen levels may be required for estrogen replacement therapy not to negatively influence spatial learning and memory.

Sex steroids might contribute to the sexually dimorphic performance in spatial learning and memory. In newborn female rodents, administration of testosterone or 17-β estradiol results in spatial learning curves similar to those of males *(53)*. During perinatal development, the hippocampus transiently expresses both estrogen receptors *(54)* and the aromatase that converts testosterone to estradiol *(53)*. In males, estradiol could lead to sexual differentiation of the hippocampus.

Indeed, in water maze experiments, male rodents castrated at birth have learning curves resembling those of females, and the administration of testosterone or estradiol to newborn female rodents produces learning curves resembling those of males *(7)*. In adulthood, testosterone *(55)*, but not 17-β estradiol *(53)*, enhances aspects of cognition. However, brain areas containing sex steroid receptors but not affected by sex steroids in development or adulthood and lacking gender-dependent changes might also mediate the potential effects of sex steroids on aspects of cognition.

POTENTIAL ROLE OF AR IN SPATIAL LEARNING AND MEMORY

Do androgen receptors play a role in spatial learning and memory? Both appear to be impaired in AD. To address this question, we started to study mutant mice with a naturally occurring defect in the AR gene (testicular feminization mutant, or *tfm*) *(56,57)*. Because the trait in *tfm* mice is X-linked, males are completely androgen-insensitive and females are partially insensitive. If ARs are important for spatial learning and memory, female *tfm* carrier mice would be expected to outperform *tfm* male mice in spatial learning and memory tests.

To assess spatial learning and memory, 6- to 8-month-old mice were tested in the water maze (Fig. 2A). The *tfm* female and male mice improved their performance over the visible and hidden platform sessions ($p < 0.01$). Although there was no difference in the ability of the *tfm* female and male mice to locate the visible platform location, *tfm* female were better than *tfm* male mice in locating the hidden platform location (acquisition, $p < 0.01$ [Tukey-Kramer]). Both groups of mice swam continuously and in similar patterns; there were no significant periods of passive floating. In the probe trial, both groups showed spatial memory retention and spent more time in the target quadrant than in any of the other quadrants ($p < 0.01$ [Tukey-Kramer]), but *tfm* female mice spent more time in the target quadrant than *tfm* male mice ($p < 0.05$ [Tukey-Kramer]). We excluded that potential differences in sensorimotor function (Fig. 2B) or anxiety levels (Fig. 2C) contributed to the differences in water maze performance. These data show that ARs are important for spatial learning and memory, as female *tfm* carrier mice outperformed *tfm* male mice in this test.

POTENTIAL NEUROPROTECTIVE MECHANISMS

How can testosterone and ARs be neuroprotective? Testosterone is not an antioxidant by itself, as it lacks the phenol group present in 17-β estradiol, but decreases susceptibility to oxidative stress *(58,59)*. Testosterone might be neuroprotective by inhibiting the stress response, which is enhanced in AD; testosterone deficiency increases the sensitivity to glucocorticoid-induced structural damage in the hippocampus and memory deficits, which can be antagonized by treatment with testosterone.

Testosterone might also be neuroprotective by interacting with AD-related factors. Selected potential neuroprotective mechanisms of testosterone are illustrated in Fig. 3 and described in the remaining sections of the chapter.

AR and β-Catenin

Increasing evidence indicates a link between AR and β-catenin *(60–62)*. β-Catenin is involved in cell adhesion and Wnt (based on the sequence similarity with the *Drosophila* Armadillo protein), which is a component of the wingless signaling pathway. Based on these functions, β-catenin is localized

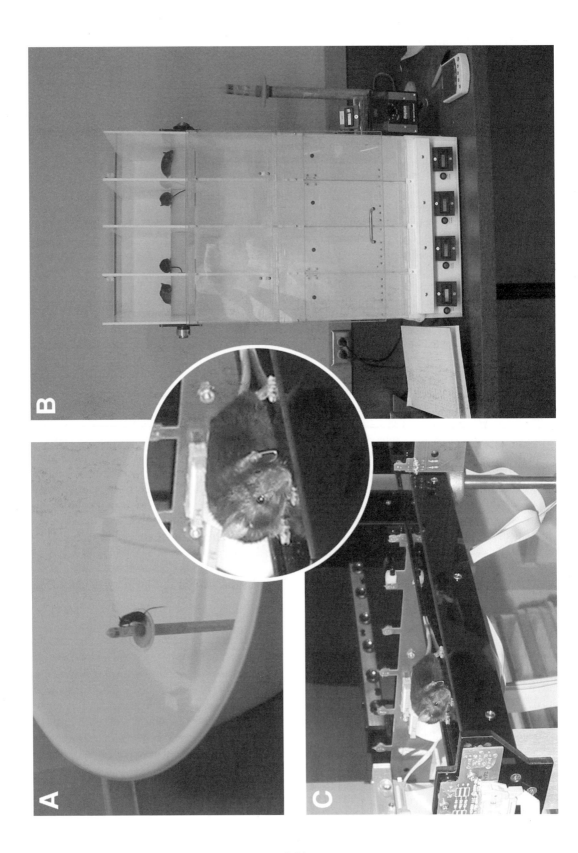

in the cell membrane for regulating cell–cell contacts and in the nucleus and plasma membrane for regulating wnt signaling. In the nucleus, β-catenin forms a complex with the T-cell factor/lyphoid enhancer factor family of transcription factors to stimulate transcriptional activation. In the absence of signaling stabilizing cytoplasmic β-catenin, it gets phosphorylated by glycogen synthase kinase-3β (GSK-3β) and subsequently undergoes proteosomal degradation.

β-Catenin lacks a nuclear localization signal required for nuclear translocation and accessory proteins are required to chaperone β-catenin into the nucleus. Interestingly, agonist, but not antagonist, -bound AR was shown to bind β-catenin *(60)*, suggesting that ARs may chaperone β-catenin. Compared to full-length AR, truncated AR mutants lacking the C-terminal ligand-binding domain showed enhanced nuclear localization of β-catenin in the absence of 5α-DHT, but incomplete nuclear localization in the presence of 5α-DHT. These data indicate that the carboxyl terminus of AR is required for complete β-catenin nuclear co-localization. In neuronal cells, hormone-bound AR co-localized to

----

Fig. 2. *(see facing page)* Behavioral tests to evaluate spatial learning and memory **(A)**, sensorimotor function **(B)**, and anxiety levels **(C)** in mice. **(A)** In the water maze, a pool (diameter 140 cm) is filled with opaque water (24°C), and mice are first trained to locate a visible platform (days 1–3), then a submerged hidden platform (days 4–7) in 2 daily sessions 3.5 hours apart, each consisting of three 60-seconds trials (10-minutes intertrial intervals). Mice that fail to find the hidden platform within 60 seconds are put on it for 15 seconds. For analysis of data, the pool is divided into four quadrants. During the visible platform training, the platform is moved to a different quadrant for each session. During the hidden platform training, the platform location is kept constant for each mouse (in the center of the target quadrant). The starting point, at which the mouse is placed into the water, is changed for each trial. Time to reach the platform (latency), path length, and swim speed are recorded with a video tracking system. Since there were significant differences in average swim speeds between the groups (*tfm* females, 9.6–0.3 cm/second, $n = 12$; *tfm* males, 8.0–0.3 cm/second, $n = 12$, $p < 0.05$ [Tukey-Kramer] during the visible platform sessions, the distance moved to locate the platform (cm) was used as the main measure for analysis. The distance moved values in all trials in which the mice did not find the platform were selected; an average distance moved for these trials was calculated to normalize and used for all trials in which the platform was not located. A 60-seconds probe trial (platform removed) was carried out 1 hour after the last hidden platform session.

(B) The rotorod test is used to screen for motor deficits that might influence performance in learning and memory tests. In this test, the mouse must balance on a rotating rod, which requires a variety of proprioceptive, vestibular, and fine-tuned motor abilities. Untreated, naive mice can remain on the rotating rod for an average of 135–177 seconds during a 180-seconds test. This task has been used successfully to detect significant alterations in motor coordination. Performance can be evaluated in trials of fixed speed; however, a slow acceleration (20 rpm) during the test session limits interindividual variability in performance. The amount of time the mouse remains on the rod is recorded automatically. The *tfm* female and male mice improved their rotorod performance with training ($p < 0.01$), but there was no group difference in their performance.

(C) Anxiety levels can be assessed with an elevated, plus-shaped maze consisting of two open arms and two closed arms, equipped with rows of infrared photocells interfaced with a computer. Rodents avoid the elevated open arms of the plus maze, so decreases in time spent in and entries into the open arms reflect enhanced anxiety. Mice are placed individually in the center of the maze and allowed free access for 10 minutes. They can spend their time either in a closed safe area (closed arms) or in an open area (open arms). Recorded beam brakes are used to calculate the time spent in the open arms, the distance moved in the open arms, and the number of times the mice extend over the edges of the open arms. Reductions in these variables indicate increased anxiety.

The *tfm* female and male traveled similar distances (*tfm* females, 172–37 cm, $n = 11$; *tfm* males, 122–29 cm, $n = 13$), spent similar amounts of time (*tfm* females, 29–6 seconds, $n = 11$; *tfm* males: 22–4 seconds, $n = 13$); rested similar amounts of time (*tfm* females, 13–2 seconds, $n = 11$; *tfm* males, 9–2 seconds, $n = 13$), and extended similar numbers of times over the edges (*tfm* females, 5.2–0.9 times, $n = 11$; *tfm* males: 4.1–0.8 times, $n = 13$) of the anxiety-provoking open arms of the plus maze.

These data show that there are no differences in anxiety levels in *tfm* female and male mice.

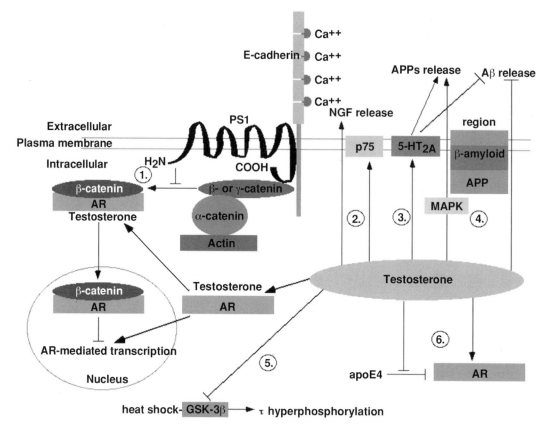

Fig. 3. Potential pathways mediating the neuroprotective effects of testosterone in aging and AD.

the nucleus with β-catenin repressed its transcriptional activity. Conversely, β-catenin repressed AR stimulation of ARE-mediated transcriptional activation. In contrast to the neuronal cells, β-catenin binds and co-activates Ars in AR-positive prostate cancer cells.

Nuclear receptors other than ARs also interact with β-catenin. ERs also modulate the activity of β-catenin, but not as ARs by interacting with it but by interacting with the T-cell factor/lymphoid enhancer factor family of transcription factors. Depending on the factors present, ER transcriptional activity is either enhanced or repressed.

In addition to nuclear factors, the transmembrane protein presenilin-1 (PS1) is also associated with β-catenin *(63,64)*. Importantly, PS1 mutations are responsible for most cases of early-onset autosomal dominant familial AD. PS1 was shown to reduce the stability and transcriptional activity of β-catenin, while PS1 containing familial AD mutations were less able to do so. Consistent with these data, lack of PS1 expression was associated with increased stability of cytosolic β-catenin. However, other studies reported that PS1 increased the stability of β-catenin. As β-catenin antagonizes the actions of ARs in the nucleus, PS1 might reduce AR function and in this way contribute to AD. Thus, the balance between AR and β-catenin may be important under both physiological and pathological conditions.

Nerve Growth Factor Neurotransmission

Impaired nerve growth factor (NGF) signaling has been proposed as mechanism contributing to AD. Testosterone might improve NGF signaling, as it increases the release of the trophic NGF and upregulates the p75 NGF receptor in brain areas relevant for cognition, including the hippocampus.

Testosterone and Serotonin

Altered serotonin 5-HT$_{2A}$ receptor signaling might be pertinent to amyloid-beta (Aβ) plaque formation, as activation of 5-HT$_{2A}$ receptors increases APP (amyloid precursor protein) and reduces Aβ formation in brain slices and cultured cells *(65)*.

The age-related decline in free plasma testosterone might be associated with changes in mood and contribute to some of the noncognitive behavioral alterations in AD. Some studies suggest that testosterone replacement therapy improves mood in hypogonadal men *(66)* and surgically menopausal women *(67)*. However, additional (placebo-controlled) studies are required to determine the potential association of testosterone with mood.

Altered serotonin signaling might contribute to this potential association *(68)*. Testosterone and estrogen, but not DHT, increase the transcription of the 5-HT$_{2A}$ receptor and serotonin transporter in the forebrain *(69)*. The lack of an effect of DHT and of testosterone on the transcription of the 5-HT$_{2A}$ receptor and serotonin transporter in the caudate putamen, a brain area that has little aromatase activity, indicates that conversion of testosterone to estrogen is required for these effects.

Testosterone, APP, and Aβ Peptides

The deposition of senile plaques made of Abeta, dystrophic neuritis, reactive glial cells, and neurofibrillary tangles made of bundles of abnormal paired-helical filaments mainly containing hyperphosphorylated tau, are hallmarks of AD. Cleavage of APP by α-secretase results in formation of the nonamyloidogenic soluble (s) α-APP (sAPPα). Cleavage of APP by β-secretase results in the formation of soluble β APP (sAPPβ). Subsequent cleavage by γ-secretase following β cleavage results in the formation of the insoluble amyloidogenic Aβ. A single or repeated dose of testosterone increases the neurotrophic sAPP secretion, mostly containing sAPPα—through a mechanism involving mitogen-activated protein kinase (MAP kinase) pathway *(70)*. The AR blockers flutamide and cypterone acetate fail to determine conclusively whether ARs are required for the effect of testosterone on sAPP secretion, which might relate to the fact that flutamide fails to block or even mimic some nongenomic effects of ARs *(71,72)*. Aromatase inhibition suppresses the effect of testosterone on sAPP secretion, indicating that at least part of the effect is mediated by conversion of testosterone to estrogen, which also increases sAPPα secretion through a mechanism involving MAP kinase. In addition to increasing the release of sAPPα, testosterone may be neuroprotective by reducing the secretion of Aβ peptides and Aβ-induced toxicity in hippocampal neurons *(73,74)*.

Testosterone and Tau Phosphorylation

The tau gene encodes multiple phosphorylated and thermostable proteins by alternative splicing. The dephosphorylation-hyperphosphorylation leading to paired helical filament tau are unknown but are suggested to represent a defense against stressors. For example, heat shock induces hyperphosphorylation of tau, which involves glycogen synthase kinase-3β (GSK-3β). Testosterone, but not 17β-estradiol, inhibits heat shock-induced hyperphosphorylation of tau by preventing overactivation of GSK-3β *(75)*. Interestingly, GSK-3β is a pro-apoptotic kinase, which inhibits the protective effects of the heat-shock response. Thus, testosterone might be neuroprotective by inhibiting the phosphorylation of tau.

AR and ApoE4

Apolipoprotein E (ApoE) plays an important role in the metabolism and redistribution of lipoproteins and cholesterol. Distinct alleles (ε2, ε3, and ε4) encode human ApoE isoforms. In the brain, ApoE has been implicated in development, regeneration, neurite outgrowth, and neuroprotection *(76)*. Compared with ApoE2 and ApoE3, ApoE4 increases the risk of AD. About 60% of AD patients carry at least one ApoE ε4-allele *(77)*. ApoE4 interacts with female gender, further increasing AD risk and decreasing treatment response.

Female mice are also more susceptible to ApoE4-induced impairments of spatial learning and memory than male mice. Using mice deficient in mouse ApoE (Apoe$^{-/-}$) and expressing human ApoE4 or ApoE3 in the brain at comparable levels, we showed that ApoE4 expression in female and male mice reduced cytosolic AR levels in the neocortex. Androgens and AR-dependent pathways protected against detrimental effects of ApoE4 on learning and memory in female mice, consistent with the positive regulation of ARs by androgens in wild-type brains *(78,79)*.

Improved memory in androgen-treated female ApoE4 mice was associated with increased cytosolic AR levels, suggesting that ApoE4 contributes to cognitive decline by reducing AR levels in the brain and that stimulating AR-dependent pathways can reverse ApoE4-induced cognitive deficits. Male ApoE4 mice might be less susceptible to ApoE4-induced AR reductions because of their higher circulating levels of endogenous androgens. The data indicate that testosterone might be neuroprotective by inhibiting the detrimental effects of ApoE4 on cytosolic AR levels.

ARs and ApoE4 might also be involved in the alterations in the cholinergic basal forebrain in aging and AD *(80)*. The major cholinergic nuclei of the basal forebrain, the vertical limb of the diagonal band of Broca and the nucleus basalis of Meynert, are affected in AD. Interestingly, the intensity of cytoplasmic AR staining in these nuclei is lower in older AD and control subjects (over 56 years of age) than in younger subjects (20–39 years of age). In addition, the proportion of neurons with cytoplasmic AR expression is lower in control aged men than control aged women and lower in AD women than control women, but not lower in AD men than control men. In women, but not in men, the presence of AD and the presence of an ApoE4-allele is negatively correlated with the percentage of AR-positive neurons in the diagonal band of Broca. In women, not in men, the presence of AD, but not the presence of an ApoE4-allele, is negatively correlated with the percentage of AR-positive neurons in the nucleus basalis of Meynert. These data indicate that there might be complex associations of ARs, gender, and ApoE4 in the cholinergic basal forebrain. Testosterone treatment might be neuroprotective by increasing cytoplasmic AR levels in this brain region.

SUMMARY

About 50% of people over 85 years of age show cognitive deficits. Reduced androgen levels and AR-mediated signaling may contribute to these deficits in the elderly and AD patients. Increasing evidence suggests that testosterone might enhance aspects of cognitive function and antagonize the detrimental effects of the AD-related factors Aβ, hyperphosphorylated tau, PS1, and ApoE4. The potential beneficial effects of testosterone may be mediated by ARs and/or ERs. Increased research efforts are needed to determine which receptors mediate these effects and to develop SARMs lacking the increased risk of developing cancer. Our next challenge will be to test the efficacy and determine the exact modes of action of androgens and SARMs in related tissue culture and animal models and ultimately in humans.

REFERENCES

1. Tan, R.S. et al.: The andropause and memory loss: is there a link between androgen decline and dementia in the aging male? Asian J Androl 2001; 3: 169–174.
2. Shealy, C.N. et al.: A review of dehydroepiandrosterone (DHEA). Integr Physiol Behav Sci 1995; 30: 308–313.
3. Vermeulen, A. et al.: Testosterone, body composition and aging. J Endocrinol Invest 1999; 22: 110–116.
4. LeBlanc, E.S. et al.: Hormone replacement therapy and cognition: systematic review and meta-analysis. JAMA 2001285: 1489–1499.
5. Janowsky, J. et al.: Sex steroids modify working memory. J Cogn Neurosci (2000; 12: 407–414.
6. Beatty, W.W.: Gonadal hormones and sex differences in nonreproductive behaviors in rodents: organizational and activational influences. Horm Behav 1979; 12: 112–163.
7. Joseph, R. et al.: Effects of hormone manipulations and exploration on sex differences in maze learning. Behav Biol 1978; 24: 364–377.
8. Falkenstein, E. et al.: Multiple actions of steroid hormones—a focus on rapid, nongenomic effects. Pharmacol Rev 2000; 52: 513–555.

9. Frye, C.A. et al.: Behavioral effects of 3 alpha-androstanediol. II: Hypothalamic and preoptic area actions via a GABAergic mechanism. Behav Brain Res 1996; 79: 119–130.

10. Lambert, J.J. et al.: Neurosteroids and GABAA receptor function. Trends Pharmacol Sci 1995; 16: 295–303.

11. Kousteni, S. et al.: Nongenotropic, sex-nonspecific signaling through the estrogen or androgen receptors: dissociation from transcriptional activity. Cell 2001; 104: 719–730.

12. Beyer, C. et al.: Androgens influence sex differentiation of developing hypothalamic aromatase neurons in vitro. Endocrinology 1994; 135: 1220–1226.

13. Beyer, C. et al.: Androgens stimulate the morphological maturation of embryonic hypothalamic aromatase-immunoreactive neurons in the mouse. Brain Res 1997; 98: 74–81.

14. Lustig, R.H. et al.: An in vitro model for the effects of androgen on neurons employing androgen receptor-transfected PC12 cells. Mol Cell Neurosci 1994; 5: 587–596.

15. Keast, J.R. et al.: Testosterone has potent, selective effects on the morphology of pelvic autonomic neurons, which control the bladder, lower bowel and internal reproductive organs of the male rat. Neuroscience 1998; 85: 543–556.

16. Matsumoto, A. et al.: Hormonally induced neuronal plasticity in the adult motorneurons. Brain Res Bull 1997; 44: 539–547.

17. Hawkins, T. et al.: The effect of neonatal sex hormone manipulation on the incidence of diabetes in nonobese diabetic mice. Proc Soc Exp Biol Med (1993); 202: 201–205.

18. Green, P.S. et al.: Neuroprotective effects of estrogens: potential mechanisms of action. Int J Dev Neurosci 2000; 18: 347–358.

19. Henderson, V.W. et al.: Estrogen for Alzheimer's disease in women. Randomized, double-blind, placebo-controlled trial. Neurology 2000; 54: 295–301.

20. Yaffe, K. et al.: Estrogen use, ApoE, and cognitive decline: evidence of gene-environment interaction. Neurology 2000; 54: 1949–1954.

21. Barrett-Connor, E. et al.: Cognitive function and endogenous sex hormones in older women. J Am Geriatr Soc 1999; 47: 1289–1293.

22. Sherwin, B.B.: Estrogen and/or androgen replacement therapy and cognitive functioning in surgically menopausal women. Psychoneuroendocrinonology 1988; 13: 345–357.

23. Simental, J.A. et al.: Domain functions of the androgen receptor. J Steroid Biochem Mol Biol 1992; 43: 37–41.

24. Quigley, C.A. et al.: Androgen receptor defects: historical, clinical, and molecular perspectives. Endocr Rev 1995; 16: 271–321.

25. Brinkmann., A.O. et al.: Androgen receptor mutations. J Steroid Biochem Mol Biol 1995; 53: 443–448.

26. Nucifora, F.C. et al.: Interference by huntingtin and atrophin-1 with CBP-mediated transcription leading to cellular toxicity. Science 2001; 291: 2423–2428.

27. Robyr, D. et al.: Nuclear hormone receptor coregulators in action: diversity for shared tasks. Mol Endocrinol 2000; 14: 329–347.

28. McKenna, N.J. et al.: Nuclear receptor coregulators: cellular and molecular biology. Endocr Rev 1999; 20: 321–344.

29. Umesono, K. et al.: Determinants of target gene specificity for steroid/thyroid hormone receptors. Cell 1989; 57: 1139–1146.

30. Ueda, T. et al.: Ligand-independent activation of the androgen receptor by interleukin 6 and the role of steroid receptor coactivator-1 in prostate cancer cells. J Biol Chem 2002; 277: 38078–38094.

31. Roof, R.L. et al.: Testosterone improves maze performance and induces development of a male hippocampus in females. Brain Res 1992; 572: 310–313.

32. Berger-Sweeney, J. et al.: Sex difference in learning and memory in mice: effects of sequence of testing and cholinergic blockade. Behav Neurosci 1995; 109: 859–873.

33. Reinisch, J.M. et al.: Hormonal contributions to sexually dimorphic behavioral development in humans. Psychoneuroendocrinology 1991; 16: 213–278.

34. van Haaren, F. et al.: Behavioral differences between male and female rats: effects of gonadal hormones on learning and memory. Neurosci Biobehav Rev 1990; 14: 23–33.

35. McNemar, Q. et al.: Sex difference in rats on three learning tasks. J Comp Psychol 1932; 14: 171–180.

36. Bucci, D.J. et al.: Spatial learning in male and female Long-Evans rats. Behav Neurosci 1995; 109: 180–183.

37. Einon, D. et al.: Spatial memory and response strategies in rats: age, sex, and rearing differences in performance. J Exp Psychol 1980; 32: 473–489.

38. Joseph, R. et al.: Gender and early environmental influences on activity, overresponsiveness, and exploration. Dev Psychol 1980; 13: 527–544.

39. Luine, V.N. et al.: Sex-dependent differences in estrogen regulation of choline acetyltransferase are altered by neonatal treatments. Endocrinology 1986; 119: 527–544.

40. McEwen, B.S. et al.: Action of sex hormones on the brain: organization and activation in relation to functional teratology. Prog Brain Res 1988; 73: 121–134.

41. Means, L.W. et al.: The effects of number of trials per day, retention interval, gender and time of day on acquisition of a two-choice, win-stay, water-escape working memory task in the rat. J Neurosci Meth 1991; 39: 77–87.

42. Roof, R.L. et al.: Gender-specific impairment on Morris water maze task after entorhinal cortex lesion. Behav Brain Res 1993; 57: 47–51.

43. Frye, C.A.: Estrus-associated decrements in a water maze task are limited to acquisition. Physiol Behav 1994; 57: 5–14.

44. Kolb, B. et al.: Sex-related differences in cortical function after medial frontal lesions in rats. Behav Neurosci 1996; 110: 1271–1281.

45. Hürtnagl, H. et al.: Sex differences and estrous cycle-variations in the Af64A-induced cholinergic deficit in the rat hippocampus. Brain Res Bull 1993; 31: 129–134.

46. Olton, D.S. et al.: Spatial correlates of hippocampal unit activity. Exp Neurol 1978; 58: 387–409.

47. Kesner, R.P. et al.: Memory for spatial locations, motor responses, and objects: triple dissociation among the hippocampus, caudate nucleus, and extrastriate visual cortex. Exp Brain Res 1993; 93: 462–470.

48. McEwen, B.S. et al.: Ovarian steroids and the brain: Implications for cognition and aging. Neurology 1997; 48: S8–S15.

49. Woolley, C.S. et al.: Naturally occurring fluctuation in dendritic spine density on adult hippocampal pyramidal neurons. J Neurosci 1990; 10: 4035–4039.

50. Gibbs, R.B. et al.: Expression of estrogen receptor-like immunoreactivity by different subgroups of basal forebrain cholinergic neurons in gonadectomized male and female rats. Brain Res 1996; 720: 61–68.

51. Berry, B. et al.: Spatial learning and memory at defined points of the estrous cycle: effects on performance of a hippocampal-dependent task. Behav Neurosci 1997; 111: 267–274.

52. Marriott, L.K. et al.: Long-term estrogen therapy worsens the behavioral and neuropathological consequences of chronic brain inflammation. Behav Neurosci 2002; 116: 902–911.

53. MacLusky, N.J. et al.: Estrogen formation in the mammalian brain: possible role of aromatase in sexual differentiation of the hippocampus and neocortex. Steroids 1987; 50: 4–6.

54. O'Keefe, J.A. et al.: Estrogen receptor mRNA alterations in the developing rat hippocampus. Mol Brain Res 1995; 30: 115–124.

55. Janowsky, J.S. et al.: Testosterone influences spatial cognition in older men. Behav Neurosci 1994; 108: 325–332.

56. Tabibnia, G. et al.: Sex difference and laterality in the volume of mouse dentate gyrus granule cell layer. Brain Res 1999; 827: 41–45.

57. Couse, J.F. et al.: Exploring the role of sex steroids through studies of receptor deficient mice. J Mol Med 1998; 76: 497–511.

58. Ahlbom, E. et al.: Androgen treatment of neonatal rats decreases susceptibility of cerebellar granule neurons to oxidative stress in vitro. Eur J Neurosci 1999; 11: 1285–1291.

59. Ahlbom, E. et al.: Testosterone protects cerebellar granule cells from oxidative stress-induced cell death through a receptor mediated mechanism. Brain Res 2001; 892: 255–262.

60. Pawlowski, J.E. et al.: Liganded androgen receptor interaction with β-catenin. J Biol Chem 2002; 277: 20702–20710.

61. Yang, F. et al.: Linking beta-catenin to androgen-signaling pathway. J Biol Chem 2002; 277: 11336–11344.

62. Sharma, M. et al.: Phosphatidylinositol 3-kinase/Akt stimulates androgen pathway through GSK3beta and nuclear beta-catenin accumulation. J Biol Chem 2002; 277: 30935–30941.

63. Georgakopoulos, A. et al.: Presenilin-1 is a regulatory component of the cadherin cell adhesion complex: implications for Alzheimer's disease. In: Iqbal, K.; Sisodia, S.S.; Winblad, B. (eds.): Alzheimer's disease: advances in etiology, pathogenesis and therapeutics. Wiley, New York, 2001: 521–530.

64. Soriano, S. et al.: Functional consequences of the association of PS-1 with b-catenin. In: Iqbal, K.; Sisodia, S.S.; Winblad, B. (eds.): Alzheimer's disease: advances in etiology, pathogenesis and therapeutics. Wiley, New York, 2001: 531–540.

65. Nitsch, R.M. et al.: Serotonin 5-HT$_{2A}$ and 5HT$_{2C}$ receptors stimulate amyloid precursor protein ectodomain secretion. J Biol Chem 1996; 271: 4188–4194.

66. Wang, C.: Testosterone replacement therapy improves mood in hypogonadal men—a clinical research center study. J Clin Endocrinol Metab 1996; 81: 3578–3583.

67. Sherwin, B.B. et al.: Differential symptom response to parental estrogen and/or androgen administration in the surgical menopause. Am J Obstet Gynecol 1985; 151: 153–160.

68. Fink, G. et al.: Androgens action on central serotonin neurotransmission: relevance for mood, mental state and memory. Behav Brain Res 1999; 105: 53–68.

69. Sumner, B. et al.: Testosterone as well as estrogen increases serotonin$_{1A}$ receptor mRNA and binding site densities in the male rat brain. Mol Brain Res 1998; 59: 205–214.

70. Goodenough, S. et al.: Testosterone stimulates rapid secretory amyloid precursor protein release from rat hypothalamic cells via the activation of the mitogen-activated protein kinase pathway. Neurosci Lett 2000; 296: 49–52.

71. Evangelou, A. et al.: Down regulation of transforming growth factor beta receptors by androgen in ovarian cancer cells. Cancer Res 2000; 60: 929–935.

72. Peterziel, H. et al.: Rapid signaling by androgen receptor in prostate cancer cells. Oncogene 1999; 18: 6322–6329.

73. Gouras, G.K. et al.: Testosterone reduces neuronal secretion of Alzheimer's b-amyloid peptides. Proc Natl Acad Sci USA 2000; 97: 1202–1205.

74. Pike, C.J. et al.: Testosterone attenuates β-amyloid toxicity in cultured hippocampal neurons. Brain Res 2001; 919: 160–165.
75. Papasozomenos, S.C. et al.: Testosterone prevents the heat shock-induced overactivation of glycogen synthase kinase-3b but not of cyclin-dependent kinase 5 and c-Jun NH$_2$-terminal kinase and concomitantly abolishes hyperphosphorylation of tau: implications for Alzheimer's disease. Proc Natl Acad Sci USA 2002; 99: 1140–1145.
76. Weisgraber, K.H. et al.: Human apolipoprotein E: the Alzheimer's disease connection. FASEB J 1996; 10: 1485–1494.
77. Farrer, L.A. et al.: Effects of age, sex, and ethnicity on the association between apolipoprotein E genotype and Alzheimer disease. A meta-analysis. ApoE and Alzheimer Disease Meta Analysis Consortium. JAMA 1997; 278: 1349–1356.
78. Lu, S.F. et al.: Androgen receptor in mouse brain: sex differences and similarities in autoregulation. Endrocrinology 1998; 139: 1594–1601.
79. Lu, S. et al.: Neural androgen receptor regulation: effects of androgen and antiandrogen. J Neurobiol 1999; 41: 505–512.
80. Ishunina, T.A. et al.: Sex differences in androgen receptor immunoreactivity in basal forebrain nuclei of elderly and Alzheimer patients. Exp Neurol 2002; 176: 122–132.

31

Role of Nutrition in Prevention or Delay of Alzheimer's Disease

Hannes B. Staehelin

INTRODUCTION

Dementia, the major health challenge of the twenty-first century, is the result of a sum of complex genetic and environmental interactions. Among these factors, nutrition plays an important role. This chapter explores to what extent healthy nutrition may prevent or delay the onset of Alzheimer's disease (AD) and related dementias, and how to advise caregivers and patients suffering from AD or other forms of dementia with regard to eating and nutrition.

AD prevalence and incidence studies consistently depict a single exponential increase with age (1). These findings indicate that a large number of factors contribute to the development of the disease. Its late onset is consistent with the theory that genetic controls diminish with advancing age and the impact of external factors becomes more prominent (2,3). Among these factors, nutrition is intimately linked to aging. Indeed, the word *old* (German: *alt*) is derived from the Latin verb *alere*—to nourish, to bring up—and the Latin word *altus* means tall, well grown, well nourished. However, the rather similar prevalence and incidence over a large spectrum of different dietary habits and social settings in different societies—at least in the industrialized world—suggest that diet and nutritional habits may have only a small effect on the manifestation of the disease. It also supports the notion of a rather unspecific response of the aging brain to the accumulating stress load of endogenous origins, such as free radicals generated during mitochondrial energy production and by exogenous factors (4).

The elucidation of the mechanism leading to the hallmarks of AD—the loss of synapses, the formation of amyloid plaques and fibrillary tangles—should yield valuable hypotheses as to how nutrients, life-style factors, or drugs might modify this otherwise largely intrinsic process linked to aging (5).

Key messages: Understanding AD and related disorders yields cues how to prevent these disorders in old age. The usual diet has a long lasting but low impact on brain aging, hence prevention should be life long.

PATHOPHYSIOLOGICAL BASIS OF NUTRIENT–DISEASE INTERACTION

AD is considered to be a proteinopathy with amyloid-beta-42 ($A\beta_{42}$) as a key factor leading to neurodegeneration, particularly in areas important for memory formation as well as memory processing and thus brain plasticity (5,6). Hence mechanisms of brain plasticity may give clues how, over time, neuronal dysfunction impairs the acquisition of new information, the key symptom of AD. Several lines of evidence point to oxidative stress as one of the primary steps leading to neurodegeneration. Brain metabolism requires a high and constant energy supply by mitochondria, leading to a constant load of free radical formation. This suggests that a high antioxidant intake by nutrients in food and beverages might be protective. Insulin seems to improve energy supply to the brain and enhance brain function.

From: *Current Clinical Neurology,*
Alzheimer's Disease: A Physician's Guide to Practical Management
Edited by: R. W. Richter and B. Zoeller Richter © Humana Press Inc., Totowa, NJ

High glucose levels and hyperinsulinemia indicate insulin resistance and the formation of advanced glycation end products (AGE) that contribute by itself to radical formation with detrimental consequences to nerve cells and blood vessels. Thus obesity is a risk factor. Caloric restriction, on the other hand, stimulates the formation of brain-derived neural growth factor and enhances brain plasticity (7–9)—phylogenetically sensible because the search for food requires adaptive cognitive functions.

The formation of Aβ from amyloid precursor protein (APP) is also to some extent influenced by nutrients. APP is processed by proteases leading to fragments that support neuronal sprouting if processed by α-secretase or amyloid formation if processed by β-secretase (BACE). Aβ fragments were shown to impair neuronal function. A recent fascinating finding showed that the membrane cholesterol content, which is dependent on the cholesterol ester content of the cell, modulates the activation of α-secretase (if cholesterol is low) or β-secretase (if cholesterol is high). In the central nervous system (CNS), apolipoprotein E (ApoE) appears to be a major cholesterol carrier. The affinity of the different ApoE alleles—e2, e4—determine among other factors the cholesterol content in the brain. Thus, genetically determined factors of lipid metabolism interact with life style and nutrition as well as brain amyloid formation (10,11).

Not only is cholesterol of importance, the highly unsaturated long-chain fatty acids, such as arachidonic acid, eicosapentaenoic acid (EPA), and docosahexaenoic acid (DHA), modulate membrane fluidity and lipid metabolism. They are also precursors for cytokines, thus modulating the immune system. The inflammatory response of the microglia is thought to enhance the development and progression of AD.

The complex signaling system is disrupted in neurodegenerative disorders. Thus AD is characterized by a deficiency of acetylcholine and (to a lesser extent) of serotonin or noradrenaline (12). Another well-known example is the dopamine deficiency in Parkinson's disease. Thus, substances such as micronutrients, B vitamins, or phytochemicals with hormonal actions such as are found in soy proteins, and those substances that interfere with the synthesis, release, and degradation of these neurotransmitters may modulate onset and manifestation of the disease.

In summary, multiple factors related to nutrition as well as essential and nonessential food components including a growing list of bioactive secondary plant components over a long period of time may modify neuronal function and regeneration in a subtle but important way, either directly or by slowing or accelerating cerebrovascular disease.

Key messages: Antioxidants may diminish oxidative stress. Fatty acids affect intracellular and extracellular signalling by cytokines. Cholesterol influences the Aβ formation related to AD.

NUTRIENTS AS PROTECTIVE FACTORS AND AS RISK FACTORS

Longitudinal studies assessing the development of dementia with reliable dietary data are rare. Most studies focus on cardiovascular disease or cancer, or target younger age groups. Cognitive function is assessed only in subsequent follow-ups limited by diagnostic problems and selection bias. The analysis of differences observed in comparing prevalence or incidence findings in different regions of the world has to be seen also in the light of substitute morbidity or mortality, and classifying systems. Cerebrovascular pathology, for example, is much more common in Japan compared to the United States or Europe. This epidemiological finding suggests that Western diet favors atherosclerosis of the large arteries, with the development of coronary heart disease, ischemic stroke, and colon cancer, whereas the traditional salty fish diet (w-3-rich, low-fat) favors hypertension and brain hemorrhage as well as stomach cancer.

Hypocaloric nutrition with adequate micronutrient supply slows the aging process by affecting a vast array of gene expressions (13). The other extreme, overfeeding leading to overweight, type 2 diabetes mellitus, and the production of AGE products, clearly triggers and maintains atherogenic and neurotoxic mechanisms (14).

To answer the question of whether a change in body weight has an impact on cognition, an analysis of the "Basel Study on the Elderly" (BASEL) was undertaken. It revealed that constant body weight over a 10-year period in healthy subjects was associated with a significantly lower risk for memory impairment than weight change (either gain or loss). This was independent of the body mass index (BMI), casting doubt on a rigid enforcement of public health measures without taking into consideration the individual risk.

Weight loss is a sign of neurodegeneration. Balance studies could not link it to an altered energy metabolism. In the light of the observation that carriers of ApoE4-allele respond more strongly to weight change with alteration in cognition suggests that neurodegeneration is the common underlying process leading to cognitive decline and loss of weight control *(15)*.

Key messages: Weight loss, weight gain, and obesity appear to be associated with poorer cognitive function in old age. Stable bodyweight is desirable. Prevalent cardiovascular risk factors have to be treated.

MICRONUTRIENTS

Micronutrients (Table 1) are essential for growth and function. Their metabolic effects were elucidated during the last century by investigating nutritional deficiency states. In this context, iodine deficiency leading to goiter and cretinism, but also other vitamins, were recognized as affecting brain function. Subsequently, regulatory agencies set the recommended daily intake at a level to prevent signs and symptoms related to this deficiency. There is evidence that higher iodine intake might be beneficial.

Another, more recent case in point is the intake of folic acid, vitamin B6, and vitamin B12. Low intake—particularly of folate—is associated with a higher homocysteine plasma level. A high homocysteine level is a well-established risk factor for atherosclerosis and probably has neurotoxic potential. High homocysteine appears to be associated with dementia, particular AD *(16–18)*. Probably as important is the DNA-stabilizing effect of folic acid by supporting methylation processes. Determined in part by genetically regulated enzymes and by micronutrients involved in the methyl–carbon cycle, especially folic acid, B12, and B6, is an important example of gene nutrient interaction with far reaching consequences. By eating meals including ample fruits and vegetables, but also sufficient protein from meat and fish, an adequate intake of these substances can best be achieved. Micronutrients, the antioxidants in nutrition, particularly vitamins C and E, but also the carotenoids, such as lycopene, show strong correlation between intake, plasma level, and cognitive function in epidemiological studies *(19–21)*.

Key messages: Regular intake of fruits and vegetables (several times a day) is an excellent source of micronutrients with protective properties. In the elderly nutritional supplements serve as a valuable alternative. Regular meat intake (albeit in small quantities) and fish consumption is important and beneficial.

TOXIC EFFECTS OF NUTRIENTS

One of the hallmarks of AD is the trapping of heavy metals in amyloid deposits. Thus the intake of aluminum or a high intake of iron, and exposure to mercury in the environment (amalgam in teeth fillings are of minor importance) is inculpated by some as a cause of AD *(22,23)*. However, these metals, albeit neurotoxic, may enhance the neurotoxic effects of Aβ deposits and support the generation of free oxygen radicals. Nevertheless, it seems to be prudent to avoid excessive red meat intake and an unnecessary exposure to high amounts of aluminum in drinking water.

Key messages: The exposure to toxic metals, e.g., aluminum, mercury, in food and drinking water and other environmental hazards should be kept at a minimum.

Table 1
Suggested Intake of Micronutrients for Institutionalized or Community-Living Elderly People

Micronutrient	DRI[a] for age > 70 (mg/d)[a] Females	Males	Upper Safe Limit (mg/d)
Vitamin A	0.7	0.9	3
Vitamin D3	0.015	0.015	0.05
Vitamin E	10	15	1000[b]
Vitamin B1	0.6	1.1	—
Vitamin B2	0.7	1.3	—
Biotin	0.03	0.03	—
Panthothenic acid	5	5	—
Niacin	14	16	35
Vitamin B6	1.5	1.7	100
Folic acid	0.4	0.4	1
Vitamin B12	0.0024	0.0024	—
Vitamin C	75	90	2000
Choline	425	550	3500
Vitamin K (menadione)	0.09	0.12	
Zinc (Zn)	8	11	40
Copper (Cu)	0.9	0.9	10
Fluorine (F)	3	4	10
Manganese (Mn)	1.8	2.3	11
Chromium (Cr)	0.02	0.03	—
Molybdenum (Mo)	0.045	0.045	2
Selenium (Se)	0.055	0.055	0.400
Iodine (I)	0.15	0.15	1.1
Iron (Fe)	8	8	45
Calcium (Ca)	1200[c]	1200[c]	2500
Phosphorus (P)	700	700	3000
Magnesium (Mg)	320	420	—
Potassium (K)	2000	2000	Estimated minimum requirement
Sodium (Na)	500	500	Estimated minimum requirement
Chlorine (Cl)	750	750	Estimated minimum requirement

[a]DRI, daily recommended intake.
[b]Intake of high amounts of antioxidants may be safe but is not yet proven to be effective.
[c]Calcium intake of 500 mg is the estimated minimum requirement to ensure optimal action of vitamin D.

NUTRITION IN SECONDARY PREVENTION OF AD

Even if a clear distinction between primary and secondary prevention is not possible (since the onset of AD takes place long before its clinical manifestation), we speak here about secondary prevention, starting with the period when first signs of cognitive impairment are noticed by the patient or his or her entourage.

The close link of cardiovascular risk factors to AD, particularly in ApoE4 carriers, makes it advisable that these risk factors should be treated medically and by diet. The question of whether high doses of antioxidants, which may be ingested by numbers of elderly people, will prevent or reverse Alzheimer changes in the brain remains controversial. The results of a rather recent study with vitamin E point to a pharmacological action of very high amounts of α-tocopherol, probably inducing choline acetyl transferase (ChAT) and boosting the synthesis of acetylcholine or having a beneficial effect on microcirculation *(24)*. The results of the hypertension trial on dementia point toward a beneficial effect of blood pressure lowering by diet *(25)*. Physical exercise—sufficient but not exhaustive—is an important adjunct measure to diet *(26)*.

Key message: Vigorous treatment of cardiovascular risk factors is important.

SUPPLEMENTS: YES OR NO?

In general, we observe a decrease in body weight with old age. One aspect of this phenomenon is related to aging per se. Thus the threshold for taste and smell increases, the kinetics of the stomach change, it becomes less compliant, and the feeling of a full stomach is felt earlier than before, thus leading to a secretion of CCK (cholecystokinin) and the sensation of (early) satiety.

There are good arguments for the recommendation of nutritional supplements for the elderly population. Diminished energy requirements as well as changes in body perception of thirst and hunger can easily lead to a situation of slight to substantial malnutrition. The intake of supplements may be an easy way to secure adequate micronutrient supply. In the case of folic acid and vitamin B12, but also of ubiquinone, there are even good arguments for amounts higher than are recommended for daily intake to lower elevated homocysteine levels or to slow down the neurodegenerative process as in the case of Parkinson's disease and ubiquinone *(27–30)*.

Key messages: Supplements of micronutrients are recommended. There is no evidence of the effectiveness of high dosages of antioxidants in the prevention of neurodegenerative diseases.

WEIGHT LOSS IN ALZHEIMER'S DISEASE

Patients suffering from AD tend to lose weight. Whether maintaining body weight slows progression of cognitive decline is still controversial *(31–33)*. There is no question, however, that malnutrition is an important co-morbidity factor. By preventing malnutrition during the early stages of AD, general health and thus mental function may be better preserved. An adequate diet sufficient in energy, essential macronutrients, and micronutrients is strongly advised.

Some AD patients develop preferences for certain foods, e.g., sugar craving. It was shown that glucose—probably via insulin actions—enhances brain function. Thus it may be advisable not to fight these desires but channel it instead toward eating, e.g., chocolate or other food with additional nutritional benefits.

A major challenge for caregivers and family members as well as fellow patients are poor eating habits. If a patient feels uncomfortably stressed, he or she becomes even more handicapped. It is therefore important to provide an appropriate setting for dining. If a demented person tends to get up and wander around, it becomes difficult to dine out. Thus isolation and loneliness of the caregiver might increase. Simple arrangements may do the trick and allow better socializing, such as sitting the patient on a bench behind the table, where it becomes more difficult to get up and stroll to other tables bothering other people. Patients experiencing difficulties using cutlery may be offered finger food. This could ensure a pleasurable experience of eating, while requiring less assistance during the meals. It is principally important for the AD patient to prepare and provide the various foods in manageable pieces.

Key messages: Provide a quiet environment and limit distractions for meal times. Provide only small amounts and one food at a time in advanced disease states. Provide high calorie nutrient dense food. Good company stimulates appetite the best.

NUTRITIONAL GUIDELINES FOR DEMENTED PATIENTS

The diminished perception of thirst and hunger with advancing age even in healthy old people makes it important that eating and drinking habits are fixed by habits and stimulated by company. Demented patients need additional special care to maintain an adequate diet. The risk of malnutrition is high in patients with early dementia who are living alone. Caloric intake should be calculated in order to maintain body weight. Energy expenditure varies along with physical activity; patients who wander a lot require more than sedentary subjects. Supplements with micronutrients are advisable, since it may be difficult always to maintain ample fruit and vegetable intake. Protein intake in the form of fish and meat but also of eggs, cheese, and other milk products also is important. A well-balanced diet will be an effective measure for secondary prevention and help diminish the risk of dehydration, infections, and frailty.

If patients have difficulties chewing and swallowing, their food should be of soft consistency. Gustatory sense and olfaction decline with age and in relation to illness (particularly in AD). Thus it is wise to experiment with spices and flavors when preparing meals.

Anorexia must be evaluated carefully. It might be a sign of the underlying disease, of badly fitted teeth, of an acute illness, or acute pain which cannot be verbalized by the patient, but it can also be a symptom of stomach or duodenal ulcer. With increasing age, visceral pain is much less well perceived compared to pain of musculo-skeletal origin. The differential diagnosis of anorexia may require gastroscopy if no other underlying cause can be identified. Ulcers should be treated by standard medical therapies, regardless of the degree of dementia.

If neurological reasons prevent proper swallowing and the patient expresses hunger and thirst, tube feeding has to be considered. It should be emphasized that tube feeding does not protect from aspiration, even though placing of a PEG (percutaneous endoscopic gastrostomy) tube is possible with minimal risks and usually is well tolerated. The endoscopic approach may visualize gastrointestinal pathology that is common in the old. Nutrition by PEG-placed tubes allows for easy and rather safe nutrition in appropriate cases. Total parenteral nutrition is almost never indicated in the long-term management of demented patients.

Key messages: Anorexia may be a sign of underlying disease. Food has to be adapted to the needs and the still preserved skills of the patient.

TO FEED OR NOT TO FEED

One of the most difficult decisions is whether a demented patient who refuses to eat, does not open the mouth, or does not swallow, expresses his will or is victim of the disease and needs artificial, e.g., tube feeding *(34)*. It is our practice to respect the patient's behavior and to refrain from forced feeding in these cases *(35–37)*. The order reads: The patient may eat and drink as much as he/she wishes. It is, however, of greatest importance, that regular offerings of drinks and food are made by the caregiver and that oral hygiene with moistening and cleaning of the mouth is assured. This is particularly important when a living will exists indicating that the patient does not wish CPR, intensive care, or artificial feeding in case of advanced dementia. If the patient swallows and drinks offered food, withdrawing nutrition would be against his present will.

Another problem arises when concurrent illness leads to anorexia and aggravates the already poor status of a demented patient. In such a case it depends critically on the concurrent disease whether food and fluids are continued or kept to a minimum in the sense of palliative medicine.

Thus, in the stages of severe dementia (FAST 6 or 7), an acute pneumonia not treated with antibiotics or congestive heart failure not responding to conventional treatment should lead to the (re)evaluation of the current nutritional strategy. Cessation of feeding and fluid administration should be considered. The decision depends on the overall prognosis, the remaining therapeutic options, and the will of the patient.

Key messages: Anorexia in the final stage of dementia is common and should be respected. Other causes leading to anorexia have to be ruled out. Tube feeding by PEG is seldom justified.

REFERENCES

1. Jorm, A.F.; Jolley, D.: The incidence of dementia: a meta-analysis. Neurology 1998; 51: 728–733.
2. Baltes, P.B.: Age and aging as incomplete architecture of human ontogenesis. Z Gerontol Geriatr 1999; 32: 433–448.

3. The Canadian Study of Health and Aging Working Group: The incidence of dementia in Canada. Neurology 2000; 55: 66–73.

4. Orth, M.; Schapira, A.H.: Mitochondria and degenerative disorders. Am J Med Genet 2001; 106: 27–36.

5. Hardy, J.; Selkoe, D.J.: The amyloid hypothesis of Alzheimer's disease: progress and problems on the road to therapeutics. Science 2002; 297: 353–356.

6. Selkoe, D.J.; Schenk, D.: Alzheimer's disease: molecular understanding predicts amyloid-based therapeutics. Annu Rev Pharmacol Toxicol 2002; 4: 4.

7. Roberts, S.B. et al.: Physiologic effects of lowering caloric intake in non-human primates and non-obese humans. J Gerontol A Biol Sci Med Sci 2001; 56 Spec No 1: 66–75.

8. Tong, L. et al.: Beta-amyloid-(1-42) impairs activity-dependent cAMP-response element-binding protein signalling in neurons at concentrations in which cell survival is not compromised. J Biol Chem 2001; 276: 17301–17306.

9. Duan, W. et al.: Dietary restriction stimulates BDNF production in the brain and thereby protects neurons against excitotoxic injury. J Mol Neurosci 2001; 16: 1–12.

10. Barres, B.A.; Smith, S.J.: Neurobiology. Cholesterol—making or breaking the synapse. Science 2001; 294: 1296–1297.

11. Mauch, D.H. et al.: CNS synaptogenesis promoted by glia-derived cholesterol. Science 2001; 294: 1354–1357.

12. Rehman, H.U.; Masson, E.A.: Neuroendocrinology of ageing. Age Ageing 2001; 30: 279–287.

13. Prolla, T.A.: DNA microarray analysis of the aging brain. Chem Senses 2002; 27: 299–306.

14. Golden, S.H. et al.: Risk factor groupings related to insulin resistance and their synergistic effects on subclinical atherosclerosis: the atherosclerosis risk in communities study. Diabetes 2002; 51: 3069–3076.

15. Luchsinger, J.A. et al.: Caloric intake and the risk of Alzheimer disease. Arch Neurol 2002; 59: 1258–1263.

16. Seshadri, S. et al.: Plasma homocysteine as a risk factor for dementia and Alzheimer's disease. N Engl J Med 2002; 346: 476–483.

17. Fenech, M.: The role of folic acid and vitamin B12 in genomic stability of human cells. Mutat Res 2001; 475: 57–67.

18. Johnson, M.A. et al.: Hyperhomocysteinemia and vitamin B12 deficiency in elderly using title IIIc nutrition services. Am J Clin Nutr 2003; 77: 211–220.

19. La Rue, A. et al.: Nutritional status and cognitive functioning in a normally aging sample: a 6-year assessment. Am J Clin Nutr 1997; 65: 20–29.

20. Masaki, K.H. et al. Association of vitamin E and C supplement use with cognitive function and dementia in elderly men. Neurology 2000; 54: 1265–1272.

21. Haller, J. et al.: Mental health: mini mental state examination and geriatric depression score of elderly Europeans in the SENECA study of 1993. Eur J Clin Nutr 1996; 50 (suppl 2): S112–S116.

22. Bolger, P.M.; Schwetz, B.A.: Mercury and health. N Engl J Med 2002; 347: 1735–1736.

23. Mendez-Alvarez, E. et al.: Effects of aluminium and zinc on the oxidative stress caused by 6-hydroxydopamine autoxidation: relevance for the pathogenesis of Parkinson's disease. Biochim Biophys Acta 2002; 1586: 155–168.

24. Sano, M. et al.: A controlled trial of selegiline, alpha-tocopherol, or both as treatment for Alzheimer's disease. The Alzheimer's Disease Cooperative Study. N Engl J Med 1997; 336: 1216–1222.

25. Posner, H.B. et al.: The relationship of hypertension in the elderly to AD, vascular dementia, and cognitive function. Neurology 2002; 58: 1175–1181.

26. Lindsay, J. et al.: Risk factors for Alzheimer's disease: a prospective analysis from the Canadian Study of Health and Aging. Am J Epidemiol 2002; 156: 445–453.

27. Shults, C.W. et al.: Effects of coenzyme Q10 in early Parkinson disease: evidence of slowing of the functional decline. Arch Neurol 2002; 59: 1541–1550.

28. Willett, W.C.; Stampfer, M.J.: Clinical practice. What vitamins should I be taking, doctor? N Engl J Med 2001; 345: 1819–1824.

29. Tabet, N. et al.: Vitamins, trace elements, and antioxidant status in dementia disorders. Int Psychogeriatr 2001; 13: 265–275.

30. Oakley, G.P. Jr.: Eat right and take a multivitamin *(editorial; comment)*. N Engl J Med 1998; 338: 1060–1061.

31. Shatenstein, B.; Kergoat, M.J.; Nadon, S.: Anthropometric changes over 5 years in elderly Canadians by age, gender, and cognitive status. J Gerontol A Biol Sci Med Sci 2001; 56: M483–M488.

32. Poehlman, E.T.; Dvorak, R.V.: Energy expenditure, energy intake, and weight loss in Alzheimer disease. Am J Clin Nutr 2000; 71: 650S–655S.

33. Gillette-Guyonnet, S. et al.: Weight loss in Alzheimer disease. Am J Clin Nutr 2000; 71: 637S–642S.

34. Li, I.: Feeding tubes in patients with severe dementia. Am Fam Physician 2002; 65: 1605–1610, 1515.

35. Dharmarajan, T.S.; Unnikrishnan, D.; Pitchumoni, C.S.: Percutaneous endoscopic gastrostomy and outcome in dementia. Am J Gastroenterol 2001; 96: 2556–2563.

36. Post, S.G.: Tube feeding and advanced progressive dementia. Hastings Cent Rep 2001; 31: 36–42.

37. Kim, Y.I.: To feed or not to feed: tube feeding in patients with advanced dementia. Nutr Rev 2001; 59 (3 Pt 1): 86–88.

32

Impact of Physical Activity on Prevention of Alzheimer's Disease

Danielle Laurin, René Verreault, and Joan Lindsay

INTRODUCTION

Much support for the role of physical fitness or physical activity in the prevention of dementia and Alzheimer's disease (AD), the most common type, comes from the identification of a number of mechanisms in experimental and clinical studies. One of the most accepted mechanisms, which may underlie the potentially protective effects of physical activity on cognitive performance, is sustenance of cerebral blood flow. As a result of exercise, there is an increase of blood circulation and energy supply throughout the body, including the brain. Vascular risk factors have been implicated in the pathogenesis of vascular dementia and cognitive impairment as well as in AD *(1)*.

In a 4-year prospective study, designed to evaluate the effects of three levels of physical activity on cerebral perfusion after retirement in three groups of 30 elderly volunteers, only cerebral blood flow levels of retired-inactive subjects decreased significantly over time. This was in contrast to working and retired-active subjects, whose values did not change *(2)*. Results also showed that retired-inactive subjects had significantly lower cognitive performance compared to working and retired-active subjects at the end of follow-up, but cognitive function was not assessed at baseline, which may bias the temporal association between cause and effect.

HOW PHYSICAL ACTIVITY PROTECTS THE BRAIN

Physical activity could contribute to sustain optimal cerebral perfusion by decreasing blood pressure in hypertensive subjects, which has been documented as a risk factor for vascular dementia and cognitive impairment *(3)*. Data from population-based prospective studies with long periods of follow-up have indicated the presence of high blood pressure several years prior to the onset of AD in association with an increased risk for AD *(4,5)*. In addition, physical activity may act on cerebral blood perfusion by reducing the concentration of low-density lipoproteins *(6)*. There is evidence pointing to endurance exercise training as an independent but complementary effect to hormone replacement therapy on serum lipid profiles in healthy postmenopausal women *(7)*. Moreover, physical activity can inhibit platelet aggregation and enhance cerebral metabolic demands *(2,8)*.

Reduced cerebral oxygenation is another mechanism that could be related to the neuropsychological function. Even though oxygen may not play the key role in brain function, it has been associated with changes that occur with aging in brain chemistry. It has been suggested that an exercise program could improve aerobic capacity and nutrient supply to the brain. Better scores on several neuropsychological tasks were obtained following a 4-month aerobic exercise program in three groups of 13–15 older sedentary volunteers *(9)*. These improvements could be attributable to the observed increase in transport and utilization of oxygen in the brain and tissues following the exercise program.

From: *Current Clinical Neurology,*
Alzheimer's Disease: A Physician's Guide to Practical Management
Edited by: R. W. Richter and B. Zoeller Richter © Humana Press Inc., Totowa, NJ

In contrast, increased aerobic metabolism during and after physical activity has also been reported to be a source of oxidative stress *(10)*. Strenuous exercise has been found to promote the production of reactive oxygen species, which lead to apoptotic (programmed) cell death *(11)*. Although this area needs further clarification, it is believed that exercise-induced apoptosis ensures an optimal body function that serves to eliminate specific damaged cells without any marked inflammatory responses *(12)*.

On a molecular basis, given their roles in promoting cell growth and neuronal function, growth factors were mentioned as stimulating protective mechanisms in the brain during exercise. Experimental studies in rodents have indicated that exercise may regulate the expression of fibroblast growth factor, which suggests that growth factors could be mediators of the effects of exercise on the brain *(13)*. Combined antidepressant treatment and physical activity led to the potentiation of brain-derived neurotrophic factor expression of the rat hippocampus, the most widely distributed growth factor within the brain that influences the function of several neurotransmitter systems *(14)*.

Finally, release of endorphins by exercise represents another psychobiochemical mechanism that could explain the improvement following exercise, inasmuch as exercise is associated with increased concentrations of endorphins, which in turn are related to reduced depression and anxiety *(15)*.

The experimental and clinical literature has proposed several mechanisms that support the hypothesis that exercise could play a role in the preservation of cognitive function. The next section will overview some of the studies that examined the associations between physical activity and cognitive performance.

PHYSICAL ACTIVITY AND COGNITIVE FUNCTION

In clinical studies, several authors have first been interested in the role of physical activity in relation to simple cognitive tasks. Improved performance following training has been observed in many of them. In a large-scale random sample of 6979 British adults aged between 18 and 94 years, the interactions of age, self-rated health, and walking activity with cognitive function were evaluated *(16)*. Cognitive testing included two measures of reaction time, a measure of incidental memory, and a measure of spatial reasoning. Cross-sectional analysis indicated that walking activity was related to the choice reaction time, which indicated that exercise could attenuate the age-related slowing of the speed of reaction. Of note, walking could modify health-related and age-related variations in cognitive function.

Positive results were also reported in more rigorous study designs. Fluid intelligence, as measured by the "culture fair intelligence test," was associated with physical fitness and age after a 4-month physical training in 36 adult men *(17)*. Regardless of age, the high-fit group scored significantly better than the low-fit group. Similarly, regardless of physical condition, the youngest group scored significantly better than the oldest group. Crystallized intelligence, however, was related to neither age nor physical activity.

In a large, randomized, controlled trial carried out in 187 older community-dwelling women, significant improvements in memory span and well-being were associated with concomitant improvements in both reaction time and muscle strength after 12 months of training *(18)*. Moreover, improvements in postural control as demonstrated by the "timed up & go test" and functional reach scores were also observed following an exercise program *(19)*. These results were achieved using a randomized, controlled trial, with 6 months of follow-up in a small group of 42 healthy elderly persons more than 75 years of age living in the community on cognitive and neurobehavioral function. The program consisted of light aerobic exercise, stretching, neuromotor coordination, and muscle-strengthening exercise. This study also indicated the acceptability of physical training in a cohort of very old subjects.

No benefits were reported in other investigations. The effects of a 12-week aerobic exercise program on psychological well-being and cognitive function were examined by comparing an exercise group (*n* = 14) with a control group (*n* = 24) in a population of community-dwelling elderly adults

(20). Results showed little change in psychological well-being and no overall change on four cognitive measures (digit symbol, digit span, copying words, copying numbers) in the exercise and control groups. Compliance problems within the groups were mentioned by the authors of the study.

Some positive effects of physical activity were reported in frail institutionalized psychogeriatric patients. The effects of mild exercise were investigated in a small group of 30 elderly subjects *(21)*. Improvements on two out of three cognitive tests (progressive matrices test and Wechsler memory scale) were found after 12 weeks of exercise therapy compared to the control group.

On the other hand, the effects of a 3-month program of light exercises, designed to improve strength and balance without increasing aerobic fitness, on the neuropsychological function of 45 elderly institutionalized women by way of a randomized controlled trial revealed no significant differences on a series of neuropsychological tests—except for the word fluency test *(22)*. According to the authors, the absence of any acute effects could be explained by the fact that neuropsychological testing was realized 3–7 days after the end of the training. These authors had previously observed a markedly improved neuropsychological function after exercise in a younger and more fit group of older persons *(23)*.

The role of physical activity in relation to cognitive performance has been studied in a series of investigations regrouping cross-sectional and more rigorous clinical trials, the majority of which included small numbers of subjects. There is substantial evidence suggesting a beneficial association between exercise and cognitive function. However, to assess more accurately the effect of physical activity on cognitive function, comprehensive extensive neuropsychological assessment, using recognized diagnostic criteria, are needed. A brief review of some of the studies interested in the effects of physical activity and dementia as the outcome is given below.

PHYSICAL ACTIVITY AND DEMENTIA

The effects of physical activity on the risk of dementia, and more particularly AD, were investigated in cross-sectional and prospective epidemiological studies. In one of the earliest case control studies of AD, conducted in a group of subjects including 85 matched pairs of cases and controls aged 52–96 years, underactivity in both the recent and more distant past was reported to be significantly associated with the risk for AD by three- and sixfold, respectively *(24)*. However, the frequency exposure contributing to AD was low, and information about risk factors came from informants, who may have recalled differently exposures of cases and controls.

In contrast, no differences between 138 cases of AD and 193 controls in the frequency of current and past athletic activity was found among community-dwelling older persons, but this latter analysis was not designed specifically to examine the relationship *(25)*.

Prospective studies gave somewhat more positive results. Li et al. conducted a 3-year follow-up study of 1090 persons aged 60 years or more, living in the community. They found a relative risk of dementia of 8.7 in subjects limited to indoor activities compared with those without such limitations, and a relative risk of 4.9 after adjustment for age *(26)*. This study, however, was based on only 13 incident cases of dementia.

In another prospective study of 828 initially nondemented subjects aged 65 years or older followed for 7 years, moderate physical activity was associated with a reduced risk for dementia *(27)*. The active group was defined as those including daily exercise during the leisure period or moderate to strenuous physical activity at work. Exercise was associated with a significant 80% reduction in risk for AD ($n = 42$) after adjustment for age and sex and initial screening score, but no positive effect of exercise was observed for the vascular dementia (VaD) group, which comprised 50 cases.

In a shorter prospective study including 327 subjects aged 75 years or more, free of dementia at baseline, no association was reported between either incident dementia ($n = 47$) or AD ($n = 29$) and exercise after 3 years *(28)*. Physical activity was assessed by asking subjects about the number of times per month they were working in the garden or yard, doing active sports or exercises, and going for walks. Associations were adjusted for age, sex, and education.

Table 1
Associations Between Physical Activity and Risk for Alzheimer's Disease,
Vascular Dementia, and All Types of Dementia

	Alzheimer's disease		Vascular dementia		Dementia	
	No. of cases/Total	OR (95% CI)[a]	No. of cases/Total	OR (95% CI)	No. of cases/Total	OR (95% CI)
Physical activity						
None	80/1183	1.00	23/1126	1.00	110/1213	1.00
Low	21/506	0.67 (0.39–1.14)	5/490	0.54 (0.20–1.44)	28/513	0.64 (0.41–1.02)
Moderate	52/1412	0.67 (0.46–0.98)	18/1378	0.70 (0.37–1.31)	79/1439	0.69 (0.50–0.95)
High	16/747	0.50 (0.28–0.90)	8/739	0.63 (0.27–1.44)	31/762	0.63 (0.40–0.98)
Test for trend	$p = 0.02$		$p = 0.46$		$p = 0.04$	

[a]OR indicates odds ratio adjusted for age, sex, and education; CI, confidence interval.

More recently, results from a large-scale, multicenter, 5-year prospective cohort study showed significant protective effects of regular physical activity on the risk of dementia, particularly AD, in a representative sample of the Canadian elderly population aged 65 and older *(29)*. The effect of physical activity was analyzed using a case control approach including information from 3894 controls and 285 incident cases of dementia, of which 194 were diagnosed with AD and 61 with VaD. Physical activity was measured at baseline by combining two questions regarding frequency and intensity of regular physical activity. A 4-level composite score rating physical activity was created and validated. Moderate and high levels of physical activity were associated with significantly lower risks for AD and dementia, by 30–50% (Table 1). Furthermore, these associations were significant mainly in women, and revealed a significant dose–response relationship—showing decreasing risk with increasing level of physical activity. A similar but nonsignificant effect was observed with VaD. In addition, there was a lower risk for cognitive loss associated with high physical activity among women who remained cognitively normal during the study period. The possibility of a selection bias due to survival was considered by the creation of a variable using information from death certificates, proxies, and a logistic regression model estimating the probability of death due to dementia. Revised analyses showed that the exclusion of deceased subjects from the analysis had little effect on the results. The potentially confounding effect of several variables related to health status was also investigated, and risk estimates remained essentially unchanged. This study suggested that regular practice of physical activity might delay or prevent the onset of cognitive impairment, AD, and dementia in an older population.

Finally, in a 7-year longitudinal cohort study of 801 older nuns, priests, and brothers, frequency of participation in physical activities was found to be inversely associated, although not significantly, with the risk for AD *(30)*. Higher quartiles of physical activity were associated with 30–40% lower risk of AD relative to the lowest quartile of physical activity. This study was originally carried out to test the relation between cognitive activities to incident dementia and AD. Participation in physical activities was roughly estimated according to the participation to a series of exercises (walking, gardening or yardwork, calisthenics or general exercise, bicycle riding, and swimming or water exercise), and if so, the number of occasions and average minutes per occasion, as well as the total weekly hours in all analyses. One important limitation of this analysis is that the cohort was selected and participants may therefore have differed from older persons in the general population in education and lifestyle.

Studies (mostly longitudinal) that focused on the association between physical activity and dementia or AD tended to observe a protective effect in the development of the disease. Further research, including the design of clinical trials, is warranted on the effects of physical activity on the onset and progression of the disease in order to verify the relationship more rigorously.

IMPLICATIONS AND RECOMMENDATIONS

AD and other forms of dementia represent major health problems in our aging societies, and are expected to become one of the most important challenges in health services for the coming decades. Despite extensive efforts directed at a better understanding of the pathogenesis of dementing illnesses, few risk factors and even fewer protective factors have been related to these degenerative diseases. The common finding of improved cognitive function or delayed risk of onset of AD or dementia with the practice of physical activity suggests that physical fitness does have some arousal effects on cognition in older persons. Benefits of physical training interventions have been reported in older people, even in the very old, healthy or frail, living in the community or in institutions. Some of these results have suggested that even a simple walking program would be a safe form of activity to recommend. This recommendation could be easily implemented in the everyday life of the majority of older people. Among other health benefits, regular practice of physical activity could thus represent a potent protective factor for cognitive impairment, AD, and other dementia in the elderly population.

SUMMARY

Several pathways have been identified in experimental studies through which the practice of physical activity could affect cognitive function and reduce the risk for dementia and AD in later life. In clinical settings, many specific beneficial effects of physical intervention programs on memory and cognitive performance have been documented in older persons. Even though epidemiological studies are just beginning to evaluate the impact of physical activity on the onset and progression of dementia and AD, results so far tend to support the presence of some positive effects. In this chapter, a brief overview has been given of the hypotheses underlying the relationship between physical activity and dementia, including AD. The existing literature is also reviewed and examined in the light of their methodological limitations. Finally, suggestions for guidelines intended to physicians regarding the recommendation of physical activity are provided.

REFERENCES

1. Launer, L.J.: Demonstrating the case that AD is a vascular disease: epidemiologic evidence. Ageing Res Rev 2002; 1: 61–77.
2. Rogers, R.L. et al.: After reaching retirement age physical activity sustains cerebral perfusion and cognition. J Am Geriatr Soc 1990; 38: 123–128.
3. Whelton, S.P. et al.: Effect of aerobic exercise on blood pressure: a meta-analysis of randomized, controlled trials. Ann Intern Med 2002; 136: 493–503.
4. Skoog, I. et al.: 15-Year longitudinal study of blood pressure and dementia. Lancet 1996; 347: 1141–1145.
5. Launer, L.J. et al.: Midlife blood pressure and dementia: the Honolulu Asia Aging Study. Neurobiol Aging 2000; 21: 49–55.
6. Stefanick, M.L. et al.: Effects of diet and exercise in men and postmenopausal women with low levels of HDL cholesterol and high levels of LDL cholesterol. N Engl J Med 1998; 339: 12–20.
7. Binder, E.F. et al.: Effects of endurance exercise and hormone replacement therapy on serum lipids in older women. J Am Geriatr Soc 1996; 44: 231–236.
8. Rauramaa, R. et al.: Inhibition of platelet aggregability by moderate-intensity physical exercise: a randomized clinical trial in overweight men. Circulation 1986; 74: 939–944.
9. Dustman, R.E. et al.: Aerobic exercise training and improved neuropsychological function of older individuals. Neurobiol Aging 1984; 5: 35–42.
10. Leeuwenburgh, C. et al.: Oxidative stress and antioxidants in exercise. Curr Med Chem 2001; 8: 829–838.
11. Bejma, J. et al.: Aging and acute exercise enhance free radical generation in rat skeletal muscle. J Appl Physiol 1999; 87: 465–470.
12. Phaneuf, S. et al.: Apoptosis and exercise. Med Sci Sports Exerc 2001; 33: 393–396.
13. Gómez-Pinilla, F. et al.: Physical exercise induces FGF-2 and its mRNA in the hippocampus. Bain Res 1997; 764: 1–8.
14. Russo-Neustadt, A. et al.: Exercise, antidepressant medications, and enhanced brain derived neurotrophic factor expression. Neuropsychopharmacol 1999; 21: 679–682.
15. Biddle, S.J.H. et al.: Exercise and health psychology: emerging relationship. Br J Med Psychol 1989; 62 (pt 3): 205–216.
16. Emery, C.F. et al.: Relationships among age, exercise, health, and cognitive function in a British sample. Gerontologist 1995; 35: 378–385.

17. Elsayed, M. et al.: Intellectual differences of adult men related to age and physical fitness before and after an exercise program. J Gerontol 1980; 3: 383–387.
18. Williams, P. et al.: Effects of group exercise on cognitive functioning and mood in older women. ANZ J Public Health 1997; 21: 45–52.
19. Okumiya, K. et al.: Effects of exercise on neurobehavioral function in community-dwelling older people more than 75 years of age. J Am Geriatr Soc 1996; 44: 569–572.
20. Emery, C.F. et al.: Psychological and cognitive effects of an exercise program for community-residing older adults. Gerontologist 1990; 30: 184–188.
21. Powell, R.R: Psychological effects of exercise therapy upon institutionalized geriatric mental patients. J Gerontol 1974; 29: 157–161.
22. Molloy, D.W. et al.: The effects of a three-month exercise programme on neuropsychological function in elderly institutionalized women: a randomized controlled trial. Age Ageing 1988; 17: 303–310.
23. Molloy, D.W. et al.: Acute effects of exercise on neuropsychological function in elderly subjects. J Am Geriatr Soc 1988; 36: 29–33.
24. Broe, G.A. et al.: A case-control study of Alzheimer's disease in Australia. Neurology 1990; 40: 1698–1707.
25. Mayeux, R. et al.: Genetic susceptibility and head injury as risk factors for Alzheimer's disease among community-dwelling elderly persons and their first-degree relatives. Ann Neurol 1993; 33: 494–501.
26. Li, G. et al.: A three-year follow-up study of age-related dementia in an urban area of Beijing. Acta Psychiatr Scand 1991; 83: 99–104.
27. Yoshitake, T. et al.: Incidence and risk factors of vascular dementia and Alzheimer's disease in a defined elderly Japanese population: The Hisayama Study. Neurology 1995; 45: 1161–1168.
28. Broe, G.A. et al.: Health habits and risk of cognitive impairment and dementia in old age: a prospective study on the effects of exercise, smoking and alcohol consumption. ANZ J Public Health 1998; 22: 621–623.
29. Laurin, D. et al.: Physical activity and risk of cognitive impairment and dementia in elderly persons. Arch Neurol 2001; 58: 498–504.
30. Wilson, R.S. et al.: Participation in cognitively stimulating activities and risk of incident Alzheimer disease. JAMA 2002; 287: 742–748.

VIII Future Developments

33

Stem Cell Therapy for Alzheimer's Disease

Kiminobu Sugaya

INTRODUCTION

Neural tissue transplantation therapy for neurodegenerative diseases is not a novel idea. Because of its specific loss of large neurons in the substantia nigra, which sends dopaminergic projections to the striatum, Parkinson's disease has been a good target for transplantation therapy. Since a conventional treatment for Parkinson's disease was L-DOPA augmentation of the dopamine content in the striatum, transplantation of dopaminergic fetal tissue into the striatum has been tested for many years. Although these neural tissue transplantations are not neuroreplacement therapies for degenerating neurons in the substantia nigra, many of the clinical trials significantly ameliorated the behavioral deficits in Parkinson's disease. A similar approach for treatment of Alzheimer's disease (AD) has been discussed. However, the use of human fetal neuronal tissue not only raises ethical concerns but also is impractical, because tissue from a single fetus is not sufficient to treat each patient. Thus, we must seek alternatives to fetal tissue in the treatment of neurodegenerative diseases.

Recent advances in stem cell technology are expanding our ability to replace many types of tissue throughout the body. In the past, cognitive impairment caused by degeneration of neuronal cells had been considered incurable because of the long-held truism that neurons do not regenerate during adulthood. However, this statement has been challenged, and we have found new evidence that neurons do indeed have the potential to be renewed after maturation. The discovery of multipotent neural stem cells (NSC) in the adult brain has brought revolutionary changes in the theory of neurogenesis, which currently postulates that regeneration of neurons can occur throughout life, thus opening a door for the development of novel therapies to treat neurodegenerative diseases—including AD—by neuronal regeneration using stem cell transplantation *(1,2)*.

This chapter reviews possible strategies for AD therapy using current stem cell technologies and discusses issues that need to be addressed before considering its clinical applications.

NEURAL STEM CELLS AS TRANSPLANTATION MATERIAL FOR NEUROREPLACEMENT THERAPY

Although stem cells are often defined as self-renewing and multipotent, the types of cells produced from stem cells are limited by their tissue-specific character. Each stem cell contains specific information that will allow it to become a special type of cell. In other words, these cells are at least partially committed to become a certain type of stem cell in a tissue-specific manner. Neural stem cells, capable of spontaneously differentiating into neurons and glia, are the most promising candidate for neuroreplacement therapies. Neural stem cells have been isolated from the embryonic and adult mammalian and human central nervous system (CNS) and propagated in vitro in a variety of culture systems *(3–6)*.

From: *Current Clinical Neurology,*
Alzheimer's Disease: A Physician's Guide to Practical Management
Edited by: R. W. Richter and B. Zoeller Richter © Humana Press Inc., Totowa, NJ

Immortalized mouse fetal neural stem cells have been studied for years *(7)*. However, current interest is focused on the ability to proliferate populations of human neural stem cells as an in vitro source of tissue for brain repair. Since successful neuroreplacement by stem cell transplantation is dependent on these capacities—as the ability of these cells to migrate and to integrate within the host CNS—the source and culture conditions of stem cells are crucial factors. The inability to grow NSC in vitro in the absence of complex and undefined biological fluids (serums) has long been a major obstacle in understanding the biology of these cells. Now, however, NSCs can be maintained or expanded in serum-free medium containing the basic fibroblast growth factor (bFGF) and the epidermal growth factor (EGF) *(8,9)*.

Nonetheless, there have been reports showing that human neural precursor cells express almost non-detectable telomerase after certain passages. These human cells also have significantly shorter telomeres than their rodent counterparts *(10)*. Some researchers have been able to continuously expand these cells in vitro *(8)*. After long-term culturing, human neural stem cells (hNSC) differentiate into cells that are immunopositive for the neuronal marker—βIII-tubulin—and the astrocyte marker—glial fibrillary acidic protein (GFAP)—in an unsupplemented medium, suggesting that the genesis of neurons or astrocytes can take place without the addition of exogenous differentiation factors.

Thus, it appears that hNSC are capable of producing the endogenous factors necessary for their own differentiation and survival, which encouraged us to investigate transplantation of hNSC in the aged animal model. This ability to expand multipotent hNSC in vitro offers a well-characterized and efficient source of transplantable cell types.

IMPROVEMENT OF COGNITIVE FUNCTION IN THE AGED RAT BY TRANSPLANTATION OF HUMAN NSC

The successful transplantation of human NSCs (hNSC) into aged rats with subsequent improvement of cognitive function reported by Qu and colleagues reinforces the potential feasibility of hNSC transplantation therapy *(11)*. In this study, hNSC, expanded without differentiation under the influence of mitogenic factors in supplemented serum-free media and labeled by the incorporation of bromo-deoxy-uridine (BrdU) into the nucleus DNA, were injected into the lateral ventricle of mature (6-month-old) and aged (24-month-old) rats. Cognitive function of the animals was assessed by the Morris water maze, both before and 4 weeks after the transplantation of hNSC.

Before hNSC transplantation, some aged animals (aged memory-unimpaired animals) functioned cognitively in the range of mature animals, while others (aged memory-impaired animals) functioned entirely below the cognitive range of the mature animals. After hNSC transplantation, most aged animals had cognitive function in the range of the mature animals. Strikingly, one of the aged memory-impaired animals showed dramatic improvement in behavior—functioning even better than the mature animals. Statistical analysis showed that cognitive function was significantly improved in both mature and aged memory-impaired animals. These behavioral results show the beneficial effects of hNSC transplantation into the host brain in most animals tested.

After the second water maze task, postmortem brains were further analyzed by immunohistochemistry for βIII-tubulin and GFAP, markers for neurons and astrocytes, respectively. There was no sign of ventricular distortion and no evidence of tumor formation. Further, no strong host antigraft immunoreactivity was observed. Intensely and extensively stained with βIII-tubulin, neurons with BrdU-positive nuclei were found in bilateral cingulate and parietal cortices and in the hippocampus. The βIII-tubulin-positive neurons found in the cerebral cortex were typified by a dendrite pointing to the edge of the cortex. In the hippocampus, donor-derived neurons exhibited multiple morphology, varying in cellular size and shape and in one or more processes and branching.

Generally, GFAP-positive astrocytes were localized near the area where neuronal cells were found. These astrocytes were larger than the host glia and also displayed thick processes. Some of these astrocytes had a unilateral morphology (asymmetric), and immunostaining formed a thin ring around the nucleus.

CONSIDERATIONS FOR NEUROREPLACEMENT THERAPIES

Even after Qu's study *(11)*, many researchers are still trying to differentiate stem cells into certain type of neuronal cells in vitro and then transplant them into the target area of brain tissue *(12)*. This approach seems natural, similar to the process in which we are transplanting fetal dopaminergic tissue into basal ganglia to increase their dopamine content in the patients with Parkinson's disease. However, we must further consider several crucial issues. First, fully differentiated neuronal cells do not migrate, meaning they do not integrate with the host brain. Second, a cure for neurodegenerative disease is conceivable only if we replace degenerating neurons in the brain. For example, dopaminergic neurons transplanted to the basal ganglia may not be functionally regulated by the host brain, and may cause side effects *(13)*. Third, if an injection is made into the brain, concomitant tissue destruction will cause monocyte recruitment, and the ensuing immune response will eliminate the transplanted cells. To avoid these problems, I suggest injecting undifferentiated stem cells directly into the brain ventricle.

Human NSC may be the most promising candidate for neuroreplacement therapy. However, ethical issues and risk of immunological rejection limit their value. Although tissue rejection may not be particularly problematic for use in neuroreplacement strategies, since the brain does not produce an immune response unless traumatic damage has occurred, an ideal biological source of cells for replacement therapies would be autologous transplantation of stem cells derived from the patient's own tissues. It is also not known whether a large volume of heterologous neuronal transplantation could change the character or personality of an individual. Some patients might also have psychological difficulties accepting brain tissue from outside sources.

Some researchers are trying to find autologous transplantable cell source in embryonic stem cells (ESCs) which proliferate extensively and theoretically can differentiate into any type of somatic cells. By cloning, these cells can also be modified into cells possessing the same genetic material as the patient. On the other hand, we must develop methods of enriching the cells of interest, because ESCs do not have the information necessary to become certain types of cells that may be needed in specific cases. In other words, ESCs are not committed to become neural cells as are NSCs.

Recently, McKay's group reported that highly enriched populations of midbrain NSC can be derived from mouse ESC. In this report, dopamine neurons generated by these stem cells show the electrophysiological and behavioral properties expected of neurons from the midbrain. This finding is encouraging us to consider the use of ESCs in cell replacement therapy for Parkinson's disease.

After this successful experiment, we still have a barrier in addition to the ethical issue of using human embryonic tissue, which has to be overcome before developing an autologous cell therapy using ESCs: that is, tissue-specific epigenetical modification. Cloning by nuclear transfer is an inefficient process in which most clones die before birth and survivors often display growth abnormalities *(14)*. This may be due to the tissue-specific DNA methylation pattern from somatic nuclei used in cloning *(15)*. Thus, cloned ESC may also receive the tissue-specific epigenetic modification and may not function fully as neural cells.

NEURAL DIFFERENTIATION OF MESENCHYMAL STEM CELLS

Bone marrow contains stemlike cells used not only for hematopoiesis but also for production of a variety of nonhematopoietic tissues. A subset of stromal cells in bone marrow, which has been referred to as mesenchymal stem cells (MeSC), is capable of producing multiple mesenchymal cell lineages, including bone, cartilage, fat, tendons, and other connective tissues *(16–19)*.

Recent reports show that human MeSC (hMeSC) also have the ability to differentiate into a diverse family of cell types that may be unrelated to their phenotypical embryonic origin, including muscle and heptocytes *(20–25)*. Although adult stem cells continue to possess some multipotency, cell types produced from adult stem cells are limited by their tissue-specific character. To overcome this barrier of stem cell lineage, alterations are necessary. However, the regulation mechanisms of tissue-specific stem cell fate decisions remain unclear. Thus, to differentiate MeSC into neural cells, alteration of their epigenetic information before transplantation may be necessary. Nonetheless, neuroreplacement therapy by MeSC transplantation must clear some hurdles before it can be considered for clinical use.

The potential therapeutic use of hMeSC in the CNS has been discussed *(26,27)*, and several in vivo transplantation studies showed neural and glial differentiation of hMeSCs *(28–32)*. Nonetheless, technologies to induce neural lineage from hMeSCs are not fully established. Verfaillie's group recently identified multipotent progenitor cells that co-purify with MeSC in adult bone marrow *(33)*. They claim that these cells contribute to most, if not all, somatic cell types. Thus, this subpopulation of hMeSC may be primarily responsible for the neural differentiation.

To investigate the neural differentiation of hMeSC in vivo, we injected hMeSC expanded without differentiation and labeled (by the incorporation of BrdU into nuclear DNA) into the lateral ventricle of mature mice. Four to six weeks after transplantation, mice brains were analyzed by immunohisto-chemistry for human-specific βIII-tubulin and GFAP, markers for neurons and astrocytes, respectively. Migration and differentiation patterns of transplanted hMeSC were quite similar to our previous results with hNSC transplanted into rats. The main difference was the size of the donor cells compared to the host cells, which were in the order of humans > rats > mice. Intensely and extensively stained with βIII-tubulin neurons, BrdU-positive nuclei were found in the bilateral cingulate and parietal cortices and in the hippocampus. The βIII-tubulin-positive neurons found in the cerebral cortex typically demonstrated a dendrite pointing to the edge of the cortex. In the hippocampus, donor-derived neurons exhibited multiple morphology and varied in size and shape, with one or more processes and branching.

Recently, two different groups reported spontaneous fusion of stem cells *(34,35)*. In these reports, the authors found that stem cells acquired phenotypes from other cells by fusion, which may occur when these stem cells directly touch other cells after transplantation. To investigate the possibility of the neural differentiation of hMeSC without fusion, we co-cultured BrdU-labeled hMeSC with differentiated hNSC. The hNSC were differentiated in 12-well tissue culture plates under the basal media condition. Then the hMeSC were transferred onto a tissue-culture 0.4-μm membrane insert and placed on top of the differentiated hNSC under the basal media condition.

Immunocytochemical examination 7 days post-co-culture revealed that hMeSC differentiated into βIII-tubulin-immunopositive small bipolar and unipolar cells (approximately 40% of the total), and GFAP-immunopositive large flattened multipolar cells (approximately 60% of the total). Thus, most hMeSC were converted into neural cells, indicating that all hMeSC can differentiate into neural cells under this condition. The general cell morphology in both hNSC and hMeSC differentiated cultures were similar.

This result indicates that hMeSC are capable of becoming neurons and astrocytes when co-cultured with differentiated NSCs. Since no exogenous differentiation factors, such as retinoic acid and BDNF, were added and no cell-to-cell contact existed in this co-culture system, it is reasonable to hypothesize that the membrane-permeable endogenous factor(s) released from differentiating hNSC altered the cell fate decisions of hMeSC. In our in vitro experiment, hMeSC were cultured on the membrane insert and were kept totally separated from the hNSC. Thus, the possibility of fusion between hMeSC and hNSC can be excluded in this study.

These results indicate that the brain environment may produce factor(s) that allow the differentiation of not only NSCs but also MeSC into neurons, and suggest that hMeSC may serve as an alternative to hNSC for potential therapeutic use in neuroreplacement.

PARTICULAR ISSUES FOR STEM CELL THERAPY FOR AD

Qu and colleagues have succeeded in recovering cognitive function in aged rats by intraventricular injection of NSCs. Nonetheless, this work did not take into account the effect of pathological changes that may occur in the diseased brain and that may prevent the regular differentiation or migration of stem cells. For example, in thinking about neuroreplacement therapy for AD, we must consider several relevant issues.

In AD, memory deterioration involves the degeneration of basal forebrain (BF) cholinergic neurons, so it is this neuron population that should be replaced. Their long projections and expression of nerve growth factor receptor make cholinergic neurons phenotypically different from dopaminergic neurons. This fact has led some researchers to declare BF cholinergic neurons irreplaceable. However, it has since been shown that BF cholinergic neurons transplanted into the striatum and nucleus basalis of Meynert (NBM, which provides major cholinergic input to the neocortex) of adult rat brain survived and expressed the cholinergic phenotype *(36)*. Furthermore, engrafted cholinergic-rich (but not noncholinergic) cell suspensions reversed the deficits in radial-arm maze performance previously caused by NBM excitotoxic lesions *(7)*. Although these results hint that it may be possible to replace BF cholinergic neurons, we must prove that degenerating BF cholinergic neurons in AD can be replaced by hNSC transplantation.

APP FUNCTION IN STEM CELL BIOLOGY

The prevalence of the beta-amyloid (Aβ) neurotoxicity theory in AD pathology and the absence of a phenotype in the Abeta protein precursor (APP) knockout mouse tend to limit our focus on the physiological functions of APP. Previous studies have shown that APP may be involved in neurite outgrowth *(37,38)*, cell proliferation *(39–41)*, neuronal migration *(42)*, and neuronal differentiation *(43)*. APP expression is increased by brain injury *(44,45)* and amyloidogenic secretions increase in apoptotic cells *(46)*. APP may also be involved in cell survival *(47–49)*. Although these facts may indicate the involvement of APP in neuroplasticity, the physiological functions of APP are not clear.

It is well established that the olfactory sensory pathway is pathologically affected in AD, and it has been suggested that this may serve as a tool to differentiate AD from other types of dementia *(50)*. Severe loss (as much as 75%) of the anterior olfactory nuclei neurons in early-onset AD has been reported *(51)*. Significant impairment in olfactory function has been reported in AD and Down's syndrome patients *(52)*. Even normal control patients, who tested positive for the ApoE4-allele, a known risk factor for AD, showed impaired odor identification compared to allele-negative subjects *(53)*.

Because of their vulnerability to toxic substances in the environment, olfactory sensory neurons readily degenerate and are replenished continuously from a population of NSCs at the base of the olfactory epithelium. It has been shown that sensory neurons born in the olfactory epithelium of adults retain the ability to differentiate and establish synaptic contact with target cells in the mature olfactory bulb *(54)*. Stem cells originating from the subventricular zone are known to migrate into the olfactory system *(55)*. Furthermore, these NSCs migrate into the hippocampus and other parts of the brain, which may be important for proper maintenance of cognitive function *(9,56)*. Thus, deficits in adult neurogenesis by NSCs may be implicated in a cascade of impairments in olfactory and cognitive function, as observed in AD.

We have previously shown that under serum-free unsupplemented media conditions, hNSC grown as neurospheres migrate and differentiate into βIII-tubulin-, GFAP-, and O4-immunopositive cells, markers for neurons, astrocytes, and oligodendrocytes, respectively *(8)*. These results suggest that hNSC are capable of producing endogenous factors necessary for their own differentiation in vitro.

To assess the migration and differentiation process in more detail, we employed a time-lapse video microscopic study. During the early stages (1–3 days in vitro, DIV) of serum-free differentiation, many hNSC exhibited the same type of shrunken morphology that cells undergoing apoptotic cell death display. To further assess the type of cell death, we used the TUNEL assay to detect in situ DNA fragmentation, an early marker of apoptosis, in hNSC differentiated in serum or in serum-free media. Many cells were positive for the TUNEL signal under serum-free differentiation conditions and displayed somal shrinkage followed by cell detachment from the culture plates. In contrast, only a few TUNEL-positive cells were detected under serum differentiation conditions. Since neurons are known to undergo apoptosis after serum deprivation, and B27 (cell culture supplement) is reported to prevent neuronal death in cultured cortical tissue, apoptosis of hNSC in serum-free differentiation conditions may be due to supplement deprivation *(57,58)*. Our time-lapse video microscopic study of hNSC plated in serum-free unsupplemented media for 1 DIV revealed that differentiating hNSC appear to reach out to the nearby morphologically apoptotic cells described above.

These results suggest that hNSC initially become apoptotic under serum-free differentiation conditions and subsequently express migration and/or differentiation factors to influence the fate of neighboring cells.

While many factors are released following apoptotic cell death, several studies point to an important correlation between apoptosis and the APP. Damaged neurons and neurons committed to apoptosis demonstrate signals strongly immunopositive for APP *(59,60)*. Moreover, amyloidogenic fragments produced from APP are reported to be released into the extracellular space from neuronal cells under serum-deprived conditions *(61)*. The expression of APP is also reported to increase during retinoic acid-induced neuronal differentiation *(62)*. The mRNA expression of β-amyloid precursor-like proteins (APLP-1 and APLP-2) is also upregulated during retinoic acid-induced differentiation of human SH-SY5Y neuroblastoma cells *(63)*. The increase in APP expression levels during neuronal differentiation in various cell culture systems suggests an important cellular function for APP during the differentiation process.

From these observations, we hypothesized that under serum-free differentiation conditions, APP fragments released from apoptotic cells serve as regulation and differentiation factors for neighboring hNSC. A combination of immunocytochemistry with 22C11, a monoclonal antibody recognizing the N′-terminal domain of APP, and the TUNEL assay revealed a marked increase of APP immunoreactivity in the TUNEL signal-positive cells under serum-free differentiation conditions compared to the background levels of APP found in neighboring hNSC. This result not only confirms previous findings, that APP expression is elevated in apoptotic cells, but more important, it suggests that one factor produced in apoptotic cells, which influences the differentiation of neighboring cells, could be the N′-terminal fragment of APP.

APP is also known to be upregulated during development and after brain damage *(64,45)*, events that involve migration and differentiation of NSCs. Secreted APP (sAPP) has also been reported to produce protein kinase C and synaptogenesis in cultured neurons, in addition to significantly enhancing proliferation and growth of NCSs *(65,66)*. Moreover, it has been shown that sAPP is able to activate mitogen-activated protein kinase (MAPK) (ERK) in PC12 cells via the Ras pathway *(67)*. Since MAPK activation can induce proliferation or differentiation, it is possible that sAPP activates this pathway in hNSC and induces cell differentiation.

These facts, together with our findings, indicate that one of APP's physiological functions may be the regulation of NSC biology to allow for the successful formation and replacement of crucial structures and neuronal circuits. A possible scenario to reconstruct neuronal circuits under the guidance of NSC could be that sAPP released from damaged or dying cells may preferentially induce glial differentiation of a population of NSCs. These NSC-derived glial cells can then produce factors that may support surrounding damaged cells and promote neuronal migration and differentiation of other NSCs in this area *(68)*.

This scenario fits nicely with our in vitro observations that the initial apoptotic cell death-induced glial differentiation was followed by neuronal differentiation *(8)*. Thus, under normal physiological conditions, APP may be necessary to recover from brain damage. In the cases of familial AD and Down's syndrome, the increased levels of APP fragments produced in the brains of these patients may modify the biological equilibrium of hNSC in such a way that a pathological shift toward premature differentiation of hNSC will occur, thereby exhausting the hNSC population. Since the effective natural replacement of degenerating neurons in the adult brain during aging or disease processes may be important in maintaining normal brain function, hNSC population exhaustion would pose serious problems.

THE IMPACT OF GENE MUTATIONS

Following some early findings of APP mutations in familial AD (FAD) *(69,70)*, it has been well recognized that the total number of FAD cases is far greater than could be accounted for by mutations in the APP gene, which led to investigations into other genes. Mutations of the presenilin 1 (PS1) gene located on chromosome 14 were found to be responsible for about 70% of FAD cases *(71)*. Additionally, a mutation of presenilin 2 (PS2) located on chromosome 1, which was identified by its homology to PS1, has been reported *(72)*.

Dominant mutations in either of these two PS genes appear to increase the amount of Aβ peptide fragments in vitro and in vivo *(72,73)*. Aβ peptide, which is heavily deposited in the brains of AD patients, is derived from APP as a result of cleavage by β- and γ-secretases. APP is a type-I integral-membrane protein that spans from the endoplasmic reticulum and Golgi apparatus to the cell surface and undergoes proteolytic processing. Cleavage by β-secretase occurs in the extracellular domain, producing a soluble membrane-associated carboxy-terminal ectodomain fragment; heterogeneous γ-secretase catalyzes an intramembranous cleavage of this fragment, resulting in the generation of Aβ and the production of a C-terminal fragment of APP. In recent studies, mice with a null allele of PS1 are reported to display selectively lower γ-secretase activity *(74)*. These observations indicate that PS either regulates the activity of γ-secretase or is itself a component of γ-secretase.

PS1-deficient mice also show developmental abnormalities and reduced NSC populations by premature differentiation of these cells, consistent with altered Notch signaling *(75)*. Furthermore, genetic interactions between the Notch homologs glp-1 and lin-12 and the PS homologs sel-12 and hop-1 in *Caenorhabditis elegans* (a small soil nematode) indicate the involvement of presenilin in the Notch signaling pathway *(76)*.

Notch is involved in critical intercellular signaling in a wide array of developmental processes that control the patterning of tissues. As an embryo develops, progenitor cells must differentiate and acquire distinct responsibilities, a process that involves communication and coordination among the emerging cells. The Notch family of genes encodes large proteins that contain segments within the membrane of the cell. These proteins act as receptors for extracellular ligands that specify cell fate, leading to tissue organization during development. Notch undergoes proteolytic processing similar to the β- and γ-secretase cleavages of APP. Notch is synthesized as a type-I integral-membrane protein with a relative molecular mass of 300 kDa, which is cleaved by a furin-like protease in the Golgi apparatus during movement to the cell surface. Signaling through Notch requires a ligand-induced cleavage occurring within the transmembrane domain that releases the Notch intracellular domain (NICD). NICD translocates to the nucleus, modifies the transcription of the target genes, and regulates the differentiation of NSC *(77)*. Thus, if a deficiency of adult neurogenesis is a factor in AD pathology, the role of FAD-linked PS mutations in the regulation of NSC biology should be considered.

We have also found evidence that APP signaling may be one of the regulatory systems involved in the differentiation of NSCs and that the pathological alteration of APP metabolism in AD may induce glial differentiation of NSCs and lead to the exhaustion of the stem cell population. This may be an important function in the ongoing neurogenesis of the adult brain.

In our study, the addition of recombinant sAPP to cell culture media dose-dependently differentiated hNSC under serum-free differentiation conditions. We also characterized the cell population of sAPP-treated hNSC at 5 DIV under the serum-free differentiation condition by double immunofluorescence labeling of GFAP and βIII-tubulin. Treatment with sAPP dose-dependently (25, 50,

100 ng/mL) increased the population of GFAP-positive cells from an average of 45% in controls (no sAPP) to an average of 83% using the highest concentration of sAPP (100 ng/mL at 5 DIV). Interestingly, it was observed that the lowest dose of sAPP treatment (25 ng/mL) also increased neuronal differentiation. However, higher doses of sAPP (50 and 100 ng/mL) dose-dependently decreased βIII-tubulin-positive neurons in the total population of differentiated hNSC. These results indicate that sAPP released from dying cells promotes differentiation of hNSC, while it causes gliogenesis at higher doses.

To confirm the glial differentiation-promoting effect of sAPP, hNSC were transfected with mammalian expression vectors containing genes for either wild-type APP or sAPP and differentiated under serum-free unsupplemented conditions. Human NSC transfected with wild-type APP revealed a significantly higher level of glial differentiation than hNSC transfected with the vector alone, at 5 DIV. These results indicate that, in addition to an excess of sAPP, wild-type APP overexpression can also induce glial differentiation of hNSC. These results indicate that released APP fragment(s) increased hNSC differentiation into glial cells, and overexpression of APP in hNSC by transfection with wild-type APP also induced glial differentiation, possibly contributing to the gliogenesis seen in AD.

Recently, Bahn and colleagues reported that stem cells from Down's syndrome subjects differentiated into astrocytes rather than neurons *(78)*. Since these patients have inherited three copies of APP (which reside on chromosome 21), this abnormal differentiation may result from an overdose of APP *(79)*. In addition to characteristic physical manifestations, Down's syndrome patients often exhibit early-onset AD. Arai and colleagues suggested that APP plays a role in neuronal development and that the earlier appearance of AD in adult Down's syndrome patients is associated with an abnormal regeneration process related to aging *(80)*. Thus, we speculate that transplantation therapy of AD with hNSC may not be effective in an environment in which APP metabolism is altered, since it might lead to excessive gliogenesis.

It is not clear whether adult neurogenesis is essential for normal cognitive function in aging. Nonetheless, it is tempting to hypothesize that pathologically altered APP metabolism could impair NSC migration and differentiation into a proper ratio of neurons and glia in AD. Aged transgenic APP mice exhibit neuronal loss and extensive gliogenesis in the neocortex *(81)*. Although the rate of endogenous neuroregeneration in the adult brain may be minimal, in the long run, a defect in this process might significantly harm normal brain function and also prevent successful neuroreplacement therapy for AD using NSCs, by shifting the differentiation pattern of the transplanted cells to glial cells rather than to neurons.

Incidentally, this possibility raises the question of whether Aβ immunization, which may also reduce APP fragments, is helpful for maintaining stem cell function in AD. My opinion is that it is not helpful because hNSC transplanted into APP-knockout mice do not migrate or effectively differentiate into neurons in the cerebral cortex. We have seen beautiful neural differentiation of transplanted hNSC in the cerebral cortex of wild-type mice in our studies. Human NSCs may play an important role in neuroregeneration—and if APP is, indeed, involved in the regulation of hNSC as we propose, destruction of the APP system may jeopardize the maintenance of normal brain function.

We further investigated the regulatory effect of APP on hNSC biology in vivo by transplanting hNSC into the brains of APP-knockout mice at 2 months of age *(82)*. Immunohistochemical examination of wild-type brain sections 4 weeks after transplantation revealed migration and differentiation patterns similar to our previous study with hNSC transplantation to aged memory-impaired rats *(11)*. Although hNSC transplanted into APP-knockout mice also differentiated into βIII-tubulin- and GFAP-positive cells, distribution and migration patterns were not symmetric and the number of the differentiated cells was lower than in control wild-type mice. Despite the rather uniform βIII-tubulin-positive cell distribution and structure in the hippocampus of APP-knockout mice, βIII-tubulin-positive hNSC almost did not exist in the cortex and these cells lacked apical dendrites. Although it is conceivable that the APP expression of transplanted hNSC can partially compensate for the APP deficit in the host brain, it is quite apparent that the level of compensation is negligible and that the absence of environmental

APP clearly alters the migration pattern of transplanted hNSC.

APP is part of a larger family comprising similar proteins, such as APLP1 and APLP2. Evolutionary studies have revealed a remarkable homology between these proteins, specifically in the N-terminal and C-terminal domains *(83,84)*. Additionally, double knockouts of both APP and APLP2 result in 80% death in the first week of life *(85)*. It is therefore possible that APLPs may compensate for the lack of APP. The successful migration of transplanted hNSC into the hippocampus of APP-knockout mice may thus be explained both by the compensatory APP function of APLPs and by the finding that APLP1 and APLP2 mRNA are highly abundant in granule cells of dentate gyrus in the hippocampus *(86)*. However, it appears that APLP function may not sufficiently replace APP, since the processes of transplanted hNSC in the hippocampus were haphazardly oriented compared with wild-type mice. These results indicate that there were insufficient environmental factors to properly guide the migration and differentiation of hNSC in APP-knockout mice, and that environmental or secreted APP may be important in regulating cell fate and migration of hNSC in vivo.

DOES APP REGULATE THE BIOLOGY OF NSCS?

These findings also indicate that one of the physiological functions of APP may be the regulation of NSC biology to allow for the successful formation and replacement of damaged structures and neuronal circuits. A possible scenario to reconstruct neuronal circuits under the guidance of NSCs could be that sAPP released from damaged or dying cells may preferentially induce glial differentiation of a specific population of NSCs. These NSC-derived glial cells can then produce factors that may support surrounding damaged cells and promote neuronal migration and differentiation of other NSCs in this area *(68)*.

This scenario fits nicely with our in vitro observations that initially, apoptotic cell death-induced glial differentiation was followed by neuronal differentiation *(8)*. Thus, under normal physiological conditions, APP may be necessary to recover from brain damage. In the cases of FAD and Down's syndrome, the increased levels of APP fragments produced in the brains of these patients may modify the biological equilibrium of hNSC in such a way that a pathological shift toward premature differentiation of hNSC will occur, thereby exhausting the hNSC population. Since the effective natural replacement of degenerating neurons in the adult brain during aging or the disease process may be important in maintaining normal brain function, exhaustion of the hNSC population would pose serious problems.

CONCLUSION

Clinical trials of NSC transplantation for AD seem to be around the corner. This approach, however, will take time to be established as a potential therapeutic option for AD. We need to know the effects NSC will have in the AD brain and how AD brain environment affects NSC biology. I personally hope our efforts in stem cell and AD research will reduce the time needed to develop better treatments for AD.

SUMMARY

The discovery of multipotent stem cells in the adult brain has brought about revolutionary changes in neurogenesis theory, which now suggests that neuronal regeneration can occur throughout life. The use of stem cells for neuroreplacement therapy is no longer science fiction—it is science fact. We have seen the improvement of cognitive function in a memory-impaired aged animal model following neural stem cell transplantation, suggesting a potential for neuroreplacement therapies in aged subjects. We are also able to produce neurons and glias from adult human mesenchymal stem cells, allowing us to perform autologus transplantation. Although these results may promise a bright future for stem cell strategies in AD therapy, we must address and weigh the factors that may affect stem cell biology under the pathological condition of this disease before we proceed to clinical applications of this technology. Here, we not only show the potential for therapeutic applications for stem cell strategies in AD therapy, we also discuss the effects on the biology of stem cells by those factors that are altered under the disease conditions.

REFERENCES

1. Alvarez-Buylla, A.; Kirn, J.R.: Birth, migration, incorporation, and death of vocal control neurons in adult songbirds. J Neurobiol 1997; 33: 585–601.
2. Gould, E. et al.: Hippocampal neurogenesis in adult Old World primates. Proc Natl Acad Sci USA 1999; 96: 5263–5267.
3. Doetsch, F. et al.: Subventricular zone astrocytes are neural stem cells in the adult mammalian brain. Cell 1999; 97: 703–716.
4. Johansson, C.B. et al.: Neural stem cells in the adult human brain. Exp Cell Res 1999; 253: 733–736.
5. Johansson, C.B. et al.: Identification of a neural stem cell in the adult mammalian central nervous system. Cell 1999; 96: 25–34.
6. Svendsen, C.N. et al.: A new method for the rapid and long-term growth of human neural precursor cells. J Neurosci Meth 1998; 85: 141–152.
7. Sinden, J.D. et al.: Functional repair with neural stem cells. Novartis Found Symp 2000; 231: 270–283.
8. Brannen, C.L.; Sugaya, K.: In vitro differentiation of multipotent human neural progenitors in serum-free medium. Neuroreport 2000; 11: 1123–1128.
9. Fricker, R.A. et al.: Site-specific migration and neuronal differentiation of human neural progenitor cells after transplantation in the adult rat brain. J Neurosci 1999; 19: 5990–6005.
10. Ostenfeld, T. et al.: Human neural precursor cells express low levels of telomerase in vitro and show diminishing cell proliferation with extensive axonal outgrowth following transplantation. Exp Neurol 2000; 164: 215–226.
11. Qu, T. et al.: Human neural stem cells improve cognitive function of aged brain. Neuroreport 2001; 12: 1127–1132.
12. Clarkson, E.D.: Fetal tissue transplantation for patients with Parkinson's disease: a database of published clinical results. Drugs Aging 2001; 18: 773–785.
13. Freed, C.R. et al.: Transplantation of embryonic dopamine neurons for severe Parkinson's disease. N Engl J Med 2001; 344: 710–719.
14. Rideout, W.M. 3rd; Eggan, K.; Jaenisch, R.: Nuclear cloning and epigenetic reprogramming of the genome. Science 2001; 293: 1093–1098.
15. Humpherys, D. et al.: Epigenetic instability in ES cells and cloned mice. Science 2001; 293: 95–97.
16. Majumdar, M.K. et al.: Phenotypic and functional comparison of cultures of marrow-derived mesenchymal stem cells (MSCs) and stromal cells. J Cell Physiol 1998; 176: 57–66.
17. Pereira, R.F. et al.: Cultured adherent cells from marrow can serve as long-lasting precursor cells for bone, cartilage, and lung in irradiated mice. Proc Natl Acad Sci USA 1995; 92: 4857–4861.
18. Prockop, D.J.: Marrow stromal cells as stem cells for nonhematopoietic tissues. Science 1997; 276: 71–74.
19. Pittenger, M.F. et al.: Multilineage potential of adult human mesenchymal stem cells. Science 1999; 284: 143–147.
20. Ferrari, G. et al.: Muscle regeneration by bone marrow-derived myogenic progenitors. Science 1998; 279: 1528–1530.
21. Makino, S. et al.: Cardiomyocytes can be generated from marrow stromal cells in vitro. J Clin Invest 1999; 103: 697–705.
22. Petersen, B.E. et al.: Bone marrow as a potential source of hepatic oval cells. Science 1999; 284: 1168–1170.
23. Mackenzie, T.C.; Flake, A.W.: Human mesenchymal stem cells persist, demonstrate site-specific multipotential differentiation, and are present in sites of wound healing and tissue regeneration after transplantation into fetal sheep. Blood Cells Mol Dis 2001; 27: 601–604.
24. Imasawa, T. et al.: The potential of bone marrow-derived cells to differentiate to glomerular mesangial cells. J Am Soc Nephrol 2001; 12: 1401–1409.
25. Liechty, K.W. et al.: Human mesenchymal stem cells engraft and demonstrate site-specific differentiation after in utero transplantation in sheep. Nat Med 2000; 6: 1282–1286.
26. Prockop, D.J. et al.: Potential use of marrow stromal cells as therapeutic vectors for diseases of the central nervous system. Prog Brain Res 2000; 128: 293–297.
27. Bianco, P. et al.: Bone marrow stromal stem cells: nature, biology, and potential applications. Stem Cells 2001; 19: 180–192.
28. Schwarz, E.J. et al.: Multipotential marrow stromal cells transduced to produce L-DOPA: engraftment in a rat model of Parkinson disease. Hum Gene Ther 1999; 10: 2539–2549.
29. Chopp, M. et al.: Spinal cord injury in rat: treatment with bone marrow stromal cell transplantation. Neuroreport 2000; 11: 3001–3005.
30. Chen, J.; Li, Y.; Chopp, M.: Intracerebral transplantation of bone marrow with BDNF after MCAo in rat. Neuropharmacology 2000; 39: 711–716.
31. Li, Y. et al.: Intrastriatal transplantation of bone marrow nonhematopoietic cells improves functional recovery after stroke in adult mice. J Cereb Blood Flow Metab 2000; 20: 1311–1319.

32. Kopen, G.C.; Prockop, D.J.; Phinney, D.G.: Marrow stromal cells migrate throughout forebrain and cerebellum, and they differentiate into astrocytes after injection into neonatal mouse brains. Proc Natl Acad Sci USA 1999; 96: 10711–10716.

33. Jiang, Y. et al.: Pluripotency of mesenchymal stem cells derived from adult marrow. Nature 2002; 418: 41–49.

34. Terada, N. et al.: Bone marrow cells adopt the phenotype of other cells by spontaneous cell fusion. Nature 2002; 416: 542–545.

35. Ying, Q.L. et al.: Changing potency by spontaneous fusion. Nature 2002; 416: 545–548.

36. Martinez-Serrano, A.; Hantzopoulos, P.A.; Bjorklund, A.: Ex vivo gene transfer of brain-derived neurotrophic factor to the intact rat forebrain: neurotrophic effects on cholinergic neurons. Eur J Neurosci 1996; 8: 727–735.

37. Roch, J.M. et al.: Biologically active domain of the secreted form of the amyloid beta/A4 protein precursor. Ann N Y Acad Sci 1993; 695: 149–157.

38. Salinero, O.; Moreno-Flores, M.T.; Wandosell, F.: Increasing neurite outgrowth capacity of beta-amyloid precursor protein proteoglycan in Alzheimer's disease. J Neurosci Res 2000; 60: 87–97.

39. Hayashi, Y. et al.: Alzheimer amyloid protein precursor enhances proliferation of neural stem cells from fetal rat brain. Biochem Biophys Res Commun 1994; 205: 936–943.

40. Hoffmann, J. et al.: A possible role for the Alzheimer amyloid precursor protein in the regulation of epidermal basal cell proliferation. Eur J Cell Biol 2000; 79: 905–914.

41. Ohsawa, I. et al.: Amino-terminal region of secreted form of amyloid precursor protein stimulates proliferation of neural stem cells. Eur J Neurosci 1999; 11: 1907–1913.

42. De Strooper, B.; Annaert, W.: Proteolytic processing and cell biological functions of the amyloid precursor protein. J Cell Sci 2000; 113 (pt 11): 1857–1870.

43. Ando, K. et al.: Role of phosphorylation of Alzheimer's amyloid precursor protein during neuronal differentiation. J Neurosci 1999; 19: 4421–4427.

44. Koszyca, B. et al.: Widespread axonal injury in gunshot wounds to the head using amyloid precursor protein as a marker. J Neurotrauma 1998; 15: 675–683.

45. Murakami, N. et al.: Experimental brain injury induces expression of amyloid precursor protein, which may be related to neuronal loss in the hippocampus. J Neurotrauma 1998; 15: 993–1003.

46. Galli, C. et al.: Increased amyloidogenic secretion in cerebellar granule cells undergoing apoptosis. Proc Natl Acad Sci USA 1998; 95: 1247–1252.

47. Rohn, T.T. et al.: A monoclonal antibody to amyloid precursor protein induces neuronal apoptosis. J Neurochem 2000; 74: 2331–2342.

48. Wallace, W.C. et al.: Amyloid precursor protein requires the insulin signaling pathway for neurotrophic activity. Brain Res Mol Brain Res 1997; 52: 213–227.

49. Wang, C.; Wurtman, R.J.; Lee, R.K.: Amyloid precursor protein and membrane phospholipids in primary cortical neurons increase with development, or after exposure to nerve growth factor or Abeta (1-40). Brain Res 2000; 865: 157–167.

50. Serby, M.: Olfaction and Alzheimer's disease. Prog Neuropsychopharmacol Biol Psychiatry 1986; 10: 579–586.

51. Bacon Moore, A.S.; Paulsen, J.S.; Murphy, C.: A test of odor fluency in patients with Alzheimer's and Huntington's disease. J Clin Exp Neuropsychol 1999; 21: 341–351.

52. Murphy, C.; Jinich, S.: Olfactory dysfunction in Down's syndrome. Neurobiol Aging 1996; 17: 631–637.

53. Murphy, C.: Loss of olfactory function in dementing disease. Physiol Behav 1999; 66: 177–182.

54. Crews, L.; Hunter, D.: Neurogenesis in the olfactory epithelium. Perspect Dev Neurobiol 1994; 2: 151–161.

55. Yi, M. et al.: Evidence that the Igkappa gene MAR regulates the probability of premature V-J joining and somatic hypermutation. J Immunol 1999; 162: 6029–6039.

56. Alonso, G.; Prieto, M.; Chauvet, N.: Tangential migration of young neurons arising from the subventricular zone of adult rats is impaired by surgical lesions passing through their natural migratory pathway. J Comp Neurol 1999; 405: 508–528.

57. LeBlanc, A.: Increased production of 4 kDa amyloid beta peptide in serum deprived human primary neuron cultures: possible involvement of apoptosis. J Neurosci 1995; 15: 7837–7846.

58. Huang, H.M.; Ou, H.C.; Hsieh, S.J.: Antioxidants prevent amyloid peptide-induced apoptosis and alteration of calcium homeostasis in cultured cortical neurons. Life Sci 2000; 66: 1879–1892.

59. LeBlanc, A. et al.: Caspase-6 role in apoptosis of human neurons, amyloidogenesis, and Alzheimer's disease. J Biol Chem 1999; 274: 23426–23436.

60. Piccini, A. et al.: Endogenous APP derivatives oppositely modulate apoptosis through an autocrine loop. Neuroreport 2000; 11: 1375–1379.

61. Hugon, J. et al.: Toxic neuronal apoptosis and modifications of tau and APP gene and protein expressions. Drug Metab Rev 1999; 31: 635–647.

62. Hung, A.Y. et al.: Increased expression of beta-amyloid precursor protein during neuronal differentiation is not accompanied by secretory cleavage. Proc Natl Acad Sci USA 1992; 89: 9439–9443.

63. Beckman, M.; Iverfeldt, K.: Increased gene expression of beta-amyloid precursor protein and its homologues APLP1 and APLP2 in human neuroblastoma cells in response to retinoic acid. Neurosci Lett 1997; 221: 73–76.

64. Kirazov, E. et al.: Ontogenetic changes in protein level of amyloid precursor protein (APP) in growth cones and synaptosomes from rat brain and prenatal expression pattern of APP mRNA isoforms in developing rat embryo. Int J Dev Neurosci 2001; 19: 287–296.

65. Ishiguro, M. et al.: Secreted form of beta-amyloid precursor protein activates protein kinase C and phospholipase Cgamma1 in cultured embryonic rat neocortical cells. Brain Res Mol Brain Res 1998; 53: 24–32.

66. Ohsawa, I.: Takamura, C.; Kohsaka, S.: Fibulin-1 binds the amino-terminal head of beta-amyloid precursor protein and modulates its physiological function. J Neurochem 2001; 76: 1411–1420.

67. Greenberg, S.M. et al.: Secreted beta-amyloid precursor protein stimulates mitogen-activated protein kinase and enhances tau phosphorylation. Proc Natl Acad Sci USA 1994; 91: 7104–7108.

68. Miyachi, T. et al.: Interleukin-1beta induces the expression of lipocortin 1 mRNA in cultured rat cortical astrocytes. Neurosci Res 2001; 40: 53–60.

69. Sorbi, S.; Forleo, P.; Nacmias, B.: Alzheimer's disease: phenotypes and genotypes. Funct Neurol 1997; 12: 147–151.

70. Karran, E.H. et al.: Presenilins—in search of functionality. Biochem Soc Trans 1998; 26: 491–496.

71. Clark, R.F. et al.: The role of presenilin 1 in the genetics of Alzheimer's disease. Cold Spring Harb Symp Quant Biol 1996; 61: 551–558.

72. Levy-Lahad, E. et al.: A familial Alzheimer's disease locus on chromosome 1. Science 1995; 269: 970–973.

73. Duff, K. et al.: Increased amyloid-beta42(43) in brains of mice expressing mutant presenilin 1. Nature 1996; 383: 710–713.

74. Steiner, H.; Pesold, B.; Haass, C.: An in vivo assay for the identification of target proteases, which cleave membrane-associated substrates. FEBS Lett 1999; 463: 245–249.

75. Yang, X.; Handler, M.; Shen, J.: Role of presenilin-1 in murine neural development. Ann N Y Acad Sci 2000; 920: 165–170.

76. Ray, W.J. et al.: Evidence for a physical interaction between presenilin and Notch. Proc Natl Acad Sci USA 1999; 96: 3263–3268.

77. Schuldt, A.J.; Brand, A.H.: Mastermind acts downstream of notch to specify neuronal cell fates in the *Drosophila* central nervous system. Dev Biol 1999; 205: 287–295.

78. Bahn, S. et al.: Neuronal target genes of the neuron-restrictive silencer factor in neurospheres derived from fetuses with Down's syndrome: a gene expression study. Lancet 2002; 359: 310–315.

79. Sawa, A.: Neuronal cell death in Down's syndrome. J Neural Transm Suppl 1999; 57: 87–97.

80. Arai, Y. et al.: Developmental and aging changes in the expression of amyloid precursor protein in Down's syndrome brains. Brain Dev 1997; 19: 290–294.

81. Bondolfi, L. et al.: Amyloid-associated neuron loss and gliogenesis in the neocortex of amyloid precursor protein transgenic mice. J Neurosci 2002; 22: 515–522.

82. White, A.R. et al.: Survival of cultured neurons from amyloid precursor protein knock-out mice against Alzheimer's amyloid-beta toxicity and oxidative stress. J Neurosci 1998; 18: 6207–6217.

83. Coulson, E.J. et al.: What the evolution of the amyloid protein precursor supergene family tells us about its function. Neurochem Int 2000; 36: 175–184.

84. Wasco, W. et al.: Identification of a mouse brain cDNA that encodes a protein related to the Alzheimer disease-associated amyloid beta protein precursor. Proc Natl Acad Sci USA 1992; 89: 10758–10762.

85. Von Koch, C.S. et al.: Generation of APLP2 KO mice and early postnatal lethality in APLP2/APP double KO mice. Neurobiol Aging 1997; 18: 661–669.

86. McNamara, M.J. et al.: Immunohistochemical and in situ analysis of amyloid precursor-like protein-1 and amyloid precursor-like protein-2 expression in Alzheimer disease and aged control brains. Brain Res 1998; 804: 45–51.

34

Secretases as Potential Targets for Treatment of Alzheimer's Disease

Weiming Xia

INTRODUCTION

Brains of patients with Alzheimer's disease (AD) are characteristic of amyloid plaques and neurofibrillary tangles. Neurofibrillary tangles are found in select neuronal cell bodies, and these intraneuronal paired helical filaments are composed of hyperphosphorylated forms of tau protein. Amyloid plaques are extracellular fibrils composed of amyloid β-protein (Aβ). The well-defined neuritic plaques are closely associated with dystrophic dendrites and axons, suggesting an intimate connection of Aβ and neuronal toxicity. Results from extensive studies on Aβ metabolism strongly support the hypothesis that gradual accumulation of Aβ in brains is the main contributor to the neuropathogenesis of AD *(1)*.

THE ROLE OF Aβ IN AD PATHOGENESIS

Amyloid precursor protein (APP) occurs in three alternative spliced forms—695-, 751-, and 770-residue polypeptides. APP is mainly cleaved by α-secretase to generate a soluble N-terminal fragment of APP (APPsα) and an 83-residue C-terminal fragment (C83) (Fig. 1). Alternatively, a small portion of APP is cleaved by β-secretase to produce a slightly shorter N-terminal fragment of APP (APPsβ) and a 99-residue C-terminal fragment (C99). Both C83 and C99 are subsequently cleaved by γ-secretase to generate p3 and Aβ, respectively *(2)*. The other peptide derived from γ-secretase cleavage of C83/C99 is called amyloid intracellular domain (AICD), and has been shown to translocate into the nucleus and regulate downstream gene expression *(3)*. Since α-secretase cleaves APP at the site corresponding to the middle of the Aβ region, APP molecules undergoing α-secretase cleavage do not lead to the formation of Aβ (nonamyloidogenic pathway). Theoretically, enhancing α-secretase activity could divert APP from its amyloidogenic pathway (β-secretase cleavage of APP) and reduce the production of Aβ. However, increasing a protease activity has rarely been a successful therapeutic approach, due mainly to nonspecific proteolysis of other biologically critical proteins. Currently, there is no ongoing clinical trial on an α-secretase enhancer.

Soluble Aβ exists in both intracellular compartments and extracellular space. A portion of soluble Aβ species undergo oligomerization, a process that may initiate inside of cells *(4)*. These small-molecular-weight oligomers further aggregate to protofibrils *(5)*, the intermediate Aβ species that gradually transform to mature amyloid fibrils. All three forms of Aβ have been reported to cause neuronal toxicity in vivo or in cultured primary neurons derived from embryonic tissues.

Recent studies have shown that cell-derived oligomeric Aβ species are able to inhibit hippocampal long-term potentiation in rats in vivo *(6)*. The protofibril Aβ converted from synthetic Aβ peptides has been found to severely change the electrical activity of neurons and gradually cause neuronal loss

From: *Current Clinical Neurology,*
Alzheimer's Disease: A Physician's Guide to Practical Management
Edited by: R. W. Richter and B. Zoeller Richter © Humana Press Inc., Totowa, NJ

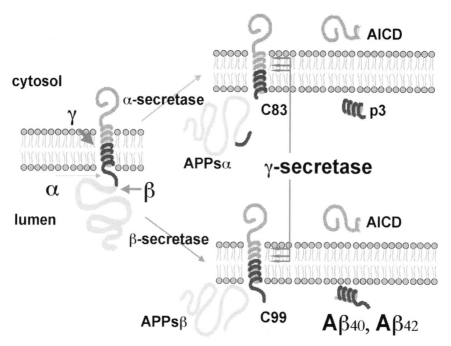

Fig. 1. Proteolytic processing of β-amyloid precursor protein by secretases. APP mainly undergoes a non-amyloidogenic pathway and is cleaved by α-secretase to generate a soluble N-terminal fragment of APP (APPsα) and an 83-residue C-terminal fragment (C83). Alternatively, APP undergoes an amyloidogenic pathway and is cleaved by β-secretase to produce a shorter N-terminal fragment of APP (APPsβ) and a 99-residue C-terminal fragment (C99). Both C83 and C99 are subsequently cleaved by γ-secretase at multiple sites to generate p3, Aβ, and amyloid intracellular domain (AICD). The 40- and 42-residue Aβ peptides (Aβ40 and Aβ42) are the major components of amyloid plaques found in brains of AD patients.

(7). Earlier studies have shown that aggregated fibril Aβ has a clear neurotoxic effect on cultured neurons. Quantitation of immunohistochemical staining of thioflavin S-positive fibrillar Aβ and closely associated neurons in AD and transgenic mouse brain tissues also shows that fibrillar Aβ is toxic to neurons *(8)*.

Analysis of proteins encoded by four genes genetically linked to AD further strengthens the implication of Aβ in pathogenesis of AD. Missense mutations in APP, presenilin 1 (PS1), and PS2 genes account for more than 50% of early-onset familial AD cases, and a polymorphism of the apolipoprotein E (ApoE) gene (e4) has been demonstrated to be a major risk factor for sporadic AD. Studies using cultured cells and transgenic mice overexpressing a mutant APP or PS gene all show a uniform increase of the 42-residue of Aβ, and in some cases (Swedish mutation of APP) an increase of all forms of Aβ *(2)*. Patients carrying the ApoEe4-allele have shown an increase of Aβ plaques *(9)*. These results, along with other studies, clearly suggest that gradual deposition of Aβ in brains is one of the main causes of AD. Therefore, interfering with Aβ-generating secretases is one of the primary approaches to prevent Aβ deposition and delay the onset of AD.

β-SECRETASE

Multiple approaches have been applied to search for the major secretase that controls the levels of Aβ generation, β-secretase. Expression cloning *(10)*, protease purification *(11)*, and aspartyl protease motif search in database *(12,13)*, carried out by several groups, led to the identification of an aspartyl protease, BACE1, which is responsible for the β-secretase cleavage of APP.

BACE1 is a 501-amino acid protein containing a single transmembrane (TM) domain. It is highly expressed in all brain regions, whereas the pancreas is the only peripheral tissue that expresses high levels of BACE1. A signal peptide of BACE1 is cleaved after synthesis, and the precursor of BACE1, proBACE1, is further cleaved by a furin-like convertase after exiting the endoplasmic reticulum (ER) *(14)*. Intracellularly, BACE1 is localized to the Golgi, trans-Golgi network (TGN), secretory vesicles, cell surface, and endosomes *(10,15)*.

One of the most exciting findings in targeting secretases for reducing Aβ came from studies using mice deficient in the BACE1 gene *(16,17)*. As expected, levels of Aβ in brains of these mice drop to almost undetectable amounts, demonstrating a major role of BACE1 for producing Aβ. These mice do not show any abnormal phenotype, predicting a lack of severe contraindication if BACE1 is targeted for inhibition. Surprisingly, a highly homologous protease of BACE1—BACE2—does not compensate for the loss of BACE1 to actively cleave APP to generate Aβ.

Although BACE2 was found to cleave APP at Asp1 of Aβ (like BACE1) and in the middle of the Aβ region (Phe19 and Phe20 of Aβ, an activity similar to α-secretase) *(18,19)*, it does not function as the major β-secretase to cleave APP at Asp 1 of Aβ. Consistent with high expression levels of BACE2 in the heart, kidney, and placenta but low levels in the brain *(20)*, BACE2 is unlikely to contribute to Aβ generation in brains.

Purified, soluble BACE1 fused to immunoglobulin G from mammalian cells is able to cleave synthetic peptide substrates in vitro, suggesting that BACE1 dose not need to anchor to the membrane for its proteolytic activity *(10)*. The C-terminal region of BACE1 is likewise not required, as the C-terminal truncated BACE1 from *Escherichia coli* shows specific cleavage of peptide substrates *(13)*. In a complex with an inhibitor, the crystal structure of soluble BACE1 (without TM and cytosolic domain) has been determined, which has opened up the venue to design specific BACE1 inhibitors to target this rate-limiting secretase for Aβ generation *(21)*.

γ-SECRETASE

Conversion of C99 into Aβ by γ-secretase cleavage occurs in the middle region of the APP transmembrane domain. Additional cleavage of C99 at a site 9 residues downstream of the Aβ-40 cleavage site is also mediated by γ-secretase, but it is not clear whether this cleavage of C99 contributes to Aβ generation *(22–24)*. It has been demonstrated that PS1, and its homolog, PS2, are required for γ-secretase activity. In primary neurons cultured from PS-knockout embryos, Aβ production was completely eliminated *(25,26)*. In the brains of conditional PS-knockout mice, levels of Aβ were also significantly reduced *(27)*.

In cultured cells, generation of Aβ is blocked when two critical aspartate residues in transmembrane domains 6 and 7 of PS1 are mutated *(28)*. Mutation of these two conserved aspartate residues in PS2 similarly block Aβ generation *(29,30)*, and overexpression of both aspartate mutant PS1 and PS2 decreases generation of Aβ to undetectable levels *(30)*.

Recent studies suggest that γ-secretase is actually a high-molecular-weight complex containing multiple components that include PS1, nicastrin, APH-1, and PEN-2 *(31–34)*. Because PS1 and PS1 homologs have nonclassic protease motifs conserved from bacteria to human *(35,36)*, including a recently identified signal peptide peptidase *(37,38)*, PS1 most likely contains the active site of γ-secretase.

In contrast to BACE1-knockout mice, deletion of PS1 in mice is lethal, with a major disruption of somite segmentation *(39,40)*. Neurogenesis is impaired and massive neuronal loss is observed in specific regions *(39)*. Although the molecular mechanisms for causing these defects are not completely understood, a lack of proteolysis of several biologically important molecules in the absence of PS1 may contribute to the phenotype of PS1-knockout mice. In addition to APP and its homologs APLP1 and APLP2, an increasing number of γ-secretase substrates are reported, including Notch *(41)*, low-density lipoprotein receptor-related protein (LRP) *(42)*, ErbB-4 *(43)*, E-cadherin *(44)*, CD44 *(45)*, and nectin1α *(46)*.

Notch is known to be critically involved in cell fate decisions during development, and ErbB-4 is a transmembrane receptor tyrosine kinase that regulates cell proliferation and differentiation. LRP is a cell surface receptor that interacts through its cytoplasmic tail with adaptor and scaffold proteins that participate in cellular signaling. E-cadherin controls cell–cell adhesion, differentiation, and tissue development, and CD44 is also a cell-surface adhesion protein. Nectin-1α is an immunoglobulin-like receptor and a Ca^{2+}-independent adherens junction protein involved in the formation of synapses.

These substrates are involved in diverse pathways related to many fundamental cellular processes. Apparently, designing a compound that can specifically block the γ-secretase cleavage of APP without affecting these substrates remains a huge challenge.

β-SECRETASE INHIBITORS

An inhibitor of BACE1, based on the sequence of the APP cleavage site, was used for initial purification of BACE1 from the human brain *(11)*. The IC_{50} of this inhibitor was found at 30 n*M* when used in an in vitro BACE1 activity assay. Another inhibitor containing isostere hydroxyethylene in EVNL*AAEF (sequence of Swedish mutant APP except Asp 1 was replaced with Ala) was able to form a complex with the catalytic domain of BACE1 for determination of the crystal structure *(21)*. A modified, more potent inhibitor, ELDL*AVEF *(47)*, was conjugated to a carrier peptide that facilitates penetration of the cell membrane, eliminating Aβ production in cells stably expressing BACE1 and the substrate Swedish mutant APP. The carrier peptide used here was a relative large peptide of nine D-Arg *(48)*.

It appears that easy delivery of the membrane permeable BACE1 inhibitor to the proper subcellular location should be considered during drug screening. In this regard, a cell-based screening system should have an advantage over the system using an in vitro BACE1 activity assay. Cells expressing a fusion protein containing the secreted form of alkaline phosphatase and the APP C-terminal fragment with a mutated α-secretase cleavage site were reported for screening a library of compounds for direct and indirect inhibition of BACE1. Levels of secreted alkaline phosphatase activity corresponded directly to the cleavage of APP by BACE1 *(49)*.

Once a membrane-permeable drug is found from cell-based assay, it should be analyzed for its capability to cross the blood–brain barrier. Theoretically, to make it much easier to cross the blood–brain barrier, an ideal small-molecular-weight drug should be lipophilic and smaller than 700 Da *(21)*. To block the large open active site of BACE1 (two aspartate residue-containing motifs—D(T/S)G(T/S)—corresponding to residues 93–96 and 289–292) with a small-molecule-weight drug, additional modification of currently available compounds is necessary, for example, elimination of noncritical residues in peptidomimetic compounds. Because the crystal structure of BACE1 is available, molecular modeling of the protease with putative inhibitors will likely overcome these difficulties. In light of the normal phenotype of BACE1-knockout mice *(16,17)*, in vivo testing of BACE1 inhibitors will not lead to foreseeable defects. Therefore, inhibiting BACE1 holds great promise in reducing Aβ burden in AD.

γ-SECRETASE INHIBITOR

Compared to the wealth of information of β-secretase (cloning of BACE1, purification of the soluble form of the active enzyme, crystallization of BACE1/inhibitor complex), our understanding of γ-secretase is not definitive. Several γ-secretase inhibitors, under the definition of blocking Aβ production without inhibiting β-secretase, have been successfully utilized to characterize the biochemical properties of γ-secretase.

For example, a γ-secretase inhibitor can specifically block *de novo* Aβ generation in the Golgi/TGN-enriched vesicles *(50)*, where PS1 and PS2 bind to C99/C83 *(51)*. Aspartyl protease transition-state analog inhibitors of γ-secretase bind directly to PS1 N-terminal fragment (NTF) and C-terminal fragment (CTF) (the functional form of PS1 derived from endoproteolysis of full-length PS1 by an unidentified protease activity named presenilinase) *(52)*, suggesting that the protease active site lies between the PS NTF and CTF *(53–55)*.

Whether PS1 should be the target for blocking γ-secretase activity is unclear. It has been reported that certain γ-secretase inhibitors can block presenilinase-mediated conversion of full-length PS1 into functional NTF and CTF in vivo and in vitro *(56,57)*. Some inhibitors are more potent in blocking presenilinase than γ-secretase *(58)*. Because of the defective phenotypes of PS1-knockout mice, completely blocking PS1 activity through inhibitor binding may not be the perfect choice.

Other than its direct participation in γ-secretase cleavage of many biological important substrates including Notch, PS1 may be involved in other metabolic processes, such as the β-catenin-mediated signaling pathway *(59,60)*. Interfering with these pathways potentially introduces new risk factors. For example, a known γ-secretase inhibitor has been shown to repress thymocyte development *(61)*. To overcome these limitations, treatment with a γ-secretase inhibitor should only be considered at a postdevelopmental stage and at concentrations that do not affect Notch and other important signaling molecules, while still partially reducing Aβ generation.

Apparently, testing γ-secretase inhibitors in vivo can address most of these concerns. A recent report has shown that treatment of APP transgenic mice close to 7 months of age with a γ-secretase inhibitor reduces brain Aβ levels within 3 hours *(62)*; chronic treatment up to 3 months results in 80–90% reduction in both total Aβ and Aβ42 levels *(63)*. In the absence of any gross pathological changes observed at necropsy, specific neuritic pathology and glial inflammatory response were suppressed by chronic treatment *(63)*.

When another γ-secretase inhibitor was used to treat transgenic mice, plasma Aβ levels were rapidly reduced within 1 hour of treatment; brain Aβ levels were also reduced at a later time (8 hours) after a higher dose of compound E was used *(64)*.

These data suggest that reduction of plasma Aβ precedes the clearance of Aβ in the brain in the presence of a γ-secretase inhibitor. Plasma Aβ42 might serve as a biological marker to track the efficacy of γ-secretase inhibitors for future clinical trials, in addition to its previously reported use as a surrogate to search for AD risk genes *(65)*.

Currently, a large number of γ-secretase inhibitors are being explored to specifically reduce Aβ generation and Aβ-associated pathological changes without causing major side effects. A functional γ-secretase inhibitor does not need to completely block Aβ generation. As long as the levels of Aβ are reduced, Aβ-associated pathology might be attenuated, which may lead to a delay of the onset of disease.

One class of promising inhibitors that may directly affect γ-secretase is nonsteroidal antiinflammatory drugs (NSAIDs) *(66)*. NSAIDs were shown to reduce Aβ42 more efficiently in cells overexpressing FAD (familial AD) mutant PS1 than that of wild-type PS1, suggesting that NSAIDs may directly affect the conformation of PS1 in the γ-secretase complex *(67)*. Furthermore, NSAIDs were found to decrease Aβ42 production in an in vitro γ-secretase assay, excluding the possibility that NSAIDs reduce Aβ42 production by activation of receptor-mediated pathways, such as the one involving peroxisome proliferator-activated receptors (PPAR) *(67)*.

Using NSAIDs to lower Aβ42 generation may avoid a contraindication, since these NSAIDs have been widely used for many years. Clinical trials of NSAIDs are actively pursued to examine whether they can be used for the treatment of AD.

SUMMARY OF CURRENT KNOWLEDGE AND IMPLICATIONS

Experimental data generated from genetic and epidemiological studies have been the base of several hypotheses on the pathogenesis of AD. The amyloid hypothesis predicts that the gradual deposition of Aβ is the primary cause of AD, and any increase of Aβ production and/or reduction of Aβ clearance leads to plaque formation as well as other pathological alterations including formation of neurofibrillary tangles. Because of a large body of evidence supporting this hypothesis, two secretases, β- and γ-secretases—responsible for the cleavage of APP and generation of Aβ—become primary therapeutic targets.

Although γ-secretase is not definitively identified, PS1 is an indispensable component of a large γ-secretase complex and likely contains the active site of γ-secretase. Mice lacking PS1 do not survive after birth—in part due to the requirement of PS1 for γ-secretase cleavages of multiple biologically important molecules. A compound that partially reduces γ-secretase activity and decreases Aβ production without affecting the cleavage of other substrates would be ideal, as a slight reduction of Aβ deposition could potentially postpone the onset of AD by a number of years.

BACE1, the aspartyl protease responsible for β-secretase activity, has been cloned, and crystal structure of BACE1 complexing with an inhibitor has revealed a large open active site. Despite the challenge of identifying blood–brain barrier-permeable small-molecule drugs, the findings that mice deficient in BACE1 gene lack Aβ production and do not have any abnormal phenotype clearly make BACE1 a superb target for therapeutic intervention.

SUMMARY

Amyloid plaques and neurofibrillary tangles are invariable neuropathological features of Alzheimer's disease. Amyloid plaques are composed of amyloid β-protein (Aβ), a 40- or 42-amino acid peptide derived from two sequential proteolytic cleavages of β-amyloid precursor protein (APP) by a recently cloned aspartyl protease, BACE1, and an elusive γ-secretase activity. Findings from genetic, biochemical, and immunohistochemical studies suggest that accumulation of Aβ in AD brains could be one of the primary causes of AD pathology. Since levels of Aβ are regulated by both BACE1 and γ-secretases, potential candidates to block BACE1 and γ-secretase are actively pursued. Currently, no U.S. Food and Drug Administration (FDA)-approved drug is available to target these two proteases.

REFERENCES

1. Hardy, J. et al.: The amyloid hypothesis of Alzheimer's disease: progress and problems on the road to therapeutics. Science 2002; 297: 353–356.
2. Selkoe, D.J.: Translating cell biology into therapeutic advances in Alzheimer's disease. Nature 1999; 399 (suppl): A23–A31.
3. Cao, X. et al.: A transcriptionally active complex of APP with Fe65 and histone acetyltransferase Tip60. Science 2001; 293: 115–120.
4. Walsh, D.M. et al.: Detection of intracellular oligomers of amyloid β-protein in cells derived from human brain. Biochemistry 2000; 39: 10831–10839.
5. Harper, J.D. et al.: Assembly of Aβ amyloid protofibrils: an in vitro model for a possible early event in Alzheimer's disease. Biochem 1999; 38: 8972–8980.
6. Walsh, DM. et al.: Naturally secreted oligomers of amyloid β protein potently inhibit hippocampal long-term potentiation in vivo. Nature 2002; 416: 535–539.
7. Hartley, D. et al.: Protofibrillar intermediates of amyloid β-protein induce acute electrophysiological changes and progressive neurotoxicity in cortical neurons. J. Neurosci 1999; 19: 8876–8884.
8. Urbanc, B. et al.: Neurotoxic effects of thioflavin S-positive amyloid deposits in transgenic mice and Alzheimer's disease. Proc Natl Acad Sci USA 2002; 99: 13990–13995.
9. Schmechel, D.E. et al.: Increased amyloid β-peptide deposition in cerebral cortex as a consequence of apolipoprotein E genotype in late-onset Alzheimer disease. Proc Natl Acad Sci USA 1993; 90: 9649–9653.
10. Vassar, R. et al.: β-secretase cleavage of Alzheimer's amyloid precursor protein by the transmembrane aspartic protease BACE. Science 1999; 286: 735–741.
11. Sinha, S. et al.: Purification and cloning of amyloid precursor protein β-secretase from human brain. Nature 1999; 402: 537–540.
12. Yan, R. et al.: Membrane-anchored aspartyl protease with Alzheimer's disease β-secretase activity. Nature 1999; 402: 533–537.
13. Lin, X. et al.: Human aspartic protease memapsin 2 cleaves the β-secretase site of β-amyloid precursor protein. Proc Natl Acad Sci USA 2000; 97: 1456–1460.

14. Bennett, B.D. et al.: A furin-like convertase mediates propeptide cleavage of BACE, the Alzheimer's β-secretase. J Biol Chem 2000; 275: 37712–37717.

15. Huse, J.T. et al.: Maturation and endosomal targeting of BACE: the Alzheimer's disease β-secretase. J Biol Chem 2000; 275: 33729–33737.

16. Cai, H. et al.: BACE1 is the major β-secretase for generation of Aβ peptides by neurons. Nat Neurosci 2001; 4: 233–234.

17. Luo, Y. et al.: Mice deficient in BACE1, the Alzheimer's β-secretase, have normal phenotype and abolished β-amyloid generation. Nat Neurosci 2001; 4: 231–232.

18. Farzan, M. et al.: BACE2, a β-secretase homolog, cleaves at the beta site and within the amyloid-β region of the amyloid-β precursor protein. Proc Natl Acad Sci USA 2000; 97: 9712–9717.

19. Yan, R. et al.: BACE2 functions as an alternative α-secretase in cells. J Biol Chem 2001; 276: 34019–34027.

20. Bennett, B.D. et al.: Expression analysis of BACE2 in brain and peripheral tissues. J Biol Chem 2000; 275: 20647–20651.

21. Hong, L. et al.: Structure of the protease domain of memapsin 2 (β-secretase) complexed with inhibitor. Science 2000; 290: 150–153.

22. Sastre, M. et al.: Presenilin-dependent γ-secretase processing of β-amyloid precursor protein at a site corresponding to the S3 cleavage of Notch. EMBO Rep 2001; 2: 835–841.

23. Yu, C. et al.: Characterization of a presenilin-mediated amyloid precursor protein carboxyl-terminal fragment γ. Evidence for distinct mechanisms involved in γ-secretase processing of the APP and Notch1 transmembrane domains. J Biol Chem 2001; 276: 43756–43760.

24. Gu, Y. et al.: Distinct intramembrane cleavage of the β-amyloid precursor protein family resembling γ-secretase-like cleavage of Notch. J Biol Chem 2001; 276: 35235–35238.

25. De Strooper, B. et al.: Deficiency of presenilin-1 inhibits the normal cleavage of amyloid precursor protein. Nature 1998; 391: 387–390.

26. Herreman, A. et al.: Total inactivation of γ-secretase activity in presenilin-deficient embryonic stem cells. Nat Cell Biol 2000; 2: 461–462.

27. Yu, H. et al.: APP processing and synaptic plasticity in presenilin-1 conditional knockout mice. Neuron 2001; 31: 713–726.

28. Wolfe, M.S. et al.: Two transmembrane aspartates in presenilin-1 required for presenilin endoproteolysis and γ-secretase activity. Nature 1999; 398: 513–517.

29. Steiner, H. et al.: A loss of function mutation of presenilin-2 interferes with amyloid β-peptide production and Notch signaling. J Biol Chem 1999; 274: 28669–28673.

30. Kimberly, W.T., et al.: The transmembrane aspartates in presenilin 1 and 2 are obligatory for γ-secretase activity and amyloid β-protein generation. J Biol Chem 2000; 275: 3173–3178.

31. Goutte, C. et al.: APH-1 is a multipass membrane protein essential for the Notch signaling pathway in *Caenorhabditis elegans* embryos. Proc Natl Acad Sci USA 2002; 99: 775–779.

32. Francis, R. et al.: aph-1 and pen-2 are required for Notch pathway signaling, γ-secretase cleavage of βAPP and presenilin protein accumulation. Dev Cell 2002; 3: 85–97.

33. Steiner, H. et al.: PEN-2 is an integral component of the γ-secretase complex required for coordinated expression of presenilin and nicastrin. J Biol Chem 2002; 277: 39062–39065.

34. Lee, S. et al.: Mammalian APH-1 interacts with presenilin and nicastrin, and is required for intramembrane proteolysis of APP and Notch. J Biol Chem 2002; 277: 45013–45019.

35. Steiner, H. et al.: Glycine 384 is required for presenilin-1 function and is conserved in bacterial polytopic aspartyl proteases. Nat Cell Biol 2000; 2: 848–851.

36. Ponting, C. et al.: Identification of a novel family of presenilin homologues. Hum Mol Genet 2002; 11: 1037–1044.

37. Weihofen, A. et al.: Identification of signal peptide peptidase, a presenilin-type aspartic protease. Science 2002; 296: 2215–2218.

38. Lemberg, M. et al.: Requirements for signal peptide peptidase-catalyzed intramembrane proteolysis. Mol Cell 2002; 10: 735–744.

39. Shen, J. et al.: Skeletal and CNS defects in presenilin-1-deficient mice. Cell 1997; 89: 629–639.

40. Wong, P.,et al.: Presenilin 1 is required for Notch 1 and Dl11 expression in the paraxial mesoderm. Nature 1997; 397: 288.

41. De Strooper, B. et al.: A presenilin-1-dependent γ-secretase-like protease mediates release of Notch intracellular domain. Nature 1999; 398: 518–522.

42. May, P. et al.: Proteolytic processing of low density lipoprotein receptor-related protein mediates regulated release of its intracellular domain. J Biol Chem 2002; 277: 18736–18743.

43. Ni, C.Y. et al.: γ-secretase cleavage and nuclear localization of ErbB-4 receptor tyrosine kinase. Science 2001; 294: 2179–2181.

44. Marambaud, P. et al.: A presenilin-1/γ-secretase cleavage releases the E-cadherin intracellular domain and regulates disassembly of adherens junctions. EMBO J 2002; 21: 1948–1956.

45. Lammich, S. et al.: Presenilin dependent intramembrane proteolysis of CD44 leads to the liberation of its intracellular domain and the secretion of an Aβ-like peptide. J Biol Chem 2002; 277: 44754–44759.

46. Kim, D. et al.: Nectin-1a, an immunoglobulin-like receptor involved in the formation of synapses, is a substrate for presenilin/γ-secretase-like cleavage. J Biol Chem 2002; 277: 49976–49981.

47. Turner, R.T. 3rd et al.: Subsite specificity of memapsin 2 (β-secretase): implications for inhibitor design. Biochem 2001; 40: 10001–10006.

48. Chang, W. et al.: In vivo inhibition of Aβ production by memapsin 2 (β-secretase) inhibitors. Neurobiol Aging 2002; 23: S134.

49. Shimabuku, A. et al.: Establishment and usefulness of a screening system for the isolation of compounds that inhibit the amyloidogenic processing of APP. Neurobiol Aging 2002; 23: S101.

50. Xia, W. et al.: FAD mutations in presenilin-1 or amyloid precursor protein decrease the efficacy of a γ-secretase inhibitor: A direct involvement of PS1 in the γ-secretase cleavage complex. Neurobiol Dis 2000; 7: 673–681.

51. Xia, W. et al.: Presenilin complexes with the C-terminal fragments of amyloid precursor protein at the sites of amyloid β-protein generation. Proc Natl Acad Sci USA 2000; 97: 9299–9304.

52. Thinakaran, G. et al.: Endoproteolysis of presenilin 1 and accumulation of processed derivatives in vivo. Neuron 1996; 17: 181–190.

53. Esler, W.P. et al.: Transition-state analogue inhibitors of γ-secretase bind directly to presenilin-1. Nat Cell Biol 2000; 2: 428–434.

54. Li, Y.-M. et al.: Photoactivated γ-secretase inhibitors directed to the active site covalently label presenilin 1. Nature 2000; 405: 689–694.

55. Seiffert, D. et al.: Presenilin-1 and -2 are molecular targets for γ-secretase inhibitors. J Biol Chem 2000;275: 34086–34091.

56. Beher, D. et al.: Pharmacological knock-down of the presenilin 1 heterodimer by a novel γ-secretase inhibitor. Implications for presenilin biology. J Biol Chem 2001; 276: 45394–45402.

57. Campbell, W. et al.: Endoproteolysis of presenilin in vitro: inhibition by γ-secretase inhibitors. Biochemistry 2002; 41: 3372–3379.

58. Campbell, W. et al.: Presenilin endoproteolysis mediated by an aspartyl protease activity pharmacologically distinct from γ-secretase. J Neurochem 2003; 85: 1563–1574.

59. Xia, X. et al.: Loss of presenilin 1 is associated with enhanced β-catenin signaling and skin tumorigenesis. Proc Natl Acad Sci USA 2001; 98: 10863–10868.

60. Kang, D. E. et al.: Presenilin couples the paired phosphorylation of β-catenin independent of axin: implications for beta-catenin activation in tumorigenesis. Cell 2002; 110: 751–762.

61. Hadland, B. et al.: γ-secretase inhibitors repress thymocyte development. Proc Natl Acad Sci USA 2001; 98: 7487–7491.

62. Dovey, H.F. et al.: Functional γ-secretase inhibitors reduce β-amyloid peptide levels in brain. J Neurochem 2001; 76: 173–181.

63. May, P.C. et al.: Chronic treatment with a functional γ-secretase inhibitor reduces Aβ burden and plaque pathology in PDAPP mice. Neurobiol Aging 2002; 23: S133.

64. Wong, G. et al.: In vivo Aβ inhibition by γ-secretase inhibitor compound E in TGCRND8 transgenic mice. Neurobiol Aging 2002; 23: S178.

65. Ertekin-Taner, N. et al.: Linkage of plasma Aβ42 to a quantitative locus on chromosome 10 in late-onset Alzheimer's disease pedigrees. Science 2000; 290: 2303–2304.

66. Weggen, S. et al.: A subset of NSAIDs lower amyloidogenic Aβ42 independently of cyclooxygenase activity. Nature 2001; 414: 212–216.

67. Weggen, S. et al.: Evidence that nonsteroidal anti-inflammatory drugs decrease Aβ42 production by direct modulation of γ-secretase activity. J Biol Chem 2003; in press.

35

AMPA Potentiation as a Treatment Option for Alzheimer's Disease

Amy S. Chappell and Michael M. Witte

INTRODUCTION

Alpha-amino-3-hydroxy-5-methyl-4-isoxazole proprionic acid (AMPA) receptor modulators, although still in their infancy from a therapeutic standpoint, have the potential to correct the deficits associated with cognitive disorders such as Alzheimer's disease (AD). This chapter reviews the AMPA receptor's role in long-term potentiation and thus in learning and memory, and describes the AMPA potentiators currently under development.

GLUTAMATE RECEPTORS AND LONG-TERM POTENTIATION

Long-lasting, activity-dependent changes in synaptic strength are thought to be responsible for learning and memory (1). Long-term potentiation (LTP), a persistent increase in synaptic strength following high-frequency stimulation of neurons, is the process by which synaptic strength is enhanced and may be a biological basis for learning and memory (2). Glutamate, as the primary excitatory transmitter in the central nervous system, is intimately involved in LTP. Glutamate mediates excitatory synaptic transmission via two ion-permeable receptors: N-methyl-D-aspartate (NMDA) and AMPA (3). AMPA receptors mediate a majority of the fast excitatory amino acid transmission in the central nervous system (CNS) (4). When activated by AMPA or glutamate, the AMPA receptor allows Na^+ and Ca^{2+} ions to flow into the cell. The influx of ions changes the membrane potential of the postsynaptic neuron, and the resulting depolarization activates the neuron. AMPA receptors also mediate cellular responses to glutamate indirectly by alleviating a magnesium block on the NMDA receptor (Fig. 1) (5).

Multiple AMPA receptor subtypes have been identified and cloned: GluR1, GluR2, GluR3, and GluR4 (6). Each receptor subunit consists of a sequence of approximately 900 amino acids. Four subunits are thought to assemble to form a tetrameric ion-channel complex. The functional properties of the ion channel complex appear to be determined by its subunit composition. Other mechanisms for increasing diversification of AMPA receptor function include structural changes of subunit proteins and amino acid sequence variations of the subunits (7). AMPA receptors have been proposed to be involved in the mechanisms explaining how neuronal activity alters the transmission properties of glutamate-responsive synapses (4). Activity-dependent changes in synaptic strength are thought to be the basis for many types of memory encryption. Increased neuronal activity has been found to cause the phosphorylation of AMPA receptor subunits, leading to an increased flow of ions through the AMPA receptor channel after stimulation by the appropriate ligand. Changes in synaptic strength could be achieved by regulating either the presynaptic neurotransmitter release or the magnitude of the post-

From: *Current Clinical Neurology,*
Alzheimer's Disease: A Physician's Guide to Practical Management
Edited by: R. W. Richter and B. Zoeller Richter © Humana Press Inc., Totowa, NJ

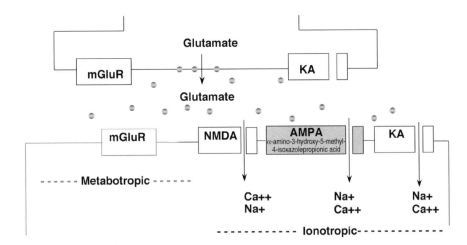

Fig. 1. Glutamate ionotropic receptors. Schematic diagram of synaptic glutamate ionotropic receptor function. Glutamate stimulation of the receptors allows the influx of Na^+ and Ca^{2+} ions, resulting in membrane depolarization. AMPA receptor activation removes a Mg^+-dependent block of the NMDA receptor. Abbreviations: AMPA, α-amino-3-hydroxy-5-methyl-4-isoxazole proprionic acid receptor; NMDA, *N*-methyl-D-aspartate receptor; KA, kainite receptor; Na^+, sodium ion; Ca^{2+}, calcium ion; Mg^+, magnesium ion; GluR1, GluR2, GluR3, GluR4, cloned AMPA receptor subtypes.

synaptic response. Increased neuronal synaptic activity leads to the insertion and accumulation of AMPA receptors at the active synapses *(8)*.

In other words, AMPA receptors undergo an activity-dependent cycle of internalization and reinsertion into the plasma membrane. The receptors move into and out of synapses as synaptic connections strengthen and weaken. Thus, data support the view that postsynaptic modifications of AMPA receptor number and/or AMPA receptor activity are primarily involved in regulating synaptic strength *(9)*.

Because AMPA receptors play an important role in strengthening synapses and in synaptic plasticity, their regulation has become a major focus of the effort to understand learning and memory. Additionally, drugs that modulate the activity of AMPA receptors are currently being studied for their potential utility in a wide range of neurological and psychiatric conditions including AD.

POSITIVE MODULATORS OF AMPA RECEPTORS

Drugs targeting the glutamatergic system, particularly NMDA antagonists, are often hampered by side effects and toxicity. One method to diminish, or even avoid, toxicity is to modulate receptor activity rather than to activate or block glutamatergic receptors directly. Positive modulators of AMPA receptors are an example of this type of mechanism (Fig. 2). Compounds that potentiate AMPA receptors (but do not activate them directly) have been shown to enhance synaptic activity in vitro and in vivo and to enhance LTP *(10–12)*. The time course of ion channel currents (measuring receptor activation) is modified by refractory states caused by excess glutamate binding (desensitization) and by the rate of glutamate removal from the ion channel binding site (deactivation). Agents that either prevent desensitization or slow deactivation rates may enhance ion flux through AMPA receptors.

These agents fall into two general chemical classes: benzothiadiazides and pyrrolidones. Benzothiadiazides include AMPA receptor potentiators, such as cyclothiazide. Pyrrolidones include aniracetam, oxiracetam, piracetam, and CX-516 (Ampalex®, Cortex Pharmaceuticals). Agents that enhance glutamate-stimulated ion influx at AMPA receptors are known as positive AMPA receptor allosteric modulators or AMPA receptor potentiators. These compounds have also been shown to enhance learning and memory in rats, monkeys, and humans *(13–19)*.

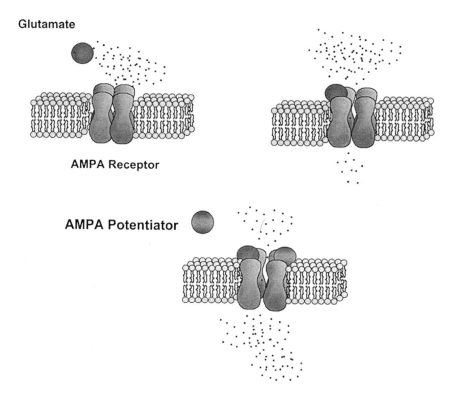

Fig. 2. Enhancement by AMPA Potentiator of ion influx through AMPA receptors.

Cyclothiazide

Cyclothiazide is a positive modulator of AMPA receptors that reduces desensitization and prolongs AMPA receptor deactivation. A cyclothiazide derivative—IDRA-21 (Fidia-Georgetown Institute for Neurosciences)—is being investigated in preclinical studies as a potential cognitive enhancer. IDRA-21 potentiates AMPA-modulated currents in cultured hippocampal neurons, but not as potently as cyclothiazide *(20)*. IDRA-21 reduces the learning deficit produced by alprazolam and scopolamine in animal models, but does not reduce the learning deficit induced by MK-801 (an NMDA antagonist under investigation at Merck) treatment. Additionally, IDRA-21 has been shown to facilitate LTP and to improve certain forms of memory in animals. However, its potency for modulating AMPA receptor function is low, with an EC_{50} value near 1 m*M*, and both, IDRA-21 and cyclothiazide produce neurotoxic effects in vitro and enhance neuronal damage during global ischemia *(21)*. These negative aspects tend to limit their usefulness as pharmaceutical agents.

CX-516

AMPA potentiators (such as CX-516, Cortex) are small molecules that exhibit acceptable safety margins and oral bioavailability, and rapidly cross the blood–brain barrier. In rat studies, CX-516 reverses memory decline due to aging and enhances learning in the spatial-maze animal model *(22)*. CX-516 and CX-691 (Servier) did not increase infarct volume and decreased the penumbral infarct area when tested in the middle cerebral artery occlusion rat model. Studies aimed at clarifying the mechanism of the neuroprotective effects of CX-516 using hippocampal cultures indicated a possible relationship to the activation of MAP (mitogen-activated protein) kinase *(23)*. CX-516 and other AMPA potentiators increase brain-derived neurotrophic factor (BDNF) expression. However, it is unclear whether the activation of BDNF is solely a secondary reaction to increased neuronal activity or a direct effect that contributes to the neuroprotective property of the molecule *(24)*.

In clinical trials, healthy young volunteers showed no signs of major toxicity at CX-516 doses of up to 900 mg; at 1200-mg doses, 7 of 12 subjects reported mild headaches beginning 2–4.5 hours after treatment. Mildly increased salivation and swallowing reactions were also observed in 3 subjects at the 900–1200-mg dose levels. CX-516 (600–1200 mg) administered to young male subjects resulted in improved recall of nonsense syllables. This effect on memory may be due to increased subject alertness or perhaps the facilitation of transient memory encoding *(25)*. In older adults (65–76 years of age), CX-516 (300–900-mg doses) was well tolerated; only one subject in the 600-mg-dose group displayed mild fatigue. In these subjects, improvement of nonsense syllable recall was seen at 75 minutes (but not at 135 minutes) after administration of 900 mg of CX-516; no effect was seen at CX-516 doses of 300 or 600 mg. No change in subject self-assessment scores were reported in this study *(26)*.

In July 2001, data concerning a pilot study of CX-516 in patients with moderate AD was reported. CX-516 was determined to be effective at an early stage of AD as measured by the CIBIC+ and ADAS-cog tests after 4 and 6 weeks, respectively *(27)*. Additional clinical trials are currently underway to examine the efficacy of CX-516 treatment in other disorders, such as mild cognitive impairment (MCI), attention deficit hyperactivity disorder (ADHD), fragile X syndrome, and autism.

LY451395

AMPA receptor modulators (including LY451395, developed by Eli Lilly and Company) are being investigated for the treatment of cognitive disorders. These compounds exhibit oral bioavailability and potentiate the effects of glutamate at AMPA receptors. In vitro studies using recombinant human glutamate receptors demonstrate that LY451395 enhances glutamate-stimulated ion influx in a concentration-dependent manner. Additional in vitro studies using rat cortical and hippocampal neurons showed that LY451395 potently enhances AMPA- and glutamate-activated ion currents in a concentration-dependent and reversible manner. LY451395 displayed a greater than 100-fold selectivity for potentiation of AMPA receptor currents vs activity at other ligand-gated and voltage-gated ion channels. In vivo studies have shown that systemic administration of LY451395 enhances AMPA receptor-mediated responses in both the hippocampus and prefrontal cortex. In the hippocampus, LY451395 also enhanced NMDA receptor-mediated responses as a consequence of AMPA receptor potentiation. Together, these results show that LY451395 is a potent and selective positive modulator of AMPA receptor function.

Animal studies were performed to determine the effects of LY451395 on memory and cognition. In rats, low oral doses of LY451395 were found to reverse memory deficits induced by pharmacological agents. Extensive neurotoxicity studies were conducted in two species to further confirm acceptable margins of safety to support continued development of the molecule.

Studies performed with LY451395 have shown no safety concerns in humans. Table 1 summarizes the clinical studies that have been completed as of December 2002. Young healthy males have tolerated single oral doses of LY451395 up to 10 mg without any adverse events. At 15- and 20-mg doses, two subjects per dose experienced adverse events with the active drug. These episodes, which occurred in supine position, included several unpleasant symptoms, such as nausea, tachycardia, malaise, and tremors (one subject with generalized tremor, one with focal tremor). No alterations of consciousness occurred, and electrocardiograms (ECG) and electroencephalograms (EEG) were normal in all subjects.

Tremor was not observed in AD patients during the multiple-dose study, in which the LY451395 dosage was slowly escalated from 5 to 18 mg twice daily. At 15 mg twice daily, 1 of 6 patients dropped out of the study, and at 18 mg, 3 of 6 patients dropped out because of dizziness and nervousness. This

Table 1
Completed Clinical Studies of LY451395 (to December 2002)

Design	Number of subjects	Subject type	Duration of treatment	Test product/Dosage
Single blind, randomized, single-dose escalation	$n = 39$	Healthy young male volunteer subjects	Single dose (Each subject received 2 single doses of LY and 1 dose of placebo)	Single oral doses of 0.05–20 mg
Double-blind, randomized, multiple-dose escalation	$n = 8$ (6 on LY; 2 on placebo) 3 (male) 3 (female)	Elderly patients with Alzheimer's disease	Multiple doses starting at 5 mg BID and escalating every 3 days to 18 mg BID (total duration of 20 d)	LY451395 multiple oral doses from 5 mg BID to 18 mg BID
Open label	$n = 6$	Young healthy subjects	Multiple doses of 1 or 5 mg BID for 7 days	LY451395, 1 or 5 mg BID

established 15 mg LY451395 twice daily as the maximum tolerated dose. A complete review of all laboratory data, vital signs, ECG, and EEG showed no clinically significant changes.

An open-label study has been conducted to determine the pharmacokinetics of LY451395 in healthy human subjects. The primary objective of this study was to measure the steady-state cerebrospinal fluid (CSF) concentration of LY451395 in 6 healthy subjects following administration of 1 mg ($n = 3$) or 5 mg ($n = 3$) twice daily (BID). The secondary objectives were as follows: to evaluate the safety of LY451395 after multiple dosing in normal healthy subjects; to determine the pharmacokinetics of LY451395 after multiple dosing in normal healthy subjects, and to determine the steady-state ratio of plasma:CSF concentration for LY451395. LY451395 (1 and 5 mg), administered as a single oral dose on days 1 and 8, with BID dosing on days 3–7, was safe and well tolerated.

The concentration of LY451395 in CSF after multiple administrations of either the 1- or 5-mg dosage was quantified. The concentration of LY451395 in CSF appeared to be linearly correlated with LY451395 concentrations in plasma. Absorption of LY451395 at both the 1- and 5-mg dosages was fairly rapid, as exemplified by t_{max} values of less than 3 hours. Mean LY451395 half-life ($t_{1/2}$) values after 1- and 5-mg single administration were 10.2 and 9.19 hours, respectively, and after multiple administrations were 11.6 and 9.92 hours, respectively.

A Phase II study to test the effects of LY451395 on cognition in patients with AD is ongoing.

SUMMARY

Alzheimer's disease is the most common form of dementia in the United States, with over 4 million Americans currently suffering from the condition. Additionally, as life expectancy continues to expand, approximately 22 million people are predicted to be afflicted with the disease around the world by the year 2025. Currently there are no curative or preventative therapies available to stop the progressive neuronal destruction associated with this disease. Only recently have we begun to piece together information from the fields of epidemiology, genetics, molecular biology, and cellular biology to identify the underlying molecular mechanisms of the disease. Current data suggest that AMPA potentiators have the potential to correct, or at least to delay, the cognitive dysfunction afflicting patients with Alzheimer's disease.

REFERENCES

1. Bliss, T.P.; Collingridge, G.L.: A synaptic model memory; long-term potentiation in the hippocampus. Nature 1993; 361: 31–39.
2. Greenmyre, J.T.: The role of glutamate in neurotransmission and in neurologic disease. Arch Neurol 1986; 43: 1058–1062.
3. Dingledine, R. et al.: The glutamate receptor ion channels. Pharmacol Rev 1999; 51: 7–61.
4. Burrone, J.; Murthy, V.N.: Synaptic plasticity: rush hour traffic in the AMPA lanes. Curr Biol 2001; 11: R274–R277.
5. Nowak, L. et al.: Magnesium gates glutamate-activated channels in mouse central neurons. Nature 1984; 307: 462–465.
6. Hollmann, M.; Heinemann, S.: Cloned glutamate receptors. Ann Rev Neurosci 1994; 17: 31–108.
7. Bleakman, D.; Lodge, D.: Neuropharmacology of AMPA and kainate receptors. Neuropharmacology 1998; 37: 1187–1204.
8. Beattie, E.C. et al.: Regulation of AMPA receptor endocytosis by a signaling mechanism shared with LTD. Nat Neurosci 2000; 3: 12.
9. Löscher, C.; Frerking, M.: Restless AMPA receptors: implications for synaptic transmission and plasticity. Trends Neurosci 2001; 24: 11.
10. Ito, I. et al.: Allosteric potentiation of quisqualate receptors by a nootropic drug aniracetam. J Physiol 1990; 424: 533–543.
11. Copani, A. et al.: Nootropic drugs positively modulate α-amino-3-hydroxy-5-methyl-4-isoxazolepropionic acid-sensitive glutamate receptors in neuronal cultures. J Neurochem 1992; 58: 1199–1204.
12. Zivkovic. I. et al.: 7-Chloro-3-methyl-3-4-dihydro-2H-1,2,4 benzothiadiazine S,S-dioxide (IDRA 21): a benzothiadiazine derivative that enhances cognition by attenuating DL-—amino-2,3-dihydro-5-methyl-3-oxo-4-isoxazolepropanoic acid (AMPA) receptor desensitization. J Pharmacol Exp Ther 1995; 272: 300–309.
13. Yamada, K. et al.: Prolongation of latencies for passive avoidance responses in rats treated with aniracetam or piracetam. Pharmacol Biochem Behav 1985; 22: 645–684.
14. Senin, U. et al.: Aniracetam (Ro 13-5057) in the treatment of senile dementia of Alzheimer type (SDAT): results of a placebo controlled multicentre clinical trial. Eur Neuropsychopharmacol 1991; 1: 511–517.
15. Maina, G. et al.: Oxiracetam in the treatment of primary degenerative and multi-infarct dementia: a double-blind, placebo-controlled study. Neuropsychobiology 1989; 21: 141–145.
16. Petkov, V.D. et al.: Age-related differences in memory and in the memory effects of nootropic drugs. Acta Physiol Pharmacol Bulgarica 1990; 16: 28–36.
17. Staubli, U.; Rogers, G.; Lynch, G: Facilitation of glutamate receptors enhances memory. Proc Natl Acad Sci USA 1994; 91: 777–781.
18. Thompson, D.M. et al.: 7-Chloro-3-methyl-3-4-dihydro-2H-1,2,4 benzothiadiazine S,S-dioxide (IDRA-21), a cogener of aniracetam, potently abates pharmacologically-induced cognitive impairments in patas monkeys. Proc Natl Acad Sci USA 1995; 92: 7667–7671.
19. Gouliaev, A.H.; Senning, A.: Piracetam and other structurally related nootropics. Brain Res Rev. 1994; 19: 180–222.
20. Szabadits, P.; Mike, A.; Vizi, E.S.: Modulation of agonist-evoked responses of hippocampal AMPA receptors by IDRA 21 and cyclothiazide (abstr 143.8). World Congr Pharmacol 2002.
21. Yamada, K.A.: AMPA receptor activation potentiated by the AMPA modulator 1-BCP is toxic to cultured rat hippocampal neurons. Neurosci Lett 1998; 249: 119–122.
22. Granger, R. et al.: A drug that facilitates glutamatergic transmission reduces exploratory activity and improves performance in a learning-dependent task. Synapse 1993; 15: 326–329.
23. Bahr, B.A. et al.: Survival signaling and selective neuroprotection through glutamatergic neurotransmission. Exp Neurol 2002; 174: 37–47.
24. Lauterborn, J.C. et al.: Positive modulation of AMPA receptors increases neurotrophin expression by hippocampal and cortical neurons. J Neurosci 2000; 20: 8–21.
25. Ingvar, M. et al.: Enhancement by an ampakine of memory encoding in humans. Exp Neurol 1997; 146: 553–559.
26. Lynch, G. et al.: Evidence that a positive modulator of AMPA-type glutamate receptors improves delayed recall in aged humans. Exp Neurobiol 1997; 145: 89–92.
27. Urbanics, R.: Neurodegenerative Drug Discovery and Development—New Directions. IDDB Meeting Report, July 18–19, 2001, London, UK.

36

Glycosaminoglycans as Potential Future Treatment of Alzheimer's Disease

Umberto Cornelli

INTRODUCTION

Alzheimer's disease (AD) is characterized by extracellular deposits of amyloid and neurofibrillar degeneration in the brain *(1–3)*. The amyloid forms senile plaques (SP, containing extracellular amyloid) and vascular amyloidosis. The neurofibrillary pathology consists of neurofilament proteins (NFs), and an abnormally phosphorylated protein tau forming paired helical filaments (PHFs), which represent the main constituents of the neurofibrillary tangles (NFTs). Amyloid, NFs, and NFTs remain in the extracellular space in different combinations following the degeneration of affected neurons. Neocortical areas of the brain are particularly susceptible, whereas primary motor and sensory areas are less susceptible. Pyramidal neurons of the layers I, III, and IV, which use excitatory aminoacids as transmitters, show a high degree of vulnerability *(4,5)*. Medial temporal lobe regions are affected early, and the disease leads to gradual degeneration of other neocortical areas *(6)*.

A modification of brain vessels is also present according to the degree of AD, as was described in the first cases observed by Aloys Alzheimer and Perusini in 1907. Altered angio-architecture in AD brains was documented quantitatively in basal forebrain and hippocampus, showing a strong reduction of the vascular density and an increase of looped vessels *(7)*.

A central issue in AD research is the relationship between pathological hallmarks and the selected population of neurons that is affected. The so-called "Baptists" show clinical and experimental arguments in favor of the amyloid cascade hypothesis, whereas the "Tauists" have clinical and experimental evidence that tau protein and NFTs are more involved *(8,9)*. However, there are also convincible hypotheses that the amyloid deposition is necessary but not sufficient factor to the pathogenesis of AD *(1)*. There is also evidence that all the three major determinants of AD—amyloid, NFTs, and vessels—show a direct or indirect relationship with proteoglycans (PGs) and glycosaminoglycans (GAGs).

GLYCOSAMINOGLYCANS AND PROTEOGLYCANS

The amount of chemical and biological literature on glycosaminoglycans and proteoglycans is abundant. Some authors have reviewed the most important issues related to GAGs and PGs characteristics *(10–13)*. Only some and fundamental aspects will be reported in this chapter.

GAGs are linear heteropolysaccharides consisting of hexosamine (D-glucosamine [GlcN] or D-galactosamine [GalN]) as well as either hexuronic acid (D-glucuronic acid [GlcA] or L-iduronic acid [IdoA]) or galactose, disposed in disaccharide units carried on sulfate substituents *(10–12)*. Usually GAGs form long chains, which consist of up to 50 disaccharides units, with molecular weight frequently between 10 and 40 kDa. The different disaccharide combinations may form various GAGs such as heparin (HEP), heparan sulfate (HS), dermatan sulfate (DS), and chondroitin sulfate (CS). The

From: *Current Clinical Neurology,*
Alzheimer's Disease: A Physician's Guide to Practical Management
Edited by: R. W. Richter and B. Zoeller Richter © Humana Press Inc., Totowa, NJ

best-documented activities of GAGs are considered to be dependent on their ability to bind specific proteinic ligands (for example, antithrombin or lipoproteinlipase). Their biological activity is frequently attributed to four different characteristics: molecular weight, density of charge, degree of sulfation, and the type of disaccharide units *(14)*. A fifth factor, difficult to standardize experimentally, and fundamental to hamper GAGs' activity and expression, is the biological environment. GAGs are not produced on a template base, and their polymorphism may be related to the necessity of a rapid reaction to the modification of the environment. Thus it is not surprising that GAGs may have an opposite activity in relation to their concentration in a biological system *(15)*.

Most of the GAGs present in humans derive from PGs. Under normal physiological conditions they are synthesized on a matrix constituted by a core protein *(10)*. This is assembled as a protein, and subsequently the glycosilation process adds the saccharidic units. Most of the subsequent enzymatic reactions to the final molecules take place in the Golgi apparatus *(10,16,17)*.

There are many different PGs—hyaluronic acid PGs, heparin PGs, dermatan sulfate PGs, heparan sulfate PG (HSPGs), keratan sulfate PGs, and chondroitin sulfate PGs. They are composed of a protein, which usually is very large, and GAGs (from 2 up to 100) of the same type or heterologous. PGs are among the most represented structures on the cellular surface. It has been tried to divide them in families according to a few common features, such as the type of GAG or the localization within the biological matrix *(10)*.

Many attempts have been made to understand why cells synthesize specific core proteins and which are the signals determining the choice of GAGs to complete the molecule assembling, but in general the results are merely speculative. There are not even common structural features that clearly distinguish core proteins from any other protein. PGs seem to be influenced by the template autonomy of GAGs, and their large heterogenicity derives from their adaptability and plasticity under a variety of influences. That is why physiological, pathological, or therapeutical aspects of either PGs or GAGs are practically hardly definable.

APOLIPOPROTEIN E, PROTEOGLYCANS, AND GLYCOSAMINOGLYCANS

Apolipoprotein E (ApoE) is one of the most documented risk factors for AD. It shows a peculiar relationship with PGs and GAGs. In the context of lipoproteins related to the human brain, ApoE is considered one of the key elements. ApoE is a 34-kDa protein associated with the transport of lipoprotein particles and chylomicrons *(18)*. It is of polymorphic nature, with three major isoforms, referred to as Apo E2, E3, and E4, which are products of three alleles at a single gene locus on chromosome 19. In the brain, ApoE is synthesized by astrocytes and microglia, where it may have either the usual role in cholesterol redistribution or in neuronal repair *(19,20)*.

The relationship between HSPGs and ApoE has been studied in various cell cultures. The findings indicate that HSPGs facilitate the linkage of the ApoE-enriched remnant lipoproteins to the low-density lipoprotein receptor protein (LRP) receptor. The hypothesis is that HSPGs serve as the initial binding site of ApoE, presenting the remnants to LRP; the following step is the internalization of the complex. These data are related to the HSPGs of cell membranes; the secreted HSPGs may not change this process or could delay it competing with the HSPGs on the membrane. A different picture can be determined with GAGs: they may interact with LRP receptors, making more difficult the internalization of the complex formed by ApoE-enriched remnant lipoproteins and HSPGs.

An alternative hypothesis is that Apo E, especially the ApoE4 isoform, contributes directly to neuropathology through a neurotoxic effect. Since HSPGs are involved in the internalization of ApoE through a binding step, compounds disrupting this binding, such as GAGs, could be effective inhibitors of ApoE toxicity *(25)*. While the role of HSPGs is convincing, the role of GAGs is more complex. They interact with LRP receptors (at least indirectly via HSPGs). Furthermore, they show similarities with the low-density lipo-protein (LDL) receptor *(21)*. In other terms, some GAGs, such as HEP, may reduce the binding of ApoE with its natural receptor or act as a trap keeping ApoE inactive.

Indirectly, HEP, activating lipoprotein lipase, increases the availability of ApoE, because the lipidic particles lose their ApoE as soon as they reach the stage of LDL. HEP accelerates this process.

ApoE4 is considered a risk factor in AD, whereas ApoE2 may provide protection from AD and even better memory performance *(22–24,26)*. Lipoproteins associated with ApoE4 are cleared more efficient than ApoE3 and E2 *(18)*. This means that the capacity of the body to internalize remnant lipoproteins may emerge as a disadvantage.

AMYLOID, PROTEOGLYCANS, AND GLYCOSAMINOGLYCANS

The initial definition of amyloid belongs to Virchow (1851), who identified with this name an abnormal deposit of substance present in many tissues or organs (such as skin, kidney, spleen, heart) in the course of a variety of chronic disorders. It was also found in brains of patients suffering from dementia. Despite the striking morphological uniformity, it was discovered that the substance was formed by different chemical entities, glucidic and protidic, that were in part aggregated as fibrils with a β-plated sheet conformation. The amyloid deposit in AD, either in senile plaques (SP) or in brain vessels (vascular amyloid), is composed of a 4.2-kDa peptide termed beta-amyloid (Aβ). This peptide is heterogeneous, being formed predominately of 39/40 residues in vessel amyloid and of 42–44 residues in SP *(27–31)*.

It is now evident that soluble Aβ can cross the blood–brain barrier, as it can be detected in cerebrospinal fluid (CSF); this means that some of it can circulate freely *(32)*. Aβ is supposed to derive from a precursor protein (β-APP or β-amyloid protein precursor) composed from a set of 677–770 amino acids. The observation that AD develops in patients suffering from trisomy 21 together with the localization of the (β-APP gene to chromosome 21 provided the first evidence of amyloid as one of the major determinants of AD.

It is well documented that Aβ is released through a cleavage of β-APP by a β-secretase (and also γ-secretase), but the main metabolic pathway is the cleavage within the Aβ sequence *(33)*.

Fibril formation is one of the key issues. In vitro, many Aβ of different lengths form fibrils, and it is easy to believe that the aggregation may depend on acidic pH, which in vivo can be found in lysosomes only. There is unquestionable evidence that in amyloid plaques (vascular and/or extravascular) ApoE, α1-antichimotripsin (ACT), HSPGs, acetylcholinesterase (AChE) and butyrilcholinestearase (BChE), and several complement proteins are present *(34–40)*. These substances are supposed to trigger the fibril formation, to reduce their possible toxic effect or to carry on some proteolytic activity as lysosomal proteases normally do *(40)*. On the other hand, in CSF, substances are present with such a high affinity for Aβ, such as ApoJ or transtyretin, that were shown to reduce fibril formation *(41)*. These last factors might not be sufficiently represented in amyloid plaques.

One possible cause for fibril formation was identified in HSPGs *(42)*. The content of CS, HA, and HS in amyloid fibrils was defined in the 1960s, but not much attention was paid to these findings until the 1980s, when Snow and colleagues started to conduct experimental studies on amyloid, in order to define its relation with GAGs/PGs *(43–45)*. Sulfated GAGs were detected in experimental amyloid as well as in all human amyloids, including neuritic, vascular plaques, and neurofibrillary tangles in AD *(46,47)*. Also, in brain tissue isolated from human cases of Gerstman-Straussler syndrome and Creutzfeld-Jakob disease, a significant amount of HSPGs were found, thus confirming that PGs are present in other CNS amyloids *(48)*.

At least two different basement membrane HSPGs were detected in either vascular or nonvascular amyloid *(49)*. It was presumed that—because of the linkage of HSPGs core protein with all the known β-APP within the Aβ area—the α-secretase could not be active, and the β-APP cleavage had to be accomplished by other proteases (β-, for instance) thus leading to amyloidogenic or neurotoxic fragments.

Experimental findings demonstrate that HSPGs may bind both, β-APP and Aβ, while GAGs inhibit this binding, probably in relation to their molecular weight and charge density. Moreover, the affinity between HSPGs and β-APP can be reduced despite the fact that the binding region is located on the polypeptide chain of the core protein and not on the carbohydrate moiety. On the other hand, HSPGs are also able to bind Aβ peptides with the carbohydrate chains. This was claimed as one of the causes of fibril formation because it might stabilize them and protect them from proteolysis *(50)*. The charges on saccharide chains of GAGs may provide sites for lateral and axial aggregation of fibrils *(51,52)*.

In conclusion, amyloid is composed of a number of compounds that are not entirely defined in either quantity or type. From the most complex organic molecules to the simplest inorganic ions, such as calcium and aluminum, every entity can trigger fibril formation. The human brain seems to be unable to eliminate this burden and reacts by creating barriers to isolate amyloid from this context. The amyloid deposit is caused not only by something that crosses the blood–brain barrier but also by something that cannot be cleared out. While PGs contribute to amyloidogenesis by increasing the polymerization of fibrils either as precursor or modifying the β-APP cleavage, GAGs may be active in counteracting fibril formation and/or toxicity in vivo.

NEUROFIBRILLARY TANGLES, PGS, AND GAGS

Up to the final stage of dementia, the cognitive deterioration is supposed to be positively correlated with the number of neurofibrillary tangles (NFTs) in the association cortex, whereas this correlation is not evidenced by the number of senile plaques *(53–58)*. In the typically affected areas of the brain there are clusters of neurons containing NFTs and a considerably more abundant amount of dystrophic neurites, which are considered to be typical markers of AD.

The core of NFTs is constituted by paired helical filaments (PHFs). Immunochemical and histochemical studies have shown that the major component of PHFs is the microtubule-associated protein tau, aggregated in a highly phosphorylated state *(59–61)*. Tau proteins are a group of at least six proteins that stabilize the microtubule network (MT) in the polymerized state so as to facilitate the polymerization of tubulin into the MT *(62)*. In the AD brain all six tau proteins are present, but they are abnormally phosphorylated at specific residues (^{396}Ser) and tend to form PHFs, which represent the dominant part of NFTs *(63)*.

Aggregation of tau into PHFs can be reconstructed in vitro, but the in vivo environment is very different, because the large number of antigenic molecules that are detectable within the NFTs might cause aggregation *(64)*. Some of these are: basic fibroblast growth factor (FGF), HSPGs, tropomyosin, ubiquitin, AChE, β-APP, and ApoE *(65–70)*. Most of these compounds could theoretically interact with tau protein, forming fibrils after the dissociation of tau from microtubules. The presence of HSPGs in NFTs is interpreted as one of the causes of PHF polymerization *(66)* because of their capacity to react either with the protein core or the carbohydrate moiety, thus creating a bridge within PHFs and other close macromolecules. In this case the presence of GAGs competing with HSPGs would probably reduce the polymerization process. However, the molecular weight of GAGs is important *(71)*, since a high molecular weight has the same effect as HSPGs, whereas a very low molecular weight may have an opposite effect.

BRAIN VESSELS, PGS, AND GAGS

A profound modification of brain vessels related to the severity of the disease is one of the main features of a brain affected by AD. Different areas of the brain were analyzed to determine the difference between patients suffering from AD and matched controls, such as hippocampus and basal forebrain *(7)*. These observations mean that a strong rheological impact is foreseeable for both endothelium and blood cells in AD brains. The investigation with magnetic resonance imaging (MRI) in some AD patients was not able to detect any atherosclerosis, but it pointed out a significant increase in the thickness of adventitia of arteries in the deep white matter *(72)*. In patients with advanced dementia, a global depression in both cerebral blood flow (CBF) and cerebral metabolism regional oxygen (CMRO$_2$) was found, while metabolic deficiencies were detected much earlier *(73,74)*. The available findings suggest that metabolic changes precede CBF modifications, and that the blood–brain barrier may have an aging-associated or stress-induced continuous silent leakage, which impairs the nutrient transport to the brain.

PGs, particularly HSPGs, are important to maintain the basement membrane function, and the removal of GAGs in general enhance the permeability of the basement membrane *(75)*. Aging has a known effect on the efficiency of the blood–brain barrier (BBB) *(76)*. Even though no specific studies have been conducted on brain vessels of AD patients, they contain large amount of HSPGs and GAGs, in all vessels, and the general reduction of GAGs is one of the features of brains affected by AD *(111)*.

THE POSSIBLE ROLE OF GAGS

The possible role of GAGs in the development of amyloid, NFTs, as well as vascular impairment involves the following considerations.

1. PGs, HSPGs particularly, seem to play an important role in amyloid deposition and in NFTs formation because of their ability to bridge among macromolecules, thus creating insoluble macrocomplexes or protecting some of them from proteolysis. The administration of exogenous GAGs could make them available to compete with PGs and reduce the macromolecular complex formation, the extracellular matrix (ECM) engorgement, and the amyloid fibril toxicity.
2. Alteration of the basement membrane may not offer the possibility to many molecules (macrocomplexes or mediate molecules) to get out of the brain. The administration of GAGs may improve the charge-dependent traffic, and give time to the basement membrane repair mechanism to replace the lamina.
3. Some GAGs increase the half-life of FGF, which is important in the brain for cellular repair. In AD patients FGF is irreversibly entrapped in the ECM.

Glycosaminoglycan Polysulfate (GAP)

The development of the glycosamynoglycan hypothesis started in the late 1970s and early 1980s as a consequence of the clinical observation that patients treated with a mixture of GAGs showed an improvement of symptoms related to the so-called cerebral atherosclerosis. The then-used GAG complex was composed of HEP (10–20%), HS (40–60%), DS (20–35%), and CS (2–8%). It was accepted for human use in Italy (Ateroid®) and in a few other countries as an antithombotic and hypolipemic drug *(115)*. The product was extracted from swine mucosa as a by-product of HEP according to a standardized method, and it is reported here with the name glycosamnioglycan polysulfate (GAP).

GAP *(77)* has shown to have hypolipemic activity and a protective effect on the development of experimental atherosclerotic lesions, both stimulating the endothelial cell proliferation and reducing the growth of arterial smooth muscle cells. The rearrangement of plasma lipoproteins was tested in rabbits. All typical parameters, such as cholesterol, tryglicerides, phospholipids, and proteins of very-low-density lipoproteins (VLDL) and LDL were reduced by this treatment *(78)*.

The pharmacokinetics of GAP were studied in animals using specific markers (tritium for the oral route and fluorescin for intravenous administration). In both cases, markers were detected in an amount compatible to a pharmacological activity. The entire molecules, however, were hardly detected. A positive correlation was found between the level of markers and lipoproteinlipase activity *(79,80)*.

The components of GAP also have antithrombotic activity. This anticoagulant activity, particularly the one related to the presence of HEP, was found to be minimal after intravenous injection and irrelevant or absent after oral administration.

An interesting study was conducted by Lorens on aged rats *(81)*. He showed a significant partial reversal of age-related deficit in animals through a conditioned one-way and two-way avoidance test, following GAP administration in drinking water for 12 weeks. A normalization of stress-induced corticosteroid secretion was also reported. Furthermore, GAP counteracted the age-related reduction of

DOPAC (3,4-dihydroxyphenyl acetic acid) and HVA (homovanillic acid) in the nucleus accumbens but did not counteract the age-related modification of HVA and 5-HIAA (5-hydroxyindoleacetic acid) in the neostriatum. Thus the behavioral effect observed may be due to GAP influence on dopamine neurotransmission.

Clinical pharmacology and Phase III trials conducted in humans confirmed the activity of GAP for the treatment of arteriosclerosis *(82)*. Many observations were spontaneously reported from medical general practitioners, indicating that patients suffering from cerebral atherosclerosis showed improvement of symptoms during GAP treatment.

After some tentative trials to understand the validity of these observations, a preliminary program was undertaken to study GAP in primary dementias. Multi-infarct dementia (MID) can take advantage from GAP because the product has been shown to increase fibrinolysis and to reduce lipid contents and platelet aggregation. Blood viscosity, increased platelet aggregability, elevated blood fibrinogen, and hyperlipidemia are among the most frequent factors determining MID *(83)*. The main goal, however, was to verify GAP activity on SDAT (senile dementia of Alzheimer's type, today simply referred to as AD).

Phase II Studies

The first clinical trial to determine the activity of GAP in primary dementia was a single-blind multicenter study comparing two dosages of GAP on 39 patients (26 suffering from SDAT and 13 suffering form MID). After a washout/run-in period of 2 weeks, patients were randomized to either 250 LRU (lipasemic releasing unit; 50 lipasemic units correspond to 6 mg) or 500 LRU administered im once a day for 12 weeks *(84)*. The admission criteria were referred to DSM-III; other admission criteria included Hachinski ischemia score (HIS), Pfeiffer questionnaire (PSPMQS), and Sandoz Clinical Assessment Geriatric scale (SCAG). Assessments were obtained after a series of interviews, examinations, and laboratory testing recorded according to an adaptation of the Early Clinical Drug Evaluation (ECDEU), the Biomedical Laboratory Information Process (BLIPS), and the Manual for the Documentation of Psychopathology in Geropsychiatry (AGP). Complete psychiatric and psychogeriatric test batteries were applied before and after the placebo washout and after 4, 8, and 12 weeks of treatment.

The treatment with GAP resulted in significant improvements in objective performance, psychopathology, and social behavior. Improvements were consistently greater in the group with SDAT than in the one with MID, and no consistent differences in therapeutic effect between the two doses were observed. The drug was well tolerated, side effects were mild and infrequent, and clinically significant laboratory abnormalities did not occur.

A pilot study was conducted in 12 SDAT patients to check monoamino oxidase type B (MAO-B) activity in platelets and 3-methoxy-4-hydroxy-phenylglycol (MHPG), homovanillic acid (HVA), and 5-hydroxy-indolacetic acid (5-HIAA) levels in CSF *(85)*. These compounds are main metabolites of norepinephrine, dopamine, and serotonin, respectively. In SDAT patients the average levels of MAO-B in platelets are significantly higher than those in normal individuals, whereas CSF average levels of MHPG, HVA, and 5-HIAA are definitely lower *(86–88)*. GAP was administered by a 1000-LRU once-a-day im injection for a period of 30 days. The treatment reduced significantly the MAO-B activity in platelets, and it increased the levels of 5-HIAA, HVA, and MHPG; thus the entire scenario of these parameters was reassessed toward normal values. The authors suggest that these activities of GAP are determined by its contribution to the maintenance of endothelial integrity.

A double-blind clinical trial in MID was conducted on 30 patients *(89)*. Patients over 70 years of age were admitted to the trial according to Hachinski (index ≥ 7) and DSM-III criteria. After a washout period of 2 weeks, patients were treated by oral route either with placebo or GAP at the dosage of 200 LRU three times a day for a period of 8 weeks. The results were assessed in terms of somatic, psychic, and neuropsychiatric symptoms. A battery of psychometric tests was administered to patients before, during, and after the treatment. The behavioral and psychometric evaluation consisted of

Stuard Hospital Geriatric Rating Scale (SHGRS), Gottfreis Rating Scale of Dementia, Nowlis' Scale, digit repetition from the Wechsler Adult Intelligence Scale (WAIS), and Corsi's test. All assessments were made before and after 4 and 8 weeks of treatment. The results showed that GAP was significantly more active than placebo, particularly in the SHGRS cluster of parameters related to cooperation, inadequacy, and cleanliness. Overall clinical impressions expressed by physicians and by caregivers agreed with the results of the psychometric tests.

Phase III Study

An international multicenter double-blind clinical study was conducted in 155 patients suffering from primary dementia *(90)*. Inclusion criteria were based on DSM-III and HIS to separate diagnosis of SDAT and MID. Only patients with moderate to severe cognitive decline (Global Determination Scale, GDS) were included in the study. The cohort of eligible subjects consisted of 71 patients suffering from SDAT and 77 suffering from MID. The patients included in the trial were randomly assigned to one of the treatment groups, which consisted of an oral intake (three times daily) of tablets containing either GAP 200 LRU or placebo. The treatment duration was 12 weeks. The clinical assessment was based on psychiatric, psychogeriatric, psychometric, physical, and laboratory analysis. The treatment with GAP was effective in controlling psychopathological symptoms. A significant improvement was also seen on social behavior as reflected in the CGI (Clinical Global Impression) scale and on cognition as reflected by the MMSE (Mini-Mental State Examination). The SCAG detected improvements in depression, agitation/irritability, and cognitive dysfunction. Treatment-emergent symptoms and toxic effects were infrequent and mild.

Phase IV Studies

Phase IV studies were also conducted in order to give support to potential GAP benefit. GAP was compared with some of the common therapies available for general practitioners. These studies gave little more information than a placebo-controlled study *(91–93)*. A special Phase IV study was then conducted *(114)*. Patient enrolment was based on mental and behavioral performances tested with a simple rating scale of six items (loss of memory, degree of mental confusion, loss of self-care, loss of sociability, depressed mood, and dizziness). Each item was scored from 1 (absent) to 5 (very severe). This rating scale was applied to patients at study entry and after 3 months of oral treatment with GAP (200 LRU three times daily). The multicenter study involved 8776 patients. The results indicated that GAP considerably alleviates the severity of symptoms. Mild and transient side effects were reported in 146 cases (1.6%). The test treatment was withdrawn in 23 cases.

Why was this drug not developed further for the indication of AD? At that time the product could not be standardized appropriately, in particular for the content of HS. However, GAP was accepted as a prototype for the development of GAGs for the treatment of AD, and led to the discovery of a heparin-derived oligosaccharide (HDO) called C3 with the particular advantage of a low molecular weight.

HEPARIN-DERIVED OLIGOSACCHARIDES (HDOS)

Oligosaccharides derived from highly sulfated GAGs maintain a high affinity for β-amyloid. The affinity for fibrillar amyloid is higher for hexasaccharides, whereas the affinity for nonfibrillar amyloid is more evident with oligomers that contain a greater number of saccharides. Oligomers with less than four saccharide units have much lower affinity for amyloid *(94,95)*. Acidic and basic fibroblast growth factors (FGFs) also seem to require a similar type and number of saccharides *(96,97)*. HDOs with 4 to 12 saccharide units may be necessary to maintain the affinity for amyloid peptide and FGFs.

C3 is the HDO we have isolated and on which we have focused our efforts. It is obtained by physical depolymerization of HEP (irradiation by γ-rays). This process generates fragments that lose the anticoagulant activity of HEP and maintain other important binding characteristics of HEP. C3 contains more than 60% of oligomers between 6 and 8 saccharides. More than 90% of the oligomers range between 4 and 12 saccharides. The residual oligomers are less than 4 (about 4%) and more than12 (approximately 6%), respectively. These characteristics are standardized in such a way that only minimal changes are detectable in the different batches of C3 that are produced. Among the HDOs, C3 has a much narrower molecular distribution than any other known low-molecular-weight heparin (LMWH). C3 is practically devoid of any anticoagulant activity *(98)*.

The pharmacokinetics of C3 have been studied in rats administered intravenously (iv) and subcutaneously (sc) at a dosage of 10 mg/kg, and orally (po) at a dosage of 25 mg/kg. Plasma levels were determined indirectly through the evaluation of anti-factor X activator (AXa) activity *(99)*. A standard curve in rat plasma indicates a very high correlation between AXa activity and plasma levels of C3. On the basis of this correlation, pharmacokinetic parameters were calculated according to a noncompartmental model. The data show that sc administration has a higher bioavailability than iv administration (due to the very rapid renal elimination). The high values of clearance found after oral administration in some animals are related to poor absorption and not to an increase in elimination. The fraction of absorption is about 10%, and in these animals the clearance is similar to that of the animals treated sc. C3 plasma levels after oral administration were highly variable. Oral administration seems to drastically change the mean residence time (MRT). However, this is due to the delay in absorption, such that MRT does not represent elimination. After oral administration, C3 behaves according to the slow-release formula of a sc or iv administered drug *(100)*.

Since its central nervous system (CNS) activity is related to the amount that crosses the blood–brain barrier, the AXa activity also was determined in cerebrospinal fluid (CSF). CSF samples were taken at different times for the three routes of administration: 45 min following iv and sc administration; and 2 hours following oral administration. Despite the consistent variation among animals after the same route of administration, it is evident that the transport index (CSF/plasma) is higher after oral and sc than after iv administration.

C3 AND NEUROPROTECTION

Intra-amygdaloid injection of Aβ25-35 in the rat induces a progressive hippocampal expression of tau-2 protein and astrogliosis, as well as strain-dependent behavioral dysfunctions *(101–103)*. C3 (2.5 mg/kg, sc, twice daily for 32 consecutive days) or saline was administered to rats starting immediately before the intra-amygdaloid Aβ25-35 or vehicle injections. The results of this study indicate that C3 significantly reduces the induction in the hippocampal formation of tau-2 protein immunoreactivity (IR) and astrogliosis as revealed by glial fibrillary acidic protein (GFAP). These results have not only been replicated, it has been observed that oral treatment with C3 (25 mg/day for 14 days) also attenuates the neuropathology induced by the intra-amygdaloid injection of Aβ25-35 in rats *(104)*. In the same test, oligomers with much lower molecular weight than C3, even though they were produced using a different process of depolymerization, were found to be practically inactive *(105)*.

The dendritic length of hippocampal neurons in Golgi-impregnated brain slices was analyzed morphometrically *(106)*. Although Aβ25-35 injection failed to alter dendritic length, the administration of C3 to vehicle-treated animals led to an increase in dendritic length that was greater than 30%, suggesting that C3 has neurotrophic activity.

C3 also was studied for its neuroprotective effects against the cholinotoxin AF64A *(107)*. Intraventricular administration of AF64A selectively damages septo-hippocampal cholinergic neurons in a dose-dependent manner and induces behavioral dysfunctions. AF64A-induced damage can be quantified both, morphologically by counting septal choline acetyltransferase (ChAT) IR neurons, and neurochemically by analyzing septo-hippocampal acetylcholinesterase (AChE) and ChAT enzymatic activities. C3 was administered orally at the dosage of 25 mg/kg starting 7 days before AF64A infusion and for 7 days postinjection. The results demonstrate the neuroprotective effect of C3 in this model of cholinergic dysfunction on both AChE and ChAT.

The same model has been used to test other GAGs deriving from DS, HS, and CS. All GAGs were prepared through γ-irradiation of the high-molecular-weight parent compound and were coded respectively D3, HS3, CS3. The average molecular weight was determined by GPC-HPLC after the fractionation and happened to be between 1900 and 2900 Da. Groups of at least 8 rats were administered with the different compounds in comparison to C3 at the dosage of 25 mg/kg (once daily for 7 days before and 7 days after the injection of AF64A). The results show that C3 > HS > DS = CS *(108)*.

HDOs of different molecular weights were also tested in the same model to determine the impact of the fraction at high molecular weight in the determination of the activity of C3. Two different types of HDO were used, C3 and C3$_{high}$. The difference: C3$_{high}$ contained a larger percentage of dodecasaccharides and a lower percentage of hexasaccharides, so as a consequence the average molecular weight was > 2600 Da. C3$_{high}$ was found much less effective (internal data), indicating the importance of the oligomers between hexa- and decasaccharides for the activity of C3.

CONCLUSIONS AND IMPLICATIONS

New treatment compounds are required that address the pathogenesis of AD. HDOs have a high probability of leading to one of these therapies. Some important aspects emerged during the development of HDO:

1. β-APP is widely distributed in the body, particularly in the human gastrointestinal tract, in the peripheral neuronal system (PNS), and in non-neuronal tissue *(109)*. Severe dysfunction of the gut, however, is very rare in SD.
2. In senile plaques and NFTs an extremely abundant array of substances has been detected, such as apolipoproteins, complement fractions, growth hormones, enzymes, matrix proteins, proteoglycans, cytoskeletron proteins, Aβ peptides, fibrillary amyloid, and trace and ultratrace metals.
3. Survival of living hippocampal neurons on brain slices deriving from AD patients is possible *(110)*.

These elements indicate that the repair process in the PNS is efficient, even when the amyloid burden is very high, whereas in the CNS it ends up with an abortion, particularly when the amyloid production for whatsoever reason is high. One of the reasons for this difference is the complexity of the interconnections of the CNS. The repair processes, which may be helpful for one set of cells, does not fit the needs of the closest dendrites (neurons) or the foot process of connecting cells (migroglia or astrocytes) or of the endothelial cell of the vessel nearby. With time (aging) and persistence of the noxious stimuli a vicious circle takes place, which has the consistence of a localized chronic process.

A significant increase of hyaluronic acid (HA) (known as a structural GAG) was found in temporal lobes of AD patients. In the same set of data a 40% reduction of the ratio between sulfate GAGs and HA in AD temporal lobes was found. On the basis of these results one may suggest the existence of a relative lack of GAGs in early-affected areas of the brain *(111)*.

An analysis of HS structure of AD and normal brains has shown no relevant differences between them *(112)*. However, brain HS has peculiar characteristics as compared to HS, which reflects mainly a difference in the degree of sulfation and adaptation of the GAG chain to the ligands (probably determined by the quantity and position of the uronic acid moieties).

HEP is present in every tissue, but it is not a compound that can stay on a cellular membrane, as can other GAGs. It is produced through serglicin, a PG that is stored in mast celles or basofils and secreted when necessary. HEP is so heavily charged that it can compete for any anionic compound, from calcium to a multimeric protein. His duty seems to be to take as soon as possible the ligand in the place where it can be processed or utilized. For these reasons, the highest quantity of HEP is found in those parts of the body that are in contact to the environment, such as gut, lungs, and skin, whereas liver and kidneys do not contain large amounts of it, even though they were the first organs in which it was found by McLean in 1916.

The activity of GAGs in the treatment of AD has been tested clinically with similar compounds, composed of different GAG mixtures, and has been found to be clinically relevant *(113)*. Among the possible active ingredients of GAP, C3 seems to be the most promising. C3 is an HDO, and its molecular-weight distribution has the narrowest spectrum among the heparin derivatives. Heparin depolymerization by γ-irradiation reliably reproduces C3 such that variation among batches is minimal. Other GAGs derived from HS, DS, and CS and treated with γ-irradiation to obtain fragments similar to C3 are much less active in preventing CNS damage caused by a cholinotoxine. Likewise, HDOs containing two to four saccharides are inactive against the neuronal toxicity induced by intramygdaloid injection of amyloid *(105)*.

AXa activity is important for the reduction of amyloid peptide toxicity and enhanced neuroplasticity. HDO with less than five saccharides are devoid of AXa activity. The data, nevertheless, indicate that C3 crosses the blood–brain barrier, as AXa activity was detected in both CSF and brain tissue. The bioavailability of C3 after oral administration is variable, suggesting that it may be necessary to develop a specialized formulation for oral use in order to improve its absorption.

C3 protects hippocampal neurons against amyloid peptides injected directly into the amygdala or cerebral ventricles, and septo-hippocampal cholinergic neurons against the cholinotoxin AF64A, injected intracerebroventricularly. Thus, C3 shows a nonspecific neuroprotective action, which may be due to an increase of the availability of FGF. It is known that FGF is mobilized by GAGs, depending on the degree of their sulfation and number of saccharides. C3, like HEP, is a polycomponent drug that behaves like that part of HEP that does not affect blood fluidity (coagulation). As a consequence, it is difficult to focus on a single mechanism of action of C3.

Since different complement fractions have affinity for GAGs, one possible mechanism of action could be the inhibition of the complement cascade. This possibility is excluded because high HDO oligomers (>12 saccharides) are much more active as inhibitors of the complement, whereas the $C3_{high}$ substantially loses its activity in the test of AF64 after both oral and sc injection for 14 days.

Another hypothesis, which has to be excluded, is the reduction of the amyloid deposit. Animal injected intracerebrally with Aβ25-35 do not show any modification of the amyloid deposit into the amygdala, whereas the reaction to the amyloid (the tau reaction and gliosis) in the upper CA1 region is significantly reduced. This means that C3 may reduce the reactive production of amyloid or the amyloid toxicity, but not the amyloid deposit once it is formed.

Pharmacological tests have shown that C3 reduces the toxicity of amyloid on CA1 neurons, consequently its action is directed to the protection of glutamatergic neurons. It is active also against damage by the cholinotoxine AF64A, which may preserve cholinergic neurons. The mobilization of FGF and the increase of its half-life seem to be one of the most convincing mechanisms of action of C3.

Further studies related to the activity of C3 have shown that it increases the plasma levels of tissue factor pathway inhibitor (TFPI) in nonhuman primates. TFPI is released by endothelial cells and is known to have anti-inflammatory activity. Pharmacokinetic studies in nonhuman primates, either sc or iv, at different dosages, after single and repeated administration, have shown that C3 does not accumulate in the blood even though its mean residence time is much higher than in rats (internal data).

Studies on behavior in old rats, after chronic ingestion of 25 mg/kg for 40–42 days, have confirmed similar activity as was found after GAP administration in reversing the age-related deficit *(114)*.

Toxicological and phase I studies suggest that C3 is well tolerated by animals and humans. These findings indicate that C3 is a promising candidate for an effective and safe therapy for patients suffering from AD and other age-related neurological disorders.

SUMMARY

The hypothesis of the role of glycosaminoglycans (GAGs) in the treatment of senile dementia/AD derives from clinical observations made in the late 1970s, when it was found that a mixture of GAGs was active in the treatment of cerebral atherosclerosis. These data were confirmed in ad-hoc clinical trials on senile dementia, in which the product was administered by oral route. These positive results indicate that glycosaminoglycan polysulfate (GAP) probably contained some very active component, which was orally bioavailable. Here we report the basic theory of the role of GAGs in the pathophysiology of dementia and AD, and the rational to isolate C3, a heparin-derived oligosaccharide (HDO), which has been found active in experimental models that reproduce some of the characteristic neuronal damages of senile dementia/AD.

REFERENCES

1. Selkoe, D.J.: Alzheimer's Disease: a central role for amyloid. J Neuropathol Exp Neurol 1995; 53: 438–447.
2. Dickson, D.W.: The pathogenesis of senile plaques. J Neuropathol Exp Neurol 1997; 56: 321–339.
3. Vickers, J.C. et al.: The cause of neuronal degeneration in Alzheimer's disease. Progr Neurobiol 2000; 60: 139–165.
4. Pearson, R.C.A.; Powell, T.P.S.: The neuroanatomy of Alzheimer's disease. Rev Neurosci 1989; 2: 101–122.
5. Hof, P.R.; Cox, C.; Morrison, J.H.: Quantitative analysis of a vulnerable subset of pyramidal neurons in Alzheimer's disease: I. Superior frontal and inferior temporal cortex. J Comp Neurol 1990; 301: 44–55.
6. Smith, A.D.; Jobst, K.A.: Use of structural imaging to study the progression of Alzheimer's disease. Br Med Bull 1996; 52: 575–586.
7. Fischer, V.W.; Siddiqi, A.; Yusufaly, Y.: Altered angioarchitecture in selected areas of brains with Alzheimer's disease. Acta Neuropathol 1990; 79: 672–679.
8. Troncoso, J.C. et al.: Neuropathology of preclinical and clinical late-onset Alzheimer's disease. Ann Neurol 1998; 43: 673–676.
9. Neve, R.L.; Robakis, N.K.: A re-examination of amyloid hypothesis. Trends Neurosci 1998; 21: 15–19.
10. Kiellen, L.; Lindahal, U.: Proteoglycans: structures and interactions. Annu Rev Biochem 1991; 60: 443–475.
11. Bantdlow, C.E.; Zimmermann, D.R.: Proteoglycans in the developing brain: new conceptual insights of old proteins. Physiol Rev 2000; 80: 1267–1290.
12. Casu, B.: Structure and biological activity of heparin. In: Tipson, R.S.; Horton, D. (eds.): Advances in carbohydrate chemistry and biochemistry, vol. 43, Academic Press, New York, 1985; 51–127.
13. Casu, B.: Heparin and heparin-like polysaccharides. In: Dumitriu, S.: Polymeric biomaterials. Marcel Dekker, New York, 1994: 159–177.
14. Casu, B.: Structure and biological activity of mammalian glycosaminoglycans. In: Ban, T.A.; Lehman, H.E. (eds.): Diagnosis and treatment of old age dementias. Karger, Basel, 1989; 23: 55–67.
15. Kouzi-Koliakos, K. et al.: Mapping of three major heparin-binding sites on laminin and identification of a novel heparin-binding site on the B1 chain. J Biol Chem 1989; 264: 17971–17978.
16. Gallager, J.T.; Lyon, M.; Steward, W.P.: Structure and function of heparan sulfate proteoglycans. Biochem J 1988; 250: 719–726.
17. Poole, A.R.: Proteoglycans in health and disease: structure and functions. Biochem J 1988; 250: 719–726.
18. Mahley, R.W.: Apolipoprotein E: cholesterol transport protein with expanding role in cell biology. Science 1988; 240: 622–630.
19. Pitas, R.E. et al.: Astrocytes synthesize apolipoprotein E and metabolize apolipoprotein E-containing lipoprotein. Biochem Biophys Acta 1987; 917: 148–161.
20. Strittmatter, W.J. et al.: Binding of human apolipoprotein E to synthetic amyloid β peptide: isoform-specific event and implications for late-onset Alzheimer disease. Proc Natl Acad Sci USA 1993; 90: 8098–8102.
21. Cardin, A.D. et al.: Binding of a high reactive heparin to human apolipoprotein E: identification of two heparin binding domains. Biochem Biophys Res Commun 1986; 134: 783–789.
22. Petersen R.C. et al.: Apolipoprotein E status as a predictor of the development of Alzheimer's disease in memory-impaired individuals. JAMA 1995; 273: 1274–1278.
23. Corder, E.H. et al: Gene dose of apolipoprotein E type 4 allele and the risk of Alzheimer's disease in late onset families. Science 1993; 261: 921–923.
24. Corder, E.H. et al.: Apolipoprotein E type 2 allele decreases the risk for late onset Alzheimer's disease. Nat Genet 1994; 7: 180–184.
25. Bazin, H.G. et al.: Inhibition of apolipoprotein E-related toxicity by glycosaminoglycans and their oligosaccharides. Biochemistry 2002; 41: 8203–8211.
26. Helkala E.L. et al.: The association of apolipoprotein polymorphism with memory: a population based study. Neurosci Lett 1995; 191: 141–144.
27. Glenner, G.G.; Wong, C.W.: Alzheimer's disease: initial report of the purification and characterization of a novel cerebrovascular amyloid protein. Biochem Biophys Res Commun 1984; 120: 885–890.
28. Masters, C.L. et al.: Amyloid plaque core protein in Alzheimer disease and Down syndrome. Proc Natl Acad Sci USA 1985; 82: 4245–4249.

29. Kang, J. et al.: The precursor of Alzheimer's disease amyloid A4 protein resembles a cell-surface receptor. Nature 1987; 325: 733–736.

30. Smith, C.; Anderton, B.H.: The molecular pathology of Alzheimer's disease: are we any closer to understanding the neurodegenerative process? Neuropathol Appl Neurobiol 1994; 20: 322–338.

31. Wisniewski, T. et al.: The amino acid sequence of neuritic plaque amyloid from a familial Alzeimer's disease patient. Ann Neurol 1994; 35: 245–246.

32. Golabek, A. et al.: Amyloid beta binding proteins in vitro and in normal human cerebrospinal fluid. Neurosci Lett 1995; 191: 79–82.

33. Sisodia, S.S. et al.: Evidence that beta amyloid protein in Alzheimer's disease is not derived by normal processing. Science 1990; 248: 492–496.

34. Ma, J. et al.: The amyloid associated α 1-chimotrypsin and apolipoprotein E promote the assembly of Alzheimer's β-protein into filaments. Nature 1994; 372: 92–94.

35. Strittmatter, W.J.: Apolipoprotein E: high-avidity binding to β amyloid and increased frequency of type 4 allele in late-onset familial Alzheimer's disease. Proc Natl Acad Sci USA 1993; 90: 1977–1981.

36. Das, S.; Potter, H.: Expression of the Alzheimer's amyloid-promoting factor antichymotrypsin is induced in human astrocytes by IL-1. Neuron 1995; 14: 447–456.

37. Cataldo, A.M.; Nixon, R.A.: Enzymatically active lysosomial proteases are associated with amyloid deposits in Alzheimer brain. Proc Natl Acad Sci USA 1990; 87: 3861–3865.

38. Mesulam, M.M.; Moran, M.A.: Cholinesterase within neurofibrillary tangles related to age and Alzheimer's patients. Nature 1985; 314: 90–92.

39. Guela, C.; Mesulam, M.M.: Special properties of cholinesterases in the cerebral cortex of Alzheimer's disease. Brain Res 1989; 498: 185–189.

40. Neuroinflammatory Working Group, Akiyama, H. et al.: Inflammation and Alzheimer's disease. Neurobiol Aging 2000; 21: 383–342.

41. Schwarman, A.L. et al.: Transthyretin sequesters amyloid β protein and prevents amyloid formation. Proc Natl Acad Sci USA 1994; 91: 8368–8372.

42. Snow, A,D. et al.: A characteristic binding affinity between heparan sulfate proteoglycans and A4 amyloid protein of Alzheimer's disease. J Neuropathol Exp Neurol 1989; 48: 352–361.

43. Bitter, T.; Muir, H.: Mucopolysaccharides of whole human spleen in generalized amyloidosis. J Clin Invest 1996; 45: 963–971.

44. Pennock, C.A.: Association of acidic mucopolysaccharides with isolated amyloid fibrils. Nature 1968; 217: 753–754.

45. Snow, A.D.; Kisilewsky, R.: Temporal relationship between glycosaminoglycans accumulation and amyloid deposition during experimental amyloidosis. Lab Invest 1985; 53: 37–44.

46. Willmer, J.P.; Snow, A.D.; Kisilewsky, R.: The demonstration of sulfate glycosaminoglycans in association with the amyloidoic lesions in Alzheimer's disease. J Neuropathol Exp Neurol 1986; 45: 340–346.

47. Snow, A.D.; Willmer, J.; Kisilewsky, R.: Sulfated glycosaminoglycans: a common constituent of all amyloidosis? Lab Invest 1987; 56: 665–675.

48. Snow, D.A. et al.: Immunolocalization of heparan sulfate proteoglycans to prion protein amyloid placques of Gerstmann-Straussler syndrome, Creutzfeld-Jakob disease and Scrapie. Lab Invest 1990; 63: 601–611.

49. Buée, L. et al.: Binding of vascular heparan sulfate proteoglycan to Alzheimer's amyloid precursor protein is mediated in part by the N-terminal region of A4 peptide. Brain Res 1993; 627: 199–204.

50. Fredrickson, R.C.A.: Astroglia in Alzheimer's disease. Neurobiol Aging 1991; 13: 239–253.

51. Fraser, P.E. et al.: Effect of sulfate ions on Alzheimer β/A4 peptide assemblies: implication for amyloid fibril-proteoglycan interaction. J Neurochem 1992; 59: 1531–1540.

52. Brunden K.R. et al.: pH dependent binding of synthetic β-amyloid peptides to glycosaminoglycans. J Neurochem 1993; 61: 2147–2154.

53. Arriagada, P.V. et al.: Neurofibrillary tangles but not senile plaques parallel duration and severity of Alzheimer's disease. Neurology 1992; 42: 631–639.

54. Berg, L. et al.: Neuropathological indices of Alzheimer's disease in demented and non demented person aged 80 and older. Arch Neurol 1993; 50: 349–358.

55. Hyman, B.T.: Studying the Alzheimer's disease brain. Insights, puzzels, and opportunities. Neurobiol Aging 1994; 15 (suppl 2): S79–S83.

56. Arnold, S.E. et al.: The topographical and neuroanatomical distribution of neurofibrillary tangles and neuritic plaques in cerebral cortex of patients with Alzheimer's disease. Cereb Cortex 1991; 1: 103–116.

57. Bouras, C. et al.: Regional distribution of neurofibrillary tangles and senile plaques in the cerebral cortex of elderly patients. A quantitative evaluation of one-year autopsy population in a geriatric hospital. Cereb Cortex 1994; 4: 138–150.

58. Hyman, B.T.; Tanzi, R.E.: Amyloid, dementia and Alzheimer's disease. Curr Opin Neurol Neurosurg 1992; 5: 88–93.

59. DeLacourte, A.; Defossez, A.: Alzheimer's disease: tau proteins, the promoting factors of microtubule assembly, are major components of paired helical filaments. J Neurol Sci 1986; 76: 173–186.

60. Grundke-Iqbal, I. et al.: Microtubule-associated protein tau: a component of Alzheimer paired helical filaments. J Biol Chem 1986; 261: 6084–6089.
61. Kosik, K.S. et al.: Epitopes that span the tau molecule are shared with paired helical filaments. Neuron 1988; 1: 817–825.
62. Weingarten, M.D. et al.: A protein factor essential for microtubule assembly. Proc Natl Acad Sci USA 1975; 72: 1858–1867.
63. Lee, V.M.-Y.; Daughenbaugh, R.; Trojanowski, J.Q.: Microtubule stabilizing drugs for the treatment of Alzheimer's disease. Neurobiol Aging 1994; 15 (suppl 2): S87–S89.
64. Wille, H. et al.: Alzheimer-like paired helical filaments and antiparallel dimers formed from microtubule-associated protein tau in vitro. J Cell Biol 1992; 118: 573–584.
65. Perry, G. et al.: Neurofibrillary tangles, neuropil threads and senile plaques all contain abundant binding sites for basic fibroblastic growth factor (β-FGF). J Neuropathol Exp Neurol 1990; 49: 318.
66. Perry, G. et al.: Association of heparan sulfate proteoglycan with neurofibrillary tangles of Alzheimer's disease. J Neurosci 1991; 11: 3679–3683.
67. Galloway, P.G. et al.: Immunochemical demonstration of tropomyosin in the neurofibrillary pathology of Alzheimer disease. Am J Pathol 1990; 137: 291–300.
68. Tabaton, M. et al.: Influence of neuronal location on antigenic properties of neurofibrillary tangles. Ann Neurol 1988; 23: 604–610.
69. Mesulam, M.M.; Moran, M.A.: Cholinesterases within neurofibrillary tangles related to age and Alzheimer's disease. Ann Neurol 1987; 22: 223–228.
70. Klier, F.G. et al.: Amyloid β-protein precursor is associated with extracellular matrix. Brain Res 1990; 515: 336–342.
71. Goedert, M. et al.: Assembly of microtubule-associated protein tau into Alzheimer-like filaments induced by sulfated glycosaminoglycans. Nature 1996; 383: 550–553.
72. Scheltens, P. et al.: Histopathologic correlates of white matter changes on MRI in Alzheimer's disease and normal aging. Neurology 1985; 45: 883–888.
73. Cutler, N.R. et al.: Clinical history, brain metabolism, and neuropsychological function in Alzheimer's disease. Ann Neurol 1985; 18: 298–309.
74. Haxby, J.V. et al.: Relation between neurophysiological and cerebral metabolic asymmetries in early Alzheimer's disease. J Cereb Blood Flow Metab 1985; 5: 193–200.
75. Rosenzweigh, L.J.; Kanvar, Y.S.: Removal of sulfated (heparan sulfate) or non-sulfated (hyaluronic acid) glycosaminoglycans results in increased permeability of the glomerular basement membrane to ^{125}I-bovine serum albumin. Lab Invest 1982; 47: 177–184.
76. Stewart, P.A. et al.: A quantitative analysis of blood brain barrier in the aging human. Miscrovasc Res 1987; 33: 270–282.
77. Prino, G: Pharmacological profile of ateroid. In: Ban, T.A.; Lehmann, H.E. (eds.): Diagnosis and treatment of old age dementias. Karger, Basel, 1989; 23: 68–75.
78. Pescador, R.; Mantovani, M.; Niada, R.: Plasma lipoprotein rearrangement in the rabbit induced by mucopolysaccharides from mammalian tissue (Ateroid). Atherogenese 1979; 4 (suppl IV): 210–216.
79. Pescador, R. et al.: Absorption by rat intestinal tract of fluorescin-labelled pig duodenal glycosaminoglycans. Arzneimittel-Forsch 1980; 30: 1893–1896.
80. Pescador, R.; Madonna, M.: Pharmacokinetics of fluorescin-labelled glycosaminoglycans and their lipoprotein lipase-inducing activity in the rat. Arzneimittel-Forsch 1982; 32: 819–824.
81. Lorens, S. et al.: Behavioral, endocrine, and neurochemical effects of sulfomucopolysaccharide treatment in the aged Fisher 344 male rat. Semin Thromb Haemost 1991; 17 (suppl 2): 164–173.
82. Strano, A.; Novo, S.; Davi, G.: Hypolipemic action of sulfomucopolysaccharides: clinical results and future prospects. In: Ricci, G. et al.: Therapeutic selectivity and risk/benefit assessment of hypolipemic drugs. Raven Press, New York, 1982.
83. Passeri, M.; Cucinotta, D.: Ateroid in the clinical treatment of multi-infarct dementia. In: Ban, T.A.; Lehmann, H.E. (eds.): Diagnosis and treatment of old age dementias. Karger, Basel, 1989; 23: 85–94.
84. Conti, L. et al.: Treatment of primary degenerative dementia and multi-infarct dementia with glycosaminoglycan polysulfate: a comparison of two diagnoses and two doses. Curr Ther Res 1993; 54: 44–64.
85. Parnetti, L.; Ban, T.A.; Senin, U.: Glycosaminoglycan polysulfate in primary degenerative dementia (pilot study of biologic and clinical effects). Neuropsychobiology 1995; 31: 76–80.
86. Oreland, L.; Gottfries, C.G.: Brain monoamine oxidase in aging and dementia of Alzheimer's type. Prog Neuropsychopharm Biol Psychiatry 1986; 10: 533–549.
87. Parnetti, L. et al.: Monoamines and their metabolites in cerebrospinal fluid of patients with senile dementia of Alzheimer type using high performance liquid chromatography-mass spectrometry. Acta Psychiatr Scand 1987; 75: 542–548.
88. Soininen, H. et al.: Homovanillic acid and 5-hydroxy-indolacetic acid levels in cerebrospinal fluid of patients with senile dementia of Alzheimer type. Acta Neurol Scand 1981; 64: 101–107.
89. Conti, L.; Pacidi, G.F.; Cassano, G.: Ateroid in the treatment of dementia: results of a clinical trial. In: Ban, T.A.; Lehmann, H.E. (eds.): Diagnosis and treatment of old age dementias. Karger, Basel, 1989; 23: 76–84.
90. Ban, T.A. et al.: Glycosaminoglycan polysulphate in the treatment of old age dementias. Prog Neuro-Psychopharmacol Biol Psychiatry 1991; 15: 323–342.

91. Astengo, F. et al.: Confronto in doppio cieco fra mucopolisaccaride solforato e placebo nel trattamento di pazienti con insufficienza cerebrovascolare. Clin Ter 1987; 120: 219–226.

92. Bardin, P.; Campo, R.: Studio clinico controllato doppio cieco sull'impiego di Ateroid 200 nel trattamento di pazienti anziani con vasculopatia cerebrale. Clin Ter 1987; 120: 111–118.

93. Perussia, M.; De Jacobis, M.: Studio doppio cieco controllato per il confronto tra il trattamento con sulfomucopolisaccaridi (600 LRU/die) e placebo in pazienti anziani con insufficienza cerebrovascolare. Farmaci 1986; 10 : 255–229.

94. Leveugle, B. et al.: Heparin oligosaccharides that pass the blood brain barrier inhibit beta-amyloid precursor protein secretion and heparin binding to beta-amyloid peptide. J Neurochem 1998; 70: 736–744.

95. Lindahl, B. et al.: Common binding sites for beta-amyloid fibrils and fibroblast growth factor-2 in heparan sulfate from human cerebral cortex. J Biol Chem 1999; 274: 30631–30635.

96. Casu, B.; Lindahal, U.: Structure and biological interactions of heparin and heparan sulfate. In: Advances in carbohydrate chemistry and biochemistry. Academic Press, San Diego, CA, 2001; 57: 159–204.

97. Barzu, T. et al.: Heparin-derived oligosaccharides: affinity for acidic fibroblast growth factor and effects on its growth promoting activity for human endothelial cells. J Cell Physiol 1989; 140: 538–548.

98. Quing, M. et al.: Molecular and biochemical profiling of a heparin-derived oligosaccharide, C3. Thromb Res 2002; 105: 303–309.

99. Quing, M. et al.: The blood-brain barrier accessibility of a heparin derived oligosaccharide C3. Thromb Res 2002; 105: 447–453.

100. Cornelli, U. et al.: Heparin derived oligosaccharides, Alzheimer's disease, and other age related neurological disorders. In: Vossougi, J. et al.: Thrombosis research and treatment: bench to bedside. Medical and Engineering Publishers, Washington, DC, 2003, in press.

101. Sigurdsson, E.M. et al.: Local and distant histopathological effect of unilateral amyloid-beta 25-35 injection into the amygdala of young F344 rats. Neurobiol Aging 1997; 17: 893–901.

102. Sigurdsson, E.M. et al.: Bilateral injections of amyloid-(25-35) into the amygdala of young Fischer rats: behavioral, neurochemical, and time dependent histopathological effects. Neurobiol Aging 1997; 18: 591–560.

103. Sigurdsson, E.M. et al.: Laterality in the histological effects of injection of amyloid-beta 25-35 into the amygdala of young Fisher rats. J Neuropathol Exp Neurol 1997; 56: 714–721.

104. Dudas, B. et al.: Oral and subcutaneous administratrion of glycosaminoglycan C3 attenuates amyloid-beta (25-35) induced abnormal tau protein immunoreactivity in rat brain. Neurobiol Aging 2002; 23: 97–104.

105. Walzer, M. et al.: Low molecular weight glycosaminoglycan blockade of β-amyloid induced neuropathology. Eur J Pharm 2002; 445: 211–220.

106. Mervis, R.F. et al.: Neurotrophic effects of the glycosaminoglycan C3 on dendritic arborization and spines in the adult rat hippocampus: a quantitative Golgi study. CNS Drug Rev 2002; 6 (Suppl 1): 44–46.

107. Rose, M.B. et al.: Protective effect of glycosaminoglycan C3 on AF64A-induced cholinergic lesion in rats. Neurobiol Aging 2003; 24: 481–490.

108. Dudas, B.; Cornelli, U. et al.: Low molecular weight (LMW) glycosaminoglycans (GAGs) protect against AF64A-induced cholinergic lesion in rat brain. Soc Neurosci Abs; November; Society for Neuroscience Meeting, Orlando, FL, 2002.

109. Cabal, A. et al.: β-Amyloid precursor protein (βAPP) in human gut with special reference to enteric nervous system. Brain Res Bull 1995; 38: 417–433.

110. Carpenter, M.R.; Crutcher, K.A.; Kater, S.B.: An analysis of the effect of Alzheimer's plaques on living neurons. Neurobiol Aging 1993; 14: 207–215.

111. Jenkins, H.G.; Bachelard, H.S.: Glycosaminoglycans in cortical autopsy samples from Alzheimer brain. J Neurochem 1988; 51: 1641–1645.

112. Lindahal, B.; Eriksson, L.; Lindahal, U.: Structure of heparan sulfate from human brain, with special regard to Alzheimer's disease. Biochem J 1995; 306: 177–184.

113. Parnetti, L. et al.: Vascular dementia Italian sulodexide study (VADISS). Clinical and biological results. Thromb Res 1997; 87: 225–233.

114. Lorens, S.A. et al.: A heparin derived oligosaccharide normalizes the fear response of old brown rats. Behav Brain Res 2003, in press.

115. Santini, V.A.: General practice trial of ateroid 200 in 8776 patients with chronic senile cerebral insufficiency. In: Ban, T.A.; Lehmann, H.E. (eds.): Diagnosis and treatment of old age dementias. Karger, Basel, 1989; 23: 95–100.

37

Implications of Research for Management of AD

Peter J. Whitehouse

INTRODUCTION

Considerable enthusiasm exists in the research community about the development of more effective treatments for Alzheimer's disease (AD) and related conditions. Although we can celebrate our modest success in translational research, expectations of major breakthroughs have not yet been realized. Moreover, there is much exaggeration in the field about rapid advances in diagnosis and therapeutics. We are also recognizing that the development of more powerful therapies is expensive and therefore issues of pharmacoeconomics are becoming more critical. As we examine the implications of the research in dementia for the development of future treatments, we must keep a balanced perspective about the goals of our work and the challenges of providing genuine hope but not false expectation.

One aspect of Alzheimer's disease is that its features overlap extensively with other neurodegenerative dementias, such as those of Parkinson's disease and Lewy body dementia, which share pathological and clinical features with each other and with AD *(1)*. Vascular dementia is now also being examined more intensively, having formerly been in the shadow of AD and more nosological challenges are emerging. One of the results of this investigation is that we find there is more overlap between vascular dementia and AD than was originally thought. In fact, our simplistic notions of separating the two conditions cleanly have fallen by the wayside.

In this chapter we will review research on dementia and its clinical implications from biological, clinical, social, and ethical perspectives. We will conclude by providing some guidance to primary-care providers as they evaluate the emerging research in AD and its implications for treatment.

MOLECULAR BIOLOGY AND GENETIC RESEARCH

Probably most research on AD continues to be associated with the genetic aspects. The situation has become enormously more complicated since the original discoveries of autosomal dominant mutations on chromosome 21 in the gene for the amyloid precursor protein (APP). Mutations also occur on chromosome 1 and 14 in association with abnormalities in presenilin, which was found to be involved in amyloid processing (*see* Chapter 1, p. 3 ff). Thus, genetic clues point to the possibility that amyloid is central to the pathogenesis of AD. AD can be inherited as an autosomal dominant, although in a very low percentage of cases of AD. Autosomal genetic abnormalities have been found in some patients with frontal lobe dementia that affect tau, a protein involved in the structure of neurofibrillary tangles. We have limited knowledge about how plaques and tangles form and how these two features relate to each.

Other genetic factors in addition to autosomal dominant mutations modify the course of AD. Apolipoprotein E (ApoE) is a susceptibility factor that has received considerable attention. Individuals with ApoEe4 alleles are more likely to develop AD than those with ApoEe3 and e2-alleles (which may

From: *Current Clinical Neurology,*
Alzheimer's Disease: A Physician's Guide to Practical Management
Edited by: R. W. Richter and B. Zoeller Richter © Humana Press Inc., Totowa, NJ

be protective). Despite many claims to the contrary, no other genes have been conclusively identified as susceptibility factors. Although ApoE modifies the risk for AD and the likelihood of an AD diagnosis, the information is not precise enough to recommend the use of this test in clinical practice.

Ultimately, the clinical symptoms in AD and related disorders relate to neuronal dysfunction and eventual cell death. We still do not have a clear understanding of how plaques and tangles relate to cell death, although tangles as intracellular structures are associated with populations of cells that eventually die. Moreover, components of APP appear to be toxic to cells. Much of the therapeutic energy has been focused on trying to prevent the cerebral accumulation of amyloid (*see* Chapter 2, pp. 21 ff).

Another major area of work on the biology of AD is the development of animal models. There are no natural or experimental models that closely mimic AD. Currently, the most widely explored models are transgenic or knockout mice, in which genes have been added or subtracted respectively. Several interventions promote the removal of amyloid in transgenic mice that were created to overexpress amyloid. However, it is not clear that therapeutic effects in these models translate into human benefits. For example, the amyloid vaccine developed by Elan appeared to work well in several transgenic mouse models *(2)*, but was not clearly helpful in that it produced a presumed allergic encephalitis in some subjects in the initial clinical trials, which were then halted.

CLINICAL RESEARCH: FROM EPIDEMIOLOGY TO CLINICAL TRIALS

Clinical research makes major contributions in several different ways to our understanding of AD and related dementias as well as to the development of more effective therapies. Epidemiologists study populations of people affected by AD. Clinicians also continue to define and refine diagnostic categories. For example, the concept of mild cognitive impairment (MCI) has recently emerged *(3)*. MCI is defined by arbitrary research criteria that can lead to labeling greater or fewer numbers of people, because it is defined in statistical terms in relation to normal population aging. The appropriateness of MCI as a clinical label needs to be questioned, however. Although, the term allows clinicians a gentler way of diagnosing or at least labeling a patient without using the name "Alzheimer's," it can result in considerable confusion. If a person is labeled as having MCI, does he or she have early AD or not, or does it mean that her or she will or may develop AD?

Epidemiological studies have also tried to identify risk and preventative factors for AD. Unfortunately, many of these trials are retrospective case control studies that have fundamental scientific limitations. Nevertheless, a variety of drugs have claimed to possibly prevent AD, including antioxidants, nonsteroidal anti-inflammatory agents (NSAIDs), estrogens, and statins. However, when randomized controlled studies have evaluated these agents, they have as yet not been found to show protection. Studies that provide evidence that education, low-fat diets, and enhanced activity may prevent AD are often prone to biases. In general, the conclusion from these studies is that leading a healthy life, getting a good education, having enough money, keeping active, eating more fruits and vegetables, and taking the prescribed drugs would seem the best way to prevent AD. It may be that people born smarter do these things and develop less AD by virtue of their better original brain endowment, however.

The contributions with the most specific impact that clinicians make to treatment development are randomized controlled studies. We now have four cholinesterase inhibitors (AChEIs) approved in the United States for the treatment of mild to moderate AD *(4)*. The first one, tacrine, is no longer used, because of its need to be administered 4 times a day and its frequent (reversible) liver toxicity. Donepezil, which is the easiest to take, because it is administered once a day and has few side effects, is currently the most widely sold medication. Galantamine, to be taken twice a day, is a little less convenient but also has a manageable side-effect profile. Rivastigmine has more severe gastrointestinal side effects, and a warning label by the U.S. Food and Drug Administration (FDA) points out that it can cause significant weight loss. Studies have shown that these drugs may produce modest effects on cognition, perhaps through effects on attention, but they may also improve behavior. Symptoms of apathy and hallucinations may be particularly likely to be affected, although the clinical benefits are in my opinion usually rather minor. Studies are ongoing to determine whether AChEIs may be useful in both milder and more severe dementia, and whether they might modify the course of the disease. Memantine, a glutamate receptor antagonist, was recently approved in Europe, and a New Drug Application has been submitted to the FDA *(5)*. The drug is likely to be able to be administered in combination with AChEIs, because it works through a different mechanism (*see* Chapter 23, pp. 203 ff).

We still do not have a consensus on how to conduct clinical trials that would allow a claim for disease modification *(6)*. However, protocols have been developed to examine if drugs can delay the diagnosis of AD. So far, results have not been encouraging and no consensus has been achieved about appropriate study design. One of the limitations is that we have no biological marker for AD, so considerable effort is being expended to develop blood, cerebrospinal fluid (CSF), or imaging markers. Most energy has been focused on the development of neuroimaging—either structural to measure brain atrophy or functional with positron emission tomography—to investigate certain aspects of the biology. The problem that biological marker studies pose is that there exists a continuum between normal aging and AD. On any measure to date there is a need for arbitrary criteria to distinguish normal aging from AD.

Thus, our abilities to diagnose AD will continue to depend on clinical judgment, which allows considerable margin for variation even among experts. Neuropsychological studies contribute by trying to identify the earliest cognitive deficits. The discussion of MCI above demonstrates how arbitrary and problematic the labeling of people with memory problems with different terms can be.

Vitamin E in high doses (1000–2000 IU) is recommended by experts to attempt to delay progression of diseases, based on basic and epidemiological data and on one not clearly interpretable randomized controlled study *(7)*. Until further studies and data analysis are completed, it cannot be considered unreasonable to recommend this rather cheap and safe intervention.

The future of biological research will likely remain focused on molecular pathogenesis. The search for agents that lower the amyloid burden continues. Drugs to prevent formation or aggregation as well as enhance clearance based on a better understanding of amyloid formation and function may emerge from various laboratories. Better symptom-treating drugs may also become available. More selective agents that stimulate or modify nicotinic cholinergic receptors offer the promise of great improvement in cognition with fewer side effects. Drugs that affect other neurotransmitter systems besides acetylcholine are reported to improve cognition in animals and might make it into the clinic in large trials in humans.

SOCIAL RESEARCH: TOWARD A BIO-PSYCHOSOCIAL MODEL

Clearly, in the future we need to integrate the use of medications with educational and social interventions. In fact, in clinical practice today, most of the benefit (and sometimes harm) that patients receive from physicians has to do with their relationship and with their doctor's referrals for additional help. It is important, for example, that people are referred to the Alzheimer's Association and to community-based services, such as day care and home care. Research on these interventions has not demonstrated clear benefit however, which probably relates to the fact that caring is complex and/or we do not have the right outcome measures *(8)*. Giving advice about long-term financial and legal planning (advance directives) for possible institutional long-term and end-of-life care is also essential.

Social researchers also spend a considerable amount of effort studying the characteristics of caregivers and caregiver stress. There is no question that caregiving can be a burden. However, it is important to look at the positive aspects of caregiving as well. Caregivers can be categorized into informal and formal caregivers. We need to understand better the stresses and strains on formal caregivers, particularly in long-term care. Many nursing homes now have special care units, which provide a more social model of care than regular nursing home units. It has been difficult, however, to demonstrate the specific value of these special care units on residents, families, or staff.

BETTER OUTCOME MEASURES ARE NEEDED

In biological, clinical, as well as in social areas, we need to develop better outcome measures. Quality of life represents the most integrative goal for therapy, and considerable work has been done to develop more reliable and valid ways of measuring quality of life *(9,10)*. This area was poorly developed in dementia, in part because of the early concern that quality of life is subjective and that patients with memory and language problems may have a difficult time evaluating their own quality of life (QOL). However, scales such as the QOL-AD can obtain reliable measures in people with mild to moderate dementia *(11)*. Caregiver rating scales of QOL can be used with subjects who have more severe cognitive problems. Assessing QOL of caregivers themselves is also key.

A focus on quality of life also allows us to recognize that there are many nonmedical interventions that may be important for health care providers to consider. As mentioned above, keeping mentally and physically active is particularly important after the onset of cognitive impairment. The use of computers to assist the person with cognitive problems and their caregivers is another area in which new technology may improve functionality and quality of life *(12)*. In addition, spiritual beliefs play a significant role in maintaining quality of life as some people progress into dementia *(13)*.

It is of utmost importance to focus on improving quality of life and reducing stress on caregivers. New research suggests that specific interventions, such as education, support groups, and counseling, aid caregivers *(14)*. However, the specific aspects of assistance programs that benefit caregivers in particular vary considerably.

Assessment of quality of life is also part of the discipline of health economics. Cost/utility analysis allows us to compare the effects of an intervention on outcomes that people value in relationship to cost. The cost of medications is an increasing concern around the world, and it is clear that we need more research to demonstrate the relative value of medications and psychosocial interventions *(15,16)*.

Moreover, treatment of persons with memory problems today and in the future will continue to include several components. Better integration of different approaches may allow better outcomes. Evaluating so-called complementary and alternative therapies should continue, as people currently spend considerable amounts of out-of-pocket funds on herbals, nutraceuticals, homeopathic, and other therapies *(17)*. Learning why people are attracted to these approaches is also critical. The focus on prevention, personal responsibility for health, perceived safety, and more "nature-friendly" techniques in many of these alternative health traditions is likely part of the broad appeal.

ETHICAL ISSUES IN RESEARCH

The list of ethical issues in conducting research in people with cognitive impairment is enormous *(18)*. Starting even before the diagnosis, we have the challenge of genetic testing. In the autosomal dominant forms of AD, family members who are at risk can be told whether they carry the particular gene. If they carry the gene, they also have an almost 100% certainty that if they live long enough they will develop the illness. We also have concerns about who has access to such information (for example, insurance carriers). We spend much of the time talking about diagnostic disclosure. Certainly, people should be informed honestly about their condition, but as mentioned above, the label MCI calls into question the fundamental categorical nature of age-related dementia. Moreover, we must recognize that when we provide information, a diagnostic label such as AD means different things to different people. A doctor's conceptions of AD may be quite different from that of the patient.

When we are conducting clinical research, there are a number of those major issues with regard to informed consent. How do we assess the capacity to provide informed consent? Who are the legally authorized representatives of patients to make substituted judgments? What degree of risk is appropriate for people at different stages of illness? Moreover, in research design there are some fundamental ethical issues, for example, under which conditions it is not appropriate to use placebo for control, now that there are some—albeit modestly effective—therapies available *(19)*?

Finally, we must recognize that many people will die with cognitive impairment. Thus, we need to address the ethical issues of end-of-life care *(20)*. What could be the appropriate use of a feeding tube, given that research demonstrates this measure does not prevent malnutrition and aspiration pneumonia? Feeding tubes should perhaps not be offered under circumstances that relate to the dementia, but be used only in the context of another evolving acute illness for which hydration is required. Whether it is early diagnosis or end-of-life care, we need to attend to the wide range of ethical issues that can affect our clinical and research enterprise.

IMPLICATIONS FOR THE HEALTH CARE PRACTITIONER

Research in AD attracts considerable attention. In an era when universities are trying to make money by transferring biotechnology into practice, breakthroughs are described with increasing frequency and sometimes with lack of critical appraisal. It is difficult for the health care practitioner to assess the relative value of different claims. Many basic animal observations are claimed to have important implications for human therapies. These assertions in fact are frequently overblown. Similarly, claims have been made that biological markers can be useful diagnostic tests. Many such claims are never replicated and are challenged fundamentally by the basic fuzziness of the relationship between normal aging and AD.

Scientific research is an exciting enterprise. To be at the forefront of the creation of knowledge about the global challenge of age-related cognitive impairment is exciting. We have to make sure, however, that we are responsible to our patients and to our colleagues who are not as directly involved in such research enterprises as we are. Frankly, we have gone overboard in creating concern about AD and the likelihood of profound therapeutic interventions.

Despite the fact that therapeutic claims are exaggerated, primary-care providers do need to maintain a sense of hope. Research does offer the promise in the future of more effective biological treatments. The danger is that those promises may distort our values and turn our attention away from the many things that we can do to provide care that is based on our relationship. Providing people a perspective based on sharing successes and challenges with other people affected by the same condition, and providing education that allows a balanced perspective on the illness, are two critical aspects of maintaining hope.

REFERENCES

1. Ritchie, K.; Lovestone, S.: The dementias. Lancet 2002; 360: 1759–1766.
2. Schenk, D. et al.: Immunization with amyloid-beta attenuates Alzheimer-disease-like pathology in the PDAPP mouse. Nature 1999; 400: 173–177.
3. Petersen, R.C. (ed.): Mild cognitive impairment: aging to Alzheimer's disease. Oxford University Press, Oxford, UK, 2003.
4. Mayeux, R.; Sano, M.: Drug therapy: treatment of Alzheimer's disease. N Engl J Med 1999; 341: 1670–1679.
5. Winblad, B.; Portiris, N.: Memantine in severe dementia: results of the M-Best Study (benefit and efficacy in severely demented patients during treatment with memantine). Int J Geriatr Psychiatry 1999; 14: 135–146.
6. The Disease Progression Sub-Group: Bodick, N.; Forette, F.; Hadler, D.; Harvey, R.; Leber, P.; McKeith, I.G,; Riekkinen, P.; Rossor, M.N.; Scheltens, P.; Shimohama, S.; Spiegel, R.; Tanaka, S.; Thal, L.J.; Urata, Y.; Whitehouse, P.J.; Wilcock, G.: Protocols to demonstrate slowing of Alzheimer disease progression. Alz Dis Assoc Disord 1997; 11 (suppl 3): S50–S53.
7. Sano, M. et al.: A controlled trial of selegiline, alpha-tocopherol, or both as treatment for Alzheimer's disease. N Engl J Med 1997; 336: 1216–1222.
8. Brodaty, H. et al.: Towards harmonization of caregiver outcome measures. Brain Aging 2002; 2:4: 3–12.
9. Whitehouse, P.J.; Rabins, P.V.: Quality of life and dementia. Alz Dis Assoc Disord 1992; 6: 135–138.
10. Dawson, N.V. et al.: Treatment goals in dementia: quality of life and ethics. In: Vellas, B.; Grundman; Feldman, H.; Fitten, L.J.; Winblad, B.; Giacobini, E. (eds.): Research and Practice in Alzheimer's Disease, vol. 8. France, Serdi (Submitted for publication, 2003).
11. Logsdon, R.G. et al.: Quality of life in Alzheimer's disease: and caregiver reports. In: Albert, S.M.; Logsdon, R.G. (eds.): Assessing quality of life in Alzheimer's disease: Springer, New York, 2000: 17–30.

12. Whitehouse, P.J.; Marling, C.; Harvey, R.: Can a computer be a caregiver? American Association for Artificial Intelligence, 2002; 103–107 (www.aaai.org).

13. Stuckey, J.C. et al.: Alzheimer's disease, religion, and the ethics of respect for spirituality: a community dialogue. Alz Care Quart 2002; 3: 199–207.

14. Mittelman, M.S. et al.: A family intervention to delay nursing home placement of patients with Alzheimer's disease. A randomized, controlled trial. JAMA 1996; 276: 1725–1731.

15. Whitehouse, P.J. et al.: First international pharmacoeconomic conference on Alzheimer's disease: report and summary. Alz Dis Assoc Disord 1998, 12: 266–280.

16. Jonsson, L. et al.: Second international pharmacoeconomic conference on Alzheimer's disease. Alz Dis Assoc Disord 2000, 14: 137–140.

17. Whitehouse, P.J.; Edwards, T.I.: Complementary and alternative medicine. In: Sugarman, J. (ed.): 20 common ethical problems in primary care. McGraw-Hill New York, 2000, pp. 27–38.

18. Whitehouse, P.J.: Ethical issues in dementia. Dialogues in clinical neuroscience 2000; 2: 165–170.

19. Kawas, C.H. et al.: Clinical trials in Alzheimer's disease: debate on the use of placebo controls. Alz Dis Assoc Disord 1999; 13: 124–129.

20. Post, S.G.; Whitehouse, P.J.: The moral basis for limiting treatment: hospice and advanced progressive dementia.In: Volicer, L.; Hurley, A. (eds.): Hospice care for patients with advanced progressive dementia. Springer New York, 1998: 117–131.

IX Treatment Outcome Measurement

38

Rating Scales and Outcome Variables Used in Clinical Trials*

Lon S. Schneider

INTRODUCTION

A basic screening of the patient's mental and functional status is part of the diagnostic assessment of dementia. Some of the same assessment measures used clinically are used as outcomes in clinical trials. Cognitive deficits are both core features of the dementia syndrome and progress over time. It is therefore important for both clinicians and clinical investigators to be able to quantify this change over time as well as possible improvements with treatment.

Because of the clinical, biological, and genetic heterogeneity of Alzheimer's disease (AD), combined with the progressive deteriorating course of untreated patients, specific treatments will be helpful for only a subset of patients. Some will respond dramatically, but many more will respond only modestly. It is therefore important to be able to assess a range of treatment responses in both individuals and groups of patients, and to identify treatment responders clearly.

Lastly, it is important that similar outcomes are used among clinical trials so that clinicians can gain a general appreciation of relative efficacy of medication from study to study and be able to compare documented effects.

The international consensus for assessments in studies with AD patients nowadays includes four domains: cognition, global clinical changes, activities of daily living (ADL), and behavior. Many experts also recommend quality of life (QOL) and resource utilization or health economics measures.

TYPES OF RATING SCALES

The types of rating scales or outcome measures generally used for AD and dementia clinical trials can be categorized into several groups:

1. Cognitive tests
2. Clinician's global assessment of severity
3. Clinician's global assessment of change
4. Behavioral ratings
5. Functional assessment

*Adapted from: Schneider, L.S.: An overview of rating scales used in dementia research. Alzheimer Insights, June 1997; Special Edition (www.alzheimer-insights.com), and from Schneider, L.S.: Assessing outcomes in Alzheimer's disease. Alz Dis Assoc Dis 2001; 15 (suppl 1): S8–S18.

From: *Current Clinical Neurology,*
Alzheimer's Disease: A Physician's Guide to Practical Management
Edited by: R. W. Richter and B. Zoeller Richter © Humana Press Inc., Totowa, NJ

COGNITIVE TESTS

The cognitive/neuropsychological test is the primary measure of efficacy in clinical trials. Instruments include the Mini-Mental State Examination (MMSE), the Alzheimer's Disease Assessment Scale cognitive subscale (ADAS-cog), the Syndrom Kurztest (SKT), the Information-Concentration-Memory subtests (ICM) of the Blessed-Roth Dementia Scale *(1)*, the Mattis Dementia Rating Scale (DRS) *(2)*, and the Severe Impairment Battery (SIB) *(3–5)*.

MMSE

The Mini-Mental State Examination (MMSE) has probably become the most widely used brief mental state examination used in both clinical practice and clinical trials *(6)*. It is a brief, structured test that takes only 5–10 minutes to perform. The MMSE addresses the following cognitive areas: orientation, memory, attention (and calculation), recall, and language. The test scoring has a range of 30 points, from normal (30) to severe impairment (0). One-third of the scoring is in orientation, nearly one-third in language, and one-sixth in attention. Registration and delayed recall are relatively underweighted. It is useful in clinical trials as a rough measure of cognitive severity and as an inclusion criterion for trials, as well as for measuring the onset, progression, and severity of AD, and the outcome of clinical trials. The average yearly change in patients with AD reaches 3 points but is highly variable depending on severity at baseline and other factors.

The advantage of instruments such as the MMSE is also the possibility of predicting the future course of the disease. A low score at baseline or a rapid fall in an unusually short period of time is an unfavorable prognostic sign. On the other hand, early cognitive deterioration cannot be easily recognized by the MMSE, because of a ceiling effect at the higher end of the scale and social and educational influences on scores.

Despite these limitations, and because it is broadly accepted and easy to administer, the MMSE is often used as a secondary measure of cognitive function in clinical trials. Typically, patients with scores between 10 and 26 are eligible for enrollment in trials of patients with "mild to moderate" dementia. Surprisingly, this test, initially often considered insensitive, has proven to be sensitive to the effects of cholinesterase inhibitors compared with placebo, when sample sizes are large enough, and correlates with change in various biological characteristics of dementia. A standardized version of the MMSE also has been used in clinical trials *(7)*.

ADAS–cog

The vast majority of clinical trials for AD have used the Alzheimer's Disease Assessment Scale—cognitive subscale (ADAS-cog) as the index of cognitive change *(8,9)*. The battery was developed to sample cognitive functions typically impaired in AD and to express an overall summary score. The test is more sensitive than the MMSE and has been shown to be valid in clinical trials by revealing significant drug–placebo differences with at least six acetylcholinesterase inhibitors and several other drugs, in nearly 30 clinical trials. Although regulatory authorities do not require that the ADAS-cog be used, it has nevertheless become a *de facto* standard.

The ADAS-cog consists of a battery of brief individual tests, which require approximately 1 hour to administer. It includes word recall, naming, commands, constructional and ideational praxis, orientation, word recognition, spoken language and comprehension, word finding, and recall of test instructions. It has a range of 70 points, from normal (0) to severe impairment (70). The average yearly change in untreated patients with AD reaches 5–8 points, although placebo-treated patients in many 1-year-long clinical trials show about a 3–4-point change.

Syndrom Kurztest (SKT)

The SKT has been used extensively in clinical trials, especially in German-speaking countries. It is a brief, time-based, and scored instrument that can be administered in less than 15 minutes and ultimately assesses attention and aspects of memory *(10,11)*. The SKT has been used as a cognitive outcome measure in trials of various cognition-enhancing drugs, especially during early development in Europe, and has demonstrated validity in clinical trials. The SKT includes nine performance subtests, each limited to 1 minute, including naming objects and numerals, reversal naming, immediate and delayed recall, recognition memory, arranging and replacing blocks, and counting symbols, which define two factors of memory and attention deficit.

Information-Concentration-Memory (ICM) Test

The ICM consists of 27 questions assessing orientation, long-term memory, recall, concentration, and performance *(1)*. It requires 20–30 minutes to administer. Scores range from 0 to 37. It can be looked upon as a somewhat expanded MMSE with respect to measures of attention and memory, and supplemented by questions about knowledge. Assessment of language is not as strong.

Mattis Dementia Rating Scale

The Mattis Dementia Rating Scale evaluates attention, perseveration, praxis, abstraction, verbal and nonverbal recent memory *(2)*. The scores range from 0 to 144 (perfect).

Severe Impairment Battery (SIB)

The SIB can be used to assess patients who cannot complete conventional testing *(3–5)*. Items are single words or one-step commands combined with gestures. The test is noteworthy because most patients who are beyond moderate-severely impaired (e.g., MMSE less than 8–10) cannot complete cognitive testing with an instrument such as the ADAS-cog because of progressive deterioration in expressive and receptive language. Thus they have been excluded from many clinical trials.

The SIB measures nine different cognitive domains as well as behavioral responses. Nine areas are assessed: social interaction, memory, orientation, language, attention, praxis, visuospatial ability, construction, and orientation to name. The scores range from 0 to 100. The SIB is useful, sensitive to change, and has been validated in patients with MMSE scores between 0 and 21. Hence, despite its name it can be used in moderately and mildly impaired patients *(5)*.

The SIB has been used as the primary cognitive outcome measure in one placebo-controlled trial of donepezil in AD patients with MMSE scores at baseline from 5 to 17 *(12)*, and in two published placebo-controlled trials of memantine in AD patients with MMSE scores at baseline from 3 to 14 *(13,14)*.

GLOBAL INTERVIEW-BASED SEVERITY SCALES

Examples of severity rating scales are the Clinician's Global Impressions—Severity of Illness Scale (CGIS) *(15)*, the Clinical Dementia Rating Scale (CDR) *(16)*, and the Global Deterioration Scale (GDS) *(17)*. Item 19 of the Sandoz Clinical Assessment Geriatric (SCAG) *(18)*, completed after addressing the previous 18 items and part II of the Behave-AD *(19)*, also represents a kind of global severity rating used in several clinical dementia trials.

Clinician's Global Impressions—Severity of Illness Scale (CGIS)

The CGIS *(15)* is an unanchored 7-point scale, performed by an experienced clinician. The patient is rated on the scale ranging from 1 (normal) through 4 (moderately ill) to 7 (among the most extremely ill).

Clinical Dementia Rating Scale (CDR)

The CDR can be utilized from the time of the clinical manifestation of the disease (rating 0.5). It provides a 5-point ordinal scale ranging from 0 = no impairment, 0.5 questionable dementia, 1 = mild, 2 = moderate, and to 3 = severe dementia *(16)*. The score is based on a comprehensive structured interview using worksheets. The CDR determines the stage of AD by scoring six cognitive areas: memory, orientation, judgment and problem solving, community affairs, home and hobbies, and personal care. The information derives from an interview with the patient and the caregiver. The CDR structured interview can be used as a diagnostic tool as well, as it is modeled on the way a clinician might perform an interview. By the time a patient reaches score 1.0 on the CDR, there is no doubt about the diagnosis of dementia. In some clinical trials the CDR is used as a more quantitative sum-of-the-boxes numerical score of outcome. In this case the 0–3 score for each of the six areas is summed, yielding a possible range from 0 to 18.

Global Deterioration Scale (GDS)

The GDS rates seven potential levels of dementia severity, scored from 1 = none, 3 = late confusion, 5 = middle dementia, to 7 = very severe *(17)*. A clinician who has access to all sources of information assesses the progressive cognitive, functional, and behavioral decline. The GDS does not require a structured interview. For each score there is a paragraph describing the characteristics of a patient who would be rated at that level.

Sandoz Clinical Assessment Geriatric—Item 19 (SCAG)

The SCAG includes 18 cardinal signs and symptoms of dementia. The last item consists of a 7-point severity rating *(18)*.

GLOBAL SEVERITY MEASURES IN CLINICAL PRACTICE AND RESEARCH

Severity measures help to provide a structure by which the clinician can assess a patient's dementia. Staging a dementia on the basis of severity alone, however, does not necessarily assist management or predict future course. For example, although increased severity of dementia correlates with institutionalization, it is not its sole predictor. Assessing dementia severity might help the physician to understand when particular symptoms might be expected or have prognostic importance. For example, Forstl was able to show through severity ratings that AD patients with hallucinations and delusions, who were more mildly impaired, had more rapid progression. By contrast, hallucinations and delusions occurring in more severe stages did not have prognostic significance *(20)*.

This example also illustrates the difficulty of assessing dementia severity with these instruments: the large degree of clinical heterogeneity among AD patients and the most likely presence of subtypes or subgroups influence the rating. On the other hand, global severity measures may be useful in diagnosis when they are structured, such as the CDR, or in clinical trials that follow patients for 1 year or longer, since change in severity may be more reliably appreciated over a longer time course. As a method of tracking disease progression, global severity measures are broader in range than neuropsychological tests, such as the MMSE or ADAS-cog, and are less subject to bottoming or topping out.

Mean differences on severity scales between one time point and another may also be difficult to interpret clinically. As examples, approximately 6-month-long clinical trials showed statistically significant 0.2-point advantages on the GDS for both tacrine and rivastigmine compared with placebo *(21–23)*, and a significant 0.6-point advantage on the CDR sum-of-the-boxes measure for donepezil compared with placebo *(24)*. The clinical meanings of these average differences are unclear. However, when these severity outcomes are assessed within the context of the outcome of other measures, including cognitive and global change scales, or with respect to expected change over 6 months, their significance becomes clearer.

GLOBAL INTERVIEW-BASED CHANGE SCALES

The broad category of global interview-based change scales for clinical assessment of change includes among others the Clinician's Global Impression of Change (CGIC), the Clinician's Interview-Based Impression of Change (CIBIC), and the CIBIC+. Global change scales have been used extensively as primary outcome criteria in clinical trials for antidementia drugs *(25–27)*. The rationale for their use is that a skilled clinician should be able to see the clinical effect of a treatment after a brief interview. Any such observed changed must be considered to be clinically meaningful *(28,29)*.

Clinician's Global Impression of Change (CGIC)

The CGIC is rated by the clinician, based on interviews with or without a collateral source, with or without reference to mental status examination, and with or without reference to cognitive assessment results *(15)*. The rating consists of seven points: 1 = very much improved, 2 = much improved, 3 = minimally improved, 4 = no change, 5 = minimally worse, 6 = much worse, 7 = very much worse. The original CGIC used in dementia trials showed little sensitivity to the treatment effects of putatively effective medications. In their newer incarnations, CGICs are important efficacy measures in neuropsychopharmacological clinical trials. The CGIC is intended to determine whether the effect of a drug is large enough to allow its detection by an experienced clinician.

Clinician's Interview-Based Impression of Change (CIBIC)

FDA modifications to the CGIC suggested that clinical change should be based on a patient interview only, without input from third parties. Access to other sources of information is prevented to minimize bias and maintain independence. During a 10-minute interview, the clinician should systematically assess the domains ordinarily considered part of a clinical examination *(25)*. The rationale for this is, if an experienced clinician can perceive clinical change on the basis of an interview, then such change is likely to be clinically meaningful. The ratings are done on the same unanchored 7-point scale as used for the CGIC.

Clinician's Interview-Based Impression of Change-Plus (CIBIC+)

The measurement of global change utilizing CIBIC+ is performed by the clinician and requires additionally the input of the caregiver *(26,27)*. The score range is form 1 to 7; scores 1, 2, and 3 = improvement, 4 = no change, 5, 6, 7 = deterioration. CIBIC+ measures the effect on global functioning, including cognition, functional stage, and behavior.

CIBI (Parke-Davis)

Parke-Davis Pharmaceuticals, Inc., in cooperation with the FDA, modified the CGIC to create the Clinical Interview-Based Impression *(25)*. Thorough interviews of the patient and the caregiver by a clinician experienced in managing AD patients require that eight specific items be addressed, including assessment of mental status. A follow-up interview takes place solely with the patient prior to making a change in rating. The rating is made on a 7-point ordinal scale similar to the CGIC. The interviewer is required to assess the patient's history, strengths and weaknesses, language, behaviors sensitive to change, motivation, activities of daily living, and anything else of apparent importance. Statistically significant effects for both the CIBI and ADAS-cog in a 30-week trial of tacrine *(21)* as well as results of previous trials, led to the approval of tacrine in the United States.

As it happened, the CIBI or CIBIC was used only in that trial. Subsequent clinical trials of drugs in development for AD used a CIBIC+, requiring caregiver input. It was generally believed that obtaining information only from the patient was too stringent a test, and that information from an informant was essential in estimating clinically significant change.

ADCS-CGIC

The most common method for employing a CIBIC+ has been the ADCS-CGIC. The AD Cooperative Study—Clinical Global Impression of Change (ADCS-CGIC) was developed for the National Institutes on Aging (NIA) AD Cooperative Study (ADCS) instrument development project as a method to examine the processes and determinants of making change scores *(27)*. It consists of a format with which a clinician may address clinically relevant overall change, including 15 areas under the domains of cognition, behavior, and social and daily functioning.

The ADCS-CGIC is a process, rather than a rating scale, for obtaining an assessment of meaningful clinical changes over time. It is a systematic method for assessing clinically significant change in a clinical trial as viewed by an independent skilled and experienced clinician. The ADCS-CGIC focuses on the clinician's observations of change in the patient's cognitive, functional, and behavioral performance since the beginning of a trial. It relies on both direct examination of the patient and interviews of informants. Unlike a targeted symptom scale, it takes into account a subject's overall function in the cognitive, behavioral, and functional activity domains.

A trained clinician who is blind to treatment assignment completes the ADCS-CGIC, using a 7-point ordinal scale to rate each patient along a continuum from "very much worse" to "very much improved." Scoring is based on an interview with the caregiver and examination of the patient by an independent evaluator, without consulting other objective measures, such as cognitive test results.

NYU-CIBIC+

This CGIC was developed by New York University and Novartis Pharmaceuticals and represents another attempt to enhance the CGIC by providing a semistructured interview with the patient and the caregiver, standardized guidelines for the assessment of change, and modest anchoring to the 7-point scale (Ferris, unpublished). The interview is semistructured and relies on descriptors from the BEHAVE-AD *(19)* and in FAST *(48)*. It was used in a series of placebo-controlled trials for rivastigmine *(22,23)*, and of memantine *(13)*.

Limitations of CGIC Ratings

The construct underlying a CGIC score is that it is an instrument whose intended use is to measure clinically meaningful change, as distinct from an instrument's use to assess any change. CGIC scales are not intended as sensitive measures of small changes that are unlikely to be clinically meaningful. In principle, a clinician rating a subject as changed on a global change scale is determining clinically meaningful and distinct change. Therefore, any change recorded on a CGIC is considered clinically significant by definition.

Although a CGIC is simpler to interpret than highly sensitive psychometric instruments, its inherent lack of structure limits the precision with which ratings can be made. Also, by definition, a CGIC rating has limited external validity. A skilled examiner is asked to make his or her own individual, unanchored rating of change, based on his or her own experience. Despite these disadvantages, there is a general opinion that CGIC ratings are potentially more sensitive to clinically meaningful effects. Indeed, in numerous trials of cholinesterase inhibitors, CGIC scales have proven sensitive enough to detect clinical effects.

BEHAVIORAL SCALES

Behavioral signs and symptoms such as depression, delusions, hallucinations, and agitation occur in the vast majority of AD patients during the course of illness. In early AD trials, the most commonly used behavioral rating was the ADAS—Non-Cognitive Subscale *(8)*. Assessing behavior has become more important as clinical trials become longer. This interest in specifically evaluating drugs such as cholinesterase inhibitors for psychosis, depression, and agitation in dementia has led to a renewed emphasis on behavioral rating scales. Selected scales are discussed below. They are each designed for different purposes, rate frequency or severity of behaviors, or require caregivers or physicians to make ratings.

ADAS—Non-Cognitive Subscale

The ADAS—Non-Cognitive Subscale assesses the following areas: tearfulness, depression, concentration, uncooperativeness, delusions, hallucinations, pacing, motor activity, tremor, and appetite on a 6-point (0–5) severity scale. Usually the ADAS—non-cog is rated by the cognitive tester; essentially limited for behavior during test taking. Scores range from 50 (more severe) to 0. It was used as an outcome measure mainly in tacrine and velnacrine trials, but is no longer employed for this purpose in regulatory trials.

Behavior Rating Scale for Dementia of the Consortium to Establish a Registry for AD (CERAD)

This instrument provides a standardized, reliable semistructured interview that is administered to caregivers based on the frequency of adverse behavior *(30)*. Eight factors map onto clinically relevant domains in AD: depressive, psychotic features, defective self-regulation, irritability/agitation, vegetative features, apathy, aggression, and affective lability. It is comprehensive in scope but not frequently used in trials.

Behavioral Pathology in AD Scale (BEHAVE-AD)

The BEHAVE-AD assesses 25 well-defined behaviors in seven areas: paranoid and delusional ideation, hallucinations, activity disturbances, aggressiveness, diurnal rhythm disturbances, affective disturbance, and anxieties and phobias *(19)*. If present, behavior is rated as mild, moderate, or severe, relying on certain anchors, individualized for each question. There is a part II that requires the examiner to rate overall clinical severity on a 0–3 scale. The BEHAVE-AD has been used in trials of risperidone for agitation and psychosis in dementia patients. Pparts of it were integrated into the NYU-CIBIC+. The BEHAVE-AD tends to be used in dementia clinical trials of antipsychotics, or when behavior is a primary outcome *(31)*.

Neuropsychiatric Inventory (NPI)

The Neuropsychiatric Inventory *(32)* was developed as a measure of the frequency and severity of psychiatric symptoms and behavioral disturbances in patients with dementia. In one version, it addresses 12 items in seven domains: mood changes (depression/dysphoria; euphoria/elation), agitation (agitation/aggression; aberrant motor behavior), personality alterations (apathy/indifference; irritability/lability; disinhibition), psychosis (delusions; hallucinations), anxiety, nighttime behavior (sleep), and appetite and eating disorders. The frequency (1 = occasionally, less than once per week; 4 = very frequently, once or more per day or continuously) and severity (1 = mild, 2 = moderate, 3 = severe) of each is scored based on responses from an informed caregiver involved in the patient's life using a structured interview. The overall score (range 0–144 for the 12-item version) and the score for each subscale (range 0–12) are the product of severity and frequency (i.e., the severity score is multiplied by the frequency score).

The NPI has been used with psychotic, agitated, and aggressive patients and with nonpsychotic patients with AD in clinical trials of cognitive enhancers. It has generally shown internal validity in terms of its ability to distinguish medication groups from placebo groups. It has been used as an outcome in metrifonate, galantamine, memantine, and some other trials.

Brief Psychiatric Rating Scale

The Brief Psychiatric Rating Scale (BPRS) consists of 18 items and was designed to assess drug treatment effects in a general adult psychiatric population *(33,34)*. It has been used widely in geropsychiatric research. Psychometric data have been provided that demonstrate its factor structure, reliability, and validity *(35)*. Each item is rated on a scale from 1 (symptom not present) to 7 (symptom extremely severe). Each assesses a different symptom domain. It takes a skilled interviewer about 20 min to administer.

Although the usefulness of the BPRS with AD patients has been at times questioned *(36)* because it includes items that occur uncommonly in AD, it has proven to be very useful and sensitive to change in many AD clinical trials, including those with haloperidol, olanzapine, quetiapine, and diavalproex.

For example, it was found that hostility and delusional items showed a different response pattern to quetiapine. The scale also showed item-specific responses to olanzapine *(37)*, haloperidol *(38)*, and to anticonvulsants *(39,40)*.

Some degree of training is needed to ensure that items such as conceptual disorganization and unusual thought content correctly reflect the psychosis of AD and not merely cognitive deterioration.

Cohen-Mansfield Agitation Inventory (CMAI)

The CMAI (long form) represents a nurses' rating questionnaire consisting of 29 'agitated behaviors, rated on a 7-point frequency scale (1 = never to 7 = several times per hour) *(41)*. It is often used in nursing homes. Four features are included: aggressive behavior, physically nonaggressive behavior, verbally agitated behavior, and hiding/hoarding behavior.

FUNCTIONAL SCALES

The functional abilities of a patient are assessed using outcome instruments that are often completed by relatives or caregivers. The Physical Self-Maintenance Scale (PSMS) and the instrumental Activities of Daily Living (IADL) have been used most commonly in early clinical trials to assess basic activities of daily living and more complex, instrumental activities. More recently developed instruments—such as the Progressive Deterioration Scale (PDS) and the Interview for Deterioration in Daily living activities in Dementia (IDDD)—tend to expand on these areas by increasing the number of items and the number of rating points, by removing gender bias, and by structuring the interview with the caregiver. Other instruments, such as the Disability Assessment for Dementia (DAD) *(42)*, assesses the patient's ability to initiate, plan, organize, and perform activities of daily living through interviewing the caregiver. Lately, the ADCS-ADL has been employed in 6-month-long clinical trials.

ADL and IADL

The functional assessment addresses the patient's performance regarding the activities of daily living (ADL), including bathing, eating, dressing, transferring, toileting, and continence. The so-called instrumental ADL (iADL) includes the use of the telephone, transportation, shopping, handling of finances, and medication management. iADL scores range from 4 to 30 points, rated by the caregiver *(43)*.

Progressive Deterioration Scale (PDS)

The PDS measures the patient's function in ADL or quality of life *(44)*. It is a questionnaire covering 29 items, rated by the caregiver. The possible range is 0–100; positive differences indicate improvements.

Physical Self-Maintenance Scale (PSMS)

The PSMS assesses more functional or basic daily activities, including toileting, feeding, dressing, grooming, bathing, and ambulation *(43)*. It has to be completed by a rater based on information from a caregiver. Scores range from 6 to 30 points.

Interview for Deterioration in Daily Living Activities in Dementia (IDDD)

The IDD is a 33-item structured interview of caregivers consisting of self-care items (e.g., washing, dressing, and eating) and complex activity items (e.g., shopping, writing, answering the phone) performed by both men and women *(45)*. Concrete descriptions are elicited. It identifies the frequency of assistance, rated on a 3-point scale for each item, for an overall range of 33–99 (most severe).

Disability Assessment in Dementia (DAD)

The DAD is conducted either as a questionnaire completed by a caregiver or as a structured interview of the caregiver *(42)*. It assesses in 20 min the ability to initiate and perform basic and instrumental ADL and leisure activities. It is rated by a trained observer, using information provided by an informant.

Functional Assessment Staging (FAST)

The FAST scale includes 16 items that consist of physical and instrumental ADL, intended to project the progression of loss of function in patients with AD *(46)*. The caregiver is interviewed. The FAST has been used to stage patients, as an inclusion criterion, and to assess response to treatment, for example, in a clinical trial of risperidone *(31)*.

Rapid Disability Rating Scale-2

The Rapid Disability Rating Scale-2 is an 18-item questionnaire completed by a caregiver based on observed performance, rated by frequency *(47)*. In addition to 10 areas of ADL, it also addresses communicative abilities, confusion, depression, and the cooperativeness of the AD patient.

The AD Cooperative Study-Activities of Daily Living Scale (ADCS-ADL)

The ADCS-ADL is an ADL inventory developed by the ADCS to assess functional performance in subjects with AD *(48)*. In a structured interview format that requires less than 15 min to administer, informants are queried as to whether subjects attempted each of 24 items in the inventory during the prior 4 weeks and their level of performance (the number of items vary in different versions). The ADCS-ADL scale discriminates well the stages of severity of AD patients, from very mild to severely impaired. It includes items from traditional basic ADL scales (e.g., grooming, dressing, walking, bathing, feeding, toileting) as well as iADL scales (e.g., shopping, preparing meals, using household appliances, keeping appointments, reading). The ADCS-ADL inventory is currently being used as an outcome measure in several AD clinical trials. Versions suitable for assessing very mild or very severe patients have been developed.

LIMITATIONS OF RATING SCALES

There has been controversy about the meaning of the outcomes of individual clinical trials in AD. Some critics discuss outcomes of cholinesterase inhibitor trials as being small in magnitude or lacking clinical significance, even as the results are statistically significant. This discussion and the interpretation of AD clinical trials in general could be enhanced by a better understanding of basic outcome measures and of the need to interpret the overall pattern of response.

Rating scales are useful and necessary both in clinical practice and in research. Clinicians can benefit from these tools in being able to better appreciate presentation, severity, frequency, and clinical course of the disease. However, a clinician should not become subject to the tyranny of scales and fail to thoroughly assess patients clinically. Similarly, when comparing group mean differences in rating scales between drug therapy and placebo, or between different drug treatments in clinical trials, clinicians should remember that individual patients may respond better or worse to a given drug. The average response of a group in fact can be misleading, masking individuals who respond particularly better or poorer than the group. To this end, individual patient analyses, such as the proportion who improve on a global rating or composite improvement scores, are essential in interpreting clinical effects *(49)*.

REGULATORY CONSIDERATIONS

The concerns that some pharmaceutical companies might test candidate antidementia drugs insufficiently, combined with the desire by some companies for clear standards, led the U.S. Food and Drug Administration to propose draft guidelines in 1990 for establishing whether a drug has antidementia efficacy. These draft guidelines required, in part, that:

1. Clinical trials be double-blind and placebo-controlled
2. Patients fulfill established criteria for an AD diagnosis

Table 1
Summary of EU and U.S. Regulatory Guidelines for Clinical Trials Outcomes

EMEA, European Union (1997, www.eudra.org)

Diagnosis, grading of severity, and patient selection for trials discussed

Diagnosis of dementia based on DSM or ICD. NINCDS/ADRDA criteria of probable AD considered most appropriate, but other dementias allowed.

Severity: mild to moderate.

Efficacy

Cognitive, functional, and global endpoints are required, focusing on symptomatic improvement. Statistically significant differences in two primary variables, one of which must be cognitive, followed by analysis of proportion who achieve a meaningful benefit using a composite score.

For a claim in behavioral symptoms, a specific trial required with this as the primary endpoint is required.

In moderate to severe illness, meaningful differences in functional and global endpoints might be acceptable.

Quality of life or economic evaluations are not required.

Trial design issues

Six months duration.

One year for maintenance of efficacy.

Instruments not specified, though required to be valid and reliable.

FDA, United States (www.fda.gov)

Diagnosis

Diagnosis of dementia based on accepted criteria, for AD usually NINCDS/ADRDA criteria of probable AD.

Efficacy

Statistically significant differences in two primary variables, one of which must be cognitive and the other a global assessment.

Global measure was originally a clinical interview-based impression of change, and currently a CIBIC+. Cognitive instrument not specified, though the ADAS-cog is most commonly used.

Quality of life or economic evaluations are not required.

Trial design issues

Three months duration is sufficient; however, recently approved drugs provide at least two 6-month trials.

Source: Adapted from ref. *29*. EMEA, European Agency for the Evaluation of Medicinal Products; FDA, Food and Drug Administration.

3. Studies be of sufficient length in order to appreciate a meaningful effect (now considered to be 6 months)
4. Appropriate instruments be used to document efficacy *(29)*

As cognitive impairment is a primary feature of dementia, it was reasoned that an experimental drug must show efficacy by improving cognition or retarding its deterioration. To address the concern that drug-related cognitive improvement measured by psychometric testing might be trivial, the FDA required that a clinically meaningful effect determined by a clinician independently from psychometric assessment must also be observed. Thus, the dual-outcome criterion was established and ultimately became the *de facto* standard after the marketing approval of tacrine in the United States in 1996. (In a 30-week trial, significant tacrine–placebo differences were observed for both the cognitive testing battery and a clinician's interview-based impression of change *[21]*.) The subsequent approvals of donepezil, rivastigmine, and galantamine were based on efficacy on both a global and the ADAS-cog in at least one 6-month-long trial.

Changes in other areas of functioning, such as behavior or capacity to perform ADL, have been considered of secondary importance by U.S. standards.

Limitations to the guidelines include the failure to recognize improvement in behavior or functional activities alone as legitimate therapeutic goals and the lack of guidelines for severely impaired patients, who are unable to perform standard cognitive tests.

The European Union, through the Committee for Proprietary Medicinal Products (CPMP) of the European Agency for the Evaluation of Medicinal Products (EMEA), issued subsequent dementia guidelines that also effectively required that a drug show efficacy on a functional or behavioral scale as well. Table 1 summarizes the FDA and EMEA guidelines with respect to outcomes.

Although the EMEA did not offer guidelines for severe dementia, in May 2002 it approved the marketing of memantine specifically for treatment of patients with moderately severe to severe Alzheimer's disease. The agency considered two placebo-controlled trials to be pivotal: a 12-week-long trial in a nursing home using a global and functional rating as primary endpoints *(50)*; and a confirmatory 24-week-long outpatient trial *(13)*.

In this latter home trial the primary outcomes were a clinical global and functional rating. In the latter trial of 252 outpatients with MMSE scores from 3 to 14, the primary outcome parameters included the CIBIC+, and a 19-item version of the ADCS. Cognition was assessed as a secondary endpoint using the SIB. Thus, a *de facto* standard for moderate to severe dementia has been established for the European Union. This basically includes efficacy on CIBIC+, ADL, and cognition using the SIB.

OTHER REFERENCES

Discussions and listings of these and other scales can be found in refs. *49* and *51*.

REFERENCES

1. Blessed, G.; Tomlinson, B.E.; Roth, M.: The association between quantitative measures of dementia and of senile change in the cerebral grey matter of elderly subjects. Br J Psychiatry 1968; 114: 797–811.
2. Mattis, S.: Mental status examination for organic mental syndrome in the elderly patient. In: Bellak, L.; Karasu, T.B. (eds.): Geriatric psychiatry. Grune & Stratton, New York, 1976: 77–101.
3. Saxton, J. et al.: Assessment of the severely impaired patient: description and validation of a new neuropsychological test battery. Psychol Assess: J Consult Clin Psychol 1990; 2: 298–303.
4. Panisset, M. et al.: Severe Impairment Battery: a neuropsychological test for severely demented patients. Arch Neurol 1994; 51: 41–45.
5. Schmitt, F.A. et al.: The severe impairment battery: concurrent validity and the assessment of longitudinal change in Alzheimer's disease. Alz Dis Assoc Disord 1997; 11 (suppl 2): S51–S56.
6. Folstein, M.F.; Folstein, S.E.; McHugh, P.R.: "Mini-mental state." A practical method for grading the cognitive state of patients for the clinician. J Psychiatr Res 1975; 12: 189–198.
7. Molloy, D.M.; Alemayehu, E.; Roberts, R.: Reliability of a standardized Mini-Mental State Examination compared with the traditional Mini-Mental State Examination. Am J Psychiatry 1991; 148: 102–105.
8. Rosen, W.G.; Mohs, R.C.; Davis, K.L.: A new rating scale for Alzheimer's disease. Am J Psychiatry 1984; 141: 1356–1364.
9. Mohs, R.C. et al.: Development of cognitive instruments for use in clinical trials of anti dementia drugs: additions to the Alzheimer's Disease Assessment Scale (ADAS) that broaden its scope. Alz Dis Assoc Disord 1997; 11 (suppl 2): S13–S21.
10. Overall, J.E.; Schaltenbrand, R.: The SKT neuropsychological test battery. J Geriatr Psychiatr Neurol 1992; 5: 220–227.
11. Erzigkeit, H.: The SKT: a short cognitive performance test as an instrument for the assessment of clinical efficacy of cognition enhancers. In: Bergener, M.; Reisberg, B. (eds.): Diagnosis and treatment of senile dementia. Springer-Verlag, Berlin, 1989: 164–174.
12. Feldman, H. et al.: A 24-week, randomized, double-blind study of donepezil in moderate to severe Alzheimer's disease. Neurology 2001; 57: 613–620.
13. Reisberg, B. et al. Memantine in moderate to severe Alzheimer's disease. N Engl J Med 2003; 348: 1333–1341.
14. Tariot, P. et al.: Memantine/donepezil dual-therapy is superior to placebo/donepezil therapy for treatment of moderate to severe Alzheimer's disease, Poster 181. ACNP 41st Annual Meeting, San Juan, Puerto Rico, December 9, 2002.
15. Guy, W. (ed.): Clinical Global Impressions (CGI). In: ECDEU Assessment Manual for Psychopharmacology. U.S. Department of Health and Human Services, Public Health Service, Alcohol Drug Abuse and Mental Health Administration, NIMH Psychopharmacology Research Branch, Rockville, MD; 1976: 218–222.
16. Morris, J.C.: The Clinical Dementia Rating (CDR): Current version and scoring rules. Neurology 1993; 43: 2412–2414.

17. Reisberg, B. et al.: The global deterioration scale for assessment of primary degenerative dementia. Am J Psychiatry 1982; 139: 1136–1139
18. Shader, R.L. et al.: A new scale for clinical assessment in geriatric populations: Sandoz Clinical Assessment-Geriatric (SCAG). J Am Geriatr Soc 1974; 22: 107–113.
19. Reisberg, B. et al.: Behavioral symptoms in Alzheimer's disease: phenomenology and treatment. J Clin Psychiatry 1987; 48 (suppl): 9–15.
20. Forstl, H. et al.: Psychotic features and the course of Alzheimer's disease: relationship to cognitive, electroencephalographic and computerized tomography findings. Acta Psychiatr Scand 1993; 87: 395–399.
21. Knapp, M.J. et al.: A 30-week randomized controlled trial of high-dose tacrine in patients with Alzheimer's disease. JAMA 1994; 271: 985–991.
22. Corey-Bloom, J.; Anand, R.; Veach, J.: A randomized trial evaluating the efficacy and safety of ENA 713 (rivastigmine tartrate), a new acetylcholinesterase inhibitor, in patients with mild to moderately severe Alzheimer's disease. Int J Geriatr Psychopharmacol 1998; 1: 55–65.
23. Rosler, M. et al.: Efficacy and safety of rivastigmine in patients with Alzheimer's disease: international randomized controlled trial. Br Med J 1999; 318: 633–638.
24. Rogers, S.L. et al.: A 24-week, double-blind, placebo-controlled trial of donepezil in patients with Alzheimer's disease. Donepezil Study Group. Neurology 1998; 50: 136–145.
25. Knopman, D.S. et al.: The Clinician Interview-Based Impression (CIBI): a clinician's global change rating scale in Alzheimer's disease. Neurology 1994; 44: 2315–2321.
26. Schneider, L.S.; Olin, J.T.: Clinical Global Impressions in Clinical Trials. Int Psychogeriatr 1996; 8: 277–280.
27. Schneider, L.S. et al.: Validity and reliability of the Alzheimer's disease Cooperative Study-Clinical Global Impression of Change. Alzh Dis Assoc Disord 1997; 11 (suppl 2): S22–S32.
28. Leber, P.: Guidelines for the clinical evaluation of anti-dementia drugs. 1st draft. U.S. Food and Drug Administration, Rockville, MD, 1990 (unpublished).
29. Leber, P.: Criteria used by drug regulatory authorities. In: Qizilbash, N.;Schneider, L.S.; Chui, H.; Tariot, P.; Brodaty, H.; Kaye, J.; Erkinjuntti, T. (eds.): Evidence-based dementia practice. Blackwell, Oxford, UK, 2002: 376–405.
30. Tariot, P.N. et al: The Behavior Rating Scale for Dementia of the Consortium to Establish a Registry for Alzheimer's Disease. The Behavioral Pathology Committee of the Consortium to Establish a Registry for Alzheimer's Disease. Am J Psychiatry 1995; 152: 1349–1357.
31. Katz, I.R. et al.: Comparison of risperidone and placebo for psychosis and behavioral disturbances associated with dementia: a randomized, double-blind trial. J Clin Psychiatry 1999; 60: 107–115.
32. Cummings, J.L. et al.: The Neuropsychiatric Inventory: comprehensive assessment of psychopathology in dementia. Neurology 1994; 44: 2308–2314.
33. Overall, J.E.; Gorham, D.R.: The Brief Psychiatric Rating Scale. Psychol Rep 1962; 10: 799–812.
34. Rhoades, H.M.; Overall, J.E.: The semistructured BPRS interview and rating guide. Psychopharmacol Bull 1988; 24: 101–104.
35. Beller, S.A.; Overall, J.E.: The Brief Psychiatric Rating Scale (BPRS) in geropsychiatric research: I. Factor structure on an inpatient unit. J Gerontol 1984; 39: 187–193.
36. Ownby, R.: Memory evaluation in Alzheimer's disease. Caregivers' appraisals and objective testing. Arch Neurol 1993; 50: 92–97.
37. Street, J.S. et al.: Olanzapine treatment of psychotic and behavioral symptoms in patients with Alzheimer's disease in nursing care facilities: a double-blind, randomized, placebo-controlled trial. Arch Gen Psychiatry 2000; 57: 968–976.
38. Devanand, D.P. et al.: A randomized, placebo-controlled dose-comparison trial of haloperidol for psychosis and disruptive behaviors in Alzheimer's disease. Am J Psychiatry 1998; 155: 1512–1520.
39. Tariot, P.N. et al.: Safety and tolerability of divalproex sodium in the treatment of signs and symptoms of mania associated with dementia: results of a double-blind, placebo-controlled trial. Curr Ther Res 2001; 62: 51–67.
40. Olin, J.T. et al.: A pilot randomized trial of carbamazepine for behavioral symptoms in treatment resistant outpatients with Alzheimer's disease. Am J Geriatr Psychiatry 2001; 9: 400–405.
41. Cohen-Mansfield, J. et al.: A description of agitation in a nursing home. J Gerontol 1989; 44: M77–M84.
42. Gélinas, I. et al.: Development of a functional measure for persons with Alzheimer's disease: the disability assessment for dementia. Am J Occup Ther 1999; 53: 471–481.
43. Lawton, M.; Brody, E: Assessment of older people: self-maintaining and instrumental activities of daily living. Gerontologist 1969: 179–186.
44. DeJong, R.; Osterlund, O.W.; Roy, G.W.: Measurement of quality-of-life changes in patients with Alzheimer's disease. Clin Ther 1989; 11: 545–554.
45. Teunisse, S.; Derix, M.M.A.; van Crevel, H.: Assessing the severity of dementia; patient and caregiver. Arch Neurol 1991; 48: 274–277.
46. Reisberg, B.: Functional assessment staging (FAST). Psychopharmacol Bull 1988; 24: 653–659.
47. Linn, M.W.; Linn, B.S.: The rapid disability rating scale-2. J Am Geriatr Soc 1982; 30: 378–382.

48. Galasko, D. et al.: An inventory to assess activities of daily living for clinical trials in Alzheimer's disease. Alz Dis Assoc Disord 1997; 11 (suppl 2): S33–S39.

49. Schneider, L.S.: Assessing outcomes in Alzheimer disease. Alz Dis Assoc Disord 2001; 15 (suppl 1): S8–S18.

50. Winblad, B.; Poritis, N.: Memantine in severe dementia: results of the 9M-Best Study (Benefit and efficacy in severely demented patients during treatment with memantine). Int J Geriatr Psychiatry 1999; 14: 135–146.

51. Bullock, R.: Appendix II: Dementia rating scales. In: Qizilbash, N.; Schneider, L.S.; Chui, H.; Tariot, P.; Brodaty, H.; Kaye, J.; Erkinjuntti, T. (eds.): Evidence-based dementia practice. Blackwell, Oxford, UK, 2002: 859–869.

X Neuropsychiatric Management

39

Gender Differences in Behavior of AD Patients

Brian R. Ott

INTRODUCTION

In this chapter gender is discussed as a contributing factor to some of the differences seen in behavior among Alzheimer's disease (AD) patients. The potential cognitive and neurobiological bases for such differences are discussed. Clinicians who diagnose and treat patients with AD will readily recognize that there is heterogeneity in the biological and behavioral manifestations of the disease (1). Converging evidence from recent research suggests that gender is an important modifying factor in the behavioral expression of AD. The social, developmental, hormonal, and pathological interactions that produce differences in the clinical manifestations of AD between men and women are very complex. Our understanding of these interactions is evolving. A great deal of work has been done in the study of gender differences in normal development and aging. Studies of gender differences in AD and the diseases of aging, however, are in their infancy.

GENDER DIFFERENCES IN BEHAVIOR

Clinical Features

Although changes in cognition are typically the first and most pervasive feature noted in AD, behavioral disturbances are also common. Such problems include apathy, social withdrawal, depression, psychosis, sleep disturbance, wandering, motor restlessness, aggression, inappropriate sexual behavior, hoarding, and altered eating and sleep habits. Many reports have suggested that behavioral disturbances in AD are related directly to the severity of dementia regardless of gender, but qualitative differences between men and women in the particular types of behavioral disturbance have been observed.

In one study we reported that female AD patients were more reclusive and emotionally labile. They tended to hoard for no obvious reason, refused help with personal care, refused to eat, as well as cried or laughed inappropriately. In comparison, men with AD showed more psychomotor changes and vegetative behaviors. They tended to show lack of interest in daily activities, pace, slept excessively during the day, and overate. In addition, there was an association between aggressive behaviors and male gender (2). This latter observation confirms several other reports of increased physical (3,4), verbal (5,6), and sexual (5) aggression in men compared to women. Derouesne (7) reported that men with AD were more likely than women to show changes in sexual behavior and to exhibit inappropriate sexual behaviors. The observation of increased aggression in men with AD is consistent with aggressive tendencies among male humans without AD (8) and other mammals (9).

In a more recent study (10), we examined gender differences in dementia-related behavioral problems using a cross section of nursing home residents in five U.S. states. Behavior problems documented at the first assessment of 28,367 residents with AD were evaluated. Men were more likely to exhibit any type of behavioral problem than women (59% vs 50%). Men exhibited greater specific problems

From: *Current Clinical Neurology,*
Alzheimer's Disease: A Physician's Guide to Practical Management
Edited by: R. W. Richter and B. Zoeller Richter © Humana Press Inc., Totowa, NJ

than women in wandering, verbal and physical abusiveness, and inappropriate social behavior, particularly in the more advanced stages of the disease.

Such behavioral differences may extend to other neurodegenerative diseases. In a follow-up study of Parkinson's disease patients in nursing homes, we found that wandering, verbal and physical abusiveness, and inappropriate behaviors were again more common in men, particularly those with severe cognitive impairment. The similarities in behavioral observations in these two studies may reflect the presence of combined Alzheimer and Parkinson pathology in some patients *(11)*.

Psychiatric symptoms have also been reported in AD patients; however, the relationship between gender and psychiatric disturbance is less clear. Apathy is seen more commonly in men *(2,12)*, whereas depression appears to be more prevalent in women with AD *(13–16)*. One study found that delusions and hallucinations occur at an earlier stage of disease *(17)*, and three others reported that delusions occur more frequently in women with AD *(13,18,19)*.

A more recent study examining psychosis in 329 patients with probable AD found that severity of cognitive impairment and rate of cognitive decline are strong predictors of psychotic features, such as hallucinations and delusions in patients with AD, but there was no gender difference *(20)*. We have also found no gender differences in prevalence of hallucinations, delusions, or depression among demented nursing home residents with AD *(10)*. Among cognitively impaired Parkinson patients in the nursing home, hallucinations and delusions were equally prevalent by gender; however, depression occurred more commonly in women *(11)*.

As in the case of aggressive behavior, the contribution of premorbid gender differences in psychiatric disorders should be considered in the etiology of these behavioral disturbances. The prevalence of depression in women is approximately twice that of men in the general population. Late-onset schizophrenia is seven times more common in women *(21)*. The basis for these differences is unknown. Disinhibited behavior due to cortical degeneration from AD may interact with these factors to amplify or accelerate their occurrence in women.

Cognitive Differences

To the extent that cognitive deficits in dementia may become manifest as changes in behavior, one can look to studies of cognition as a partial explanation for these gender-related observations. For example, inability to communicate due to aphasia may result in reclusive social behavior. Several studies of gender differences in cognition have pointed to a greater deficit on tests of language in women with AD as compared to men.

Naming and word recognition skills have been reported to be more adversely affected in female AD patients than in male patients, and the differences have been shown to be sustained over time *(22)*. Buckwalter and colleagues *(23,24)* have conducted a series of studies that have demonstrated differences between men and women with AD, with language skills being particularly more affected in women.

In a recent study *(25)*, semantic memory was evaluated in patients with AD and vascular dementia (VaD). Women with VaD performed worse than men on semantic memory, while women with AD showed a trend to perform worse than men on the semantic memory test. No other gender differences were reported on other tests of neuropsychological function administered. These findings suggest that semantic memory may be more impaired in women than in men with AD, as well as in VaD. McPherson and colleagues *(26)* also found gender-related cognitive deficits on semantic and episodic memory as well as tasks of confrontation naming and expressive word knowledge for women compared to men with AD.

Bayles and colleagues *(27)* performed a critical analysis of previous studies revealing several statistical limitations, including insufficient control of dementia severity, failure to correct for multiple comparisons, and inappropriate statistical comparisons. In their own study, 63 patients with AD were administered a battery of tests designed to assess language comprehension and production. Based on cross-sectional analysis of the data, no significant differences between men and women were found on any of the language measures, when controlling for dementia severity. The authors interpreted their findings as suggesting that there was no evidence that AD adversely affected language performance of women more than men.

The absence of gender-related differences in language in AD has also been reported recently by Hebert and colleagues *(28)*. Four hundred ten patients with AD were followed for up to 5 years and evaluated on a number of cognitive tests. There was no significant difference between the female and male AD patients in language decline or other measures of cognition, including memory and perception. The discrepant findings reported in these studies suggest that additional work is needed to address adequately the issue of cognitive differences between men and women with AD.

Structural Brain Differences

There have been many observations of gender differences in normal brain structure and function. Quantitative sex differences in brain aging of healthy people have been reported in a number of magnetic resonance imaging (MRI) studies. Recently, Coffey et al. reported that reduction in brain volume was greater in men in the parieto-occipital regions. No hemispheric asymmetries were noted between sexes. In their review of 19 prior studies examining radiological changes of brain aging, there were inconsistent observations on gender differences *(29)*.

There are fewer studies of the morphological and physiological differences between sexes with AD, and again, no consistent patterns of gender difference have emerged. Jack et al. reported that medial temporal atrophy measured on MRI was similar between men and women in normal aging. Furthermore, no gender effect was found for decline in medial temporal lobe volumes for those with early AD *(30)*. In a magnetic resonance spectroscopy study, phosphorus metabolism was reduced in the frontal lobes of women with AD compared to men. A similar though nonsignificant effect was seen among normal eldery *(31)*.

Functional brain imaging using positron emission tomography (PET) and single-photon emission computed tomography (SPECT) may provide more sensitive measures of physiological and pathological changes in the brain than MRI, particularly in AD, in which abnormalities have been demonstrated even in the predementia phase of the illness. Small et al. studied metabolic rates in 13 subjects with early-onset and 11 subjects with late-onset AD. Women had higher metabolic rates in all regions studied compared to men; however, the differences did not approach statistical significance *(32)*. Jagust et al., however, found that women with AD had lower metabolic rates in all regions evaluated, particularly in the visual cortex *(33)*. Such inconsistent gender effects may be related to the small sample sizes employed in earlier studies.

Based on two recent separate studies of 220 *(34)* and 300 patients *(35)*, unilateral temporo-parietal defects are seen more commonly on SPECT images of women with AD compared to men, indicating a potential gender effect on diagnostic utility. This is a finding of practical importance, because bilateral defects are regarded as the characteristic pattern in AD.

Furthermore, we have found that unilateral left hemisphere perfusion defects were more common in women compared to men, particularly for those with probable AD. In a multiple-regression model, female gender and shorter duration of disease were independent predictors of the unilateral left hemisphere pattern in those with AD. There was a nonsignificant trend indicating that this pattern was seen more often in women receiving estrogen replacement therapy *(35)*.

This evidence suggests that the left hemisphere of the female brain may be more vulnerable to AD, or that the right hemisphere may be relatively protected in some women by estrogen or other factors yet to be determined. Such hemispheric factors may affect the expression of language and mood disturbances in women with AD.

OTHER BIOLOGICAL DIFFERENCES

Differences in regional cortical brain pathology may account for behavioral heterogeneity in men and women with AD. Psychosocial factors and premorbid personality traits are other areas that have not been addressed by research to date. Proponents of gender difference in language function in AD have pointed to differing patterns of neural organization in development that may influence the course of language breakdown in the course of the disease *(22)* or to the influence of sex hormones on the brain *(36)*.

Hormonal Factors

Abnormal brain–adrenal axis function has been observed in some but not all studies of patients with AD (as evidenced by reduced cortisol suppression dexamethasone challenge), particularly among advanced dementia cases. Oxenkrug et al. demonstrated that the relationship between dementia severity and nonsuppressibility is seen in women but not men, which may explain the discrepancy among different studies *(37)*.

There is accumulating evidence that ovarian hormones may be important modulators of the cognitive effects of aging and AD expression. This subject has been reviewed elsewhere *(38–40)*.

There are a number of scientific reasons why estrogen may play a role in AD. Estrogen receptors are present in various areas of the brain, including those that are integral to AD pathology, such as hippocampus, cerebral cortex, and nuclei of the basal forebrain. Estrogen increases both, cerebral blood flow, and glucose utilization. It also has a direct neurotrophic effect, such as stimulation of neurite outgrowth. Estrogen has been shown to favorably affect amyloid precursor protein (APP) processing *(41,42)* and reduce oxidative stress *(43)*, which may confer a cytoprotective effect. In addition to possible trophic effects on cholinergic neurons, it appears to play a role in the regulation of serotonergic and catecholaminergic pathways, which may be relevant to observations of mood change in women with AD *(44)*.

For men, estrogenic influences on the development and expression of AD are less likely. Although testosterone levels drop with age in men, aromatization of testosterone and androstenedione to estrogens increases. This results in relatively stable or increased levels of estradiol in aging men *(45)*.

The potential influence of testosterone on cognition and behavior in AD is an area deserving of further exploration. Neuroprotective activity for testosterone has been shown experimentally for prevention of tau phosphorylation *(46)* as well as attenuation of beta-amyloid toxicity *(47)*. Beneficial effects of androgens on cognition have been shown for apolipoprotein E4 (ApoE4)-expressing mice *(48)*. Testosterone blockade with flutamide has been reported to result in cognitive decline in a case report of a patient with AD, consistent with previous observations of enhanced cognition in nondemented men treated with testosterone *(49)*.

Testosterone could also have a modulating effect on the presence and type of aggressive behaviors seen in men with dementia. Orengo et al. *(50)* have reported that free testosterone levels showed a significant positive correlation with measures of aggression in 50 elderly men with dementia.

Other Genetic Factors

Numerous studies have demonstrated that the presence of the ApoEe4-allele is an important risk factor for sporadic AD, the most common form of the disease. Some reports have suggested an interaction between gender and ApoE genotype, with women being more influenced by the e4 genotype than men *(51,52)*. In an experimental study of ApoE-knockout mice, the negative effect of the e4 genotype on learning behavior was seen primarily in females *(53)*.

In a study of risk factors for depression in AD, family history of mood disorders was associated with an increased risk of major depression only for women *(54)*, suggesting that genetic influences may be more important in women than in men for the expression of mood disturbances in the disease.

THERAPEUTIC IMPLICATIONS

Quantitative sex differences in cognitive function of persons with AD may reflect normal effects of estrogen on the human brain. In a review of estrogen effects on cognition in menopausal women, Sherwin concluded that there is substantial evidence that estrogen maintains memory in normal women. Studies show a positive effect of exogenous estrogen, which is relatively modest, on verbal but not visual memory *(36)*. Withdrawal of estrogen due to menopause may produce a greater vulnerability of women to the loss of verbal memory as the result of pathological processes such as AD.

The evidence that estrogen replacement therapy (ERT) may enhance cognitive function in nondemented women has been drawn from small-sized studies. Contradictory evidence of estrogen's effects on cognition has also been reported. Yaffe et al. found no relation between endogenous estrogen levels and cognitive performance or risk of cognitive decline in a cohort of 532 women over age 65 *(55)*.

Despite theoretical and epidemiological evidence for the beneficial effects of estrogen for women, there is now good evidence that ERT does not improve cognition or slow progression of dementia. Three recent prospective controlled clinical trials *(56–58)* found no benefit for estrogen treatment on cognition in women with dementia of Alzheimer type. Also, in a retrospective cohort study of 191 women estrogen users in nursing homes compared to 6663 women not using estrogen, no significant difference was seen for the rate of decline. Of interest, there was a trend toward less cognitive decline in estrogen users with minimal cognitive impairment at study entry *(59)*.

Hormonal therapies may ultimately have a role in the prevention of AD. Prospective studies are in progress to investigate the therapeutic role of estrogen in women. The Women's Health Initiative Memory Study will address the question of whether ERT can prevent or delay the development of AD in women who are initially free of dementia.

Fetal sexual differentiation appears to affect estrogen's effect on the brain. Regulation of acetylcholine activity by estrogen differs by gender. For example, in female rats, estradiol has been shown to increase the activity of the enzyme choline acetyl-transferase, but not in males *(60)*. This effect has clinical relevance to therapeutic response to cholinergic medications. In a retrospective analysis of a clinical trial, Schneider et al. found that the benefits of tacrine, as measured by cognitive tests and global clinical impression, were greater for women receiving ERT and tacrine than for those receiving tacrine alone or placebo. This observation was interpreted to suggest that ERT may enhance the response to cholinergic medications in AD patients *(61)*.

ApoE genotype and gender may affect the response to cholinergic therapy in humans. In a retrospective study of a clinical trial of tacrine, the e4 genotype exerted a negative effect on clinical response to the drug in women, but not in men *(62)*. It is unknown whether women who were ApoEe4-positive were less likely to have been on ERT in this sample. A more recent prospective open-label trial of donepezil found no effect of gender or ApoE genotype on treatment outcome *(63)*.

Research is in progress to develop nonfeminizing estrogen-like compounds that may be used in treating men with AD. Androgenic effect on AD behavior expression is another potential area of research. To date only anecdotal reports suggest beneficial effects of estrogen *(64)* and anti-androgen drugs *(65–67)* in reducing aggressive behaviors in men with dementia.

The tendency of men to exhibit more aggressive behaviors is likely to be associated with more prevalent use of major tranquilizers to treat agitated behavior. Among nursing home residents with dementia, men were found to be more likely to be treated with antipsychotic medications and less likely to be treated with antidepressants (after controlling for age and degree of cognitive impairment), even though psychosis and depression were equally prevalent between sexes *(10,11)*. The more prevalent use of major tranquilizers in men with AD might contribute to the increased mortality reported for male nursing home residents *(68)*.

Women have been reported to be more likely to respond to antidepressants for agitated behaviors than men in a double-blind, randomized, placebo-controlled crossover study of sertraline in 22 patients with severe AD *(69)*.

SUMMARY

Present knowledge about sex differences in AD patients suggests that there may be a differential vulnerability of the brains of men and women to aging and neurodegeneration processes, resulting in

Table 1
Reported Gender Differences in Alzheimer's Disease:
Aspects of Disease as They Most Closely Relate to Gender

	Female traits	Male traits
Behavior disturbances	Reclusiveness/resistiveness *(2)* Hoarding behavior *(2)* Emotional lability/depression *(2,13–16)* Psychosis *(13,17–19)*	Aggression *(2–6,10)* Apathy *(2,12)* Vegetative behavior *(2)* Inappropriate behavior *(2,10)* Wandering *(10)*
Cognitive deficits	Language *(22–26)* Semantic memory *(25,26)* Orientation *(70)* Constructions *(70)*	—
Brain structure and function	Unilateral temporoparietal reduction of cerebral perfusion *(34,35)* Reduced frontal phosphorus metabolism *(31)* Higher metabolic rate *(32)* Lower metabolic rate *(33)*	Reduced temporoparietal cerebral perfusion *(71)*
Genetics	ApoEe4 risk factor: Alzheimer's disease *(51,52,72)* Early age of onset *(73)* Poor response to cholinergic treatment *(62)* Familial depression risk factor: depression with AD *(54)*	—

Adapted with permission from J Gender Specific Med *(74)*.

a variation in clinical manifestations. Furthermore, gender may interact with other genetic risk factors in disease expression and response to treatment. It remains controversial, though, whether indeed men and women differ in the incidence of AD, as well as whether there are clearly definable and clinically relevant sex differences in cognition and behavior among those afflicted. The reported gender differences in cognition and behavior that could relate to multiple factors acting alone or in combination are summarized in Table 1. A thorough understanding of these differences is important for the sake of understanding the behavioral problems of AD and developing a more refined approach to their treatment. More research into the biological underpinnings as well as the social influences on these differences is needed. To the extent that hormonal influences may be etiologically important, new avenues to treatment may be opened. Finally, morbidity and mortality outcomes for different therapies used to treat agitated or aggressive behaviors in men and women need further study.

REFERENCES

1. Friedland, R.P. et al: Alzheimer disease: Clinical and biological heterogeneity. Ann Intern Med 1988; 109: 298–311.
2. Ott, B.R. et al.: Gender differences in the behavioral manifestations of Alzheimer's disease. J Am Geriatr Soc 1996; 44: 583–587.
3. Burns, A.; Jacoby, R.; Levy, R.: Psychiatric phenomena in Alzheimer's disease. IV: disorders of behaviour. Br J Psychiatry 1990; 15: 86–94.
4. Lyketsos, C.G. et al.: Physical aggression in dementia patients and its relationship to depression. Am J Psychiatry 1999; 156: 66–71.
5. Drachman, D.A. et al.: The caretaker obstreperous-behavior rating assessment (COBRA) scale. J Am Geriatr Soc 1992; 40: 463–480.

6. Eustace, A. et al.: Verbal aggression in Alzheimer's disease. Clinical, functional and neuropsychological correlates. Int J Geriatr Psychiatry 2001; 16: 858–861.
7. Derousne, C. et al.: Sexual behavioral changes in Alzheimer's disease. Alzheimer Dis Assoc Disord 1996; 10: 86–92.
8. Christiansen, K.; Knussmann, R.: Androgen levels and components of aggressive behavior in men. Horm Behav 1987; 21: 170–180.
9. Bouissou, W.: Androgens, aggressive behavior, and social relationships in higher mammals. Horm Res 1983; 18: 43–61.
10. Ott, B.R.; Lapane, K.L.; Gambassi, G.: Gender differences in the treatment of behavior problems in Alzheimer's disease. Neurology 2000; 54: 427–432.
11. Fernandez, H.H. et al.: Gender differences in the frequency and treatment of behavior problems in Parkinson's disease. Movement Disorders 2000; 15: 490–496.
12. Teri, L. et al.: Behavioral disturbance, cognitive dysfunction, and functional skill. J Am Geriatr Soc 1989; 37: 109–116.
13. Cohen, D.; Eisdorfer, C.; Gorelick, P.: Sex differences in the psychiatric manifestations of Alzheimer's disease. J Am Geriatr Soc 1993; 41: 229–232.
14. Reifler, B.V.; Larson, E.; Hanley, R.: Coexistence of cognitive impairment and depression in geriatric outpatients. Am J Psychiatry 1982; 139: 623–626.
15. Teri, L.; Hughes, J.P.; Larson, E.: Cognitive deterioration in Alzheimer's disease: Behavioral and health factors. J Gerontol B Psychol Sci Soc Sci 1990; 45: 58–63.
16. Lazarus, L.W.; Newton, N.; Cohler, B.: Frequency and presentation of depressive symptoms in patients with primary degenerative dementia. Am J Psychiatry 1987; 144: 41–45.
17. Jost, B.C.; Grossberg, G.T.: The evolution of psychiatric symptoms in Alzheimer's disease: A natural history study. J Am Geriatr Soc 1996; 44: 1078–1081.
18. Agniel, A. et al.: Psychiatric disorders in dementia of Alzheimer type: cognitive and hemodynamic correlates. Dementia 1990; 1: 215–221.
19. Devanand, D.P. et al.: Behavioral syndromes in Alzheimer's disease. Int Psychogeriatr 1992; 4 (suppl 2): 161–184.
20. Paulsen, J.S. et al.: Incidence of and risk factors for hallucinations and delusions in patients with probable AD. Neurology 2000; 54: 1965–1971.
21. Guarda, A.S.; Swartz, K.L.: Psychiatric disorders in women. In: Kaplan, P.W. (ed.): Neurologic disease in women. Demos Medical, New York, 1998: 379–403.
22. Ripich, D.N. et al.: Gender differences in language of AD patients: A longitudinal study. Neurology 1995; 45: 299–302.
23. Buckwalter, J.G. et al.: Gender differences on a brief measure of cognitive functioning in Alzheimer's disease. Arch Neurol 1993; 50: 757–760.
24. Henderson, V.W.; Buckwalter, J.G.: Cognitive deficits of men and women with Alzheimer's disease. Neurology 1994; 44: 90–96.
25. Buckwalter, J.G. et al.: Gender comparisons of cognitive performances among vascular dementia, Alzheimer's disease, and older adults without dementia. Arch Neurol 1996; 53: 436–439.
26. McPherson, S. et al.: Gender-related cognitive deficits in Alzheimer's disease. Int J Psychogeriatr 1999; 11: 117–122.
27. Bayles, K.A. et al.: Gender differences in language of Alzheimer disease patients revisited. Alzheimer Dis Assoc Disord 1999; 13: 138–146.
28. Hebert, L.E. et al.: Decline of language among women and men with Alzheimer's disease. J Gerontol B Psychol Sci Soc Sci 2000; 55: P354–P360.
29. Coffey, C.E. et al.: Sex differences in brain aging: a quantitative magnetic resonance imaging study. Arch Neurol 1998; 55: 169–179.
30. Jack, C.R. et al.: Medial temporal atrophy on MRI in normal aging and very mild Alzheimer's disease. Neurology 1997; 49: 786–794.
31. Smith, C.D. et al.: Frontal lobe phosphorus metabolism and neuropsychological function in aging and in Alzheimer's disease. Ann Neurol 1995; 38: 194–201.
32. Small, G.W. et al.: Cerebral glucose metabolic patterns in Alzheimer's disease: effect of gender and age at dementia onset. Arch Gen Psychiatry 1989; 46: 527–532.
33. Jagust, W.J. et al.: Functional imaging predicts cognitive decline in Alzheimer's disease. J Neuroimaging 1996; 6: 156–160.
34. Buchpiguel, N.R. et al.: SPECT in Alzheimer's disease: features associated with bilateral parietotemporal hypoperfusion. Acta Neurol Scand 2000; 101: 172–176.
35. Ott, B.R. et al.: Lateralized cortical perfusion in women with Alzheimer's disease. J Gender Specific Med 2000; 3: 29–35.
36. Sherwin, B.B.: Estrogen effects on cognition in menopausal women. Neurology 1997; 48 (suppl 7): S21–S26.
37. Oxenkrug, G.F. et al.: Correlation between brain-adrenal axis activation and cognitive impairment in Alzheimer's disease: is there a gender effect? Psychiatry Res 1989; 29: 169–175.
38. McEwen, B.S. et al.: Ovarian steroids and the brain: implications for cognition and aging. Neurology 1997; 48 (suppl 7): S8–S15.
39. Henderson, V.W.: The epidemiology of estrogen replacement therapy and Alzheimer's disease. Neurology 1997; 48 (suppl 7): S27–S35.

40. Yaffe, K. et al.: Estrogen therapy in postmenopausal women: effects on cognitive function and dementia. JAMA 1998; 279: 688–695.

41. Jaffe, A.B. et al.: Estrogen regulates metabolism of Alzheimer amyloid-precursor protein. J Biol Chem 1994; 269: 13065–13068.

42. Xu, H. et al.: Estrogen reduces neuronal generation of Alzheimer beta-amyloid peptides. Nat Med 1998; 4: 447–451.

43. Behl, C. et al.: Neuroprotection against oxidative stress by estrogens. Mol Pharmacol 1997; 51: 535–541.

44. Heritage, A.S. et al.: Brainstem catecholamine neurons are target sites for sex steroid hormones. Science 1980; 207: 1377–1380.

45. Kaiser, F.E.; Morley, J.E.: Reproductive hormonal changes in the aging male. In: Timiras, P.S.; Quag, W.D.; Vernadakis, A. (eds.): Hormones and aging. CRC Press, New York, 1995: 153–168.

46. Papasozomenos, S C.: The heat shock-induced hyperphosphorylation of tau is estrogen-independent and prevented by androgen: implications for Alzheimer's disease. Proc Natl Acad Sci USA 1997; 94: 6612–6617.

47. Pike, C.J.: Testosterone attenuates beta-amyloid toxicity in cultured hippocampal neurons. Brain Res 2001; 919: 160–165.

48. Raber, J. et al.: Androgens protect against apolipoprotein E4-induced cognitive deficits. J Neurosci 2002; 22: 5204–5209.

49. Almeida, O.P. et al.: Effect of testosterone deprivation on the cognitive performance of a patient with Alzheimer's disease. Int J Geriatr Psychiatry 2001; 16: 822–825.

49. Behl, C. et al.: Neuroprotection against oxidative stress by estrogens. Mol Pharmacol 1997; 51: 535–541.

50. Orengo, C. et al.: Do testosterone levels relate to aggression in elderly men with dementia? J Neuropsychiatry Clin Neurosci 2002; 14: 161–166.

51. Poirier, J. et al.: Apolipoprotein E polymorphism and Alzheimer's disease. Lancet 1993; 342: 697–699.

52. Payami, H. et al.: Gender differences in apolipoprotein E-associated risk for familial Alzheimer's disease: possible clue to the higher incidence of Alzheimer's disease in women. Am J Hum Genet 1996; 58: 803–811.

53. Wong, R.J. et al.: Isoform-specific effects of human apolipoprotein E on brain function revealed in ApoE knockout mice: increased susceptibility of females. Proc Natl Acad Sci USA 1998; 95: 10914–10919.

54. Lyketsos, C.G. et al.: Major depression in Alzheimer's disease. An interaction between gender and family history. Psychosomatics 1996; 37: 380–384.

55. Yaffe, K. et al.: Serum estrogen levels, cognitive performance, and risk of cognitive decline in older community women. J Am Geriatr Soc 1998; 46: 816–821.

56. Mulnard, R. et al.: Estrogen replacement therapy for treatment of mild to moderate Alzheimer's disease. 2000; JAMA 283: 1007–1015.

57. Henderson, V.W. et al.: Estrogen for Alzheimer's disease in women: randomized, double-blind, placebo-controlled trial. Neurology 2000; 54: 295–301.

58. Wang, P.N. et al.: Effects of estrogen on cognition, mood, and cerebral blood flow in AD: a controlled study. Neurology 2000; 54: 2061–2066.

59. Ott, B.R.; Belazi, D.; Lapane, K.L.: Cognitive decline among female estrogen users in nursing homes. J Gerontol A Biol Sci Med Sci 2002; 57: M594–M598.

60. Luine, V.N.: Estradiol increases choline-acetyltransferase activity in specific basal forebrain nuclei and projection areas of female rats. Exp Neurol 1985; 89: 484–490.

61. Schneider, L.S. et al.: Effects of estrogen replacement therapy on response to tacrine in patients with Alzheimer's disease. Neurology 1996; 46: 1580–1584.

62. Farlow, M.R. et al.: Treatment outcome of tacrine depends on apolipoprotein genotype and gender of the subjects with Alzheimer's disease. Neurology 1998; 50: 669–677.

63. Rigaud, A.S. et al.: Presence or absence of at least one epsilon 4 allele and gender are not predictive for the response to donepezil treatment in Alzheimer's disease. Pharmacogenetics 2002; 12: 415–420.

64. Kyomen, H.H.; Nobel, K.W.; Wei, J.Y.: The use of estrogen to decrease aggressive physical behavior in elderly men with dementia. J Am Geriatr Soc 1991; 39: 1110–1112.

65. Rich, S.S.; Ovsiew, F.: Leuprolide acetate for exhibitionism in Huntington's disease. Movement Disord 1994; 9: 353–357.

66. Ott, B.R.: Leuprolide treatment of sexual aggression in a patient with dementia and the Kluver-Bucy Syndrome. Clin Neuropharm 1995; 18: 443–447.

67. Amadeo, M.: Antiandrogen treatment of aggressivity in men suffering from dementia. J Geriatr Psychiatry Neurol 1996; 9: 142–145.

68. Lapane, K.L. et al.: Gender differences as predictors of mortality in nursing home residents with AD. Neurology 2001; 56: 650–654.

69. Lanctot, K.L. et al.: Gender, aggression and serotonergic function are associated with response to sertraline for behavioral disturbances in Alzheimer's disease. Int J Geriatr Psychiatry 2002; 17: 531–541.

70. Doraiswamy, P.M. et al.: The Alzheimer's Disease Assessment Scale: patterns and predictors of baseline cognitive performance in multicenter Alzheimer's disease trials. Neurology 1997; 48: 1511–1517.

71. Swartz, R.H. et al.: Sex and mental status, but not apolipoprotein E, correlate with parietal and temporal hypoperfusion on SPECT in Alzheimer's disease. Neurology 1998; 50: A159.

72. Kamboh, M.I. et al.: Gender-specific nonrandom association between the alpha-1-antichymotrypsin and apolipoprotein E polymorphisms in the general population and its implication for the risk of Alzheimer's disease. Genet Epidemiol 1997; 14: 169–180.
73. Duara, R. et al.: Age and sex differences in cerebral glucose consumption measured by PET using [18-F] fluoro-deoxyglucose (FDG). J Nuclear Med 1985; 26: P68.
74. Ott, B.R.: Cognition and behavior in patients with Alzheimer's disease. J Gender Specific Med 1999; 2: 63–69.

40

Management of Emotional and Behavioral Symptoms in AD

Myron F. Weiner

INTRODUCTION

Emotional and behavioral symptoms are common in patients with Alzheimer's disease (AD). Unfortunately, we have little understanding of the pathophysiology of these symptoms, which include disturbances of:

1. Ideation (suspiciousness, delusions)
2. Perception (illusions, hallucinations)
3. Mood, vegetative function (sleep/wake disturbance, appetite disturbance)
4. Executive function (apathy, irritability, disinhibition, pacing and restlessness, hoarding, rummaging, wandering, and functional incontinence)

Many of these symptoms are subsumed under the appellation of agitation—a term used to describe an array of disturbed and disturbing behaviors. It seems reasonable to assume that emotional and behavioral symptoms result from complex interactions between patients, brain disease, premorbid personality, and their interpersonal and physical environment. Caregivers can be helped to reduce these symptoms or to minimize their effects through environmental, behavioral, and psychopharmacological means.

SOME SYMPTOMS CAN BE TRACED

Appropriate treatment of emotional and behavioral symptoms depends on the cause of the symptoms (if it can be determined). A reasonable search for an etiology should be undertaken. The type of search depends on the type of symptom. In the case of depression in a person with early AD, the symptoms may be traceable to attempts at maintaining former activities, such as managing family finances and bill paying. Often, relieving the person of the mathematics and enabling the person to continue participating in the bill-paying process by signing the checks and making sure that envelopes are stamped and sealed will help restore self-esteem and improve mood.

When measures such as this do not ameliorate mood, psychopharmacological treatment may be indicated. In the case of repetitive vocalizations such as "Help me, help me!" in persons who are otherwise incapable of verbal communication, a search for potential sources of pain is warranted. Having ruled out possible etiologies such as a urinary tract infection or a fracture, an analgesic such as acetaminophen may be prescribed on a regular basis to diminish the ordinary aches and pains due to muscle stiffness and osteoarthritis in elders.

ALWAYS TO BE CONSIDERED: THE QUALITY OF LIFE

In managing emotional and behavioral symptoms, strong consideration is given to the effect of treatment on quality of life. Quality-of-life considerations relate to both patient and caregiver, and often

From: *Current Clinical Neurology,*
Alzheimer's Disease: A Physician's Guide to Practical Management
Edited by: R. W. Richter and B. Zoeller Richter © Humana Press Inc., Totowa, NJ

call for striking a balance between the needs of both. For AD patients, the side effects of medications, such as drowsiness, and their risks in terms of falls or extrapyramidal symptoms are weighed against their potential benefits. My own rule of thumb is that symptoms that are infrequent and not dangerous to patients or caregivers should be dealt with by environmental means. Thus, when a person with AD occasionally becomes angry when a caregiver insists that a bath must be taken, the caregiver is instructed to be less insistent.

By contrast, premedication is advisable when severe behavioral symptoms are a predictable outcome of specific unavoidable situations; for example, in the case of the person who always becomes combative when faced with the need to bathe. In this situation, administration of a calming agent 30 minutes before bath time might be a useful prophylactic measure. On the other hand, persons who are psychotic, depressed, or who become unpredictably assaultive should receive ongoing medication.

USEFUL QUESTIONS TO BEGIN WITH

My approach to managing emotional or behavioral disturbances begins with these questions *(1)*.

1. *What are the symptoms or behaviors?* Is there a treatable psychiatric syndrome, such as an anxiety disorder, depression, or delirium?
2. *Where, when, and with whom do symptoms/behaviors occur?* Emotional upset that occurs because patients think that television characters are actually in the room can be dealt with by turning off the television. Fear of the "stranger" seen in mirrors can be managed by covering mirrors. Problems associated with a particular activity, such as bathing, may be dealt with by reducing the frequency of baths or by sponge-bathing rather than showering. Caregiver–patient mismatches also occur. Caregivers who need to be in charge may clash with strong-willed AD patients for whom self-determination is important. Sundowning may be reduced by increasing sensory cues in the late afternoon and early evening. A primary cause of disturbed behaviors is the interaction between AD patient and caregiver or the influence of the caregiving environment. Caregivers who are tired or insensitive, as well as a noisy, crowded physical environment, are the two prime causes. Although antipsychotic medications are used frequently to control agitation, psychotic ideation does not appear to drive most of these behaviors *(2)*.
3. *With which medication or medical condition?* Increased agitation may occur with benzodiazepines, akathisia with neuroleptics or serotonin-reuptake inhibitors, and delirium may result from an occult infection. Urinary incontinence may occur when diuretics are employed to control hypertension.
4. *How often and how long?* As mentioned above, infrequent, brief, nondangerous behaviors, such as cursing or shouting, are better dealt with by psychosocial means than medication. When psychotropics are prescribed for preemptive purpose, they are often given after the behavior has already subsided. Prescribing psychotropics on a daily basis for a nondangerous behavior that occurs for a few minutes once a month is subjecting the patient to the risks of medication for little potential gain.
5. *How troubling or dangerous to patient, caregivers, or others?* A trial of drug treatment is indicated for behaviors that are dangerous or that undermine caregivers' ability to do their job.
6. *How well can the patient comprehend?* Persons who are unable to comprehend that what they are doing is dangerous or alienating cannot internalize limits, which may then be required in the form of locked doors or brief physical restraint.

Continence can be reinforced by scheduled toileting during the day (usually, every 2 hours). A means to avoid persons urinating in inappropriate places is to enable them to find toilets. This can be done with signs, well-lighted hallways, and by leaving bathroom doors open.

Good sleep hygiene (regular bedtime, keeping patient up until at least 10 p.m., no stimulants or heavy meals in the evening, moderate level of daytime activity, no or limited daytime naps) helps to prevent reversal of the disturbed sleep–wake cycle that often occurs in persons with AD.

ADAPT THE ENVIRONMENT

Behaviors best dealt with by the physical environment are wandering, pacing, rummaging, and functional incontinence. Wandering is best dealt with in home environments by creating indoor and out-of-doors wandering paths, and securing doors to unsafe areas *(3)*. In residential facilities, wandering may be minimized by concealing door handles, having no windows in doors leading to unsafe or undesirable areas, and allowing access to safe out-of-doors environments, such as enclosed yards. To reduce mistaken intrusions into others' rooms, it is useful to find means to help individuals identify their own rooms. This can be done by means of a large sign on the door, taping a large piece of colored construction paper on the door (Your room has the green door, Mr. Smith!), or by having personal memorabilia at bedroom entrances.

Pacing (except for akathisia) is best dealt with by allowing the individual adequate room to pace. Patients with AD (especially those with frontal lobe involvement) are often environmentally dependent. That is, they do what the environment dictates. If an item of clothing is in a drawer, it is put on, regardless of whether a similar article of clothing is already being worn. If a door or a drawer is at hand, they open it. Persons with AD can be allowed to open doors as long as they cannot get to a place where they could be lost or hurt. They can be allowed to open drawers as long as the drawers belong to nobody else. One means to deal with rummaging is to provide a set of drawers specifically for rummaging.

MEDICATIONS FOR THE MANAGEMENT OF EMOTIONAL AND BEHAVIORAL SYMPTOMS

The results of drug treatment of many of these symptoms are modest, at best, and do not seem to be specific to AD. Most of the behavioral and emotional symptoms for which drugs are prescribed for persons with AD are not well-defined psychiatric syndromes, such as major depression, anxiety disorder, or delirium. Psychotic symptoms tend to be intermittent, and the development of a delusional system is rare.

Depression

Caregivers often confuse apathy with depression, because their loved ones do not initiate activities they formerly found pleasurable *(4)*. The distinction of apathy from depression is that if activity is initiated by another person, the nondepressed AD patient will join in and may well enjoy it. In addition, many of the symptoms of depression overlap with those of AD, including reduced appetite, poor sleep, less pleasure from activities that were formerly pleasurable, and difficulty with concentration. Clues to the diagnosis of major depression in cognitively impaired persons include early-morning awakening with inability to return to sleep, diurnal mood variation, and lowered self-esteem. As the day goes on, such patients usually brighten, and many experience near-normalization of mood in the late afternoons.

Depression may require urgent inpatient treatment, especially if patients are suicidal or homicidal, profoundly agitated, or have rapid weight loss or marked dehydration. The treatment of choice for severe depression with rapid weight loss and suicidal acts or preoccupation is electroconvulsive therapy (ECT) performed in a psychiatric facility. ECT is safe and rapidly effective, with symptomatic relief occurring within 3 weeks. Complications of properly administered ECT are rare, and in fragile elders, ECT is safer than running the risk of cardiovascular collapse from inanition while awaiting relief from treatment with medication. ECT can also be employed to treat major depression after the failure of an adequate trial of antidepressant medication (at least 6 weeks at therapeutic doses). It is not clear whether instituting antidepressant therapy after ECT is useful in preventing relapse. In many cases, elders will require maintenance ECT. After a course of 6–9 treatments (usually given 3 times a week), sessions may be spaced out to once a week, then once every 2 weeks, and finally to every month for an indefinite period of time. Confusion is often increased during a course of ECT, but pretreatment cognitive function may improve with remission of depression *(5)*.

Due to their benign side-effect profile and their low toxicity, the first-line drugs for treatment of depression in elderly patients are the selective serotonin-reuptake inhibitors (SSRIs) fluoxetine (Prozac), sertraline (Zoloft), paroxetine (Paxil), and citalopram (Celexa). They have almost no anti-

Table 1
Selected Antidepressant Drugs and Their Dosage

Generic name	Trade name	Adult dosage (mg/day)	Geriatric dosage (mg/day)
Paroxetine	Paxil	20–40	10–40
Sertraline	Zoloft	50–200	50–100
Fluoxetine	Prozac	20–40	20–40
Citalopram	Celexa	20–40	20–40
Mirtazepine	Remeron	15–30	15–30
Venlafaxine	Effexor	75–225	37.5–225
Bupropion	Wellbutrin	75–450	75–225

cholinergic (except for paroxetine), antihistaminic, or antiadrenergic side effects. All have long half-lives. Fluoxetine and its active metabolite norfluoxetine have a total half-life of up to 12 days; sertraline and its active metabolite as long as 4 days, and paroxetine, with no active metabolite, 24 hours. Each of the drugs is dosed once a day; fluoxetine may be dosed every other day. They are administered in the morning because of their tendency to stimulate.

All of these medications may produce nausea, anxiety, restlessness, and sleep loss and are relatively nontoxic when taken in overdose. Fluoxetine may produce hyponatremia by inducing inappropriate secretion of antidiuretic hormone. SSRIs should not be administered in conjunction with monoamine oxidase (MAO) inhibitors or tryptophan. The so-called serotonergic state resulting from such combinations ranges from simple agitation to hyperthermia, muscular rigidity, delirium, coma, and death.

The dosage of SSRIs is indicated in Table 1. SSRIs may cause akathisia, restlessness, sleeplessness, and hyponatremia, the latter from inappropriate ADH secretion *(6)*.

Patients who are unable to tolerate the side effects or who fail to respond after 4–6 weeks of treatment at full doses may be tried on another SSRI. Should that fail, it is appropriate to consider another class of antidepressants (see also Table 1), or in the case of disabling depressive symptoms, ECT.

Maintenance Treatment of Patients with Major Depressive Disorders

Major depression at any age is a recurrent illness. For this reason, it is best to maintain patients for a substantial period of time (6 months to a year) on the dose of medication that was effective in relieving their symptoms. Withdrawal of medication should be gradual (over weeks or months). Patients with one or more previous episodes should be maintained on therapeutic doses of antidepressants.

Anxiety

Benzodiazepines may be useful in persons with dementia who report subjective anxiety, have symptoms of high arousal, muscular tension, and autonomic hyperactivity *(7)*. These drugs must be used cautiously because they may produce ataxia, sedation, and disinhibition. It is preferable to use benzodiazepines metabolized by conjugation rather than oxidation because of their shorter half-lives (oxazepam, lorazepam, temazepam). They should also be withdrawn gradually to prevent withdrawal symptoms.

Delirium

Most important aspect of treating delirium is the diagnosis of the precipitating condition. With the exception of withdrawal delirium, delirium in persons with dementia is ordinarily treated with antipsychotic drugs, so as to avoid the clouding of sensorium that may be produced by antianxiety drugs.

Table 2
Selected Neuroleptics and Their Dosage

Generic name	Trade name	Liquid (mg/mL)	Adult dosage (mg/day)	Geriatric dosage (mg/day)
Haloperidol	Haldol	2	4–8	0.25–6
Clozapine	Clozaril		100–900	0.625–25
Risperidone	Risperdal	1	1–6	0.5–1.5
Olanzapine	Zyprexa		5–20	2.5–10
Quetiapine	Seroquel		50–500	25–400

High-potency neuroleptics are indicated for the treatment of delirium because they lack potentially life-threatening cardiovascular effects *(8)*.

Appropriate drug management of behaviors that do not fit into clearly delineated syndromes has been problematic, and complicated by concern that psychotropic drugs may have been overused in extended-care facilities *(9)*.

Agitation and Violence

Neuroleptics have been the mainstay of drugs for the control of agitation and violence, but their effects are modest and only slightly better than diphenhydramine or oxazepam *(10–12)*. The choice among neuroleptics is governed by side-effect profile. Lower-potency drugs are avoided because of their pronounced anticholinergic and cardiovascular effects. On the other hand, many AD patients are very sensitive to the extrapyramidal effects of the high-potency drugs (Table 2).

Nevertheless, risperidone in doses of 0.25–1.0 mg twice a day is my antipsychotic drug of choice because of its low toxicity. I seldom use the drug for more than a few months, and therefore have had little difficulty with tardive dyskinesia. Among the atypical neuroleptics, Clozapine, which lacks extrapyramidal side effects, has been used in low doses to control agitation in persons with dementia, but its numerous other side effects and toxicity preclude its routine use *(13)*. Risperidone is effective in low doses, but it has significant extrapyramidal effects when administered above 1.75 mg/day *(14)*. Olanzapine appears to be effective in agitated AD patients in doses of 5–10 mg/day *(15)*. Its side effects include sedation, postural hypotension, and weight gain. Quetiapine is widely used for the control of psychotic symptoms in persons with AD and with Parkinson's disease, but no controlled study has been reported *(16)*. Many other classes of drugs have been used, including the serotonin-reuptake inhibitor trazodone, whose two principal side effects are sedation and postural hypotension. Trazodone is short-acting, lasting only 3–4 hours. The anticonvulsants carbamazepine and valproic acid have been employed *(17,18)*. These drugs require monitoring of potential toxic effects on bone marrow and liver, respectively. The serotonin-1A agonist buspirone has also been reported to be effective in a few cases *(19)*.

Sleep/Wake Disturbances

Medications used range from neuroleptics to trazodone, and include short-acting benzodiazepine hypnotics and short-acting benzodiazepine tranquilizers, such as lorazepam.

Suspiciousness, Delusions, and Hallucinations

Suspiciousness, irritability, and delusions are frequently eased by low doses of neuroleptics. Visual hallucinations are frequent in the middle stages of AD. As long as these hallucinations are not frightening to the person with dementia, they are probably best left untreated. When there are intense emotional or behavioral reactions, neuroleptics are often beneficial. Clozapine has been used for the treatment of psychotic symptoms in Parkinson's disease, but because of its toxicity, this drug has largely been supplanted by olanzapine and quetiapine for these symptoms and for treatment of psychosis in dementia with Lewy bodies *(20)*.

Inappropriate Sexuality

For persistent inappropriate sexual behavior in male patients with AD, we have found the use of intramuscular 100–150 mg of medroxyprogesterone acetate every other week to be useful *(21)*. The preparation can also be administered orally at a dose of 5 mg/day.

CONCLUSION

Using the diagnostic frame of reference suggested in the summary, below, followed by an approach that combines behavioral, environmental, and pharmacological agents, it is possible to reduce the impact of emotional and behavioral symptoms of AD by

1. Creating a tolerant interpersonal environment
2. Adding to the physical environment elements that accommodate behaviors that cannot be ameliorated by behavioral means or by drugs
3. Giving caregivers chemical means to dampen mood and psychotic symptoms as well as to avert or reduce dangerous behaviors

SUMMARY

Changes in behavior or emotional state should be attributed to AD only after other potential etiologies are considered:

1. Change in significant others (spouse' tolerance decreasing or fatigue increasing; new persons in the environment)
2. Change in relationship with significant others (reaction to increasing dependency on others, or increasing resentment by others)
3. Change in physical environment (new residence)
4. Change in health status (urinary tract infection, arthritis pain)
5. Drug toxicity (over-the-counter or prescription)
6. Multiple etiologies

Changes in behavior or emotional state are usually transient (hours to months) and do not usually require chronic psychotropic usage.

ACKNOWLEDGMENT

This work was supported in part by National Institutes on Aging grant P30 AG12300.

REFERENCES

1. Weiner, M.F.: Gray, K.F.: Balancing psychosocial and psychopharmacologic interventions in Alzheimer's disease. Am J Alzheimer Care Rel Disord Res 1994; 9: 6–12.
2. Deutsch, L.H. et al.: Psychosis and physical aggression in probable Alzheimer's disease. Am J Psychiatry 1991; 148: 1159–1163.
3. Warner, M.L.: The complete guide to Alzheimer's. Proofing your home. Purdue Univerity Press, West Lafayette, IN, 1998.
4. Levy, M.L. et al.: Apathy is not depression. J Neuropsychiatry Clin Neurosci 1998; 10: 314–319.
5. Rao, V.; Lyketsos, C.G.: The benefits and risks of ECT for patients with primary dementia who also suffer from depression. In J Geriatr Psychiatry 2000; 16: 919–920.
6. Hwang, A.S.; Magraw, R.M.: Syndrome of inappropriate secretion of antidiuretic hormone due to fluoxetine. Am J Psychiatry 1989; 146: 399.
7. Patel, S.; Tariot, P.N.: Use of benzodiazepines in behaviorally disturbed patients: risk-benefit ratio. In: Lawlor, B.A. (ed.): Behavioral complications in Alzheimer's disease. American Psychiatric Press, Washington, D.C., 1995: 153–170.

8. Weiner, M.F.; Schneider, L.S.: Pharmacologic management and treatment of dementia and secondary symptoms. In: Weiner, M.F. (ed.): The dementias: diagnosis, treatment, and research (3rd ed.). American Psychiatric Press, Washington, D.C., 2003, pp. 219–283.

9. Committee on Nursing Home Regulation. Improving the quality of care in nursing homes. National Academy of Sciences, Institute of Medicine, Washington, D.C., 1986.

10. Schneider, L.S.; Sobin, P.: Treatments for psychiatric symptoms and behavioral disturbances in dementia. In: Burns, A.; Levy, R. (eds.): Dementia. Chapman & Hall, London, UK, 1994, pp. 517–538.

11. Schneider, L.S.; Pollock, V.E.; Lyness, S.A: A metaanalysis of controlled trials of neuroleptic treatment of dementia. J Am Geriatr Soc 1990; 38: 553–563.

12. Coccaro, E.F. et al.: Pharmacologic treatment of noncognitive behavioral disturbances in elderly demented patients. Am J Psychiatry 1990; 147: 1640–1645.

13. Oberholzer, A.F. et al. Safety and effectiveness of low-dose clozapine in psychchogeriatric patients: a preliminary study. Int Psychogeriatr 1992; 4: 187–195.

14. Katz, I.R. et al.: Comparison of risperidone and placebo for psychosis and behavioral disturbances associated with dementia: a randomized, double-blind trial. J Clin Psychiatry 1999; 60: 107–115.

15. Street, J.S. et al.: Olanzapine treatment of psychotic and behavioral symptoms in patients with Alzheimer disease in nursing care facilities: a double-blind, randomized, placebo-controlled trial. Arch Gen Psychiatry 2000; 57: 968–976.

16. Fernandez, H.H. et al.: Quetiapine for psychosis in Parkinson's disease versus dementia with Lewy bodies J Clin Psychiatry 2002; 63: 513–515.

17. Tariot, P.N. et al.: Efficacy and tolerability of carbamazepine for agitation and aggression in dementia. Am J Psychiatry 1998; 155: 54–61.

18. Porsteinsson, A.P. et al.: Placebo-controlled study of divalproex sodium for agitation in dementia. Am J Geriatr Psychiatry 2001; 9: 58–66.

19. Herrmann, N.; Eryavec, G.: Buspirone in the management of agitation and aggression associated with dementia. Am J Geriatr Psychiatry 1993; 1: 249–253.

20. Cummings, J.L. et al.: Efficacy of olanzapine in the treatment of psychosis in dementia with Lewy bodies. Dement Geriatr Cognitive Disord 2002; 13: 67–73.

21. Weiner, M.F. et al.: Intramuscular medroxyprogesterone acetate for sexual aggression in elderly men. Lancet 1992; 339: 1121–1122.

41

Assessment and Treatment of Neuropsychiatric Symptoms in Alzheimer's Disease

Andrew R. Gustavson and Jeffrey L. Cummings

INTRODUCTION

Neuropsychiatric symptoms are a common feature of Alzheimer's disease (AD). The most common neuropsychiatric symptoms are apathy (72%), aggression/agitation (60%), anxiety (48%), and depression (48%) *(1)*. Patients with psychosis experience a more rapid cognitive decline. The development of these symptoms is particularly problematic for patients and caregivers, and is frequently the factor that leads to nursing home placement. Hence, psychiatric symptoms may be thought of as having a particularly ominous prognostic significance if not detected and treated. Successful complete or partial treatment may reduce patient distress and extend independent living in AD patients *(2)*. Neuropsychiatric symptoms are not always disclosed to physicians by patients or caregivers until they are intolerable, or precipitate a crisis. Routine clinical assessments may allow more proactive clinical management.

SYMPTOM EVALUATION

Several instruments have been developed to systematically evaluate the presence and severity of neuropsychiatric symptoms. These include the BEHAVE-AD, Manchester and Oxford Universities Scale for the Psychological Assessment of Dementia (MOUSEPAD), Consortium to Establish a Registry for Alzheimer s Disease (CERAD) Behavioral Rating Scale, the Neurobehavioral Rating Scale, the Dysfunctional Behavior Rating Instrument for Dementia (DBRI), and the Cornell Scale for Depression in Dementia, among others *(3–8)*. Many of these were developed in the context of clinical research, and while both reliable and valid, they are typically too time-consuming for routine use in clinical practice. Others focus on relatively specific behavioral symptom clusters. The Neuropsychiatric Inventory (NPI) was developed to evaluate the presence, frequency, and severity of the most common neuropsychiatric symptoms in dementia in a systematic and efficient manner *(9)*. It has been demonstrated to be both reliable and valid. The NPI consists of 12 items that assess for the presence of delusions, hallucinations, agitation, depression, anxiety, euphoria, apathy, disinhibition, irritability, aberrant motor behavior, nighttime behaviors, and appetite and eating disorders (Table 1). If these items elicit positive responses, then the severity and nature of the symptom is addressed individually. The severity of the symptoms is rated on a scale of 1–3, and the frequency on a scale of 1–4. The amount distress experienced by the caregiver for each symptom is rated on a scale of 1–5. For each symptom category there are four scores: frequency, severity, total (frequency × severity), and caregiver distress. By first screening and then pursuing in detail only items that elicit positive responses, considerable time can be saved. Patients without neuropsychiatric symptoms can be screened in only a few minutes, and those with problems can be quantitatively assessed in terms of

From: *Current Clinical Neurology,*
Alzheimer's Disease: A Physician's Guide to Practical Management
Edited by: R. W. Richter and B. Zoeller Richter © Humana Press Inc., Totowa, NJ

Table 1
Percentage of Patients With Neuropsychiatric
Symptoms, Scorable on the NPI (*n* = 50)

Symptom	Percentage
Delusions	21%
Hallucinations	10%
Depression	38%
Anxiety	48%
Apathy	72%
Irritability	41%
Aggression	60%
Disinhibition	36%
Aberrant motor behavior	38%

severity and caregiver distress. The clinician is free to pursue any feature with more detailed history as indicated. Table 1 lists the frequency of the most common symptoms as determined by the NPI *(1)*. These symptoms tend to cluster into three groups based on factor analysis: a mood disorder group comprised of depression and anxiety; a psychosis group comprised of agitation, hallucinations, delusions, and irritability; and a frontal behavior group consisting of disinhibition and euphoria. Apathy and aberrant motor behavior did not cluster with other symptoms.

The differential diagnosis of neuropsychiatric symptoms in patients with dementia should always include concurrent delirium due to adverse medication side effects, infections, or other systemic illness. A rapid or fluctuating decline in cognitive function with onset of hallucinations, delusions, agitation, insomnia, aggression, emotional lability, or disinhibition may be a sign of an underlying treatable medical problem. The most common cause of delirium in this context is an adverse effect of medication, especially involving compounds with anticholinergic, sedative, or psychotropic actions. Patients with dementia are at particular risk for many illnesses, such as urinary tract infections, dehydration, respiratory infections, and nutritional deficiency. All these conditions can manifest as new neuropsychiatric symptoms. For example, pain associated with a urinary tract infection may contribute to agitation and insomnia. Many of the illnesses that precipitate delirium are relatively treatable, and, if detected, can lead to resolution of neuropsychiatric symptoms by elimination of the underlying problem.

NONPHARMACOLOGICAL INTERVENTIONS

Managing the neuropsychiatric aspects of AD involves interventions in both the patient's physical and social environment. Patient and caregiver support groups are of particular value. There are several excellent community recourses available that provide education and support to both patients and caregivers. These include the Alzheimer's Association and Alzheimer's Disease International. Family members provide the majority of care for AD patients in their homes *(10)*. Providing 24-hour care for a patient with AD, especially in the context of agitation, aggression, or psychosis, represents a potentially overwhelming responsibility. The burden on caregivers should not be underestimated and is a risk for the development of clinically significant depression or other mental health problems. Although support groups are very helpful, some caregivers may themselves need referral for family counseling or psychiatric treatment.

Early detection and diagnosis of AD is important, because it allows the patient to be involved in decision-making processes before the cognitive impairment is severe. Both patients and caregivers benefit from learning coping strategies to compensate for the cognitive problems at all stages of the illness. Reactive depression and other emotional difficulties caused by the fact of diagnosis can be identified early and treated. Early education about the nature of the illness also helps patients and families prepare for the future interpersonally, psychologically, legally, and financially. Many patients are comforted by knowing that they have been involved in determining their affairs.

Involvement of frontal and limbic structures in the neurodegenerative process contributes to the development of behavioral and psychiatric symptoms. Ultimately, the biological, cognitive, psychological, family, and social aspects of the illness combine and together contribute the development and nature of neuropsychiatric problems in AD.

Nonpharmacological interventions are frequently adequate to manage neuropsychiatric symptoms and are preferred when the behavior is not dangerous or aggressive *(11,12)*. The importance of environmental interventions should not be underestimated. The cognitive deficits of AD patients can be compensated partially with careful attention to their environment. Providing visual aids such as written reminders for important daily tasks, prominent calendars to help maintain orientation, and written signs in rooms and on doorways identifying locations can be very helpful to prevent patients from wandering and getting lost. Safety measures such as having safe-return bracelets, and locked doors and gates should be used. Maintaining a constant, familiar physical living environment is helpful. A regular daily routine of activities with predictable sleep and wake times can minimize daytime napping and nighttime insomnia. Providing night lights helps patients retain orientation at night and can be useful in preventing nighttime confusion, anxiety, and hallucinations when patients awaken at night.

Medications and other substances with stimulating effects (including cholinesterase inhibitors), caffeine, and nicotine should be avoided before retiring. Fluid intake should be minimized in the hours before sleep, and diuretics given in the morning if possible.

Both family and professional caregivers benefit from education in nursing care skills, measures for effective communication, and behavioral management strategies for resistive and aggressive behavior. For example, teaching caregivers even simple strategies such as the the four Rs,

1. Reassure
2. Reorient
3. Remind
4. Redirect

can be of considerable benefit. The fact that the disturbed behaviors are caused by brain pathology and do not represent volitional acts by the patient needs to be strongly emphasized. The progressive nature of the disease necessitates ongoing education as the symptoms change, and requires alterations of expectations for the patient's abilities and needs.

GENERAL PRINCIPLES OF PHARMACOTHERAPY IN AD

Although nonpharmacological management strategies are preferred, pharmacotherapy should not be avoided on the basis of the patient's age or the presence of dementia. Both should be used concurrently as parts of a complementary overall treatment plan. Initiation of pharmacotherapy begins with medical history and physical examination. An accurate diagnosis of AD and identification of concurrent medical problems should be performed. In addition to defining the nature of the present illness and presenting problems, the history should include a thorough past medical and psychiatric history, current and past medication, and social history. The latter should include the patient's current living situation, identification of the principle caregivers, and the caregivers' expectations, as well as resources.

Based on the history, a specific target symptom should be selected for treatment, and an appropriate medication prescribed. The target symptoms should then be monitored closely for response. A partial response can be acceptable, and symptoms do not need to be completely eliminated if this would require unacceptable side effects or risks. Monotherapy is generally to be preferred.

Medications are typically started at one-third to one-half of the standard dose for adults and slowly titrated up as needed. Careful attention should be given to avoiding interactions with concomitantly taken prescription, over-the-counter, and alternative drugs. Both the patient and the caregiver should receive clear verbal and written instructions in language they are able to understand about the medication's use and side-effect profile. Medications should be tried at sufficient doses and for long enough time periods to constitute an adequate therapeutic trial before changes are made. If necessary, changes should be made one at a time, and serum drug levels should be obtained when available. Some medications are best tapered when discontinued, and beginning a new medication is delayed to avoid drug–drug interactions. Patients should be monitored closely for changes in their target symptoms, side effects, decline in cognition, concurrent medical problems, and social circumstances. All of these can change over time. Drug regimens should be simplified both in terms of the number of medications prescribed and their scheduled dosing.

Unnecessary medications should be discontinued. When multiple drug regimens are necessary, agents with complementary actions and favorable potential interaction profiles should be used together.

Acetylcholinesterase inhibitors (AChEI), particularly in combination with 2000 IU vitamin E daily, have been shown to be of benefit in treating cognitive decline, deterioration in activities of daily living (ADLs), and loss of global functioning in AD. They also may be beneficial for preventing and treating neuropsychiatric symptoms and should be considered the first agents to treat AD *(12)*. In some cases, use of psychotropic medications can be avoided. In the discussion of pharmacological therapy below it will be assumed patients have been treated with one of these agents.

No specific AChEI has been shown to be superior to the others, and choice of drug depends largely on tolerability, dose schedule, side-effect profile, and physician's preference. If one agent is not tolerated, a therapeutic trial with a different member of this class is warranted, as each of them has a unique mechanism of action, and individual responses to different agents do vary.

Donepezil (Aricept) is a piperazine AChEI, with a half-life of 70–80 hours. It is dosed once daily, typically in the morning, administered with food. The drug is started at 5 mg, and then increased to 10 mg daily after a delay of at least 4 weeks. Depression, apathy, anxiety, and agitation may improve *(13,14)*. The most common side effects are nausea, vomiting, anorexia, and diarrhea and relate to increased acetylcholine activity. Overall, it seems to be well tolerated, and side effects do not frequently cause discontinuation of therapy.

Rivastigmine (Exelon) is a carbamate that inhibits acetylcholinesterase and butyrylcholinesterase. It has a half-life of 2 hours in the serum and 8 hours in the brain. It is dosed twice daily with a starting dose of 1.5 mg twice daily for 1 month and then increased to 3 mg twice daily for another month, finally increased to 4.5 or 6 mg twice daily, depending on the response. Food delays the absorption of this compound, and administration with food may help decrease side effects. Rivastigmine has been shown to be effective in improving global function, cognition, and behavior *(15–17)*. Side effects are similar to those of donepezil. They may, however, occur somewhat more often. Weight loss can be pronounced. Slow titration to individual tolerability and taken on a full stomach help minimize side effects.

Galantamine (Reminyl) is a phenanthrene alkaloid AChEI with allosteric nicotinic-modulating properties; it has a half-life of 5–7 hours, to be dosed twice daily. The initial dose is 4 mg, then increased to 8 mg twice daily. Most patients stay at this dose. An additional increase to 12 mg twice daily can be considered in patients who do not respond well or deteriorate at some point in their illness. Food delays the absorption of the compound. Galantamine reduces behavioral symptoms present at the initiation of therapy, and ameliorates the emergence of new symptoms as well as benefiting cognition when compared to a placebo. Beneficial effects on apathy, disinhibition, anxiety, and agitation have been reported *(18,19)*. The agent has also been documented to reduce caregiver distress related to behavioral symptoms *(18)*.

AGITATION

Agitation describes disruptive, resistive, and aggressive behaviors and is typically associated with more advanced age, later onset of dementia, and more severe cognitive impairment *(1,20)*. It is a common symptom, occurring in approximately 70% of AD patients *(1,21)*. It can range from relatively mild problems, such as repeated questioning, pacing, and stereotyped behavior, to overt violent acts. Males are more likely to manifest aggression *(20–24)*. Once present, symptoms of agitation tend to persist *(25–27)*.

Neuropsychological, pathological, and brain imaging studies suggest that agitated behavior may largely arise from frontal lobe dysfunction with loss of the ability to appropriately respond to external provocations and internal emotional states arising from comorbid neuropsychiatric syndromes *(28)*. Aggressive behavior is often accompanied by other neuropsychiatric symptoms. Identifying the nature of these can help direct effective treatment to the appropriate target symptom. Common co-morbid problems include psychotic symptoms, such as delusions, hallucinations, and misidentification syndromes. Disturbances of sleep, circadian cycles, and activity also are frequently associated.

Pharmacological treatment of agitation is directed largely by the nature of the associated neuropsychiatric symptoms (Table 2). Patients with concurrent psychosis will frequently respond to low-dose atypical antipsychotics. A traditional agent, such as haloperidol, may be tried after an atypical agent has failed. Concurrent use of antipsychotics, either conventional or atypical agents, should be avoided. If monotherapy proves inadequate, addition of a mood stabilizer, such as valproate or carbamazepine, is a rational first addition. Its substitution with either trazodone or buspirone is a further alternative—as a third-line treatment approach. When anxiety is the prominent feature of agitation, buspirone appears to be a relatively safe and effective first-line agent.

Propranolol, a nonselective β-adrenergic antagonist, may also be used. This medication, however, has many known interactions, may precipitate depression, and may cause orthostatic hypotension, posing a risk for falls. If these measures have proven unsuccessful, a benzodiazepine anxiolytic may be substituted for buspirone. These medications, however, can have a disinhibiting effect and—paradoxically—produce more agitation and concurrent confusion.

Agitation concurrent with depression is managed in an analogous manner. First an antidepressant is added, usually a selective serotonin-reuptake inhibitor (SSRI). Substitution with an antidepressant of a different pharmacological profile within the class may be tried as a further measure. When sleep disturbances, abnormal circadian cycles, or nocturnal agitation are prominent, trazodone is recommended as initial therapy. This can be substituted by a nonbenzodiazepine hypnotic, such as zolpidem or zoleplon. Benzodiazepines may be necessary should the above approaches fail. They should be used in the same fashion as described below under the treatment of insomnia.

Nonspecific agitation with no specific concurrent target symptom can be managed with an atypical antipsychotic agent. Addition of a mood stabilizer is appropriate if no response is achieved. If this combination fails, substitution of the mood stabilizer with trazodone or buspirone might be tried *(28)*.

PSYCHOSIS

Delusions and hallucinations are the most common psychotic symptoms in AD patients. Together they occur with a prevalence of 40–60%. Delusions are more common (30–50%) than hallucinations (10–20%) *(29–32)*, and they tend to differ from those of primary psychiatric disorders. Specific syndromes of abnormal thought content are common. Typical delusions include the idea of infidelity of a spouse, paranoia concerning theft, misidentifications similar to Capgras syndrome, and belief that the house where they live is not their home *(3,33–38)*. Visual hallucinations are typical, but auditory hallucinations can occur. Patients with extrapyramidal symptoms (EPS) are at greater risk for experiencing hallucinations.

To be attributed to AD, psychotic symptoms should be sufficiently severe to disrupt patient function, be present for at least 1 month, and should not occur as the result of delirium, or a preexisting axis I psychotic or substance abuse disorder. The concurrent manifestation of delusions together with hallucinations can be helpful in discerning inaccurate beliefs related to memory deficits, as can persistence over time and severity of associated distress.

Table 2
Medications Commonly Used in the Treatment of Agitation

Medication (commercial name)	Usual dose (mg)	Range (mg)	Comments
Risperidone (Risperdal)	1	0.5–2	Atypical antipsychotic with minimal extrapyramidal symptoms (EPS) at low doses. Minimal anticholinergic properties.
Olanzapine (Zyprexa)	5	5–10	Atypical antipsychotic with minimal EPS at low doses; may have some antidepressant action.
Quetiapine (Seroquel)	300	50–400	Atypical antipsychotic; may produce less EPS.
Haloperidol (Haldol)	2	0.5–3	High-potency traditional antipsychotic; relatively less anticholinergic than others in class
Carbamazepine (Tegretol)	400	200–1200	Anticonvulsant with mood-stabilizing properties. Check liver function tests (LFTs), and complete blood count (CBC), electrolytes at initiation of therapy, and periodically. Autoinduces its own metabolism during initial 3–5 weeks. Serum levels widely available and should be monitored periodically.
Divalproex (Depakote)	500	250–3000	Anticonvulsant with mood-stabilizing properties. Check LFTs, CBC, prothrombin time/partial thromboplasin time (PT/PTT), and pancreatic enzymes at initiation of therapy and periodically. Serum levels widely available, and should be monitored periodically.
Trazodone (Desyrel)	100	50–400	Antidepressant thought to exert effect though serotonin-reuptake inhibition. Minimal anticholinergic properties. May have anxiolytic action.
Buspirone (Buspar)	30	15–45	Anxiolytic without benzodiazepine properties. Mechanism of action unknown, but may relate to serotonin inhibition in the dorsal raphe. Minimal sedation and not considered habit-forming.
Propranolol (Inderal)	120	40–240	Nonselective β-adrenergic antagonist. Has many known interactions. May cause orthostatic hypotension and pose a fall risk.
Lorazepam (Ativan)	1	0.5–2	Intermediate half-life (6–20 hour), high-potency benzodiazepine. Has no active metabolites, and requires no first-pass metabolism.

Psychotic symptoms tend to occur later in the disease process and are associated with more severe dementia and more rapid cognitive decline *(39–44)*. Psychotic symptoms may manifest as agitation, aggression, anxiety, and purposeless behavior *(45–48)*. Abnormalities in visual or auditory sensation can worsen both delusions and hallucinations.

Delusions and hallucinations in AD patients respond to antipsychotic medication, usually at lower dose than required for primary psychiatric diseases (Table 3). AD-related psychosis may respond to SSRIs. These antidepressants can be used as an adjuvant or an alternative to antipsychotics. Atypical antipsychotics/neuroleptics are preferred over conventional ones because of their relatively lower propensity to cause EPS.

Table 3
Medications Commonly Used in the Treatment of Psychosis

Medication (commercial name)	Usual dose (mg)	Range (mg)	Comments
Risperidone (Risperdal)	1	0.5–2	Atypical antipsychotic with minimal EPS at low doses. Minimal anticholinergic properties.
Olanzapine (Zyprexa)	5	5–10	Atypical antipsychotic, may have activating antidepressant properties.
Quetiapine (Seroquel)	300	50–400	Atypical antipsychotic, may produce less EPS.
Clozapine (Clozaril)	50	12.5–100	Atypical antipsychotic with no known EPS. Seizures can be common. Potentially fatal agranulocytosis requires special monitoring and prescribing procedures. Typically used in context of parkinsonism and psychosis.
Haloperidol (Haldol)	2	0.5–3	High-potency conventional antipsychotic. Relatively less anticholinergic than others in the same class.

Quetiapine is frequently favored clinically, as it potentially induces little or no EPS, although long-term data to support this desirable characteristic are not yet available. The other atypical agents listed in Table 3 also tend to produce little EPS at the doses used in AD.

Clozapine is a unique tricyclic atypical antipsychotic that can be effective in dementia; it has relatively few extrapyramidal side effects. However, it has been associated with potentially fatal agranulocytosis, which requires close monitoring and special prescribing procedures. Seizures are an occasional side effect. These features make it appropriate for the treatment of AD-related psychosis only under unusual and specific circumstances. Clozapine should be initiated only in consultation with a psychiatrist or neurologist familiar with its use in the geriatric population.

Haloperidol has proven efficacy in AD-related psychosis and may be beneficial for relatively rapid symptomatic relief in the context of severe agitation. It has a greater risk, however, of inducing parkinsonism, tardive dyskinesia, and other extrapyramidal disorders. Although lower-potency conventional antipsychotics are more sedating and hence may seem beneficial in patients with concurrent agitation, they should be avoided. These agents produce sedation via their strongly anticholinergic properties; they can diminish cognition and precipitate anticholinergic delirium. Dosing above the recommended ranges rarely is beneficial; it increases the risk of adverse reactions, such as EPS, and drug-induced confusion.

If agitation worsens on antipsychotics, especially conventional agents, the possibility of akathisia (an extrapyramidal disorder characterized by motor restlessness and anxiety) should be considered as a possible adverse reaction. In this case antipsychotics should be discontinued. In patients who experience a marked extrapyramidal syndrome in response to conventional dopamine-blocking agents, reassessment of the diagnosis with thought to dementia with Lewy bodies might be prudent, although such a reaction does not preclude a diagnosis of AD.

DEPRESSION

Depression is common at onset and early in the course of AD. It may even precede the diagnosis of dementia by several years *(49,50)*. As the disease progresses, depressive symptoms continue and are frequent in the late stages. There is some evidence that depression earlier in life may be a risk factor for the development of AD *(50)*. Major depressive disorder is estimated to have a prevalence of 1.5–25%, while minor depressive disorders are prevalent in 10–30% of AD patients *(51–54)*. There may be a tendency for families and caregivers to confuse symptoms of depression with signs of dementia. This can lead them to conclude that the patient is depressed more often than is accurate (55,56). A working group of the National Institute of Mental Health has developed specific criteria for the diagnosis of depression in AD (57), based on but not identical to those of the Fourth Edition of the Diagnostic and Statistical Manual of Mental Disorders (DSM-IV) (58). These criteria include the presence of depressed mood, decreased positive affect or anhedonia, and three of the following features during the same 2-week period:

1. Depressed mood
2. Decreased positive affect or diminished pleasure in response to social contacts, and usual activities, social isolation or withdrawal
3. Disruption in appetite and sleep, psychomotor agitation or retardation, irritability; fatigue or loss of energy, feelings of worthlessness or hopelessness, inappropriate or excessive worry or guilt, and recurrent thoughts of death, suicidal ideation, plan or attempt

These symptoms cannot occur solely in the presence of a delirium, cannot be better accounted for by other causes of depression, or be the direct effect of a substance. The depressive syndrome typical in AD is frequently less severe and does not necessarily meet DSM-IV criteria for a diagnosis of major depression. Depression in AD may also manifest as irritability, demanding, aggression, complaining, and dependency. Patients with depression and AD have more impairment in ADL than those without mood disorder. A related depression phenomenon is the catastrophic reaction observed in approximately 15% of AD patients. It is a syndrome of relative sudden onset, short duration, severe mood symptoms, including crying, resistive and aggressive behavior, profanity, and anxiety (59).

SSRI are the initial treatment of choice for depression (Table 4). Citalopram and sertraline are favored by many clinicians, because they are thought to be mildly sedating, have anxiolytic properties, and have few anticholinergic properties. Citalopram, uniquely, is not metabolized via the CYP2D6 isoenzyme system, minimizing potential drug-drug interactions. Sertraline has relatively limited potential for drug–drug interactions compared to other SSRIs. Fluoxetine has a tendency to be activating and may therefore be of advantage in cases where apathy is present or a prominent feature of depression. It has a higher potential for drug interactions.

It is important to allow a sufficiently long period of time to constitute a therapeutic trial before changing agents. Twenty-five percent of patients with AD will have evidence of coexisting microvascular ischemic disease or infarcts (28). The presence of lacunar infarcts or subcortical hyperintensities (on imaging studies) is correlated with reduced response to antidepressant therapy and can increase the risk of drug-related confusion (60).

Some patients who do not respond to one SSRI may respond to another. Alternatively, changing to a medication with combined transmitter effects is a rational approach (e.g., venlafaxine). Once these options have proven ineffective, a tricyclic agent may be considered. Nortriptyline is most commonly favored because it has relatively less anticholinergic activity. Another advantage is that there are established therapeutic serum levels for this medication, which can be monitored. Serum concentrations above and below the therapeutic range are not considered effective in treating depression, and levels should be maintained within this therapeutic window.

If a tricyclic agent is ineffective, augmentation with mood stabilizers or levothyroxine may be considered. Alternatively, a monoamine oxidase inhibitor (MAO-I) such as phenelzine can be used. These medications have potentially fatal interactions with both medications and foods. Special attention to patient and caregiver education is required. Prior to initiation of a MAO-I, all medications with potentially dangerous interactions should be discontinued and sufficient time (typically 5 half-lifes) allowed to pass for the serum concentrations to fall near to zero (28,60).

Patients who do not show adequate therapeutic response to tricyclic agents with augmentation or MAO-Is are considered candidates for electroconvulsive therapy (ECT). ECT is both safe and effective in patients with AD. There is a risk of worsening confusion and anterograde memory deficit during

Table 4
Medications Commonly Used in the Treatment of Depression

Medication (commercial name)	Usual dose (mg)	Range (mg)	Comments
Citalopram (Celexa)	20	10–40	SSRI with relatively simple titration and once-per-day dosing. May have less anticholinergic effects than other SSRIs. Not metabolized via CYP2D6 pathway, minimizing potential drug interactions.
Sertraline (Zoloft)	50	50–200	SSRI with mild sedating property. Once-per-day dosing. Relatively few drug interactions. Minimally anticholinergic.
Paroxetine (Paxil)	20	10–50	SSRI with mild sedating properties. Once-per-day dosing. May have more benefit in anxiety disorders.
Fluoxetine (Prozac)	20	10–40	SSRI with possible activating properties. Once-per-day dosing. Longest time available. Highest potential for drug interactions among SSRIs.
Venlafaxin (Effexor)	100	50–300	Combined serotonergic and noradrenergic-reuptake inhibitor. Limited information in geriatric population. Minimally anticholinergic. May have activating properties. Two- to three-times-per-day dosing.
Nefazadone (Serzone)	400	200–600	Atypical serotonergic antidepressant related to trazodone. Relatively complex titration and twice-per-day dosing. Strong muscarinic receptor antagonism and may cause memory impairment.
Mirtazepine (Remeron)	15	7.5–30	Noradrenergic and specific serotonergic antidepressant. Strong histaminic$_1$ receptor antagonism and may cause sedation and potentiation of CNS depression. Limited information in geriatric population.
Nortriptyline (Pamelor)	50	50–100	Tricyclic antidepressant with relative safety in geriatric population within its class. Has a therapeutic window for efficacy. Serum levels widely available and should be periodically monitored. ECG prior to initiation of therapy recommended.
Phenelzine (Nardil)	60	15–90	MAO-I. Dosage should be titrated to minimum clinically effective dose on an individual basis. Standard initial dose is 15 mg once daily. Must be used with considerable caution, as potentially fatal drug–drug and drug–food interactions are possible. Typically reserved for patients refractory to all other agents.

the period immediately after treatment. In patients with a severe or refractory depression combined with suicidal ideation or psychosis, the risks of temporary memory loss and confusion can definitely be outweighed by the benefits. Consultation with a psychiatrist familiar with the treatment of geriatric depression is recommended if ECT is considered. Some patients require a single course of treatment, while a small subset of patients requires maintenance therapy. After ECT, patients are typically

Table 5
Medications Commonly Used in the Treatment of Anxiety

Medication (commercial name)	Usual dose (mg)	Range (mg)	Comments
Oxazepam (Serax)	30	20–60	Short half-life (4–8 hour) benzodiazepine. Metabolism is via glucuronidation only and has few or no active metabolites. Elimination relatively unaffected by liver dysfunction.
Lorazepam (Ativan)	1	0.5–2	Intermediate-half-life (6–20 hour) benzodiazepine. Has few or no active metabolites, and is relatively unaffected by liver dysfunction.
Buspirone (Buspar)	30	15–45	Anxiolytic without benzodiazepine receptor activity or GABA effects. Mechanism of action unknown, but may relate to serotonin inhibition in the dorsal raphé. Minimal sedation and not considered habit-forming.

treated with an antidepressant, usually a different agent than the ones that failed previously.

Once a therapeutic response has been achieved, patients should be continued on therapy for 3–6 months before a tapered withdrawal is considered. If a patient relapses, therapy should be restarted with the previously successful measure and then the above algorithm followed *(60,61)*. Recurrent depression is common, and prolonged treatment is frequently required.

ANXIETY

Anxiety disorders occur in approximately 50% of AD patients, typically in mild to moderate severity. Anxiety is more common in patients with onset of dementia before the age of 65 years. The symptoms become more common as the disease progresses and are associated with greater disability in ADL *(62)*.

Anxiety frequently responds well to treatment with trazodone or SSRI with anxiolytic properties, such as citalopram, sertraline, and paroxetine (Table 5). Buspirone can be an effective agent and may be tried when antidepressants are not effective. Anxiety can reflect an undetected psychosis, especially in patients with severe language impairment. A trial with an atypical antipsychotic may be beneficial, particularly if anxiety manifests as agitation. Benzodiazepines can be alternatives when the above measures fail or a rapid response is necessary in the context of markedly severe anxiety with agitation. These medications carry the risk of paradoxical agitation, disinhibition, and drug-induced confusion. Agents such as lorazepam and oxazepam that are metabolized directly to inactive glucuronides are typically preferred for use in elderly patients. The use of benzodiazepines should be short-term and the need for this medication regularly reevaluated. One strategy is to use a benzodiazepine for immediate short-term relief of symptoms, while an SSRI antidepressant is allowed time to be of benefit. Once the SSRI is therapeutic, the benzodiazepine can be tapered. Medications that are strongly anti-cholinergic, such as diphenhydramine or hydroxyzine, should be avoided.

INSOMNIA

When an AD patient does not sleep, neither does the caregiver. This makes insomnia a major problem. Insomnia may be related to primary disturbance of diurnal cycles, depression, anxiety, psychosis,

Table 6
Some Suggested Nonpharmacological Interventions
for Treatment of Sleep Disturbances in AD

Maintain regular bed and wake times.
Use bedroom only for sleep.
Do not stay in bed awake.
Establish regular meal times.
Avoid caffeine, nicotine, and alcohol.
Avoid excessive evening fluid intake.
Void before retiring to bed.
Treat pain symptoms.
If awakened, do not watch television.
Seek morning sunlight exposure.
Engage in regular daily exercise.
Establish a quiet, comfortable sleep environment.

delirium, or agitation. When it is the primary target symptom, the nonpharmacological and sleep hygiene measures described above and in Table 6 should be tried first. If pharmacotherapy is necessary, sleep hygiene measures should be continued. In some patients, particularly those who nap excessively during the day, an increase in daytime activity, exercise, and a regular daily schedule may be combined with short-term pharmacological interventions in order to reestablish the circadian rhythm.

Medications commonly used in the treatment of insomnia are listed in Table 7. Sedating antidepressants, particularly trazodone, are frequently sufficient to provide relief. Nonbenzodiazepine hypnotics, such as zolpidem or zoleplon, are of second choice. These medications show a relative selective affinity for the omega-1 receptor on the α subunit of the γ-aminobutyric acid (GABA) receptor complex. This receptor selectivity is thought possibly to provide hypnotic qualities similar to benzodiazepines, but without as much the risk of unwanted side effects, such as executive system dysfunction, confusion, and amnesia. Used long-term, they can produce dependence. With refractory insomnia in particular, benzodiazepines may be warranted. Medium-duration agents, such as temazepam, are favored. There is evidence that hypnotic medications are more useful in initiating than maintaining sleep *(63)*.

OTHER BEHAVIORAL CHANGES

Apathy

Apathy is the most common neuropsychiatric symptom observed in AD, occurring in approximately 70% of patients. Patients typically lose interest in usual activities, hobbies, as well as in social and family interactions. AchEIs have stimulating properties and may provide adequate therapy *(28)*. Apathy may be part of a depressive syndrome, but might also occur independently of any mood changes *(64)*. A trial of an activating SSRI (such as fluoxetine) or tricyclic antidepressant (such as desipramine) may be warranted and sufficient (Table 8). In rare cases the problem is severe enough to warrant use of psychostimulants (including methylphenidate or dextroamphetamine). These medications can pose considerable risk of adverse reactions and confusion, and should therefore be used with caution. Modafinil relieves daytime sleepiness, so it may also be tried in cases of apathy.

Sexual Behavior Problems

The most common but rarely treated sexual symptom in AD is loss of libido. A minority of patients may become hypersexual or sexually aggressive. This appears to be more common in males than in

Table 7
Medications Commonly Used in the Treatment of Insomnia

Medication (commercial name)	Usual dose (mg)	Range (mg)	Comments
Trazodone (Desyrel)	100	50–400	Antidepressant thought to exert effect through serotonin-reuptake inhibition. Minimal anticholinergic properties. Sedating and may have anxiolytic action.
Zolpidem (Ambien)	10	5–10	Nonbenzodiazepine hypnotic thought to exert its effect through selective activity at the omega-1 receptor subtype on the α subunit of the γ-aminobutyric acid $(GABA)_A$ receptor complex.
Zoleplon (Sonata)	10	5–10	Nonbenzodiazepine hypnotic thought to exert its effect through selective activity at the omega-1 receptor subtype on the α subunit of the $GABA_A$ receptor complex.
Temazepam (Restoril)	15	15–30	Intermediate-half-life (5–8 hour) benzodiazepine. Has no active metabolites, and is relatively unaffected by liver dysfunction.

Table 8
Medications Used in the Treatment of Other Behavioral Disturbances

Target symptom	Medication	Usual dose	Range
Apathy	Antidepressants		
	Fluoxetine (Prozac)	10 mg	10–20 mg
	Desipramine (Norpramin)	50 mg	50–250 mg
	Stimulants		
	Methylphenidate (Ritalin)	10 mg	10–30 mg
	Dextroamphetamine (Dexadrine)	5 mg	5–20 mg
	Modafanil (Provigil)	200 mg	100–200 mg
Sexual aggression in males	Leuprolide (Lupron)		
	Depot intramuscular	7.5 mg/month	Same as usual dose
	Subcutaneous	1 mg	
	Medroxyprogesterone		
	intramuscular	150 mg/3 months	Same as usual dose
	oral	5 mg/day	

females. Sexual aggression in males may respond to testosterone inhibitors, such as leuprolide, or estrogenic compounds, such as medroxyprogesterone *(28)*.

SUMMARY

Neuropsychiatric symptoms are an important aspect of AD and are a significant source of distress for both patients and caregivers. With detection and accurate diagnosis, these problems can be treated effectively using a comprehensive treatment plan combining both pharmacological and nonpharmacological interventions. Important nonpharmacological interventions include support and education of both the patient and family caregivers, alterations of the patient's physical and social environment, and careful evaluation of the disease process over time. Efficacious pharmacological therapies are available and should be used when indicated. Treatment begins with cholinesterase inhibitors, which are effective in treating problems related to cognitive decline and may affect neuropsychiatric symptoms. There are rational principles of pharmacotherapy to help direct clinicians in the safe and efficacious management of medications and to provide strategies for treatment of patients with refractory symptoms. Effective management of neuropsychiatric symptoms in AD can substantially improve the quality of life for patients suffering from the disease and for family members responsible for their care.

ACKNOWLEDGMENTS

This work was supported by an Alzheimer's Disease Research Center Grant (AG16570) from the National Institutes on Aging, Alzheimer's Disease Research Center grant (AG 16570), an Alzheimer's Disease Research Center of California Grant, and the Sidell-Kagan Foundation.

REFERENCES

1. Mega, M.S. et al.: The spectrum of behavioral changes in Alzheimer's disease. Neurology 1996; 46: 130–135.
2. Steele, M.S. et al.: Psychiatric symptoms and nursing home placement of patients with Alzheimer's disease. Am J Psychiatry 1990; 147: 1049–1051.
3. Reisberg, B. et al.: Behavioral symptoms in Alzheimer's disease: phenomenology and treatment. J Clin Psychiatry 1987; 48: 9–15.
4. Allen, N.P.H. et al.: Manchester and Oxford Universities Scale for the Psychological Assessment of Dementia (MOUSEPAD). Br J Psychiatry 1996; 169: 293–307.
5. Tariot, P.N. et al.: The Behavior Rating Scale for Dementia of the Consortium to Establish a Registry for Alzheimer's Disease. Am J Psychiatry 1995; 152: 1349–1357.
6. Sultzer, D.L. et al.: Assessment of cognitive, psychiatric, and behavioral disturbances in patients with dementia. J Am Geriatr Soc 1992; 40: 549–555.
7. Molloy, D.W. et al.: Validity and reliability of the Dysfunctional Behavior Rating Instrument. Acta Psychiatr Scand 1991; 84: 103–106.
8. Alexopoulos, G.S. et al.: Cornell Scale for Depression in Dementia. Biol Psychiatry 1988; 23: 271–284.
9. Cummings, J.L. et al.: The Neuropsychiatric Inventory: comprehensive assessment of psychopathology in dementia. Neurology 1994; 44: 2308–2314.
10. Buckwalter, K.C.: Overview of psychological factors contributing to stress of family caregivers. In: Radebaugh, T.S. (ed.): Alzheimer's disease: causes, diagnosis, treatment, and care. CRC Press, New York, 1996: 305–312.
11. Cohen-Mansfield, J.: Nonpharmacological interventions for inappropriate behaviors in dementia: a review, summary, and critique. Am J Geriatr Psychiatry 2001; 9: 361–381.
12. Doody, R.S. et al.: Practice parameter: management of dementia (an evidence-based review). Report of the Quality Standards Subcommittee of the American Academy of Neurology. Neurology 2001; 56: 1154–1166.
13. Tariot, P.N. et al.: A randomized, double-blind, placebo-controlled study of the efficacy and safety of donepezil in patients with Alzheimer's disease in the nursing home setting. J Am Geriatr Soc 2001; 49: 1590–1599.
14. Feldman, H. et al.: A 24-week, randomized, double-blind study of donepezil in moderate to severe Alzheimer's disease. Neurology 2001; 57: 613–620.
15. Corey-Bloom, J.; Anand, R.; Veach, J.: A randomized trial evaluating the efficacy and safety of ENA 713 (rivastigmine tartrate), a new acetylcholinesterase inhibitor, in patients with mild to moderately severe Alzheimer's disease: The ENA 713 B352 Study Group. Int J Geriatr Psychopharmacol 1998; 1: 55–65.
16. Rosler, M. et al.: Effects of two-year treatment with the cholinesterase inhibitor rivastigmine on behavioural symptoms in Alzheimer's disease. Behav Neurol 1998/1999; 11: 211–216.
17. Rosler, M. et al.: Efficacy and safety of rivastigmine in patients with Alzheimer's disease: international randomized controlled trial. Br Med J 1999; 318: 633–640.
18. Cummings, J.; Mega, M.: Neuropsychiatry and clinical neuroscience. Oxford University Press, New York, 2003.
19. Tariot, P.N. et al.: A 5-month, randomized, placebo-controlled trial of galantamine in AD: the Galantamine USA-10 Study Group. Neurology 2000; 54: 2269–2276.
20. Tsai, S.J. et al.: Physical aggression and associated factors in probable Alzheimer disease. Alzheimer Dis Assoc Disord 1996; 10: 82–85.
21. Tractenberg, R.E.; Weiner, M.F.; Thal, L.J.: Estimating the prevalence of agitation of community-dwelling persons with Alzheimer's disease. J Neuropsychiatry Clin Neurosci 2002; 14: 11–18.
22. Eastley, R.; Wilcock, G.: Prevalence and correlates of aggressive behaviours occurring in patients with Alzheimer's disease. Int J Geriatr Psychiatry 1997; 12: 484–487.

23. Eustace, A. et al.: Verbal aggression in Alzheimer's disease: clinical, functional, and neuropsychological correlates. Int J Geriatr Psychiatry, 2001; 16: 858–861.

24. Teri, L. et al.: Behavioral disturbance, cognitive dysfunction, and functional skill: prevalence and relationship in Alzheimer's disease. J Am Geriatr Soc 1989; 37: 109–116.

25. Devanand, D.P. et al.: The course of psychopathologic features in mild to moderate Alzheimer's disease. Arch Gen Psychiatry 1997; 54: 257–263.

26. Hope, T. et al.: Natural history of behavioural changes and psychiatric symptoms in Alzheimer's disease. Br J Psychiatry 1999; 174: 39–44.

27. Keene, J. et al.: Natural history of aggressive behaviour in dementia. Int J Geriatr Psychiatry 1999; 14: 541–548.

28. Cummings, J.L.: Neuropsychiatric aspects of Alzheimer's disease and related disorders. Martin Dunitz, London, 2002.

29. Cooper, J.K. et al.: Psychotic symptoms in Alzheimer's disease. Int J Geriatr Psychiatry 1991; 6: 721–726.

30. Gormley, N.; Rizwan, M.R.: Prevalence and clinical correlates of psychotic symptoms in Alzheimer's disease. Int J Geriatr Psychiatry 1998; 13: 410–414.

31. Mendez, M.F. et al.: Psychiatric symptoms associated with Alzheimer's disease. J Neuropsychiatry Clin Neurosci 1990; 2: 28–33.

32. Ballard, C. et al.: The prevalence and phenomenology of psychotic symptoms in dementia sufferers. Int J Geriatr Psychiatry 1995; 10: 477–485.

33. Tekin, S. et al.: Activities of daily living in Alzheimer's disease: neuropsychiatric, cognitive, and medical illness influences. Am J Geriatr Psychiatry 2001; 9: 81–86.

34. Binetti, G. et al.: Delusions in Alzheimer's disease and multi-infarct dementia. Acta Neurol Scand 1993; 88: 5–9.

35. Burns, A.; Jacoby, R.; Levy, R.: Psychiatric phenomena in Alzheimer's disease. I: Disorders of thought content. II: Disorders of perception. Br J Psychiatry 1990; 157: 72–81.

36. Hwang, J.-P. et al.: Delusions of theft in dementia of the Alzheimer type: a preliminary report. Alzheimer Dis Assoc Disord 1997; 11: 110–112.

37. Mendez, M.F.: Delusional misidentification of persons in dementia. Br J Psychiatry 1992; 160: 414–416.

38. Migliorelli, R. et al.: Neuropsychiatric and neuropsychological correlates of delusions in Alzheimer's disease. Psychol Med 1995; 25: 505–513.

39. Chui, H.C. et al.: Extrapyramidal signs and psychiatric symptoms predict faster cognitive decline in Alzheimer's disease. Arch Neurol 1994; 51: 676–681.

40. Haupt, M.; Romero, B.; Kurz, A.: Delusions and hallucinations in Alzheimer's disease: results from a two-year longitudinal study. Int J Geriatr Psychiatry 1996; 11: 965–972.

41. Mortimer, J.A. et al.: Predictors of cognitive and functional progression in patients with probable Alzheimer's disease. Neurology 1992; 42: 1689–1696.

42. Paulsen, J.S. et al.: Incidence of and risk factors for hallucinations and delusions in patients with probable AD. Neurology 2000; 54: 1965–1971.

43. Stern, Y. et al.: Utility of extrapyramidal signs and psychosis as predictors of cognitive and functional decline, nursing home admission, and death in Alzheimer's disease: prospective analyses from the Predictors Study. Neurology 1994; 44: 2300–2307.

44. Wilson, R.S. et al.: Hallucinations, delusions, and cognitive decline in Alzheimer's disease. J Neurol Neurosurg Psychiatry 2000; 69: 172–177.

45. Rapoport, M.J. et al.:. Relationship of psychosis to aggression, apathy and function in dementia. Int J Geriatr Psychiatry 2001; 16: 123–130.

46. Chemerinski, E. et al.: Prevalence and correlates of aggressive behavior in Alzheimer's disease. J Neuropsychiatry Clin Neurosci 1998; 10: 421–425.

47. Deutsch, L.H. et al.: Psychosis and physical aggression in probable Alzheimer's disease. Am J Psychiatry 1991; 148: 1159–1163.

48. Flynn, F.G.; Cummings, J.L.; Gornbein, J.: Delusions in dementia syndromes: investigation of behavioral and neuropsychological correlates. J Neuropsychiatry Clin Neurosci 1991; 3: 364–370.

49. Devanand, D.P. et al.: Depressed mood in the incidence of Alzheimer's disease in the elderly living in the community. Arch Gen Psychiatry 1996; 53: 175–182.

50. Speck, C.E. et al.: History of depression as a risk factor for Alzheimer's disease. Epidemiology 1995; 6: 366–369.

51. Ballard, C. et al.: The prevalence, associations and symptoms of depression amongst dementia sufferers. J Affect Disord 1996; 36: 135–144.

52. Lyketsos, C.G. et al.: Major and minor depression in Alzheimer's disease: prevalence and impact. J Neuropsychiatry Clin Neurosci 1997; 9: 556–561.

53. Vida, S. et al.: Prevalence of depression in Alzheimer's disease and validity of research diagnostic criteria. J Geriatr Psychiatry Neurol 1994; 7: 238–244.

54. Weiner, M.F. et al.: Prevalence and incidence of major depressive disorder in Alzheimer's disease: findings from two databases. Dement Geriatr Cogn Disord 2002; 13: 8–12.

55. Burns, A.; Jacoby, R.; Levy, R.: Psychiatric phenomena in Alzheimer's disease, IV: disorders of behaviour. Br J Psychiatry 1990; 157: 86–94.
56. Mackenzie, T.B.; Robiner, W.N.; Knopman, D.: Differences between patient and family assessments of depression in Alzheimer's disease. Am J Psychiatry,1989; 146: 1174–1178.
57. Olin, J.T. et al.: National Institute of Mental Health—provisional diagnostic criteria for depression of Alzheimer disease. Am J Geriatr Psychiatry 2002; 10: 129–141.
58. American Psychiatric Association, Diagnostic and statistical manual of mental disorders: DSM-IV (4th ed). American Psychiatric Association, Washington, DC, 1994.
59. Tiberti, C. et al.: Prevalence and correlates of the catastrophic reaction in Alzheimer's disease. Neurology 1998; 50: 546–548.
60. Lavretsky, H.: Choosing appropriate treatment for geriatric depression. Clin Geriatr 2000; 9 (5): 31–46.
61. Rao, G.; Constantine, L.G.: The benefits and risks of ECT for patients with primary dementia who also suffer from depression. Int J Ger Psychiatry 2000; 15: 729–735.
62. Bliwise, D.L. et al.: Disruptive nocturnal behavior in Parkinson's disease and Alzheimer's disease. J Geriatr Psychiatry Neurol 1995; 8: 107–110.
63. Geldmacher, D.S.: Contemporary diagnosis and management of Alzheimer's disease. Handbooks in Health Care Co., Newton, PA, 2001: 200.
64. Levy, M.L. et al.: Apathy is not depression. J Neuropsychiatry Clin Neurosci 1998; 10: 314–319.

42

Neuropsychiatric Symptoms in African American Dementia Patients

Raymelle Schoos, Carl I. Cohen, and Lorna Walcott-Brown

INTRODUCTION

African Americans currently comprise 8.5% of the U.S. population aged 65 and over *(1)*, and elderly minority persons are one of the most rapidly growing segments of the U.S. population. Over the next 30 years it is predicted that there will be a threefold increase in the elderly African American population, compared to a doubling of the Caucasian elderly population *(1)*. Neuropsychiatric behaviors— e.g., depression, agitation, delusions, and hallucinations—may occur in up to 86% of patients with dementia *(2)*. Considerable research has been devoted to this subject, but disproportionately little has focused on minority patients. In this chapter we review the neuropsychiatric symptoms as it pertains to black persons with dementia.

ISSUES IN ASSESSING DEMENTIA IN BLACK POPULATIONS

Black minorities in the United States can be divided into several subgroups: African Americans born and raised in the United States, African Caribbeans, and a smaller number of blacks from Africa who have immigrated to the United States. Each group has significant cultural differences compared to the others. As H. Fabrega and colleagues noted *(3)*, "even a biologically well-defined black group is likely to contain subjects that are influenced by highly diverse (background) cultures (and national traditions) so that it naturally does not constitute a well-established 'cultural' group" (p. 286).

Most community studies have found blacks to have higher rates of dementia than whites *(4,5)*. Several factors have been identified that could account for the differences *(5–7)*:

1. Proportionately more whites are in long-term care institutions so that they are excluded from community surveys.
2. Criteria for dementia may be educationally or culturally biased, e.g., when different cutoff scores on the Mini-Mental State Examination (MMSE) were used for blacks and whites, the differences were less apparent.
3. Among some subgroups of blacks, such as Africans or Caribbeans, migratory status seems to predispose to greater rates of dementia.

RACIAL DIFFERENCES IN NEUROPSYCHIATRIC SYMPTOMS

There are a number of methodological limitations to accurately assessing racial differences in the prevalence of neuropsychiatric symptoms among dementia patients.

1. Psychometric properties of instruments for assessing neuropsychiatric symptoms have not always been tested in minority populations, although, as described below, many of the instruments probably meet minimal criteria of reliability, and to a lesser degree, validity.

From: *Current Clinical Neurology,*
Alzheimer's Disease: A Physician's Guide to Practical Management
Edited by: R. W. Richter and B. Zoeller Richter © Humana Press Inc., Totowa, NJ

2. The length and severity of illness is difficult to delineate accurately. Determination of the length of illness relies heavily on caregiver perceptions of when the patient began to show cognitive or behavioral disturbances. Cultural and educational differences influence these perceptions, although good history taking can enhance but not always overcome these obstacles.

3. Severity of illness is typically based on use of cognitive batteries that have been found to have educational and cultural biases, and consequently, minority patients may appear more severely impaired than white patients *(5)*.

4. In addition to severity and length of illness and education, a variety of other clinical and demographic factors may influence neuropsychiatric symptoms, such as sensory impairment, poor physical health, gender, income, and the interactive effects of several neuropsychiatric symptoms occurring together *(8)*.

5. As described above, black dementia patients are not a homogeneous population. Many blacks were born abroad, mostly in the Caribbean. It is estimated that there are as many as 2 million African Caribbeans living in the United States, with a great number of them in large cities in the Northeast and Florida *(9)*. As S. Gopaul-McNicol observed *(10)*, "Although black West Indians share the African legacy and the historical experience of slavery with African Americans, and although the two groups possess some cultural similarities, there are many differences . . ." (p. 60). Such differences can potentially be reflected in psychiatric symptoms, either as a result of delays in health-seeking behavior, the use of alternative treatments such as herbalists or spiritualists, or in the cultural expressions of illness.

6. Because virtually all samples are derived from dementia clinics or nursing homes, there has been considerable variability in their composition. Accessibility, referral networks, cost, attitudes about the facility, and so forth, will all determine who becomes a patient and is included in the data analysis. Moreover, some studies have looked at all dementia patients and others have looked only at Alzheimer's disease (AD) patients. Although some studies have tried to control for dementia diagnoses, the fact that there is increasing recognition that many dementia cases are really hybrids of AD and varying degrees of vascular pathology create further confusion with respect to this issue.

HIGHER PREVALENCE OF PSYCHOTIC SYMPTOMS IN BLACK DEMENTIA PATIENTS

These limitations not withstanding, some general trends have emerged concerning race and neuropsychiatric symptoms. A preponderance of studies has found black dementia patients to have a higher prevalence of psychotic symptoms—i.e., hallucinations and delusions—than white patients. In studies that have tried to control for various confounding variables, the results continued to support the finding of greater levels of psychotic symptoms among blacks. Several studies have found that both hallucinations and delusions are significantly more common among blacks *(11–15)*. Other studies that have examined either hallucinations or delusions, but not both, have found that each of these symptoms are significantly more prevalent among black patients *(16,17)*. In our own studies in an urban dementia clinic in Brooklyn, New York, we found that 77% of blacks and 69% of whites exhibited psychotic symptoms *(13)*. In contrast, in a study of three nursing homes in the same geographic area we found rates of psychoses of 22% among blacks and 25% among whites *(12)*. However, in both settings, the severity of psychotic symptoms was higher among black patients. A survey of statewide dementia centers in California found that 28% of blacks and 8% of whites had hallucinations, and 49% of blacks and 35% of whites had delusions *(15)*. Moreover, racial differences in psychotic symptoms have not always been found, especially after controlling for confounding variables. For example, the latter group initially found racial differences in psychotic symptoms, but these differences disappeared after controlling for confounding variables *(15)*. Another study that included a very small sample of black AD patients also found no racial differences *(18)*.

MORE DEPRESSION IN WHITE DEMENTIA PATIENTS

The incidence of depression has been consistently found to be higher among Caucasian than among black dementia patients. This relationship seems to persist even after controlling for confounding variables. For example, in our dementia clinic, rates of depression were 44% and 52% for blacks and whites, respectively *(13)*. The California study found that 28% of blacks and 34% of whites evidenced depression *(16)*. In our nursing home study, rates of possible depression were 19% and 34% for blacks and whites, respectively *(12)*. However, depression is often difficult to assess in more severe dementia patients. Thus, in nursing homes, some of the depression instruments have not detected racial differences *(19)*. If the incidence of depression is indeed higher in whites, this would be somewhat surprising, since greater vascular pathology is likely to be present among black dementia patients. Increased vascular pathology has been linked to depression in older persons.

RELATIONSHIP BETWEEN RACE AND BEHAVIORAL DISTURBANCES IS LESS CLEAR

Most studies have found negligible racial differences, especially after controlling for confounding variables. For example, we found a higher prevalence and severity of activity disturbance in black vs white dementia outpatients (79% vs 65%), but this difference did not persist in multivariate analysis *(13)*. The California study found essentially no difference between blacks (37%) and whites (39%) in prevalence of agitation *(15)*. However, in nursing homes, we found that whites had higher rates and severity of activity disturbance than black dementia patients (28% vs 17%). This difference persisted even after controlling for confounding variables *(8,12)*.

This racial difference between community and nursing home may reflect the way blacks and whites enter long-term-care facilities. As compared to whites, blacks more frequently enter nursing homes from an acute-care hospital, and they are more apt to have been living alone prior to their hospitalization. Admissions for whites are more planned, and caregivers difficulties in controlling agitation most likely contribute to admission *(12)*.

In looking at within-group differences, our center has found no differences in any of the neuropsychiatric symptoms between U.S.-born African Americans and African Caribbeans *(12,13)*. Thus, despite their cultural diversity, the similar socioeconomic and racial background may attenuate any potential differences.

POTENTIAL REASONS FOR RACIAL DIFFERENCES IN SYMPTOMS

There are several reasons why there may be racial differences in neuropsychiatric symptoms.

1. Studies are typically conducted in dementia clinics, so the type and intensity of neuropsychiatric symptoms may reflect the degree of severity of the dementia. Black caregivers seem to be less likely than white to identify memory problems as an illness or as a problem in the early stages of dementia. This in part reflects cultural beliefs and lower educational levels among blacks. For example, Haley and co-workers observed that black caregivers may consider the early stages of dementia as normal aging *(20)*. Moreover, black caregivers seem to find the task of caring for an elderly individual less burdensome and depressing and more satisfying than either white or Hispanic caregivers do *(21–23)*. The implications of caregiving on neuropsychiatric symptoms are described in greater detail below.
2. Black dementia patients may be more apt to suffer from vascular or mixed dementias than either whites or Hispanics *(6)*. It is well established that African Americans have a high prevalence of hypertension, diabetes, and stroke, which have been recognized not only as risk factors for vascular dementia but as factors that may worsen the course of AD *(15)*. These vascular or mixed dementias are believed by some researchers to be associated with an even higher prevalence of "psychopathology" than is observed in AD alone *(15)*. However, in our study no racial differences in neuropsychiatric symptoms were observed in an outpatient sample between persons with AD and persons with multi-infarct (vascular) dementia *(8)*.

   Presence of other conditions may further confound the presentation. A study by Akpaffiong and colleagues found African Americans to have a greater number of alcoholic dementia diagnoses than Caucasians, whereas whites had higher rates of Parkinsonian-type dementia *(24)*. Perhaps most important, compared to whites, blacks have higher rates of medical illness, with less adequate care. Their lifetime income is lower, and they are twice as likely to live in poverty. The impact of physical disease and poverty on psychiatric symptoms is well established, and it is plausible that they may shape the neuropsychiatric symptoms of dementia.

3. There may be racial differences in access to medical care and referral patterns, particularly to specialists in dementia assessment and treatment *(15)*. Consequently, blacks may enter treatment with more severe symptoms and at a later stage of illness.

4. Even when in clinical settings, blacks may be less apt to receive treatment for symptoms than are whites. For example, our group documented that approximately one-sixth of black nursing home patients with symptoms of psychoses or aggression received antipsychotic medication *(12)*. However, for the white nursing home patients, 38% with psychoses and 25% of those with aggressive behavior received antipsychotic medications. More recently, in another nursing home study, we reported that blacks were significantly less likely than whites to receive antidepressants for their mood disorder *(25)*.

5. There may be racial differences in premorbid traits or illnesses. Heurtin-Roberts and colleagues observed that the language of distress may present with different patterns of symptoms in different cultures *(26)*. There is evidence that level of paranoid ideation and psychoses is higher in nondemented community-dwelling older blacks than whites *(27)*. On the other hand, lifetime prevalence of depression is lower among blacks than whites *(28)*.

6. There may be genetic differences in the etiology of dementias such as AD or genetic differences that affect the prevalence of neuropsychiatric symptoms. For example, although research indicates that for African Americans the association between apolipoprotein E (ApoE)e4 and risk of AD is present, it is weaker than in Caucasians, and may be restricted to homozygotes as opposed to heterozygotes *(29)*. When the ApoEe4 allele was present, for example, African Americans, Hispanics, and Caucasians had a similar risk of AD up to the age of 90 years, whereas with the ApoEe4-allele absent, African Americans and Hispanics were two to four times more likely to develop AD up to the age of 90 than were Caucasians *(29)*.

There have been mixed findings with respect to the relationship between ApoEe4-alleles and depression, with most studies suggesting lower rates of depression among persons with AD and ApoEe4 and higher rates among AD patients with ApoEe2 or ApoEe3 alleles *(30)*. However, one small study found an increased risk of depression among those with one ApoEe4-allele vs those with only ApoEe3-alleles *(31)*. No association has been found with between ApoE alleles and other neuropsychiatric symptoms.

These findings are potentially relevant to the presentation of neuropsychiatric symptoms, since a study of older residents of Northern Manhattan found significantly greater ApoEe2 and ApoEe3-alleles in white than in black people (87% vs 79%), although among AD patients there were no observed differences in e2 and e3 alleles *(29)*.

Another exploratory tack has been to examine genetic polymorphisms. For example, Holmes and colleagues found an association between common polymorphic variations in serotonin receptor genes and psychotic symptoms in AD *(30)*. These same genes have been implicated in contributing to psychotic symptoms in schizophrenia and bipolar illness. To date, no studies have examined the implications of these findings with respect to racial differences in neuropsychiatric symptoms.

Finally, a greater risk of depression in AD has been linked to a family history of depression. Thus, because African Americans in the general population appear to have a lower prevalence of depression than Caucasians, it would then follow that the rates of familial depression should be lower *(28)*.

ASSESSING NEUROPSYCHIATRIC SYMPTOMS IN BLACK DEMENTIA PATIENTS

There are limited data available concerning the psychometric properties of the assessment instruments for neuropsychiatric symptoms in minority dementia patients. Our group has examined the reliability—the consistency or stability of the measurement process across patients, time, or observers—for many of these instruments for use with black patients *(12)*. One measure that we examined was internal consistency (alpha). This is a reliability measure that examines how well items of a scale measure the same theme. Values of 0.60 and above are considered acceptable. We found those two measures of behavioral disturbances, the Cohen-Mansfield Agitation

Inventory (CMAI) and the BEHAVE-AD, had internal consistency coefficients of 0.98 and 0.81, respectively *(32,33)*.

In another study in which we looked separately at subscales of the BEHAVE-AD, we found internal consistency coefficients of 0.74, 0.67, and 0.62 for psychoses, aggressiveness, and activity disturbance, respectively *(13)*. Our unpublished data using the Neuropsychiatric Inventory (NPI) with 93 black dementia outpatients (51% of whom were African Caribbean) yielded internal consistency coefficients of 0.80 for both the 10-item and the 12-item scales *(34)*. We have also examined the interrater reliability (level of agreement among raters) for all these scales except the NPI and found intraclass correlations of between 0.88 and 0.95.

For black dementia patients, our group has also confirmed strong psychometric properties for several depressive scales *(19)*. We found high internal and interrater reliabilities for the Cornell Depression Scale in Dementia and for the Geriatric Depression Rating Scale (GDRS), although the latter was only useful in early- and early-middle-stage dementia *(35,36)*. The internal reliability for both scales among black dementia patients was over 0.80, and interrater reliabilities were over 0.90 *(19)*. Looking at concurrent validity, both scales exhibited significant correlation with each other as well as with several other depression scales and with our clinical diagnosis of depression. For both scales, sensitivity was higher than 75%, but specificity was better for the Cornell Scale (73%) than for the GDRS (61%). We established cutoff scores for possible depression of 5 on the Cornell Scale and 14 on the GDRS. Therefore, we believe that the Cornell Scale is a psychometrically acceptable instrument to use with black dementia patients. The GDRS had lower specificity and should be restricted to use with persons with milder dementia.

TREATMENT OF NEUROPSYHIATRIC SYMPTOMS IN BLACK DEMENTIA PATIENTS

Although there is evidence that black patients may be undertreated with respect to various neuropsychiatric symptoms, there have been no controlled studies that have compared treatment response to medications among racial groups. An open study conducted in a Veterans Administration geropsychiatric outpatient unit found no racial differences in dementia patients' response to pharmacotherapy *(24)*. However, theoretically, there may be differential pharmacotherapeutic responses among races. Recent studies revealed that among African Americans there may be a disproportionate number of slow and nonmetabolizers of psychotropic medications *(37)*. For example, twice as many African Americans as Caucasians (25% vs 13%) show no activity of the CYP2C19 system; 25–40% of African Americans present reduced activity of the CYP2 D6 system, whereas 25% of Caucasians show no activity. The former enzyme system is involved in the metabolism of diazepam and tricyclic antidepressants (TCA). The latter system acts on various TCA, selective serotonin reuptake inhibitors (SSRIs), and antipsychotic agents. Thus, clinicians may need to consider using lower initial doses of some medications in African American than in white dementia patients, although there are no definitive clinical data to substantiate this caveat.

Moreover, it is important not to undertreat. For example, in a multiracial study in nursing homes, we found that many depressed dementia patients had not been placed on optimal dose *(25)*. Thus, one should start low, go slow, but keep going.

Despite black caregivers' greater propensity to spend more time caring for persons with more severe dysfunction than white caregivers, the former are less likely to use formal services. Some of the reasons why blacks are less apt to seek formal treatment and support services include *(21,22)*:

1. The caregiver avoids seeking help because of shame.
2. Familial obligations or duties may preclude seeking help outside the family.
3. Caregiving is seen as rewarding, as an act of love, and of positive value.

4. Formal services are not seen as culturally sensitive or relevant.
5. Situations are reframed so that outside support is not seen as an option.
6. Dementia is seen as part of normal aging, not requiring outside help.
7. Appraisal of disruptive behavior is more benign and there is higher self-efficacy in managing problems (for example, milder forms of hallucinations and paranoid ideation are twice as common in the older black than in the white community [24% vs 10%] *(27)*, so caregivers may be more apt to accept or tolerate the symptoms in persons with dementia).

Hence, studies suggest that black caregivers may not report or may minimize the extent of any memory impairment or neuropsychiatric symptom until the point when the caregiver feels unable to manage the patient due to lack of support and the ability to handle the symptoms.

Primary-care physicians must be sensitive to these cultural differences when assessing and developing a treatment plan for black dementia patients. Often, black caregivers may present with conflicting messages. On one hand, they express the need for help in dealing with behavioral symptoms, and on the other hand they are prone to minimize the extent of difficulties. Also, because minority caregivers are more often nonspouses than white caregivers (children, siblings, nieces or nephews), the competing demands of other familial obligations may conflict with cultural obligations to take care of one's kin.

SUMMARY

There are four key points for clinicians to bear in mind with respect to neuropsychiatric symptoms in black dementia patients. *First,* compared to white dementia patients, black patients have generally been found to exhibit higher rates of psychotic symptoms, such as hallucinations and delusions, and lower rates of depression. Racial differences in agitation are less clear, although it appears that blacks exhibit higher rates in outpatient settings, whereas whites exhibit higher rates in nursing homes. *Second*, although biological factors (e.g., genetics, physical disorders) may contribute to these racial differences in neuropsychiatric symptoms, cultural beliefs about symptoms, disparities in access to dementia care, and caregiver attitudes and behaviors probably have more effect on the etiology of these differences. *Third*, in contradistinction to cognitive batteries that have considerable educational and cultural biases, the Cornell Scale has acceptable psychometric properties for assessing depression in black dementia patients. The CMAI, BEHAVE-AD, and the NPI, although not fully validated, had good reliability in black subjects and appear to be suitable for assessing psychoses and agitation. *Fourth,* limited data indicate that the effectiveness of medications for the treatment of neuropsychiatric symptoms is comparable between white and black dementia patients. In both racial groups, but perhaps more so in blacks, there are theoretical reasons to start with lower doses of those medications that are metabolized through CYP2C19 and CYP2 D6 cytochrome systems, although there are currently no clinical studies to support this caveat.

REFERENCES

1. U.S. Census Bureau. Population Projection Branch, August 2, 2002.
2. Lawlor, B.A. (ed.): Behavioral complications in Alzheimer's disease. American Psychiatric Press, Washington, DC, 1995.
3. Fabrega, H.; Mezzich, J.; Ulrich, R.F.: Black-white differences in psychopathology in an urban psychiatric population. Comprehensive Psychiatry 1988; 29: 285–297.
4. Harwood, D.G.; Ownby, R.L.: Ethnicity and dementia. Curr Psychiatry Rep 2000; 2: 40–45.
5. Froehlich, T.E.; Bogardus, S.T. Jr.; Inouye, S.K.: Dementia and race: are there differences between African Americans and Caucasians? J Am Geriatr Soc 2001; 49: 477–484.
6. Gurland, B.J. et al.: Rates of dementia in three ethnoracial groups. Int J Geriatr Psychiatry 1999; 14: 481–493.
7. Livingston, G.; Leavey, G.; Kitchen, G.: Mental health of migrant elders—the Islington study. Br J Psychiatry 2001; 179: 361–366.
8. Cohen, C.I.: Racial differences in neuropsychiatric symptoms among dementia patients: a comparison of African Americans and whites. Int Psychogeriatr 2000; 12 (suppl 1): 395–402.
9. Pierre-Pierre, G.: West Indians adding clout at the ballot box. The New York Times, September 6, 1993: 17, 19.
10. Gopaul-McNicol, S.A.: Working with West Indian families. Guilford, New York, 1993.

11. Cohen, C.I.; Carlin, L.: Racial differences in clinical and social variables among patients evaluated in a dementia assessment center. J Natl Med Assoc 1993; 85: 379–394.

12. Cohen, C.I.; Hyland, K.; Magai, C.: Interracial and Intraracial differences in neuropsychiatric symptoms, sociodemography, and treatment among nursing home patients with dementia. Gerontologist 1998; 38: 353–361.

13. Cohen, C.I.; Magai, C.: Racial differences in neuropsychiatric symptoms among dementia outpatients. Am J Geriatr Psychiatry 1999; 7: 57–63.

14. Cooper, J.K.; Mungas, D.; Weiler, P.G.: Relation of cognitive status and abnormal behaviors in Alzheimer disease. J Am Geriatr Soc 1990; 38: 867–870.

15. Hargrave, R. et al.: Clinical aspects of Alzheimer's disease in black and white patients. J Natl Med Assoc 1998; 90: 78–84.

16. Bassiony, M.M. et al.: Isolated hallucinosis in Alzheimer's disease is associated with African-American race. Int J Geriatr Psychiatry 2002; 17: 205–210.

17. Deutsch, L.H. et al.: Psychosis and physical aggression in probable Alzheimer's disease. Am J Psychiatry 1991; 148: 1159–1163.

18. Shadlen, M.F. et al.: Alzheimer's disease symptom severity in blacks and whites. J Am Geriatr Soc 1999; 47: 482–486.

19. Cohen, C.I.; Hyland, K.; Magai, C.: Depression among African American nursing home patients with dementia. Am J Geriatr Psychiatry 1998; 6: 162–175.

20. Haley, W.E. et al.: Psychological, social, and health impact of caregiving: a comparison of black and white dementia caregivers and noncaregivers. Psychol Aging 1995; 10: 540–552.

21. Earran, C.J. et al.: Race, finding meaning, and caregiver distress. J Aging Health 1997; 9: 316–333.

22. Dilworth-Anderson, P. et al.: Issues of race, ethnicity, and culture in caregiving research: a 20-year review (1980–2000). Gerontologist 2002; 42: 237–272.

23. Lawton, M.P. et al.: The dynamics of caregiving for a demented elder among black and white families. J Gerontol Soc Sci 1992; 47: 5156–5164.

24. Akpaffiong, M. et al.: Cross-cultural differences in demented geropsychiatric inpatients with behavioral disturbances. Int J Geriatr Psychiatry 1999; 14: 845–850.

25. Cohen, C.I.; Hyland, K.; Kimhy, D.: Mandatory depression screening of dementia patients in nursing homes. Annual Meeting of American Psychiatric Association, Philadelphia, May 2002.

26. Heurtin-Roberts, S.; Snowden, L.; Miller, L.: Expressions of anxiety in African Americans: ethnography and the epidemiological Catchment area studies. Culture, Med Psychiatry 1997; 21: 337–363.

27. Cohen, C.I. et al.: Paranoid ideation and psychoses in an urban population. Annual Meeting of American Psychiatric Association, San Francisco, May 2003.

28. Weissman, M.M. et al.: Affective disorders in psychiatric disorders. In: Robins, L.N.; Regier, D.A. (eds.): Psychiatric disorders in America. American Psychiatric Press, Washington, DC, 1992, pp. 53–80.

29. Tang, M.X. et al.: The ApoE-e4 allele and the risk of Alzheimer disease among African Americans, whites, and Hispanics. JAMA 1998; 279: 751–755.

30. Holmes, C.: Contribution of genetics to the understanding of behavioral and psychological symptoms of dementia. Int Psychogeriatr 2000; 12: 83–88.

31. Ramachandran, C. et al.: A preliminary study of apolipoprotein E genotype and psychiatric manifestations of Alzheimer's disease. Neurology 1996; 47: 256–259.

32. Cohen-Mansfield, J.; Marx, M.S.; Rosenthal, A.S.: A description of agitation in a nursing home. J Gerontol 1989; 44: 77–86.

33. Reisberg, B. et al.: Stage specific incidence of potentially remediable behavioral symptoms in aging and Alzheimer's disease: A study of 120 patients using the BEHAVE-AD. Bull Clin Neurosci 1989; 54: 95–112.

34. Cummings, J.L. et al.: The Neuropsychiatric Inventory: comprehensive assessment of psychopathology in dementia. Neurology 1994; 44: 2308–2314.

35. Alexopoulos, G.S. et al.: Cornell Scale for Depression in Dementia. Biol Psychiatry 1988; 23: 271–284.

36. Yesavage, J.A. et al.: The Geriatric Depression Rating Scale: comparison with other self-report and psychiatric rating scales. In: Crook, T.; Ferris, S.; Bartus, R. (eds.): Assessment in geriatric psychopharmacology. Mark Powley, New Canaan, CT, 1983: 153–157.

37. Lin, K.M.; Smith, M.W.: Psychopharmacotherapy in the context of culture and ethnicity. In: Ruiz, P. (ed.): Ethnicity and psychopharmacology. American Psychiatric Press, Washington, DC, 2000, pp. 1–36.

43

Resource Utilization by African American Dementia Patients

Beatrice Pollock

INTRODUCTION

In March 1994, the U.S. National Institutes of Health (NIH) published its guidelines on the inclusion of women and minorities as subjects in clinical research in the *Federal Register*. The goal of this legislation is to increase opportunities for obtaining critically important information with which to enhance health and treat disease among all Americans, and to detect and account for significant differences between genders or racial and ethnic groups *(1)*.

The infamous Tuskegee Syphilis Study conducted by the U.S. Public Health Service (PHS) from 1932 to 1972 withheld treatment from 399 poor African American men suffering from syphilis. These men were sharecroppers and laborers from Macon County, Alabama *(2)*. Penicillin was not available in the 1930's. However, in the 1940's, after its use for syphilis treatment became widespread, these men were neither told of, nor treated with, penicillin. This continues to play a critical role in deterring African Americans as well as other minorities from clinical trial participation, creating mistrust of the system. Even today, this mistrust is still hard to overcome. Communication will help to eliminate the "guinea pig" feeling and foster a sense of contributing to the field of medical knowledge by participating in a trial, even if there is no apparent benefit to that person.

Minority participation by ethnic group/gender in all clinical trials must be promoted by medical personnel and all other sources. To facilitate a subject's participation, all aspects of the potential subject's life need to be examined, beginning with racial/ethnic group and cultural biases, socioeconomic and employment status, transportation, age, and gender. Communication is essential: language, education, and literacy skills need assessment. What are the community and cultural values of subject? Do they lend support? Are sites for accessing these services conveniently located? Even more basic: does someone speak their own language? How will they understand and how will they be treated? Prior studies on minority recruitment show that immigration status and the ability to speak English were important factors affecting participation *(3)*. All these are barriers, which can be insurmountable to some people.

Are clinical trials involving minorities even an option? Celia Maxwell, special assistant to the commissioner of the U.S. Food and Drug Administration (FDA) and assistant professor of medicine at Howard University Hospital, during her remarks to the Florida AIDS Education and Training Centers (FLAETC), stated that the FDA's public health mission is to ensure that drugs and other health care products used in the United States are safe and effective for all Americans, and that minority participation must be increased. She noted that, at the time of her talk, nearly one-fourth of the U.S. population are people with diverse ethnic and racial backgrounds. By 2050, nearly half (48%) will be. Yet only 5% of clinical trial participants are from minority/racial/ethnic groups *(4)*. Shavers/Lynch data

From: *Current Clinical Neurology,*
Alzheimer's Disease: A Physician's Guide to Practical Management
Edited by: R. W. Richter and B. Zoeller Richter © Humana Press Inc., Totowa, NJ

supported the finding that African Americans and whites differ in their willingness to participate in medical research. Racial differences in this willingness to participate are primarily due to the lower level of trust of medical research among African Americans, who believe they bear most of the risks (5).

A survey conducted at Rush University in Chicago showed that reasons for the lack of minority participation in clinical trials and factors influencing African American recruitment included lack of patient awareness of trials, patient mistrust of the medical community, too many additional administrative tasks associated with study participation and blinded drug/placebo arms (6).

We must continue to emphasize the need and reasons for clinical trial participation for all groups, but especially minorities. Participation in an Alzheimer's disease clinical trial may aid in early diagnosis and treatment. Why are early diagnosis and treatment important? Participation will give both the individual and their loved ones more time for adjustment and planning. The subject can participate in decision making, and some of the symptoms can also be treated (agitation, hallucinations, delusions, depression). Participation will give the caregiver and the patient insight into the question of when to consider dementia. It will alert them to warning signs, such as trouble learning and retaining new information, handling complex tasks, reasoning ability (what to do if your house is on fire), orientation to time and place, language, behavior, and changes in walking ability.

The medical/health care community contributes to knowledge, aids in diagnosis, and provides many free services at seminars, health screenings, as well as events with small co-pays. Just show up, listen, and learn. Attendance at these events is typically white, with few minorities present, due to language barriers and the feeling of being not part of the group .

The business community has begun to be involved in bettering their employees' health. Many companies sponsor health/benefit fairs, with employees encouraged to participate by awarding prizes. Get your memory checked! Have your eyes tested! Check your glucose and cholesterol! How's your blood pressure? What's your body mass index? These fairs are free of charge, fun, educational, and greatly contribute to the participants' basic medical knowledge. Since employees are racially/gender and ethnic-group diverse, these fairs can help to break down barriers. Employees see each other asking questions, getting tested, receiving information.

SUPPORT GROUPS ARE MAINLY ALL WHITE

Support groups do not retain minorities for four main reasons: language, knowledge of the disease, lack of education, and mistrust. Conversation in support groups is perceived as being all white. Minorities in these groups do not feel sufficiently at ease to participate in the conversational mix, thus depriving themselves of the offered support. Lack of knowledge of their disease contributes to minorities' lack of participation in support groups as well as in utilizing other resources. (This lack of disease knowledge is not limited to minorities.) Education must be encouraged to improve the overall quality of life. There is, as mentioned before, based on the Tuskegee experience, a general mistrust of medicine and especially of clinical trials. Statements such as "Who are you?" or "Who do you work for?" or "Why are you asking me this?" are frequently voiced by minorities as well as mentally impaired/demented individuals.

Internet use is up for all populations in the United States, but minority use still lags behind, based on cost and convenience (home use is easier than going to a library or finding an internet café, neither of which is frequently used by minorities yet).

Family and friends are the most important sources in determining what an individual does medically. Their opinions and medical knowledge are crucial. The family bases their decision on many factors, such as religious beliefs, cultural bias, access to health care, employment, and number of immediate family members (children, parents, grandparents, siblings).

The media play a crucial role in influencing people. We nowadays get a daily dose of medical news coverage with myriad facts on television, radio, movies, and in print, fed to us by responsible media. What we do with this input is crucial. Minorities do not believe the media as readily as whites, again based on the basic mistrust spawned by the Tuskegee legacy. In the past, radio, TV, movies, and the press have been guilty of reporting sensational facts, not based on medical knowledge, thus creating bad public relations (PR). Today, good PR is plentiful, and all racial/ethnic groups should partake of this free source of valuable information.

Religious affiliations historically have played an important role in everyday life of minorities, and should not be ignored. An effective means to convey knowledge and usefulness of clinical trials for example is a true and balanced presentation, even a mini-health fair.

HOW TO SUCCEED?

This question must be answered by all of us. No one person or group can do it alone. A multifront attack on education, community involvement, interpersonal relationships, and advocacy groups should be a priority. Education for the everyday citizen and medical community must be increased. Doctors and medical personnel need to learn of newer and successful treatments and use this knowledge, as well as interpersonal relationships, to encourage patients. Likewise, patients must be aware of these new advances, with the related pros and cons, inquire about them, and make an intelligent choice. The media must play a pivotal role in disseminating facts. All people must readily use this information for a common good. Advocacy groups, seen early in the war on AIDS, can be a very effective way of bringing problems to public awareness and not letting them slip below radar.

WHY PARTICIPATE IN AN AD CLINICAL TRIAL?

Alzheimer's disease (AD) does not know racial or ethnic or gender or socioeconomic status. It is an equal-opportunity disease. Participation in a clinical trial brings the latest breakthrough drugs to people years prior to being available commercially. All aspects of these trials are provided free of charge to study participants. Improving the overall quality of life for the individual, lengthening time until a skilled care or a nursing home is needed, are important goals. Delay to nursing home placement and improvement in the individual's quality of life saves precious dollars for families and government.

AD can be diagnosed and treated early. The illness causes dementia in up to 70% of elderly of all racial and ethnic groups. Early diagnosis and treatment leaves the patient and his or her family more time for adjustment and planning. The patient also can participate in the necessary decision making.

REFERENCES

1. Outreach Notebook for the NIH Guidelines on Inclusion of Women and Minorities as Subjects in Clinical Research. National Institutes of Health, Bethesda, MD, 1994.
2. Closing the Gap. A newsletter of the office of minority health. January 1998.
3. Welsh, J.L. et al.: Recruiting for a randomized controlled trial from an ethnically diverse population: lessons from the maternal and preterm labor study. J Fam Pract 2002; 51: 760.
4. Maxwell, C.: Speech to FLAETC. Posted on the Web by the Office of Special Health Issues, FDA. July 10, 1998.
5. Shavers, V.L.; Lynch, G.F.; Burmeister, L.F.: Racial differences in factors that influence the willingness to participate in medical research studies. Ann Epidemiol 2002; 12: 248–256.
6. Lynch, G.F. et al.: A pilot survey of African American physician perceptions about clinical trials. The Rush Neuroscience Institute, Rush University, Chicago, Illinois, USA. Natl Med Assoc 2001; 93 (12 suppl): 8S–13S.

44

Apathy in Alzheimer's Disease

Relationship to Executive Function

Susan McPherson

INTRODUCTION

Apathy is defined as a lack of motivation or initiation and is characterized by indifference, disengagement with passivity, and loss of enthusiasm, interest, empathy, and interpersonal involvement *(1)*. Patients with apathy exhibit a marked decrease in goal-directed behavior, and the primary clinical feature is a lack of motivation accompanied by indifference, low social engagement, poor persistence, and a lack of initiation. Apathy is a syndrome that is distinct from depression. The cardinal symptoms of depression are pervasive feelings of sadness or anhedonia, accompanied by sleep and appetite changes, feelings of hopelessness, and guilt and suicidal ideation. Furthermore, patients with apathy (with or without depression) exhibit greater deficits on measures of executive function than patients rated as dysphoric, providing additional evidence that the two disorders are distinct.

Apathy has been documented as a behavioral feature of numerous neurological disorders, including Alzheimer's disease (AD), cerebrovascular accidents, Parkinson's disease (PD), human immunodeficiency virus (HIV) encephalopathy, traumatic brain injury (TBI), and multiple sclerosis (MS). Apathy occurs in approximately 70% of cases of AD and is one of the most frequent behavioral changes *(2)*. Moreover, apathy has been linked to greater impairments in activities of daily living (ADL) and a greater degree of functional decline and is a distressing behavioral change for caregivers of patients with AD *(3,4)*.

This chapter focuses on the relationship between apathy and executive functions in AD. More specifically, this chapter will:

1. Discuss the anatomical substrates of apathy
2. Introduce the clinician to scales used to measure apathy
3. Review the relevant research conducted on apathy and executive functions
4. Discuss the impact of apathy on activities of daily living

ANATOMICAL SUBSTRATES OF APATHY

The areas of the brain most commonly implicated as a cause of apathy, when damaged, are the frontal lobes. Lesions to the anterior region of the medial frontal cortex result in profound indifference, docility, loss of motivation to engage in tasks, and lack of emotional response; lesions to the supracallosal area of the cingulate result in poor initiation of cognitive processes and an ensuing lack of cognitive initiative. Bilateral lesions to the basal ganglia, particularly the caudate, and lesions of the dorsomedial thalamic nucleus, also result in apathy.

Disruption of the anterior cingulate–subcortical circuit is associated with apathy in Alzheimer's disease and many other disorders. The anterior cingulate circuit originates in the cortex of the ante-

From: *Current Clinical Neurology,*
Alzheimer's Disease: A Physician's Guide to Practical Management
Edited by: R. W. Richter and B. Zoeller Richter © Humana Press Inc., Totowa, NJ

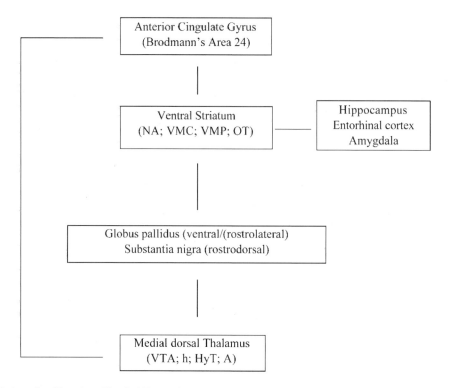

Fig. 1. Anterior Cingulate Circuit. NA, nucleus accumbens; VMC, ventromedial caudate; VMP, ventromedial putamen; OT, olfactory tubercle; VTA, ventral tegmental area; h, habenula; HyT, hypothalamus; A, amygdala.

rior cingulate gyrus (Brodmann's area 24) and projects to the ventral striatum, which is comprised of the nucleus accumbens (NA), olfactory tubercle (OT), and the ventromedial portions of the caudate (VMC) and putamen (VMP) *(5)* (Fig. 1). The ventral striatum receives projections from hippocampal, amygdala, and entorhinal cortices and sends projections to the ventral and rostrolateral globus pallidus and rostrodorsal substantia nigra. Specific regions of the medial dorsal nucleus of the thalamus, the ventral tegmental area (VTA), habenula (h), hypothalamus (HyT), and amygdala (A) receive efferents from the globus pallidus and substantia nigra. Projections from medial dorsal thalamic neurons back to the cingulate cortex complete the circuit. Evidence from imaging studies suggests that moderate to severe apathy is associated with reduced cerebral blood flow in the anterior temporal, orbitofrontal, anterior cingulate, and dorsolateral prefrontal regions.

APATHY RATING SCALES

Although apathy has been identified as one of the more common behaviors in AD, there are only a few scales designed to assess this condition. Principle scales are

1. Neuropsychiatric Inventory (NPI)
2. Apathy Evaluation Scale (AES)
3. Dementia Apathy Interview and Rating (DAIR)
4. Frontal Behavioral Inventory (FBI)

Neuropsychiatric Inventory (NPI)

The Neuropsychiatric Inventory *(6)* was developed specifically to assess psychopathology in dementia. The 10 behavioral domains evaluated by the NPI include delusions, hallucinations, agitation/aggression, dysphoria, anxiety, euphoria, apathy, disinhibition, irritability/lability, and aberrant motor behavior. Information is gathered from an informant who has daily contact with the patient and is familiar with the patient's behavior. The instrument utilizes screening questions that provide an overview of each behavioral domain, with a subset of questions that are asked only if the screen is endorsed as positive. The questions are scripted and determine if the patient's behavior has changed since the onset of disease and scores behaviors present in the past 1 month. Each of the ten behavioral features is rated by the informant for frequency and severity. The score for each domain is the product of the frequency multiplied by the severity.

The NPI has been used in numerous clinical trials to document behavioral changes in a wide variety of disorders. One of the advantages of the NPI is that it assesses depression separately from apathy, thereby allowing the clinician to differentiate between the two behavioral syndromes using just one scale. The NPI has demonstrated validity and reliability.

The Apathy subscale of the NPI consists of a screening question and eight subquestions consistent with behaviors observed in patients with apathy. Behaviors explored in the screening questions include loss of interest in the world, lack of motivation, and indifference. The subquestions focus on specific behaviors, such as lack of spontaneity and decline in usual activities, reduction in initiation of conversations, lack of emotions or reduction in affection, lack of interest in activities and plans of others, loss of interest in family and friends, loss of enthusiasm regarding usual activities, and other evidence that the patient does not care about participating in new behaviors.

Apathy Evaluation Scale (AES)

The Apathy Evaluation Scale (AES) *(7)* is an 18-item scale that has been extensively validated in the assessment of apathy. Clinician, informant, and self-rated versions of the scale have been developed, each consisting of the same 18 items. The apathy rating is based on assessment of the subject's thoughts, emotions, and activities during the previous four weeks. The scale can be subdivided into three different components of apathy: cognitive, behavioral, and emotional.

Emotional apathy is defined by items that reflect level of emotional excitement and intensity in approach to life. Behavioral apathy is defined as actual performance or engagement in a number of activities. Cognitive apathy refers to level of interest in a variety of tasks such as learning and having new experiences, self-initiation and completion of tasks, concern about one's own situation, and social interactions. Although no definitive cutoff score has been established, a score greater than 38 is indicative of apathy.

Patients are likely to minimize or underestimate the extent of their apathy, and it is recommended that a concomitant rating from either a caregiver or clinician might be obtained. The AES has been shown to discriminate among groups of subjects based on mean levels of apathy. Studying patients with AD, stroke, and major depression, Marin et al. found that AD patients and patients with right hemisphere stroke had high apathy but low depression scores, while patients with left hemisphere stroke or major depression had low apathy but high depression scores *(8)*. Apathy may be a manifestation of some depression syndromes, but the two symptoms can be distinguished.

Dementia Apathy Interview and Rating (DAIR)

The DAIR is a relatively new scale designed specifically to rate apathy in AD *(9)*. It is comprised of 16 items administered in a structured interview format and uses a 4-point scale to rate the frequency of occurrence of each behavior over the past month (e.g., indifference, spontaneity). Following the frequency rating, caregivers are asked if the behavior represents a change from behavior prior to memory loss. Total apathy score is calculated by summing all items reflecting change, divided by the number of items completed, with higher scores representing greater apathy. The scale has been found to be a valid and reliable instrument for the assessment of apathy in AD. Similar to the NPI, it focuses on determining if the onset of the behavior represents a change following the onset of the memory disorder.

One caveat of the DAIR is that it is a unidimensional scale and requires that an additional scale be administered in order to rate depression or other psychopathology.

Frontal Behavioral Inventory (FBI)

Developed specifically to identify the behavioral and personality changes associated with the onset of frontal lobe dementia (FLD), including apathy, the FBI is a 24-item informant-rated questionnaire that uses scripted questions in order to elicit responses from informants *(10)*. Scores are based on a scale of 0 to 3, with "0" as "never" and "3" as "severe or very frequent," thereby providing a quantitative measure for determining the severity of impairment and for assessing change and potential therapeutic effect. Individual questions pertaining to different components of apathy, such as amotivation, aspontaneity, indifference and inattention, are rated. The scale has been shown to differentiate AD from FLD. It has not been widely used, and studies of validity are in process.

Summary: There are four principal scales that assess apathy. Although the NPI, DAIR, and AES have been shown to be valid and reliable, the NPI is the only scale that is multidimensional and allows the concomitant assessment of apathy and dysphoria

EXECUTIVE FUNCTIONS: DEFINITION

Executive functions refer specifically to the ability to initiate, plan, sequence, and monitor behavior. Executive functions encompass those abilities that allow an individual to engage in independent, purposive, self-directed behavior as well as one's capacity for self-awareness. Executive functions require multiple self-motivated processes to organize a behavioral response and solve a complex problem. Such processes include the activation of remote memories, self-direction and independence from environmental contingencies, the ability to appropriately shift and maintain behavioral sets, the generation of motor programs, and the use of verbal skills to guide behavior *(11)*.

Measurement of executive function is predictive of functional status in higher activities of daily living, such as money management, safety, medication administration, and social functioning. Deficits in self-awareness translate into social consequences characterized by lack of empathy and social insight.

The terms *executive function* and *frontal abilities* are often used interchangeably. The frontal lobes are clearly involved in the successful performance of executive functions, but also are involved in executing a wide range of additional cognitive abilities, including selective and sustained attention, motor abilities, speech and language, verbal and nonverbal fluency, working memory, organization of information, temporal ordering, and spatial orientation. Some of these abilities represent combinations of executive and nonexecutive functions. In addition, nonfrontal areas of the frontal–subcortical circuits participate in the mediation of executive abilities.

The implications of deficits in executive functions in daily activities such as driving has recently been addressed. Daigneault et al. reported a positive correlation between the number of accidents documented for a group of nondemented elderly males with low levels of education and the number of errors on measures of response inhibition and the number of perseverative errors on a measure of set shifting *(12)*. These investigators also stated that individuals who had more accidents reported having reduced their speed as a compensatory mechanism, although Daigneault et al. cautioned that these self-reports were not corroborated by observational data. Reductions in cognitive flexibility, adaptation to environmental changes, and poor planning capacity may help explain the relationship found by these investigators between number of accidents and decreased executive function.

Summary: Executive functions are responsible for those abilities that allow an individual to engage in independent, purposive, self-directed behavior. Performances on tasks of executive function are predictive of functional status in higher activities of daily living such as money management, safety, medication administration, and social functioning

APATHY AND EXECUTIVE FUNCTIONS IN AD

The presence of apathy has been associated with greater deficits in executive function and, subsequently, greater functional impairment in activities of daily living. Patients with apathy perform more poorly on tasks of executive function than patients with depression, but no apathy. Cognitively, patients with apathy have been found to have significantly lower scores on tests of selective attention and response inhibition, cognitive flexibility and set shifting, sustained attention, and verbal fluency *(13–15)*. Apathy has been associated with deficits on tests of word-list learning, a task requiring initiation, motivation, and the ability to organize the information to be retained in a meaningful way. The relationship between apathy and poor executive function has been documented in patients with Huntington's disease, mild TBI, and PD, as well as AD.

A few studies have examined the relationship between apathy and executive frontal lobe dysfunction. Kuzis et al. studied the neuropsychological performance of four groups of subjects with AD *(13)*: (1) a control group of AD patients with neither depression nor apathy; (2) patients with AD and depression, (3) patients with AD and apathy, and (4) patients with AD with both depression and apathy.

Patients with apathy performed more poorly than AD patients without apathy on measures of verbal memory, confrontation naming, set shifting, and verbal fluency. Patients with both depression and apathy had significantly greater deficits only on a test of abstract reasoning. No significant differences were found for patients with AD and depression as compared with the control group of patients with AD without apathy or depression. The investigators concluded that apathy was associated with frontally mediated cognitive deficits. A correlation between apathy and number of errors on a measure requiring the ability to inhibit an automatic response has been found in studies of patients with PD, and in a study of HIV-positive males *(16,17)*.

Andersson and Bergedalen examined the relationship between apathy and cognitive functions in 53 patients with severe TBI *(18)*. The results revealed a significant negative correlation between performance on a measure of executive function and ratings from the clinician version of the AES. No association was found between global level of cognitive functioning and apathy rating. Factor analysis confirmed the relationship between performance on measures of executive function, psychomotor speed and acquisition, and memory and the cognitive apathy items of the AES, with the measure of executive function loading as the primary component. These results suggest that executive functions account for the majority of the variance of cognitive apathy.

A recent study revealed that AD patients with apathy performed more poorly on measures of selective attention and response inhibition, cognitive flexibility, and set shifting *(15)*. The relationship between apathy and executive dysfunction was not attributable to dysphoric mood changes. In addition, AD patients with apathy did not perform better or worse than those without apathy on tests of memory, visuo-spatial abilities, confrontation naming, or simple attention, suggesting that the results were not due solely to a reduction in level of global cognitive functioning ability.

Taken together, these data indicate that apathy is an independent dimension of behavior, not completely attributable to cognitive abnormalities. Conversely, executive abnormalities impair the processes of planning, implementing, assessing, and correcting behavior and may explain some portion of the elevated apathy subscale scores, especially those assessing cognitive apathy.

Another plausible explanation for the co-occurrence of apathy and executive dysfunction involves the overlapping but distinct anatomical circuitry mediating both behavior and cognition. Anterior cingulate lesions result in profound indifference, docility, and loss of motivation to engage in a task; lesions to the supracallosal area of the cingulate result in poor initiation of cognitive processes and an ensuing lack of cognitive motivation *(11,19)*; lesions of the dorsolateral frontal cortex impair executive functions. Thus, lesions affecting medial and lateral frontal cortex would affect both abilities.

Summary: Apathy is associated with poor performance on measures of executive function. Distinct anatomical circuitry mediates both apathy and executive functions.

IMPACT OF APATHY ON ACTIVITIES OF DAILY LIVING

Initiation, planning, and motivation play a substantial role in the ability to function independently. Patients with apathy have been found to be two to three times more impaired in basic activities of daily living (ADL) than patients without and require more support and management by caregivers. A study of elderly patients in Japan found that apathy was a powerful predictor of an elderly patient's ability to perform routine ADL *(20)*. Apathy, but not depression, was significantly correlated with greater functional impairment in ADL in AD patients *(21)*.

Ultimately, caregivers of patients with apathy report higher levels of caregiver burden, distress, and depression *(14)*. Early detection of apathy is important to determine which patients are likely to require a higher level of care and which caregivers a higher level of support.

SUMMARY

Apathy is a disorder distinct from depression and from cognitive impairment. The ability to distinguish apathy from depression has important implications in the treatment of AD patients, given that the two disorders respond to different interventions. Apathy is a common occurrence in AD and is associated with greater declines in executive functions and instrumental activities of daily living as well as higher levels of caregiver burden and distress. Early detection of apathy will allow clinicians to educate family members as to the behavioral consequences of the disease, possibly resulting in reduction of caregiver burden.

ACKNOWLEDGMENTS

This project was supported by the National Institute on Aging Alzheimer's Disease Research Center, Core grant (AG16570); an Alzheimer's Disease Research Center of California grant; and the Sidell-Kagan Foundation.

REFERENCES

1. Marin, R.S.: Differential diagnosis and classification of apathy. Am J Psychiatry 1990; 147: 22–30.
2. Mega, M.S. et al.: The spectrum of behavioral changes in Alzheimer's disease. Neurology 1996; 46: 130–135.
3. Gilley, D.W. et al.: Predictors of behavioral disturbance in Alzheimer's disease. Gerontology 1991; 46: 362–371.
4. Kaufer, D.I. et al.: Assessing the impact of neuropsychiatric symptoms in Alzheimer's disease: the Neuropsychiatric Inventory Caregiver Distress Scale. J Am Geriatr Soc 1998; 46: 210–215.
5. Cummings, J.L. Frontal-subcortical circuits and human behavior. Arch Neurol 1993; 50: 873–880.
6. Cummings, J.L. et al.: The Neuropsychiatric Inventory: comprehensive assessment of psychopathology in dementia. Neurology 1994; 44: 2308–2314.
7. Marin, R.S. et al.: Reliability and validity of the Apathy Evaluation Scale. Psychiatry Res 1991; 38: 143–162.
8. Marin, R.S. et al.: Group differences in the relationship between apathy and depression. J Nervous Mental Dis 1994; 182: 235–239.
9. Strauss, M.E.; Sperry, S.D.: An informant-based assessment of apathy in Alzheimer's disease. Neuropsych Neuropsychol Behav Neurol 2002; 15: 176–183.
10. Kertesz, A. et al.: Frontal Behavioral Inventory: diagnostic criteria for frontal lobe dementia. Can J Neurol Sci 1997; 24: 29–36.
11. Mega, M.S.; Cummings, J.L.: The cingulate and cingulate syndromes. In: M. R. Trimble, M.R.; Cummings, J.L. (eds.): Contemporary Behavioral Neurology. Butterworth-Heinemann, Boston, MA, 1997: 189–214.
12. Daigneault, G.: Executive functions in the evaluation of accident risk of older drivers. J Clin Exp Neuropsychol 2002; 24: 221–238.
13. Kuzis, G. et al.: Neuropsychological correlates of apathy and depression in patients with dementia. Neurology, 1999; 52: 1403–1407.

14. Landes, A.M. et al.: Apathy in Alzheimer's disease. J Am Geriatr Soc 2001; 49: 1700–1707.

15. McPherson, S. et al.: Apathy and executive function in Alzheimer's Disease. J Int Neuropsychol Soc 2002; 8: 373–381.

16. Aarsland, D. et al.: Range of neuropsychiatric disturbances in patients with Parkinson's disease. J Neurol Neurosurg Psychiatry 1999; 67: 492–496.

17. Castellon, S.A. et al.: Neuropsychiatric disturbance is associated with executive dysfunction in HIV-1 infection. J Int Neuropsychol Soc 2000; 6: 336–347.

18. Andersson, S.; Bergedalen, A.: Cognitive correlates of apathy in traumatic brain injury. Neuropsych Neuropsychol Behav Neurol 2002; 15: 184–191.

19. Laplane, D. et al.: Bilateral infarction of the anterior cingulate gyri and of the fornices. J Neurol Sci 1981; 51: 289–300.

20. Yamashita, K. et al.: Relationship among activities of daily living, apathy, and subjective well-being in elderly people living alone in a rural town. Gerontology 1999; 45: 279–282.

21. Tekin, S. et al.: Activities of daily living in Alzheimer's disease. Am J Geriatric Psych 2001; 9: 81–86.

45

Are Alzheimer's Patients Aware of Their Deficits?

Ben Seltzer

INTRODUCTION

It is a common clinical observation that, despite significant and often disabling cognitive dysfunction and impaired self-care abilities, patients with Alzheimer's disease (AD) frequently seem to be unaware of their deficits. In some individuals this is manifested simply by a tendency to minimize the significance of their symptoms, while at the opposite extreme, patients may positively deny the most flagrant of clinical deficits. In others, unawareness is apparent from a patient's actions, even if he or she verbally acknowledges the presence of the illness and its attendant symptoms. It is probable that—at least to some extent—virtually all individuals with established AD exhibit a deficiency in the metacognitive capacity to monitor their own physical and mental state.

This symptom has been given a number of different names. In classical neurology, anosognosia is used to describe patients who are unaware of focal neurological deficits, such as left-sided weakness or cortical blindness, but the same term is applicable to unawareness of cognitive deficits as the result of more widespread brain injury. Denial of illness is frequently used as an equivalent to anosognosia, although this term might carry the connotation of an active refusal to recognize the presence of deficits. Similarly, the alternative lack of insight might suggest a deficit in the capacity to understand the inner nature of events, an ability that is not highly developed in many individuals. Unawareness and lack of awareness are perhaps the most descriptive, and least theoretically charged, terms to describe the phenomenon under discussion.

Unawareness of deficit in AD is of interest for several reasons. First, it is of enormous practical significance. Patients with AD are often slow to recognize the development of symptoms and seek medical help. If early intervention proves beneficial in preventing, delaying, or significantly influencing the course of AD, patient unawareness will be a major obstacle to effective treatment. Even at the present time, unawareness frequently affects patient compliance with medication and other treatments. Patients who lack awareness of memory and other intellectual deficits often engage in activities that may cause physical or financial harm to themselves and others. Finally, unawareness of deficit is relevant to issues such as competence to vote, sign legal documents, and consent to participate in research. Awareness of deficit in AD is also of considerable theoretical interest. The study of this phenomenon affords an opportunity to examine the neural and psychological bases for conscious awareness. It may also contribute to an understanding of the biology of AD.

ASSESSMENT OF AWARENESS

A fundamental issue in studying unawareness of deficit in AD concerns how best to measure the symptom. Broadly speaking, three different approaches have been taken. The simplest is to question patients directly concerning their deficits, e.g., "Is there anything wrong with your memory?" "Are you able to drive a car safely?" Several scales have been developed to quantify the results obtained

From: *Current Clinical Neurology,*
Alzheimer's Disease: A Physician's Guide to Practical Management
Edited by: R. W. Richter and B. Zoeller Richter © Humana Press Inc., Totowa, NJ

by this method *(1–3)*. Although this approach is straightforward, it does not take into consideration the severity of an individual patient's symptoms. The questionnaire discrepancy (QD) technique corrects for this deficiency by examining differences between patient self-report and the report of an observer (typically a family caregiver) regarding patient abilities on questionnaires tapping symptoms commonly found in AD. Thus each patient's self-assessment is compared to an assessment of the same patient by a cognitively intact observer using the same instrument.

Although it is probably the most prevalent method of quantifying awareness used in research at the present time, the QD technique necessarily relies on the caregiver to provide the "gold standard" regarding patient functioning. Caregivers may, however, either over- or underestimate the abilities of their loved one. The QD technique is also restricted to examining patient self-awareness, not awareness of others, or global awareness.

The performance-prediction (PP) technique, in which participants (patients and caregivers) estimate their own performance and that of someone else on memory and other cognitive tasks, is a more complex methodology that does allow for such comparisons *(4–6)*. This method also permits the researcher to compare an individual's estimate of his or her own abilities against an objective measure of that function. Prior to being administered a standard neuropsychological instrument, the subjects, AD patients and their caregivers, are presented information on the scoring of the test and asked to predict both their own and the other person's performance. They are then (independently) administered the test, generating a score for each subject. Following actual testing, the subjects are asked to estimate ("post-dict") the actual score obtained by themselves and the other individual. A mathematical formula expresses the patient's accuracy in predicting and post-dicting his or her own performance and that of the caregiver compared to the caregiver's accuracy in predicting and post-dicting his or her own performance and that of the patient *(6)*. The equation also allows, for both patients and caregivers, a comparison between predicted, post-dicted, and actually obtained scores.

In addition to these three principal techniques, a variety of other methods, such as error detection, may also prove useful in measuring different facets of unawareness in AD *(7)*. Indeed, it is probable that the different methods of measurement tap different aspects of unawareness *(8)*.

It is also apparent from recent research that awareness in AD is not a unitary phenomenon. In reviewing the literature, it is important to distinguish between studies that focus on patient awareness of the dementing condition as a whole vs those that examine awareness in relation to specific domains of function, e.g., memory, mood, activities of daily living, social interaction, and emotional control, affected by the disease. Lack of awareness may vary depending on the domain assessed *(9–13)*. Another important distinction exists between the patient's awareness of his or her own deficits and the capacities of other individuals.

CLINICAL FINDINGS AND CORRELATIONS

Virtually all studies, regardless of methodology, show that AD patients, considered as a group, exhibit some degree of unawareness of their deficits Thus, Sevush and Starkstein et al., using awareness scales, demonstrated that AD patients do not show full awareness of their symptoms *(1,2)*. QD techniques consistently show that they tend to underestimate many of their deficits compared to the assessment of their caregivers *(9,10,12,13)*. The PP method also provides evidence that patients overestimate their own performance, while at the same time accurately estimating the intact abilities of their caregivers *(5,14)*. The latter finding suggests that lack of awareness in AD involves a particular problem with *self*-awareness rather than global unawareness. On the other hand, the patients' assessment of their relatives may simply be a default response, since in most instances the caregivers are in fact cognitively normal.

There would appear to be little question that, overall, and compared to controls and individuals with other neurological diseases, AD patients are unaware of the effects of their disease, but the actual prevalence of unawareness symptoms is disputed, with rates ranging from 20% to 80% of AD patients

(15–17). Such figures assume that anosognosia is a categorical symptom, with some patients aware and others unaware. More probably, lack of awareness is a continuous variable *(18)*. Many *(1,3,4,9,16,17,19–25)* but not all *(12,13,26–32)* studies demonstrate a positive correlation between unawareness and increasing severity of dementia as measured by stage of illness or by a cognitive test, such as the Mini-Mental State Examination (MMSE). The positive correlation between unawareness and duration of illness is weaker.

Does Every Patient With AD Demonstrate Anosognosia?

Given the association between unawareness and severity of dementia, one way to answer this question is to look at patients with very early AD or those with mild cognitive impairment (MCI). Deroussene et al. found that most patients with mild AD acknowledged their cognitive deficits but failed to recognize the impact of these symptoms on everyday life *(18)*. In a recent study of MCI, using an exceptionally comprehensive instrument to assess functioning, Taber et al. showed that those subjects who progressed to AD were less aware of their (comparatively minor) deficits than those who remained stable *(33)*. Thus subtle impairment in awareness seems to characterize AD from the start.

Lack of awareness has also been studied in relation to the emotional symptoms of AD, especially depression. The results are contradictory. While some authors find no significant association between awareness and depression *(12,23,27)*, others report a positive correlation *(17,19,20–22,26,34)*. That is, patients, who are relatively aware of their deficits are more likely to have depressive symptoms than those who are unaware. This has led to the common-sense conclusion that depression in AD is a psychological reaction to the perception of loss of cognitive and other abilities. While this explanation might be true in selected patients, the data do not prove a causal relationship. Other factors might explain the association. Furthermore, AD patients, who are relatively aware do not invariably have depressive symptoms, while depression can occur in patients who are unaware of their deficits. There are undoubtedly multiple reasons why AD patients become depressed.

EXPLANATIONS FOR UNAWARENESS

Because of the association between degree of unawareness and extent of cognitive deficit, investigators have sought to relate lack of awareness in AD to impairment in specific cognitive domains. The most obvious is memory. Indeed, one explanation for unawareness in AD is that patients forget their condition and its symptoms. It is unlikely, however, that memory impairment by itself can account for anosognosia in AD and other neurological conditions. Patients with dense amnesia resulting from focal cortical disease, e.g., bilateral involvement of the medial temporal lobe, often remain intensely aware of their memory deficit *(35)*. Patients with right hemisphere disease who are unaware of left-sided body weakness do not necessarily have significant amnestic symptoms. Nevertheless, memory impairment may contribute at least to some extent to the unawareness shown by AD patients.

For example, using the PP methodology, Duke et al. recently showed that, for a brief period of time immediately following the administration of a verbal learning test, AD patients corrected their overoptimistic prediction of their performance *(8)*. After a 20-minute delay, however, they reverted to underestimating the degree of their impairment. As discussed below, it is probable that anosognosia in AD is a heterogeneous phenomenon, resulting from the disruption of multiple cognitive processes, of which memory is but one domain.

Because anosognosia has been repeatedly described in relation to disease of the right parietal lobe, some investigators have suggested that unawareness in AD seems to be correlated with the degree of right parietal lobe dysfunction occurring in the disease. This has been examined using both neuropsychological and cerebral blood flow measures of focal cerebral dysfunction *(28,36)*. A more prevalent view relates unawareness in AD to frontal lobe involvement. The rationale for this theory is that unawareness is frequently observed in patients with frontal lobe disease *(37)*. Studies seeking to correlate anosognosia in AD with neuropsychological and neuroimaging evidence of frontal disease lend some support to this hypothesis *(2,15,38)*.

Motivated Denial?

The oldest theory to explain unawareness in AD attributes the symptom to motivated denial *(39,40)*. Since most studies show an association between impaired awareness and greater cognitive impairment, it seems unlikely that patients with severe brain impairment would be more capable of initiating an active coping strategy than individuals with less severe cerebral involvement. At the present time, most investigators attribute unawareness in AD to cerebral disease.

Recognizing the heterogeneity of the phenomenon and the multiple cortical areas implicated, it has been proposed that a distributed (frontal *and* parietal) cortical conscious awareness system, interacting with other neurocognitive functions, especially memory, forms the neural basis for the phenomenon of awareness *(37,41)*. Because AD pathology involves precisely these cortical areas in different patterns, patients might be predicted to exhibit various types of anosognosic symptoms.

The practical consequences of unawareness in AD, though intuitively obvious, have been little studied. As might be predicted, AD patients who are unaware of their deficits are less likely to impose driving restrictions on themselves than those who are comparatively more aware *(42)*. Patient unawareness contributes significantly to the distress experienced by AD family caregivers but, at the same time, results in a higher level of life satisfaction for the patients themselves *(24,43)*.

SUMMARY

Anosognosia is an important, and probably invariable, finding in AD. Future research is needed to examine the clinical implications of patient unawareness. Practical methods are needed to deal with this serious safety issue and obstacle to effective treatment. At the same time, future research in awareness has the potential of expanding our understanding of the basic mechanisms of cognitive functioning.

REFERENCES

1. Sevush, S.: Relationship between denial of memory deficit and dementia severity in Alzheimer disease. Neuropsych Neuropsychol Behav Neurol 1999; 12: 88–94.
2. Starkstein, S.E. et al.: Neuropsychological deficits in patients with agnosia. Neuropsych Neuropsychol Behav Neurol 1993; 6: 43–48.
3. Zanetti, O. et al: Insight in dementia: when does it occur? Evidence for a nonlinear relationship between insight and cognitive status. J Gerontol B Psychol Sci Soc Sci 1999; 54: P100–P106.
4. McGlynn, S.M.; Kaszniak, A.W: Unawareness of deficits in dementia and schizophrenia. In: Prigatano, G.P.; Schacter, D.L. (eds.): Awareness of deficit after brain injury: Clinical and theoretical issues. Grune & Stratton, New York, 1991: 77–121.
5. McGlynn, S.M.; Kaszniak, A.W.: When metacognition fails: impaired awareness of deficit in Alzheimer's disease. J Cogn Neurosci 1991; 3: 183–189.
6. Trosset, M.W.; Kaszniak, A.W: Measures of deficit unawareness for predicted performance experiments. J Int Neuropsychol Soc 1996; 2: 315–322.
7. Giovanetti, T.; Libon, D.J.; Hart, T: Awareness of naturalistic action errors in dementia. J Int Neuropsychol Soc 2002; 8: 633–644.
8. Duke, L.M. et al: Cognitive components of deficit awareness in Alzheimer's disease. Neuropsychology 2002; 16: 359–369.
9. Vasterling, J.J. et al: Unawareness of deficit in Alzheimer's disease: domain-specific differences and disease correlates. Neuropsychiatry Neurosychol Behav Neurol 1995; 8: 26–32.
10. Vasterling, J.J. et al: Unawareness of social interaction and emotional control deficits in Alzheimer's disease. Aging Neuropsych Cogn 1997; 4: 280–289.
11. Starkstein, S.E. et al: Two domains of anosognosia in Alzheimer's disease. J Neurol Neurosurg Psychiatry 1996; 61: 485–490.
12. DeBettignies B.H.; Mahurin, R.A.; Pirozzolo, F.J: Insight for impairment in independent living skills in Alzheimer's disease and multi-infarct dementia. J Clin Exp Neuropsych 1990; 12: 355–363.
13. Green, J. et al: Variable awareness of deficits in Alzheimer's disease. Neuropsychiatry Neuropsychol Behav Neurol 1993; 6: 159–165.

14. Kaszniak, A.W.; Zak, M.G: On the neuropsychology of metamemory: contributions from the study of amnesia and dementia. Learning Individual Diff 1996; 8: 355–381.

15. Seltzer, B. et al: Clinical and neuropsychological correlates of impaired awareness of deficits in Alzheimer's disease and Parkinson's disease. Neuropsych Neuropsychol Behav Neurol 2001; 14: 122–129.

16. Migliorelli, R. et al: Anosognosia in Alzheimer's disease: a study of associated factors. J Neuropsychiatry Clin Neuroscis 1995; 7: 338–344.

17. Sevush, S.; Leve, N: Denial of memory deficit in Alzheimer's disease. Am J Psychiatry 1993; 150: 748–751.

18. Derousesne C. et al: Decreased awareness of cognitive deficits in patients with mild dementia of the Alzheimer type. Int J Geriat Psychiatry 1999; 14: 1019–1030.

19. Feher, E.P. et al: Anosognosia in Alzheimer's disease. Neuropsychiatry Neuropsychol Behav Neurol 1991; 4: 136–146.

20. Mangone, C.A. et al: Impaired insight in Alzheimer's disease. J Geriatr Psychiatry Neurol 1991; 4: 189–193.

21. Seltzer, B. et al: Unawareness of memory deficit in Alzheimer's disease: relation to mood and other disease variables. Neuropsych Neuropsychol Behav Neurol 1995; 8: 176–181.

22. Seltzer, B.; Vasterling, J.J.; Buswell, A.: Awareness of deficit in Alzheimer's disease: association with psychiatric symptoms and other disease variables. J Clin Geropsychol 1995; 1: 79–87.

23. Lopez, O.L. et al: Awareness of cognitive deficits and anosognosia in Alzheimer's disease. Eur Neurol 1994; 34: 277–282.

24. Seltzer, B. et al: Awareness of deficit in Alzheimer's disease: relation to caregiver burden. Gerontologist 1997; 37: 20–24.

25. McDaniel, K.D. et al: Relationship between level of insight and severity of dementia in Alzheimer disease. Alzheimer Dis Assoc Disord 1995; 9:101–104.

26. Feher, E.P. et al: Memory self-report in Alzheimer's disease and in age-associated memory impairment. J Geriatr Psychiatry Neurol 1994; 7: 58–65.

27. Reed, B.R.; Jagust, W.J.; Coulter, L: Anosognosia in Alzheimer's disease: relationship to depression, cognitive function, and cerebral perfusion. J Clin Exp Neuropsychol 1993; 15: 231–244.

28. Auchus, A.P. et al: Unawareness of cognitive impairments in Alzheimer's disease. Neuropsych Neuropsychol Behav Neurol 1994; 7: 25–29.

29. Kotler-Cope, S.; Camp, C.J: Anosognosia in Alzheimer's disease. Alzheimer Dis Rel Disord 1995; 9: 52–56.

30. Correa, D.D.; Graves, R.E.; Costa, L: Awareness of deficit in Alzheimer's patients and memory-impaired older adults. Aging Neuropsychol Cogn 1996; 3: 215–228.

31. Almeida, O.P.; Crocco, E.I: Percepcao dos deficits cognitivos e alteracoes do comportamento em pacientes com doença de Alzheimer. Arquiv Neuro-Psiquiatria 2000; 58: 292–299.

32. Smith, C. et al: Anosognosia and Alzheimer's disease: the role of depressive symptoms in mediating impaired insight. J Clin Exp Neuropsychol 2000; 22: 437–444.

33. Taber M.H. et al: Functional deficits in patients with mild cognitive impairment: prediction of Alzheimer's disease. Neurology 2002; 58 758–764

34. Harwood, D.G.; Sultzer, D.L.; Wheatley, M.V: Impaired insight in Alzheimer's disease: association with cognitive deficits, psychiatric symptoms, and behavioral disturbances. Neuropsych Neuropsychol Behav Neurol 2000; 13: 82–88.

35. Schacter, D.L: Unawareness of deficit and unawareness of knowledge in patients with memory disorders. In: Prigatano, G.P.; Schacter, D.L. (eds.): Awareness of deficit after brain injury: clinical and theoretical issues. Grune & Stratton, New York, 1991: 127–151.

36. Ott, B.R.; Noto, R.B.; Fogel, B.S: Apathy and loss of insight in Alzheimer's disease: a SPECT imaging study. J Neuropsychiatry Clin Neurosci 1996; 8: 41–46.

37. Schacter, D.L: Toward a cognitive neuropsychology of awareness: implicit knowledge and anosognosia. J Clin Exp Neuropsychol 1990; 12: 155–178.

38. Michon, A. et al: Relation of anosognosia to frontal lobe dysfunction in Alzheimer's disease. J Neurol Neurosurg Psychiatry 1994; 57: 805–809.

39. Weinstein, E.A.; Friedland, R.P.; Wagner, E.E: Denial/unawareness of impairment and symbolic behavior in Alzheimer's disease. Neuropsychiatry Neuropsychol Behav Neurol 1994; 3: 176–184.

40. Reisberg, B. et al: Clinical symptoms accompanying progressive cognitive decline and Alzheimer's disease: relationship to denial and ability to give informed consent. In: Melnick, V.L.; Dubler, N.H. (eds.): Alzheimer's dementia, Humana Press, Totowa, NJ, 1985: 19–39.

41. Agnew, S.K.; Morris, R.G: The heterogeneity of anosognosia for memory impairment in Alzheimer's disease: a review of the literature and a proposed model. Aging Mental Health 1998; 2: 7–19.

42. Cotrell, V.; Wild, K: Longitudinal study of self-imposed driving restrictions and deficit awareness in patients with Alzheimer's disease. Alzheimer Dis Assoc Disord 1999; 13: 151–156.

43. Phinney, A.; Stewart, A.; Brod, M.: The effects of symptom awareness on dementia patients report of life satisfaction. Gerontological Society of America, Cincinnati, OH, November 1997.

XI | Family and Care Issues

46

Diagnostic Family Conference in AD

Issues and Recommendations

Paul Michael Ramirez, David Castro-Blanco, and Michelle Kehn

INTRODUCTION

The Alzheimer's Association reports that more than 70% of people with Alzheimer's disease (AD) live at home, and that almost 75% of the home care is provided by family and friends. The remainder is paid part-time care costing an average of $12,500 per year. Families pay almost all of that out of pocket. It is not uncommon for patients with dementia to live for 10–15 years or longer following onset *(1)*. For these reasons, a consensus statement of the American Association for Geriatric Psychiatry, the Alzheimer's Association, and the American Geriatrics Society states that family intervention is critical, particularly in the assessment and diagnostic process *(2)*. Recent studies agree, stressing that family caregivers need to be educated about the diagnosis and course of AD, receive counseling for emotional difficulties, be trained in behavior management, taught to implement medication and treatment schedules, and directed to outside services and means of support *(3,4)*. However, results from one study of how well clinicians are following dementia practice outlines has found that only about half of the clinicians studied actually provide caregiver support for the majority of their patients *(5)*. This chapter discusses issues regarding informing patients and their families of a diagnosis of dementia and provides recommendations that may be useful in helping them cope with this diagnosis.

THE NEED TO KNOW: SHARING THE NEWS IN THE DIAGNOSTIC FAMILY CONFERENCE

Many studies have been conducted in order to determine whether the advantages of informing patients of their diagnosis outweigh the disadvantages, particularly in cases of dementia. One survey of adults waiting to see their physician found that over 90% of those completing the survey would want to be told about their diagnosis of dementia. They went on to report that it would make them feel angry and deceived not to be told by their physician. Obviously, such an omission could very well be expected to adversely affect the therapeutic doctor–patient alliance. Some of the most frequently cited reasons patients wanted to be told of such a diagnosis included making plans for future care, obtaining a second opinion, and resolving family matters *(6)*.

In attempting to determine the advantages and disadvantages of receiving a diagnosis of Alzheimer's disease, investigators asked spouse caregivers to rate, in order of importance, their concerns about receiving their spouse's diagnosis *(3)*. The items rated most important by a large majority of the surveyed spouses included:

From: *Current Clinical Neurology,*
Alzheimer's Disease: A Physician's Guide to Practical Management
Edited by: R. W. Richter and B. Zoeller Richter © Humana Press Inc., Totowa, NJ

1. Knowing what was wrong with their spouse
2. Ruling out other causes of problems
3. Obtaining information about dementia
4. Appropriate treatment planning for the future
5. Knowing about the possibility of a hereditary condition
6. Involving the spouse in important decisions
7. Using appropriate community resources.

The most commonly cited disadvantages included the amount of time the diagnostic process takes, the expense of the process, and the minimal number of local physicians trained in diagnosing dementia.

Several impediments to obtaining a diagnosis were discussed, including finding a physician with expertise in dementia, diagnostic and assessment procedures, the manner in which the diagnosis was disclosed to the patient and family, the perceived consequences of obtaining a diagnosis, and benefits of obtaining a diagnosis. Common problems with diagnosis and assessment include the financial cost of the process, the amount of time it takes to see a doctor and to actually receive a diagnosis, and doctors leaving the family out of the process. The most common problem spouses reported regarding the manner in which patient and family were informed of the diagnosis was that the doctor was unsympathetic, uncaring, or unfeeling toward both the patient and family.

EMPATHY INSTEAD OF BLUNTED SENSITIVITY

Clinicians who deal with dementing conditions on a regular basis may become somewhat desensitized to the impact of such a diagnosis. While one may share the detection of dementia with family members several times or more per week, it is important to appreciate that each family is hearing it for the first time and probably has a sense of the progressive deterioration of this disorder. Prospective taking in psychology involves the process in which we strive to understand a situation from the perspective of others. Clinicians should strive to understand just how devastating a diagnosis of dementia invariably is for a loved one.

In a film called *The Doctor*, actor William Hurt portrayed a very ambitious and successful physician who did not have time to empathize with his patients and was totally focused on treating the illness and not the person. When he developed a growth very near his vocal cords, this physician naturally wanted the very best surgeon to treat him. Unfortunately, the best available surgeon was a woman who was very much the doctor that William Hurt had been. She gave him very little information and even less time, reminding him that he was now just a patient and should blindly follow her orders. Eventually, William Hurt became so enraged at her behavior that he stormed into her office and demanded his records. He then sought out a mild-mannered surgeon who, while a good surgeon, was a very caring individual, who listened carefully to his patients and answered their questions. These had been the qualities that had made William Hurt tease and even dislike the surgeon that he now was eager to entrust with his vocal cords.

True, that is Hollywood drama, but the message is nevertheless worthy of our attention. Patients and their families hear this diagnosis of dementia, often after having been in denial and having made excuses for the gradual deterioration that they have been witnessing in their loved one, and it is devastating.

THE DELIVERY OF THE DIAGNOSIS SETS THE STAGE
FOR THE ENTIRE COURSE

The delivery of the diagnosis essentially sets the stage for the entire course of the disease. It is from this diagnosis that the caregiver(s) will form expectations about the nature and progress of the illness. These expectations will profoundly influence the lives of the patient and caregiver alike, affecting basic assumptions and decisions about the patient's illness, care, and the prospect of hope. The doctor is finally confirming what they have suspected and feared for some time. It is difficult to hear and more difficult still to process. In fact, it is often a good practice to arrange for the patient and family to meet with other professionals for follow-up, as the information provided by the diagnosing physician may fall upon deaf ears in the wake of the shock.

As is true of many medical conditions, information can be helpful on several levels. Specifically, information can help with patient treatment compliance during the initial stages of the disorder, families can be enlisted as treatment allies and informants, and family members can benefit tremendously from support groups. A referral to a geriatric counselor, often a specialist social worker, can help the family with resources available to them in the form of entitlements and can help them with the inevitable decision making that is an unpleasant but unavoidable by-product of this disorder.

IT IS ESSENTIAL TO INCLUDE THE FAMILY

There is general agreement in the field that it is essential to include families in the diagnostic and assessment process when a patient is suspected of having a dementing illness such as AD. In one study, active and former family caregivers of patients with AD were surveyed in order to determine the information and services necessary at the time of diagnosis. It was reported that both *(4)* active and former caregivers agreed that information about AD, referral resources, caregiver training workshops, and general information about dementia were essential. Caregivers also specified in-home respite care as an important service that was not currently available to them. Many former caregivers rated training as an important service that was not available to them but would have been extremely helpful.

The results of this study emphasize the importance of education and training in providing care for patients with dementia following the diagnosis. Although physicians, for many pragmatic reasons, are usually not in the position to provide such training, referral to allied professionals who can work with the families should be included as part of any diagnostic informing session. At a minimum, information regarding dementia, listing of relevant support groups, and appropriate referrals should be provided by the physician making the diagnosis.

NO FALSE HOPES; ENCOURAGEMENT SHOULD BE PROVIDED

One of the difficult issues the informing physician faces involves questions regarding the prognosis. Although it is difficult to share a bleak prognosis and to answer questions about the course of this disorder, this is part of the responsibilities of the physician and should not be avoided. As their medical counselor, the physician is in a unique position to guide the family through the pain of an initial diagnosis and into a problem-solving mode that will be of maximum benefit to the patient. The physician needs to remind the patient and the family that, while AD is a progressive disorder, they should strive to enjoy the time they have together. There may be several years or more of relative mental clarity, and there are medications available that may, for a while, help improve the quality of life for both the patient and the family. This may seem merely a cliché, but there are clinical trials presently underway to determine the efficacy of new antidementia compounds, and the family should not give up all hope. One must, of course, guard against implanting false expectations, but there is nothing wrong with providing a little hope that the patient's quality of life will be preserved for as long as possible.

USEFUL INTERVENTIONS

Several models have been developed that describe interventions useful in the assessment and diagnostic process of patients with AD and other dementias. These interventions tend to be most beneficial if family members are involved as soon as the diagnosis is suspected. A model has been proposed that utilizes a collaborative treatment team consisting of nurses, physicians, social workers, psychiatrists, and psychologists *(7)*. They discuss the importance of being able to relate to the family and to work with their preexistent coping styles, as well as being nonjudgmental, empathetic, and knowl-edgeable about dementia.

Similar interventions for clinicians have been proposed within a more structured paradigm (8). This structural model has been empirically validated and is effective in both reducing strain on the family caregiver and avoiding inappropriate nursing home placements, thus being a cost-effective solution. Using this model, the assessment process includes a collaborative effort between physician and family in order to validate the diagnosis. The clinician also assesses the family's understanding of the disease, while identifying those presenting problems that are perceived as major stressors for the caregiver and/or family.

At this time, the clinician can also explore the family's extended network, any formal services the family may have already tried that have or have not been useful, and the level of emotional distress that the caregiver is currently experiencing.

This model also stresses the importance of being nonjudgmental and allowing the patient and family to make decisions based on their preexisting value system. Thus, the clinician should take the wishes of the patient and the family into consideration when making recommendations.

As an example, if the patient wishes to return to independent living, this may be an immediate goal (if he is able), despite the clinician knowing that in 3–6 months, the patient may no longer be able to care for himself. We, as clinicians, must appreciate the fear that the inevitable loss of control over one's life engenders in patients. For someone who may have been a very independent person, such loss can be overwhelming. While the loss is inevitable, clinicians should strive to preserve a patient's independence for as long as possible (9).

This more structured model features three primary intervention modalities: counseling the caregiver, family meetings, and support groups. These different venues are used to share information, help both the family and patient with problem solving, and provide support (8). Counseling involves providing the caregiver/family and patient with information about AD, treatment and care possibilities, and prognosis. Issues concerning the patient's safety and security, especially driving, should also be discussed (10). Given that driving is often equated with independence, particularly in areas offering minimal public transportation, the clinician will likely meet any suggestion to stop driving with significant resistance. In cases where the patient should clearly give up driving a vehicle, the family's help may be enlisted.

STRESS THE PROBLEM OF THE PATIENT'S BEHAVIOR

It is also important that the clinician be prepared with appropriate books, pamphlets, and referrals, so that all the family's needs are met. Other essential information to convey at this time includes talking about the patient's behavior in terms of the disease. It is often difficult for families to understand that the patient's actions and words are the result of the disease and not intentional. Along the same lines, it is important for the family to gain an understanding of the types of behaviors they should expect to encounter, as well as the types of interventions that might help or frustrate the situation. For example, families should be taught that confrontation is not an appropriate solution in dealing with a patient who is unaware of his or her deficits, while reinforcement might help shape behavior (11).

Psychologist Albert Ellis has developed a model of behavioral psychotherapy in which problem behaviors are conceptualized with the mnemonic A–B–C, in which A = Activating event, or precipitant, B = Behavioral response, and C = Consequences of the behavior. Using this framework, clinicians can help caregiver families to recognize and better understand the occasionally erratic behavior of their loved ones. Knowing that behavioral consultation can aid the family is an important part of the clinician's treatment and referral planning. Providing family support is also essential. Support can be obtained through the clinician within a therapeutic setting, through friends and other relatives, or in support groups (8).

Individual Counseling

An innovative structural intervention model identifies three primary dimensions, the first of which is one-on-one or individual counseling of the caregiver. The goal of this modality is to discuss ways in which the situation can be changed and/or handled to make it less stressful for the caregiver. Individual counseling is particularly important in that it provides the caregiver with a safe place in which to examine feelings and attempt to generate possible solutions to problems.

Family Meetings

Family meetings are also important in that they allow the primary caregiver a chance to address situations in which it would be most helpful to have the support of other family members, as well as to discuss issues that may be causing additional conflict in the family. It is important that the clinician takes some time with the caregiver before a family meeting in order to gain a clear understanding of the family's dynamic.

Support Groups

Finally, support groups can help to validate the feelings and frustrations of the caregiver among those with similar experiences and can provide an opportunity to learn about other channels of help available to them *(8)*.

CAUTIOUS PRESCRIPTION OF BEHAVIORAL MEDICATIONS

Physicians also treat cognitive as well as emotional dementia-related problems using cognitive-enhancing and behavioral medications for agitation and depression *(11)*. The nonspecialist physician prescribing such medication must take a complete psychiatric and medical history, including medications that the patient is currently taking as well as nonprescribed herbal remedies. Drug–drug interaction effects must be carefully considered in choosing psychotropic medication for elderly patients. The physician must also consider certain age-related issues surrounding the patient's biological processes, which are likely to affect the pharmacodynamics and pharmacokinetics of prescribed medications.

Given that the patient with dementia may not be able to give a complete or accurate history, it is important for the physician to include the caregiver and/or family members as informants. Caregivers can also be a valuable asset to the physician in determining whether a medication is actually alleviating symptoms, since the caregivers spend the most time with the patient and are able to keep track of behaviors and symptoms *(11)*.

PROVIDE GOOD INFORMATION AND BE AVAILABLE

Regardless of how far the disease has progressed when a patient is brought in for an evaluation, it is critical that clinicians and/or treatment teams follow a model in the diagnosis and assessment process to ensure that the patient's and caregiver's needs are met. The first and most basic need of the patient and family is that of obtaining information. Clinicians should be sensitive to the fact that families are often overwhelmed by the initial diagnosis and are likely not to retain all of the information provided by the physician. Thus, the clinician should be prepared with a list of informative books as well as pamphlets and other community resources, such as the phone number and Web address of their local chapter of the Alzheimer's Association.

It is also important that the clinician remain available to the patient and family throughout treatment, whether for emotional support or to provide necessary referrals. The clinician must also be prepared to maintain close and frequent contact with the family in order to ensure that the treatment plan is being followed appropriately, and to provide crisis intervention and referral as needed.

CONCLUSIONS

An important aspect of assessing and diagnosing patients suspected of having AD that is too often overlooked is the inclusion of the family and/or primary caregiver. Though it is sometimes difficult not to include the family because they often bring the patient in to be checked, many clinicians overlook the significance of the information they can elicit from family members. Throughout the assessment and diagnostic process, the clinician must be sensitive to and aware of the patient's and family's feelings surrounding this difficult process. Physicians, however, cannot do it all. Other professionals, including neuropsychologists, geriatric psychologists, social workers, and geriatric counselors, must be incorporated within a treatment team approach to be successful in helping caregivers provide loving care to the patient. In this progressively incapacitating and incurable disease process, family members are all too often unrecognized victims as well.

REFERENCES

1. Aneshensel, C.S. et al.: Profiles in caregiving: The unexpected career. Academic Press, San Diego, CA, 1995.
2. Small, G.W. et al.: Diagnosis and treatment of Alzheimer disease and related disorders: consensus statement of the American Association for Geriatric Psychiatry, the Alzheimer's Association, and the American Geriatrics Society. JAMA 1997; 278: 1363–1371.
3. Connell, C.M.; Gallant, M.P.: Spouse caregivers' attitudes toward obtaining a diagnosis of a dementing illness. J Am Geriatric Soc 1996; 44: 1003–1009.
4. Fortinsky, R.H.; Hathaway, T.J.: Information and service needs among active and former family caregivers of persons with Alzheimer's disease. Gerontologist 1990; 30: 604–609.
5. Rosen, C.S. et al.: How well are clinicians following dementia practice guidelines? Alzheimer Dis Ass Disord 2002; 16: 15–23.
6. Erde, E.I.; Nadal, E.C.; Scholl, T.O.: On truth telling and the diagnosis of Alzheimer's disease. J Family Pract 1988; 26: 401–406.
7. Keizer, J.; Feins, L.C.: Intervention strategies to use in counseling families of demented patients. J Gerontol Social Work 1991; 17: 201–216.
8. Zarit, S.H.; Zarit, J.M.: Mental disorders in older adults: fundamentals of assessment and treatment. Guilford Press, New York, NY, 1998.
9. Moskowitz, B.A.: "Do I know you?"' Living through the end of a parent's life. Kodansha International, New York, NY, 1998.
10. Larson, E.B.: An 80-year-old man with memory loss. JAMA 2000; 283: 1046–1053.
11. Weiner, M.F. (ed.): The dementias: diagnosis, management, and research. (2nd ed.). American Psychiatric Press, Washington, D.C., 1996: 233–249.

47

Care, Caregiver Issues, and Communication With the Demented Patient

Ralph W. Richter and Brigitte Zoeller Richter

INTRODUCTION

Patients with Alzheimer's disease (AD) will usually require long-term care. Initially, this care is provided mainly by relatives, especially by spouses, daughters, daughters-in-law, sons, close friends, and sometimes even supportive neighbors. As the disease worsens, AD patients require much more care, in many instances up to 24 hours a day. As many as 90% of dementia patients become institutionalized before death *(1)*. This is partly because of the progressive cognitive decline ending in severe impairment, that characterizes the degenerative disease. The main reason is the fact that the frequently occurring behavioral problems as well as the extensive nursing care requirements in the later stages of AD can no longer be managed by the caregiver at home.

ASSESSMENT OF THE CAREGIVER

Persons who serve as caregiver for an AD patient are very likely to be also well known by the family physician. Family physicians should systematically assess/reassess the degree of the caregiver burden. Because caregivers are at high risk for developing depression and other mood disorders, the family physician should regularly query the caregiver to exclude the development or presence of these disorders. The family physician and his or her staff can also assess the caregiver's skills in managing the AD patient and provide practical counseling about resources that could benefit the caregiver. Helping the caregiver learn coping strategies may reduce at least some of the stress that is associated with the long-term care of an AD patient *(2)*.

Maintaining the well-being and stability of the caregiver will strengthen his or her relationship with the patient. Life satisfaction and self-esteem of the caregiver can be considered as indicators for a better potential outcome of caregiving, as can the caregiver's subjective perception of the stability of the caregiving situation *(3)*. The results of a discriminative analysis conducted in Germany revealed the degree of cognitive impairment of the patient as a decisive parameter for the self-esteem of the caregiver. The more severe the patient's impairment was, the higher the caregiver's self-esteem was rated *(3)*.

The emotional burden for a caregiver is deeply influenced by the quality of the relationship with the patient. Caring for a spouse or parent with dementia involves loss and inevitable grieving during the course of the disease. The level of affection and the satisfaction with the relationship before the illness—the marriage, for example—appears to be inversely related to symptoms of grief *(4)*. The emotional distress a caregiver experiences thus includes reactions to the losses and deficits encountered long before the illness has created a dependent relationship of a completely different nature.

Social isolation will develop within a long period of caring for a family member with AD. Family life may also become disrupted. The perception of children within a family setting must also be con-

From: *Current Clinical Neurology,*
Alzheimer's Disease: A Physician's Guide to Practical Management
Edited by: R. W. Richter and B. Zoeller Richter © Humana Press Inc., Totowa, NJ

Table 1
Difficulties in Health Maintenance

Eating problems
Lack of physical exercise
Poor or neglected personal hygiene (grooming, dressing)
Insufficient dental hygiene
Incontinence

sidered. Young children are especially vulnerable because they lack understanding and are thus not able to cope with this disease. Here it becomes necessary to discuss honestly with them the nature and the progression of the disease *(5)*. Children generally are open to shared experiences between generations and may thus show greater understanding and natural empathy in dealing with patients than many grown-ups.

NURSING HOME PLACEMENT—A TOUGH DECISION TO BE MADE BY THE FAMILY

The decision to place a patient in a nursing home is complex. It depends partly on the sociocultural background of the caregiver on one hand, and the burden the caregiving poses on the other *(6)*. Health professionals who work with demented patients in the community are aware of the difficulties that family members are faced with when the decision is made to seek nursing home placement of their beloved one. At this point the family physician and his or her staff can offer special support.

The health status of the caregiver is a third factor that influences the timing of nursing home placement. Care of an AD patient frequently is not only personally exhausting for the caregiver but also affects family life, social contacts, job situations, and finances.

ONE AD CASE = TWO PATIENTS

One case of AD usually means that there are two patients—the demented individual and the caregiver. Health care providers must always consider not only the condition of the AD patient, but also the physical and mental health of the caregiver. Depression and loneliness are frequent features in this relationship, as reviewed in Chapter 50 *(see* pp. 449 ff).

As soon as difficulties in health maintenance are suspected or recognized (Table 1), more formal care systems must be utilized. These include day care, home health care, and other community-based services as well as long-term-care institutional facilities *(7)*. General information about these facilities may be available through the Alzheimer's Association and local health agencies.

Several basic parameters determine the maintenance of the health of a patient with AD. They have to be ensured by the caregiver in home care. These are:

1. *Nutrition.* Special attention to protein caloric and vitamin intake/absorption is required.
2. *Exercise.* Activities should be chosen depending on the patient's age and physiological capabilities as well as preferences—walking, dancing, swimming, games.
3. *Personal hygiene.* Bathing, dressing, toileting; it is important to advise family members to follow a regular daily schedule in order to decrease anxiety. Basic rule: maintain activity, but not at the cost of emotional stress.
4. *Dental hygiene. See* Chapter 48 *(see* pp. 427 ff).
5. *Incontinence.* Recognize and treat infection; establish a routine and provide frequent toileting, even if the patient feels no urge; identify patient signals.

ENVIRONMENTAL SAFETY

Patients with dementia are at increased risk for accidents and falls. From an early stage of the illness, it is important to provide a safe and simple environment and to reduce means that could cause confusion.

1. Manage wandering with the installation of special locks or electronically operated doors. Supply patients with identification and a transmitter for locating their position in case they get lost.
2. Help the patient find the bathroom with special signs; leave lights on and keep toilet seats open.
3. Secure electrical devices and equipment and put away potentially dangerous material, such as medications or cleansing agents.
4. Remove unnecessary furniture, uneven rugs, and obstacles that could facilitate stumbling, optimize lighting, and reduce noise.
5. Consider safety problems that are posed by a demented patient who continues to drive. Advise the patient not to drive. Report the unsafe driver to the state motor vehicle agency, if necessary.

HOW TO LOCATE SUPPORT SERVICES

A physician should learn which social services are available in the community for dementia patients and their caregivers. Assistance can be obtained by the physician's staff from the area agency on aging, the state office or department on aging, the local Alzheimer's Association, community mental health centers, state health departments, Eldercare, the state adult protective services division, as well as discharge planners at local hospitals or social workers in local home health care programs. These organizations are also excellent referral sources for family caregivers, who are then better enabled in tracking down their own resources.

THE PHYSICIAN IN THE NURSING HOME

Physicians will be better served if they limit the number of nursing homes to which they admit their AD patients. This will enable them to interact more effectively with and train the nursing home staff members, thereby ensuring a better quality of care for their patients.

The most common and prevalent medical problems seen in nursing home practice are incontinence and urinary infections, weight loss, falls, skin rashes and skin breakdown, behavioral manifestations of dementia, and, in the late stages of AD, pneumonia and cardiac complications. Effective nursing care requires a balance between too little and too much medical and nonmedical intervention.

Care of the patient with dementia is a particular challenge to the attending physician. Physician interventions are often needed, both directly through pharmacotherapy and indirectly through support of staff and environmental change. Beyond the treatment of excess morbidity, these patients need structure throughout the day and rely more on nonverbal cues and touch than do noncognitively impaired patients.

Most families continue to be involved in their relative's life after they decide to place the patient in a nursing facility. Physicians must appreciate that much of the stress and burden of providing care to a disabled older person continues after placement in an institution.

End-of-life issues also need to be addressed through family conferences. Hospice services may also be special help and comfort to families during the final stages of their loved one's life.

COMMUNICATION WITH THE DEMENTED PATIENT

In AD, the effect of the progressive cognitive decline on the language and the ability to express oneself verbally is profound. As the disease progresses, the patient at some point loses his or her language skills and consequently is no longer able to interact or communicate with others. This loss creates a common problem between the caregiver and a demented patient. This breakdown of communication is frustrating for both and is a major source of caregiver stress, because of the psychological and interpersonal burden it presents *(8)*.

Knowledge of these changes that occur individually at different disease stages and at different rates helps us to cope better with the deterioration and to develop new strategies for enhanced nonverbal communication. It is not only of help to make the patient comprehend what the caregiver wants him or her to understand. It is even more important to understand what the patient wants to express with his or her remaining means of communication, such as facial expression and body language, moaning or vocalizations.

How to Communicate With the Patient

The extensive, progressive deterioration in cognition affects the ability of AD patients to receive, store, retrieve, and send information. To help the demented individual to comprehend, the communication with the patient generally should be slow, simple, concrete, repetitive, and honest *(9)*. A supportive, positive approach and the use of nonverbal channels may facilitate communication with an AD patient.

As the long-term memory in AD is usually preserved for several years, patients tend to live in and talk about the past. Knowledge of a patient's biography, cultural background, and past history will help the caregiver or nursing home staff have a better understanding of the patient's attempts at communication.

The more a patient has lost his cognitive abilities and executive functions during the course of the disease—a process termed retrogenesis (a return to childhood) by psychiatrist Barry Reisberg *(10)*—the more he or she depends on emotions. At the same time there is a need for skin contact—of the same nature as a baby experiencing pleasure when being lovingly hugged and pampered by the parents. The warm human touch is an excellent way to reach an AD patient and to make him or her feel comfortable and appreciated as a human being as well as protected.

Touch and massage are well-acknowledged, viable nursing modalities with particular value for the care of demented patients. Unfortunately, in our modern Western culture they are both still underutilized and understudied *(11)*. Touch can be useful to significantly improve the health and mood status of older adults and especially for the improvement of communication with cognitively impaired older individuals.

The effects of an expressive physical touch in patients with dementia are multiple. According to a study from South Korea, an expressive touch with verbalization immediately lowers anxiety and causes decreasing episodes of dysfunctional behavior *(12)*. It need not be emphasized that this measure is extremely cost-effective and rather easy for nearly everybody to learn.

It is also very important to reassure frequently patients of their personal value and achievements during life, as they may rapidly lose self-esteem with this devastating disease right from the beginning, ending up with feelings of hopelessness, helplessness, and unworthiness.

Misunderstandings and conflicts are frequent in situations where regular communication is no longer possible. This may, however, be partly avoided with such simple measures as those listed in Table 2.

How the Patient Communicates With You

The relatively rare research that has been done in the field of communication in the demented has focused mainly on enhancing the communication from the caregiver to the patient. The content and meaning of communication received from the cognitively impaired has remained largely unexplored until recently *(13)*.

It has been demonstrated that individuals with dementia are able to transmit meaningful communication, and that this communication may with some training and experience can be interpreted by others *(13)*. Severely demented patients who lost their language ability often show emotions, needs,

Table 2
Tips for Effective Communication With the Severely Impaired AD Patient

Sit (when possible) face to face with the patient in a quiet setting.

Observe the patient's facial and body language to recognize his or her emotional state and needs.

Smile and maintain warm eye contact (without staring).

Express caring with a gentle physical touch.

Reassure the patient with calm affirming words, such as "We are very proud of you."

Complement the patient concerning special skills and achievements that he or she had in the past (try to get to know the biography). For example, "You have been a great golfer in your time."

Be patient and allow sufficient time for a possible response (even if nonverbal).

Listen to the patient, even when the words do not make sense or are repetitive.

Ask a patient with only nonverbal expressions to join you or someone else in singing the words to a song or to a hymn that the caregiver says the patient has known well.

When unable to maintain the patient's attention, try again at another time/occasion.

Always consider: It is not intelligence that declines in patients with AD, it is the cognitive function that vanishes with the progressive degenerative destruction of areas of the brain associated with this disease.

and pain in different ways, either by (unpleasant) vocalizations or moaning, or by squeezing a caregiver's arm, as well as through changes in facial expression (grimacing) and body language.

Unsuitable and unpleasant vocalizations are prevalent among cognitively impaired patients and are often considered disruptive and problematic by their families, caregivers, and nursing home staff as well as inmates. The vocalizations, however, frequently serve as a communication attempt to gain attention for the expression of an actual need, such as hunger or pain or a bad feeling. A caregiver or nurse should not get angry with the person but better find out what the patient is trying to tell. There is mostly a certain meaning underlying these vocal behaviors *(14)*. As well as a mother can differentiate the crying of her hungry or happy or pain-experiencing baby, AD patients present with different tones when they vocalize their various needs.

Even when speech is partially maintained, severely ill AD patients may withdraw into themselves and only rarely attempt to verbalize their feelings and wishes.

Communication Attempts Through Preserved Skills—Patient Vignettes

Patients may communicate feelings and emotions by exhibiting retained skills, especially in the areas of music and the creative arts. Some may find a last vehicle for expressing their emotions by taking up previously learned musical skills, dancing, or painting.

A woman who could no longer speak was able to paint beautiful paintings. She also tried to communicate feelings by patting her chest and gesturing, as if trying to release feelings from within herself.

A 69-year-old man, a retired business executive, in the late stages of AD, who exhibited periods of agitation, opened up briefly after I told him how proud I was of him for trying so hard to keep going. He then made a truly profound statement, which in fact was his last attempt at communication. Within 3 weeks he died of pneumonia. He told me:

> *My life is not up to quality. What I see is like a swinging pendulum. I feel like I want to bring things out but I can't seem to. I don't know if I can bring them out. I want to. It is like my shoe doesn't fit. I'm going to do the best and I won't let alone.*

A 74-year-old man with severe AD spoke only a few garbled words. His wife mentioned that he could still play the harmonica. At the next office visit he brought in a bag filled with harmonicas. He picked out one of the instruments and played several tunes perfectly. He was overjoyed to be able to demonstrate this retained talent.

A 66-year-old woman, a former university professor and chairperson of a business administration department, was followed through various stages to the point at which she lost comprehensible speech. She had previously lost all her computer skills. At several visits she was still, however, able to join me in singing words and music (albeit with errors) to several hymns, which she had learned in childhood. Her Sunday school class is still important to her. Class members bring a meal to her every week. The patient's husband feels that she thus bonds with the different class members.

One day the same patient noticed that her husband was using one of her briefcases. She picked it up and started carrying it, and continued to do so every day for a period of time. The husband believed that the briefcase represented an association with her past profession.

IMPLICATIONS

Communication certainly is a topic of paramount importance in the care of AD patients, which warrants more and specific training. To better meet the needs of dementia patients, caregivers should focus on recognizing and interpreting communication messages—either verbal or nonverbal—conveyed by the afflicted individuals. To learn and acquire communication techniques it is necessary to be aware of the nature and progression of the disease and to understand the needs of the patient. A recently published study revealed a lack of knowledge and training that adversely affects the quality of hospice care for demented persons *(15,16)*. Hospice teams could benefit from dementia-specific training that includes useful communication techniques for the different disease stages.

For the majority of (private) caregivers such training is neither provided nor affordable. In these cases attributes such as friendliness, empathy, and warmth should enhance and characterize the care, always bearing in mind that an AD patient remains until the very end a valuable human being, fully deserving humane and dignified treatment.

REFERENCES

1. Smith, G.E. et al.: Risk factors for nursing home placement in a population-based dementia cohort. J Am Geriatr Soc 2000; 48: 519–525.
2. Parks, S.M.; Novielli, K.D.: A practical guide to caring for caregivers. Am Fam Physician 2000; 62: 2613–2611.
3. Schacke, C.; Zank, S.: Family care of patients with dementia: differential significance of specific stress dimensions for the well-being of caregivers and the stability of the home nursing stuation. Z Gerontol Geriatr 1998; 31: 355–361.
4. Lindgren, C.L. et al.: Grief in spouse and children caregivers of dementia patients. West J Nurs Res 1999; 21: 521–537.
5. Winters, S.: Alzheimer disease from a child's perspective. Geriatr Nurs 2003; 24: 36–39.
6. Yaffe, K. et al.: Patient and caregiver characteristics and nursing home placement in patients with dementia. JAMA 2002; 287: 2090–2097.
7. Persson, D.I.; van Winkle, N.: Home and long-term care issues. In: Richter, R.W.; Blass, J.P. (eds.): Alzheimer's disease—a guide to practical management. Pt. III, Mosby, St. Louis, 1994: 141–155.
8. Hendryx-Bedalov, P.M.: Alzheimer's dementia. Coping with communication decline. J Gerontol Nurs 2000; 26: 20–24.
9. Tappen, R.M.: Alzheimer's disease: communication techniques to facilitate perioperative care. AORN J 1991; 54: 1279–1286.
10. Reisberg, B. et al.: Evidence and mechanisms of retrogenesis in Alzheimer's and other dementias: management and treatment import. Am J Alzheimer Dis Other Demen 2002; 17: 202–212.
11. Bush, E.: The use of human touch to improve the well-being of older adults. A holistic nursing intervention. J Holist Nurs 2001; 19: 256–270.
12. Kim, E.J.; Buschmann, M.T.: The effect of expressive physical touch on patients with dementia. Int J Nurs Stud 1999; 36: 235–243.
13. Acton, G.J. et al.: Communicating with individuals with dementia. The impaired person's perspective. J Gerontol Nurs 1999; 25: 6–13.
14. Clavel, D.S.: Vocalizations among cognitively impaired elders: what is your patient trying to tell you? Geriatr Nurs 1999; 20: 90–93.
15. Kirchhoff, M.: Lack of knowledge and training affects quality of hospice care for persons with dementia. Am J Hosp Palliat Care 2002; 19: 372.
16. Thompson, P.M.: Communicating with dementia patients on hospice. Am J Hosp Palliat Care 2002; 19: 263–266.

48

Dental Care of AD Patients

Christina A. Gitto, Michael J. Moroni, Geza T. Terezhalmy, and Satinderpal K. Sandu

INTRODUCTION

To provide optimal care to patients with Alzheimer's disease (AD), health care providers must understand the disease, its treatment, and the effects that both the disease and/or its treatment may have on the patient's quality of life. Physicians who treat patients with AD must better understand the role of adequate dental health care in improving the quality of life and not forget to initiate timely referral to oral health care providers. Oral health care providers, in turn, must develop preventive and therapeutic strategies compatible with the patient's physical and cognitive ability to undergo and respond to dental care. Adequate dental care is a vital aspect of a patient's well-being.

PREVALENCE OF ORAL COMPLICATIONS

To provide optimal care to patients with AD, health care providers must understand all aspects of this disease, its treatment, and the effects that both the disease and/or its treatment may have on oral health and, ultimately, on the patient's quality of life.

Odontopathic/Periodontopathic Problems

Limited data on the oral disease burden of patients suffering from AD indicate increased plaque accumulation, calculus formation, and gingival bleeding as compared to age- and sex-matched controls *(1)*. Patients with cognitive impairment also tend to have older and less clean prostheses than those without dementia *(2)*. Patients with seizures may be taking phenytoin and those with cardiovascular diseases may be on calcium channel-blocking drugs. Both of these agents have been associated with gingival hyperplasia, especially in patients with significant plaque accumulation due to poor oral hygiene. Patients with AD also experience a higher incidence of maxillofacial injuries and traumatic oral ulcerations, and often present with attrition, abrasion, and migration of the residual dentition *(3)*.

Xerostomia

Patients with AD have reduced submandibular salivary flow rates *(4)*. Four acetylcholinesterase inhibitors (AChEI) are now approved for the treatment of cognitive symptoms associated with mild to moderate dementia. Patients with AD may also need treatment for anxiety, depression, insomnia, and other systemic problems prevalent in this age group. The parasympatholytic or antimuscarinic effects of the drugs used for treating these disorders may contribute to additional qualitative and quantitative salivary changes. The lack of the antibacterial, lubricating, and buffering functions of the saliva places these patients at increased risk for caries, periodontal diseases, dysfunctional speech, chewing

From: *Current Clinical Neurology,*
Alzheimer's Disease: A Physician's Guide to Practical Management
Edited by: R. W. Richter and B. Zoeller Richter © Humana Press Inc., Totowa, NJ

and swallowing, and dysgeusia or ageusia *(1,5)*. Chronic xerostomia may result in painful (burning) oral soft tissue problems and poor tissue adaptation to prostheses. Xerostomia may also predispose to esophageal injury and contribute to nutritional deficiencies and weight loss *(6,7)*. Difficulty in swallowing, secondary to xerostomia, may cause aspiration pneumonia, a common cause of death in AD patients.

Tardive Dyskinesia

Patients with AD who experience psychotic symptoms or disruptive behavior are commonly prescribed antipsychotic/neuroleptic agents, such as haloperidol. While moderate doses appear to improve the symptoms in cognitively impaired elderly patients, the risk of extrapyramidal effects or tardive dyskinesia (TD) is high *(8)*. The estimated cumulative rates of TD after treatment with antipsychotic drugs for 1, 2, and 3 years is 20%, 30%, and 42%, respectively *(9)*. TD is characterized by rapid, jerky, writhing (twisting and turning) involuntary movements often affecting the orofacial region and distorted tonicity of the arm, leg, and trunk muscles, which appears chiefly on walking. Puckering or pouting, lip smacking, chewing, jaw clenching or mouth opening, facial grimacing, and blowing are common features. As the condition progresses, writhing of the tongue develops, which is characterized by a thrusting-out of the mouth as if fly-catching, repeatedly licking the lips, or pressing against the cheek to produce a bulge. Orofacial movements can lead to difficulty in eating or retaining dentures, and weight loss or cachexia may develop.

Bleeding

Therapeutic strategies that are frequently used in order to improve cognition in patients with AD include nonsteroidal anti-inflammatory drugs (NSAID) and extracts of *Ginkgo biloba,* available in the United States as dietary supplements *(10–13)*.One of the active ingredients of this herbal remedy, the terpenoid ginkgolide B, inhibits platelet activation and may interfere with platelet aggregation and blood clotting. Severe, spontaneous bleeding (subdural hematoma, bleeding from the iris) has been reported with *Ginkgo biloba* intake, and this adverse drug effect is potentiated when the agent is co-administered with acetylsalicylic acid (aspirin) and other NSAIDs, which preferably act as cyclooxygenase-1 (COX-1) inhibitors, or with oral and systemic anticoagulants *(14–16)*.

Hyperorality

AD patients exhibit a strong tendency to examine objects by mouth (hyperorality), characterized by licking, biting, chewing, and touching them with their lips. Placing inappropriate objects into the mouth may cause trauma to oral hard and soft tissues, lead to inadvertent swallowing or aspiration of foreign objects, and may contribute to accidental poisoning.

Hypermetamorphosis

Patients with AD may also demonstrate a tendency toward forced grasping and gripping (hypermetamorphosis). In combination with hyperorality, which may include a tendency to touch and examine the mouth, hypermetamorphosis characterized by forced grasping and gripping of teeth has been observed to lead to luxation and systematic avulsion (extraction) of teeth.

PRINCIPLES OF DENTAL MANAGEMENT

Dental management of the AD patient requires an awareness of the progressive and multidimensional nature of this neurodegenerative disorder. Cognitive, behavioral, and motor deficits cause significant decline from previous levels of functioning and are accompanied by a gradual inability to perform adequate oral hygiene *(1,5,8,17)*. AD also interferes with the patient's ability to communicate dental symptoms of pain or dysfunction, and progressive deterioration interferes with the patient's ability to participate in or tolerate most therapeutic interventions in a dental setting. When providing oral health care to AD patients, the main goal is to develop and implement timely preventive and therapeutic strategies that are compatible with the patient's physical, cognitive, and behavioral decline, that is, with his/her (remaining) ability to undergo and respond to dental care as well as with his social, psychological, and emotional needs and desires *(8,18)*. Oral health care providers must exercise empathy, congruence, and positive regard and strive to reach this goal with the same ethical, moral, and professional standards of care as may be appropriate in the management of any other patient *(19–22)*.

Rationale for Early Therapeutic Intervention

AD patients show a gradual deterioration in various features of cognition and functioning. A more rapid decline in intellectual capacity beginning with the second stage of AD underscores the patient's increasing inability (or sometimes) unwillingness to care for himself and, consequently, to perform normal oral hygiene procedures. Furthermore, AD interferes with the patient's ability to communicate dental symptoms of pain or dysfunction *(23)*. The progressive deterioration can be associated with disorientation, agitation, and inappropriate behavior in unfamiliar surroundings such as a dental office, and interfere with the patient's ability to participate in or tolerate therapeutic interventions. Since oral infections have been reported to contribute to aspiration pneumonia in the elderly, and aspiration pneumonia is a common cause of death in AD patients, a comprehensive oral rehabilitation should be implemented as early as possible following the diagnosis of AD *(19–25)*. Early therapeutic intervention minimizes the potential for odontopathic/periodontopathic pain and infection and associated systemic complications, and maximizes the potential for optimal nutritional intake.

Coordination of Care

The primary-care physician, oral health care providers, and other involved health care professionals, together with the caregiver, should discuss the patient's oral health care needs and identify risk factors that may influence proposed preventive and therapeutic strategies. They should as a team develop options on how best to manage the patient and facilitate the timing and the sequencing of dental and medical treatment, and other therapeutic activities. The oral health care provider should also provide the caregiver or the patient's family with appropriate training to facilitate the implementation of tasks required to maximize the patient's oral health, comfort, independence, and quality of life *(3,19–23)*.

Communicating With Patients

An essential element of the diagnostic and clinical process is the doctor–patient relationship. To nurture this alliance, oral health care providers should use appropriate communication techniques and recognize that AD patients lose the ability to understand speech and experience partial or total loss of speech as they progress though the stages of the disease. As long as the patient is capable of understanding, the dentist should address him or her directly. The presence of a family member or caregiver is useful to minimize the patient's anxiety and to obtain information that the patient may not be able to provide. Regardless of the state of cognitive deficiency, however, the patient should always be a part of, rather than the object of, any discussion.

Particularly helpful, when dealing with AD patients, are nonverbal communication skills. Approaching the patient with calm confidence, maintaining direct eye contact, and moving the patient into the chair by gentle body contact can make him or her feel comfortable with the unfamiliar surroundings and might have a calming effect.

Informed Consent

In the early stage of the disease, patients may experience errors in judgment and demonstrate a notable decline in personal appearance and hygiene. They, however, may still be able to comprehend oral health care instructions, participate in oral health care-related decision making, and be able to cooperate in their treatment.

As the disease progresses there is a more rapid decline in intellectual capacity and the patient may see the dental office as unfamiliar and threatening. He or she may become uncooperative, anxious, and aggressive. Hallucinations and episodes of delusional ideation may also occur. Such patients will not be able to furnish clinicians with informed consent. In such cases, dentists must obtain an informed consent for both diagnostic and therapeutic procedures from legal guardians, from other designated representatives for the patient, or from the courts *(3)*.

IMMEDIATE ASSESSMENT OF ORAL HEALTH AT TIME OF DIAGNOSIS

As soon as possible after the diagnosis of AD is made, the patient should undergo a comprehensive physical evaluation by the oral health care provider. This evaluation should include documentation of the patient's medical history with a review of organ systems, followed by a clinical and radiographic examination of the head and neck region, and oral soft and hard tissues.

Medical History

The most important component of the pretreatment evaluation of all dental patients is the establishment of a historical profile. The historical profile should identify the patient, establish the chief complaint, reveal experiential dental history; document drug allergies and other adverse drug effects; identify medications, consumption of vitamins and dietary supplements, or special diets; and provide a record of past and present illnesses, major hospitalizations, and a review of the major organ systems. An initial medical history must be obtained from all patients, and it should be updated at each subsequent appointment. A special attempt should be made when eliciting or reviewing the medical history of an AD patient to identify the current stage of the disease. The Mini-Mental Status Examination (MMSE) is a widely used instrument to categorize a patient as having mild, moderate, or severe AD *(23,26)*.

Physical Examination

The initial physical evaluation should also include an assessment and documentation of the patient's blood pressure and pulse/heart rate. Since many of the medications used to treat psychotic symptoms associated with AD can cause orthostatic hypotension, the vital signs should be reassessed at each appointment. In addition, patients with AD may lose weight because they have difficulty eating or remembering to eat. It is not clear whether subtle cognitive dysfunction somehow predisposes to weight loss, or whether poor nutrition hastens cognitive dysfunction in patients predisposed to develop AD. In any case, clinicians should consider the possibility of early AD when they encounter elderly patients with unexplained weight loss *(24)*.

An initial comprehensive regional examination of the head and neck and of oral soft and hard tissues should be conducted and the findings recorded. To complete the examination successfully, an extraoral mouth prop may be essential to help control the patient's head position and to maintain the oral opening *(23)*. Since AD patients may not be able to cooperate during radiographic examination, the use of a leaded glove and a leaded apron worn by the operator is also recommended *(23)*. Table 1 provides a checklist for an accurate assessment of risk factors that may affect strategies for enhanced oral health.

PREVENTIVE STRATEGIES

Dental management plans for patients with AD should include appropriate preventive strategies, taking into consideration the patient's physical and cognitive deficiencies. If it is within the capabilities of the patient to recall previously learned information and to learn new information, one should educate the patient to carry out his or her oral hygiene procedures. This is the best way to ensure compliance. As the mental condition deteriorates, the patient may be incapable of carrying out the dental hygiene regimen. In these cases, the education of a family member and/or caregiver is essential *(3)*.

Table 1
Oral Health Assessment of the AD Patient

1. How often does the patient visit his or her oral health-care provider?
   Emergencies only
   Bi-annually
   Annually
   Never
2. Does the patient have any of the following conditions?
   Own teeth
   Removable partial denture
   Complete denture
   Upper
   Lower
   No teeth
3. How often does the patient brush his or her own teeth?
   Once a day
   Twice a day
   Three times a day
   Occasionally
   Never
4. Are any of the following conditions noted?
   Caries
   Xerostomia
   Oral cancer
   Other adverse oral conditions
5. Which risk factors for periodontal disease are present?
   Reduced manual dexterity
   Impaired cognition
   Multiple medical conditions
   Polypharmacy
6. What other negative factors are present?
   Sensory impairment
   Lack of family support
   Restricted transportation
   Limited finances

From ref. *45*, with permission, © Quintessence International 2001.

It is important that the patient's caregivers receive appropriate training to allow them to understand and to be able to implement the preventive plan.

Information should be included in this training on the proper positioning of patients to safely implement home-care activities, the technique of inserting, removing, and caring for prostheses, and the technique for oral cancer screening. However, caregivers should only perform those oral hygiene procedures that the patient cannot implement. The need for professional supervision consisting of frequent communication with the patient's caregiver, in concert with frequent recall and office-based preventive care, should be stressed.

Plaque Removal

Elderly patients in general and AD patients in particular have demonstrated diminished manual dexterity, which limits their ability to carry out effective plaque removal on a daily basis with a conventional toothbrush and dental floss *(1,3,5)*. Consequently, preventive strategies should take into consideration toothbrush design and technology to increase the effectiveness of plaque removal in individuals with below-average manual dexterity and/or cognitive ability. It has been reported that even

Table 2
Chlorhexidine Gluconate

Chlorhexidine gluconate is a topical antimicrobial mouth rinse active against Gram-positive as well as Gram-negative aerobes and facultative anaerobes, and yeast. It binds to negatively charged bacterial cell walls and extramicrobial complexes, and precipitates the cytoplasmic content in susceptible organisms. Chlorhexidine gluconate exerts a sustained reduction of plaque-forming organisms when adsorbed on tooth surfaces, dental plaque, and oral mucosa.

1. Indications	Treatment of gingivitis.
2. Contraindications	Chlorhexidine is contraindicated in patients with known hypersensitivity to chlorhexidine gluconate.
3. Drug interactions	May precipitate a disulfiram-like effects with antabuse and metronidazole due to alcohol content.
4. Administration (route and dosage)	Oral rinse. Dosage form: 0.12% in 16-oz bottle. Rinse with 15 mL for 30 seconds bid after brushing/flossing teeth and expectorate after rinsing OR: Using a small spray bottle, gently spray the product on the oral tissues and suction excess. OR: Apply with a toothbrush, a sponge applicator, or a cotton swab while suctioning the oral cavity to remove the excess.
5. Monitor efficacy	Reduced gingivitis in association with effective reduction of plaque in the presence of mechanical plaque removal.
6. Monitor toxicity	Irritation of oral tissues, nasal congestion, dyspnea, and facial swelling.
7. Length of treatment	Indefinite.
8. Cessation	May be withdrawn immediately and completely without adverse effects.
9. Instruction to patient and/or caregiver	May alter taste, and stain oral soft tissues and permanently discolor composite restorations.

with average dexterity, no specific manual toothbrush design has been shown to be superior for plaque removal *(27)*. In both, short-term and long-term studies, electromechanical and ultrasonic/electromechanical brushes have been shown to be more effective than conventional ones in reducing plaque and gingivitis in all age groups *(28–40)*.

Regardless of the toothbrush design, care must be taken to instruct the patient and/or caregiver in proper use in order to prevent unwanted soft tissue laceration or periodontal tissue trauma. With decreasing muscle coordination and increasing motor difficulty, modification of oral hygiene aids, such as toothbrush, proxybrush, and floss handles, may also be recommended. The handles of these oral hygiene aids may be lengthened or thickened with acrylic, aluminum foil, or a tennis ball. An elastic or Velcro handle can be applied to the handle to facilitate its proper use. Patients with removable prostheses can have their denture brushes replaced with a nailbrush attached with suction cups to a sink. This enables patients to clean their denture with one hand. The goal of these modifications is to allow the patient to maintain self-care as long as possible.

Topical Rinses

The use of topical agents, such as chlorhexidine gluconate (Table 2), is helpful to combat gingivitis and other periodontal diseases that result from plaque accumulation. However, these products require the use of a swish-and-spit technique that may be beyond the capabilities of an AD patient. In such cases, a small spray bottle filled with the therapeutic agent may be used to gently deliver the

Table 3
Sodium Fluoride

Sodium fluoride promotes the remineralization of decalcified enamel. It can increase resistance to acid dissolution by forming fluorohydroxyapatite and inhibits cariogenic processes attributed to microorganisms in dental plaque.

1. Indications	Prevention of dental caries.
	Reduce dentinal hypersensitivity.
2. Contraindications	Contraindicated in patients with known hypersensitivity to fluoride or when the fluoride content of drinking water exceeds 0.7 ppm.
3. Drug interactions	Decreased effect/absorption has been reported with magnesium-, aluminum-, and calcium-containing products.
4. Administration (route and dosage)	Topical gel.
	Dosage form: 1.1% (24 g, 125 g).
	Apply thin ribbon onto toothbrush and brush all tooth surfaces for 2 minutes.
	Expectorate and refrain from rinsing, eating, or drinking for 30 minutes.
5. Monitor efficacy	Reduction in caries incidence.
6. Monitor toxicity	Rash, nausea, and vomiting.
7. Length of treatment	Treatment should be ongoing as long as the patient presents with a high caries incidence or high caries risk assessment.
8. Cessation of treatment	May be withdrawn immediately and completely without adverse effects.
9. Instructions to patient and/or caregiver	Ingestion of excessive doses may result in dental fluorosis and osseous changes.

product on the oral tissues (either by the patient or the caregiver) and the excess suctioned. When the potential for silent aspiration is a concern, a chlorhexidine gel may be applied with a toothbrush, a sponge applicator, or a cotton swab while suctioning the oral cavity to remove the excess *(1,3)*.

Fluorides

The incidence of xerostomia among AD patients is high. Since it can lead to increased caries activity, preventive modalities, such as dietary analysis, dietary counseling, and prophylaxis should be combined with over-the-counter home fluoride use. A topical fluoride, 1% NaF (Table 3), in the form of a brush on gel is more appropriate than topical solutions, since patients may not be able to adequately swish and expectorate to minimize ingestion. The use of a topical fluoride gel in a carrier is another alternative. However, more patient and caregiver cooperation is required. The application of topical fluorides, including a 5% fluoride varnish, should be part of office-based preventive care *(19–22)*.

The effectiveness of chemoprevention, using both chlorhexidine and a fluoride, has been demonstrated in patients at high risk for caries and periodontal disease *(41)*. To maximize therapeutic efficacy, it is suggested that the chlorhexidine be used first, followed 30 min later by the application of the fluoride gel *(42)*.

Sialagogues

It has been suggested that there may be an association between the neurologic changes that occur and salivary dysfunction in AD *(3,4)*. Qualitative and quantitative changes in the saliva lead to

Table 4
Pilocarpine Hydrochloride

Pilocarpine hydrochloride is a parasympathomimetic drug. It exerts a broad spectrum of pharmacologic activities, with a predominantly muscarinic-cholinergic action. It has been shown to stimulate lacrimal, salivary, gastric, intestinal, respiratory, and pancreatic secretions.

1. Indications	To stimulate salivary flow in patients with salivary gland dysfunction secondary to drug-induced xerostomia.
2. Contraindications	Known hypersensitivity to pilocarpine. Use with caution in patients with cardiovascular disease, urinary tract obstruction, and Parkinson's disease.
3. Drug interactions	Increased myopia with sympathomemetic amines; monitor patients.
4. Administration (route and dosage)	Oral. Dosage form: tablets: 5 mg. Initially give 2.5–5.0 mg tid; titration up to 30 mg/day at variable dosage intervals may be considered for patients who have not responded adequately.
5. Monitor efficacy	The primary endpoint for therapeutic efficacy is increased salivary flow, which is not necessarily accompanied by subjective improvement. It may require up to 4 weeks for peak effect. Secondary indications of efficacy of pilocarpine are diminished oral mucositis and candidiasis and improvement of dysphagia.
6. Monitor toxicity	Common adverse reactions include blurred vision, miosis, headaches, diaphoresis, and polyuria—titrate the dosage downward and/or increase the dosage interval. Symptoms of overdose include bronchospasm, bradycardia, involuntary urination, vomiting, hypotension, and tremors.
7. Length of treatment	May be continued indefinitely as long as the salivary flow continues to be stimulated and the patient experiences no serious side effects.
8. Cessation of treatment	May be withdrawn immediately and completely without adverse effects.
9. Instructions to patient and/or caregiver	Promptly report any adverse drug effect.

From ref. *45*, with permission, © Quintessence International 2001.

1. Reduced lubrication
2. Reduced antibacterial, antiviral, and antifungal activity
3. Loss of mucosal integrity
4. Loss of buffering capacity
5. Reduced lavage and cleansing of oral tissues
6. Interference with the normal remineralization of teeth
7. Altered digestion, taste, and speech

Patients with xerostomia whose salivary glands can respond to stimulation may benefit from simple dietary measures, such as eating carrots or celery, or by chewing sugarless or xylitol-containing gums. However, the prescription of cholinergic agonists, such as pilocarpine hydrochloride or cevimeline hydrochloride, may more predictably increase salivary activity (Tables 4 and 5). In those patients with no residual salivary gland function, salivary substitutes, oral moisturizers, and artificial saliva may provide some, if inadequate, relief for xerostomia.

Table 5
Cevimeline Hydrochloride

Cevimeline hydrochloride is an acetylcholine derivative. It exerts a broad spectrum of pharmacologic activities, with a predominantly muscarinic-cholinergic action. Cevimeline has been shown to stimulate lacrimal and salivary secretions.

1. Indications	To stimulate salivary flow in patients with salivary gland dysfunction secondary to drug-induced xerostomia.
2. Contraindications	Known hypersensitivity to acetylcholine. Contraindicated in patients with uncontrolled asthma, narrow-angle glaucoma, or iritis. Use with caution in patients with cardiovascular disease, urinary tract obstruction, and Parkinson's disease.
3. Drug interactions	Additive effects in slowing cardiac conduction in patients taking β-blockers. Antagonizes the effects of antimuscarinic drugs such as atropine or scopolamine.
4. Administration (route and dosage)	Oral. Dosage form: 30-mg capsules. One 30-mg capsule tid.
5. Monitor efficacy	The endpoint for therapeutic efficacy is increased salivary flow, which is not necessarily accompanied by subjective improvement. Secondary indicators of efficacy, when applicable, include diminished oral mucositis and oral candidiasis, and improvement in dysphagia.
6. Monitor toxicity	Common adverse drug effects include sweating, nausea, rhinitis, diarrhea, and visual disturbances (especially at night)—titrate dosage downward and/or increase dosage interval. Symptoms of overdose may include bronchospasm, bradycardia, involuntary urination, vomiting, hypotension, and tremors.
7. Length of treatment	May be continued indefinitely as long as the salivary flow continues to be stimulated and the patient experiences no serious adverse drug effects.
8. Cessation of treatment	May be withdrawn immediately and completely without adverse effects.
9. Instructions to patient and/or caregiver	Promptly report any adverse drug effect.

THERAPEUTIC STRATEGIES

The patient's physical and emotional state will determine whether he or she can receive treatment in the dental office. When it is not possible or it may not be in the best interest of the patient to receive treatment in a dental chair, an outpatient surgical suite or a hospital operating room should be chosen to provide for the patient's comfort and safety while allowing for the delivery of the highest-quality dental care *(20,21)*. If the patient is confined to a wheelchair, wide parking spaces and entrance ramps as well as the removal of other impediments to access of care must be considered.

Positioning of the Patient

At times, the patient's inability to cooperate with the dentist during treatment procedures is further complicated by his or her inability to maintain an open airway. The dentist must position the patient in a sitting or semireclined position (45° angle) to avoid pooling of saliva and other fluids, airway obstruction, and/or aspiration. The routine use of a rubber dam is recommended, except in those cases where the patient is unable to swallow and handle oral secretions. A rubber dam can also be beneficial in the management of patients with tardive dyskinesia.

Orthostatic hypotension, a potential adverse drug effect, is often encountered in patients with AD and must be given special consideration at the end of the appointment. The dental chair should be raised slowly and the patient allowed adequate time to adjust to the upright sitting position before being instructed to rise slowly from the chair. Orthostatic hypotension and balancing problems or disequilibrium upon standing should be anticipated, to minimize the potential of a fall.

Restraints

The judicious use of physical, mechanical, or pharmacological restraints can alleviate the problem of akathisia or constant movement by the patient, often associated with antipsychotic therapy. Physical restraint implies that a person is holding the patient to control voluntary or involuntary movements. Mechanical restraints include the use of Papoose Boards, Pedi-Wraps, tape, straps, or blankets. The use of physical and mechanical restraints should occur only when absolutely necessary, and the choice should be the least restrictive alternative. The treatment record should reflect the type of restraint used, the justification for its use, as well as the length of time that the patient was restrained *(3,20–22)*.

Pharmacological restraints imply the use of sedative agents. This approach is a viable alternative whenever physical or mechanical restraints are ineffective or are contraindicated. If the patient is not already on sedative/hypnotic agents, a short-acting benzodiazepine may be prescribed *(43)*. If the patient is already on sedative medication, the dental appointment should be coordinated with regularly scheduled dosage intervals for maximum benefit. If the patient is using anxiolytics on an as-needed basis, instruct him or her to take the medication prior to the appointment.

Older patients tend to experience longer periods of sedation, with associated prolonged cognitive, behavioral, and motor dysfunction requiring close monitoring before, during, and after treatment. When considering the use of sedation, always consult with the patient's primary-care physician and the caregiver to obtain their concurrence with the plan. As in the case of physical or mechanical restraints, the least restrictive method is the most appropriate and requires proper documentation in the treatment chart.

If the patient is able to cooperate and breathe through the nose, nitrous oxide inhalation is an effective adjunct to behavioral management. It is helpful in relaxing spastic patients, controlling the gag reflex, and increasing the patient's pain threshold. However, for those who are unable to cooperate and cannot breath through their nose, oral sedation with a short-acting benzodiazepine is more predictable. Other alternatives are intravenous and intramuscular sedation. These techniques are useful to control the uncooperative patient, but appropriately trained staff and special monitoring equipment is required. The use of general anesthesia is the technique of last resort for the uncooperative patient *(3,19,20,23)*.

Restorative Dentistry

Restorative procedures using posterior amalgam and anterior composite restorations are the accepted norm. However, for patients with poor gingival health and/or extensive caries activity, amalgam restorations may also be acceptable for the treatment of anterior teeth. The suspected association between AD and the trace element mercury, as it is found in dental amalgams in particular, has been investigated. It was concluded that there is no correlation between the number of amalgam restorations and brain concentrations of mercury *(44)*. It appears that amalgam restorations are not neurotoxic and the applied mercury does not contribute to the pathogenesis of AD.

Other options that are beneficial for patients at high risk for caries, especially in non-stress-bearing areas of teeth, include the use of resin-modified glass ionomer or compomer restorative materials. They leach fluoride and impart some caries resistance to tooth structure immediately adjacent to them. They also are recharged with fluoride from oral gel, so that the fluoride release is continuous.

When patients in the early stages of AD present with extensive loss of tooth structure, the use of stainless steel, polycarbonate, or composite crowns may be appropriate. These alternatives may allow the retention of teeth with guarded prognosis for a finite period of time and/or provide an interim solution to caries control until the patient's ability to participate in his or her oral hygiene can be better assessed or may provide long-term solutions in the management of highly debilitated patients (20).

The use of a rubber dam for isolation should be considered. However, saliva could build up excessively in the mouth under the rubber dam, which might lead to choking and aspiration, and should be guarded against. Four-handed dentistry (with an assistant to suction the saliva) is imperative.

Periodontics

Prophylaxis and scaling and root planing, at short intervals, are the cornerstones of treatment and are appropriate for periodontal maintenance. Clinicians are effective in removing plaque and calculus in shallow pockets (less than 4 mm) using nonsurgical root planning, but in deeper sites, effective calculus removal is limited. In patients with one or a few sites of deep pocketing, local antimicrobial treatment as an adjunct to proper scaling and root planing may be beneficial. However, the local delivery of antibiotics would not be appropriate for the management of localized periodontitis in AD patients who may also be immunocompromized or in patients with generalized periodontitis.

Corrective periodontal surgery is usually not an option for AD patients, because of their inability to perform the required plaque control before and after surgery. The administration of systemic antibiotics, such as metronidazole, may be justified for the treatment of acute episodes of generalized periodontitis if the disease cannot be controlled by proper home care, scaling and root planing, and surgical treatment is contraindicated.

Patients with drug-induced gingival hyperplasia (phenytoin, calcium channel blockers, cyclosporin) are candidates for a gingivoplasty. This is especially true when the tissue interferes with oral hygiene and/or the patient is experiencing pain and discomfort. Since many of these patients cannot tolerate periodontal packs, the use of either electrosurgery or laser surgery is an appropriate alternative (20).

Endodontics

Endodontic treatment is appropriate if the targeted tooth is restorable and is essential to maintain function. In addition, it may be the only option in irradiated and immunocompromised individuals, and in patients presenting with other systemic diseases that preclude extraction (20).

Prosthetic Dentistry

When patients are able to insert, remove, and maintain their dentures or when caregivers are available to provide these services, removable prostheses are appropriate to restore function (20). To minimize problems with adaptation, ill-fitting, "old-friend" prostheses should be modified or improved when possible. The use of tissue conditioners is recommended for functional relines where vertical dimension has to be changed. If the dental practitioner is providing replacement complete dentures for a person with AD, a copy/duplication technique should be used in order to retain the learned muscle control of the familiar dentures.

If planning to provide dentures for the first time, the use of overdentures should be considered, as they help to retain proprioception and maintain jaw control. For the person with early AD who requires dentures, consideration should be given to the possible role of implants or implant-retained overdentures. Although this is an expensive option, it may well be cost-effective in the long term, providing the individuals with security and helping them to preserve their self-esteem and social contacts. AD patients who experience frequent, severe seizures are not good candidates for removable prostheses.

Patients and caregivers must be informed that success with dentures depends to a large degree on appropriate muscle function, which controls and stabilizes the prosthesis during periods of rest and use. The tongue may dislodge the mandibular denture, and facial muscles that are rigid or uncontrollable may prevent a maxillary denture from maintaining a retentive seal. Even with the best technique, removable prostheses cannot be guaranteed to function properly because of the diminishing adaptive skills of the patient. All prostheses should be labeled with the owner's name and social security number for ready identification.

Oral and Maxillofacial Surgery

The prophylactic extraction of teeth to prevent odontopathic and/or periodontopathic infections or for the convenience of caregiver is inappropriate *(20)*. As long as the patient is able to undergo and respond to dental care and his or her physical well being is not compromised, oral health care providers should consider all available conservative techniques before rendering a patient edentulous.

SUMMARY

As the incidence of AD increases, oral health care providers can expect to be increasingly called upon to care for patients with this debilitating condition. To provide competent and timely care to patients with AD, clinicians must understand the disease, its treatment, and its effects on patients' physical and cognitive ability to maintain their oral health and undergo and respond to dental care. In addition, oral health care providers should be sensitive to the needs of the patient's family and caregivers.

Diminished physical and cognitive function during the course of the disease underscores the patient's inability to care for oneself and, consequently, to perform normal oral hygiene procedures. Furthermore, AD interferes with the patient's ability to communicate dental symptoms of pain or dysfunction. The progressive deterioration of cognition can cause agitation, disorientation, and inappropriate behavior in unfamiliar surroundings such as a dental office and interfere with the patient's ability to tolerate most therapeutic procedures.

Clinicians must attempt to keep odontopathic and periodontopathic problems to a minimum by implementing comprehensive oral rehabilitation as early as possible following the diagnosis of AD. The prophylactic extraction of teeth to prevent oral complications or for the convenience of caregivers is inappropriate. When treating patients with AD, clinicians must exercise empathy, congruence, a positive regard, and must strive to reach these goals with the same ethical, moral, and professional standards of care as may be appropriate in the management of any other patient.

REFERENCES

1. Ship, J.A.: Oral health of patients with Alzheimer's disease. J Am Dent Assoc 1992; 123: 53–58.
2. Wittle, J.G. et al.: The dental health of the elderly mentally ill: a preliminary report. Br Dent J 1987; 162: 381–383.
3. Henry, R.G.; Wekstein, D.R.: Providing dental care for patients diagnosed with Alzheimer's disease. Dent Clin N Am 1997; 41: 915–944.
4. Ship, J.A. et al.: Diminished submandibular salivary flow in dementia of the Alzheimer type. J Gerontol: Med Sci 1990; 45: M61–M66.
5. Jones, J. et al. Caries incidence in patients with dementia. Gerondontology 1993; 10: 76–82.
6. Jolly, D.E.; Paulson, G.W.; Pike, J.A.: Parkinson's disease: a review and recommendations for dental management. Spec Care Dent 1989; 9: 74–78.
7. Fiske, J.; Hyland, K.: Parkinson's disease sufferers. Geredontology 1998; 15: 73–78.
8. Devenand, D.P. et al.: A randomized, placebo-controlled dose-comparison trial of haloperidol for psychosis and disruptive behaviors in Alzheimer's disease. Am J Psychiatry 1998; 155: 1512–1520.
9. Woerner, M.G. et al.: Prospective study of tardive dyskinesia in the elderly: rates and risk factors. Am J Psychiatry 1998; 155: 1521–1528.
10. Stewart, W.F. et al.: Risk of Alzheimer's disease and duration of NSAID use. Neurology 1997; 48: 626–632.
11. Tariot, P.N.: Treatment strategies in Alzheimer's disease. Mediguide to Geriatr Neurol 1997; 1: 1–8.
12. Kleijnen, J.; Knipschild, P.: Ginkgo biloba. Lancet. 1992; 340: 1136–1139.
13. Le Bars, P.L. et al.: A placebo-controlled, double-blind, randomized trial of an extract of *Ginkgo biloba* for dementia. North American EGb Study Group. JAMA 1997; 278: 1327–1332.

14. Rowin, J.; Lewis, S.L.: Spontaneous bilateral subdural hematomas associated with chronic *Ginkgo biloba* ingestion. Neurology 1996; 46: 1775–1776.

15. Rosenblatt, M.; Mindel, J: Spontaneous hyphema associated with ingestion of *Ginkgo biloba* extract. N Engl J Med 1997; 336:1108.

16. Mathews, M.K. Jr.: Association of *Ginkgo biloba* with intracerebral hemorrhage. Neurology 1998; 50: 1933–1934.

17. Ship, J.A.; Puckett, S.A.: Longitudinal study on the oral health in subjects with Alzheimer's disease. J Am Geriatr Soc 1994; 42: 57–63.

18. Niessen, L.C. et al.: Dental care for the patient with Alzheimer's disease. J Am Dent Assoc 1985; 110: 207–209.

19. Carr-Hosie, M.A.: Treatment considerations for the dental professional for patients with Alzheimer's disease. Ohio Dent Assoc J 1993; Winter: 36–42.

20. ADA oral health care guidelines: patients with physical and mental disabilities. American Dental Association, Chicago, May 1991.

21. Casada, J.P.; Casada, D.B.: Guidelines for dental care for the patient with Alzheimer's disease. J Greater Houston Dent Soc 1990; Feb.: 3–5.

22. Boccia, A.: Alzheimer's disease and the dental patient: recognizing and dealing with dementia. Ontario Dentist 1992; April: 16–18.

23. Henry, R.G.: Alzheimer's disease and cognitively impaired elderly; providing dental care. CDA J 1999; 27: 709–717.

24. Barrett-Connor, E. et al.: Weight loss precedes dementia in community-dwelling older adults. J Am Geriatr Soc 1996; 44:1147–1152.

25. Navazesh, M.; Mulligan, R.: Systemic dissemination as a result of oral infection in individuals 50 years of age and older. Spec Care Dent 1995; 15: 11–19.

26. Folstein, M.F.; Folstein, S.E.; McHugh, P.R.: A practical method for grading the cognitive state of patients or the clinician. J Psychiatric Res 1975; 12: 189–198.

27. Park, K.K.; Matis, B.A.; Christen, A.G.: Choosing an effective toothbrush. Clin Prev Dent 1985; 7: 5–9.

28. Mandel, I.D.: The plaque fighters. J Am Dent Assoc 1993; 124: 71–73.

29. Youngblood, J.J. et al.: Effectiveness of a new home plaque removal instrument in removing subgingival and interproximal plaque: a preliminary in vivo report. Compend Contin Educ Dent 1985; 6: S128–S132.

30. Baab, D.A.; Johnson, R.H.: The effect of new electric toothbrush on supragingival plaque and gingivitis. J Periodontol 1989; 60: 336–341.

31. Killoy, W.J. et al.: The effectiveness of a counterrotary action powered toothbrush and conventional toothbrush on plaque removal and gingival bleeding. A short-term study. J Periodontol 1989; 60: 473–477.

32. Wilcoxon, D.B. et al.: The effectiveness of a counter-rotational action power toothbrush on plaque control in orthodontic patients. Am J Orthod Dentofac Orthop 1991; 99: 7–14.

33. Wilson, S. et al.: Effects of two toothbrushes on plaque, gingivitis, gingival abrasion and recession: a one-year longitudinal study. J Dent Res 1993; 72: 333.

34. Wilson, S. et al.: Effects of two toothbrushes on plaque, gingivitis, gingival abrasion and recession: a one-year longitudinal study. Compend Contin Educ Dent 1993; 14(suppl 16): s69–s79.

35. Yukna, R.A.; Shaklee, R.L.: Interproximal vs midradiculor effects of a counterrational powered brush during supportive periodontal therapy. Compend Contin Educ Dent 1993; 14 (suppl 16): s80–s86.

36. Love, J.W. et al.: Clinical assessment of the INTERPLAK® powered toothbrush vs a conventional brush plus floss. Compend Contin Educ Dent 1993; 14 (suppl 16): s87–s98.

37. Blahunt, P.: A clinical trial of the INTERPLAK® powered toothbrush in a geriatric population. Compend Contin Educ Dent 1993; 14 (suppl 16): s606–s610.

38. Terezhalmy, G.T. et al.: Clinical evaluation of the efficacy and safety of the UltraSoex ultrasonic toothbrush: a 30-day study. Compend Contin Educ Dent 1994; XV: 866–874.

39. Terezhalmy, G.T. et al.: Clinical evaluation of the effect of an ultrasonic toothbrush on plaque, gingivitis, and gingival bleeding: a six-month study. Prosthet Dent 1995; 73: 97–103.

40. Whitmyer, C.C. et al.: Clinical evaluation of the efficacy and safety of an ultrasonic toothbrush system in an elderly patient population. Geriatr Nurs 1998;1 9: 29–33.

41. Keltjens, H.; Schaeken, T.; van der Hoeven, H.: Preventive aspects of root caries. Int Dent J 1993; 43: 143–148.

42. Ten Cate, J.M.; Parsh, P.D.: Procedures for establishing efficacy of antimicrobial agents for chemotherapeutic caries prevention. J Dent Res 1994; 73: 695–703.

43. Matear, D.W.; Clarke, D: Considerations for the use of oral sedation in the institutionalized geriatric patient during dental interventions: a review of the literature. Spec Care Dent 1999; 19: 56–63.

44. Saxe, S.R. et al.: Alzheimer's disease, dental amalgam and mercury. J Am Dent Assoc 1999; 130: 191–199.

45. Gitto, C.A.; Moroni, M.J.; Terezhalmy, G.T.; Sandu, S.: The patient with Alzheimer's disease. Quintessence Int. 2001; 32: 221–231.

49

Long-Term Medical Care Issues

Vonda K. Gravely and Jacobo Mintzer

INTRODUCTION

This chapter focuses on the medical complications of dementia of Alzheimer's type. In addition to the syndrome of acquired and persistent impairments of cognitive function, dementia is also associated with numerous conditions that directly affect the integrity of the central nervous system. Many afflictions are more prominent in the elderly as a direct result of the changes associated with the aging process. Moreover, those who carry the diagnosis of dementia are at even greater risk of developing co-morbid medical complications. In this chapter we discuss common medical problems such as adverse drug reactions, interactions, urinary tract infections, pneumonia, as well as delirium. Other problems that are highlighted include nutritional deficits and incontinence as they relate to the development of pressure sores, as well as the increased susceptibility to falls and fractures. We conclude with a discussion of nursing home placement, signs of elder abuse, and family issues.

MEDICAL ASSESSMENT

As clinicians, we place a great responsibility on patients to describe their problems. However, patients with dementia may not be able to verbalize their complaints. Therefore, we must acquire information from other sources such as the caregiver (1). In dementia, medical conditions such as cardiovascular disease, chronic obstructive pulmonary disease, infection, anemia, and metabolic disturbances may manifest as an agitated state (2).

These issues are also important when treating patients with advanced dementia, such as a consideration of the benefit vs the burden imposed by the treatment as well as the prolongation of life in an already extremely demented patient. Therefore, decreased life expectancy should be taken into account with regard to managing chronic illnesses in this population. For example, preventive measures such as restricted diets and various screening procedures are often ordered inappropriately. Treatment of diabetes and hypertension should be more conservative and directed toward prevention of serious side effects such as postural hypotension, which can lead to falls and subsequent hip fractures (2).

Other difficulties in the evaluation include the possible absence of fever and leukocytosis in a septic patient. Therefore, a change in the mental status from an already deteriorated cognitive baseline may be the only presenting problem in an older patient with sepsis. Other signs and symptoms that may suggest an infection include tachypnea, decreased appetite, nausea, vomiting, falls, and incontinence. Only about 60% of older adults with a serious infection will develop leukocytosis; they also do not mount a great febrile response.

One of the most important factors contributing to the increased severity of infections in the elderly is the many anatomical and physiological changes that occur with age. Aging is associated with disrupted cilia movement, which may predispose to bacterial aspiration and pneumonia. Elderly men,

From: *Current Clinical Neurology,*
Alzheimer's Disease: A Physician's Guide to Practical Management
Edited by: R. W. Richter and B. Zoeller Richter © Humana Press Inc., Totowa, NJ

due to conditions such as benign prostatic hypertrophy, which obstructs urine outflow, as well as elderly woman who have lost peri-urethral host defenses, are more susceptible to urinary tract infections. The normal changes of the skin associated with aging, such as atrophy, decreased blood flow, and decreased elasticity, can increase the risk of skin and soft tissue infections.

Another challenge facing the elderly is decline in neuromuscular function, which leads to dysphasia affecting both aspiration risks as well as nutrition. Finally, the age-related deficits in T-cell-mediated immunity as well as an impairment in the serum antibody response predisposes the elderly to a host of infectious agents *(2)*.

POLYPHARMACY AND CHANGES OF AGING

One of the primary problems involving medical complications in the elderly involves medication-prescribing habits. Older Americans spend approximately $3 billion annually on prescription medications. This overutilization poses the potential problems of adverse drug events and drug–drug interactions. Adverse drug reactions are a key factor in iatrogenic illnesses. Pharmacokinetics such as absorption, distribution, metabolism, and excretion also play an important role. The following is a brief review of age-related changes in pharmacokinetics.

Absorption slows with the aging process. Medication distribution in the elderly is related to body weight and body composition. Because of changes that occur with aging, such as decreased lean muscle mass, increased fat mass, and decreased total body water, drug dosages have to be modified. Fat-soluble drugs are also given in lower dosages, as they can accumulate in fatty tissue and thus provide for a longer duration of action. Drugs are metabolized either through hepatic or renal means. Hepatic metabolism depends on liver blood flow, age, and the competition of other medications. Drug elimination is correlated to creatinine clearance, which declines with age. The serum creatinine level (Cr), however, is a poor indicator of creatinine clearance in older adults. The Cockrott-Gault formula therefore should be used to estimate creatinine clearance here and is given as the following equation:

$$140 - age \times weight\ in\ kilograms/72 \times serum\ Cr\ (\times 0.85\ for\ females)$$

Pharmacodynamics involves the sensitivity of tissues to drugs. This may increase or decrease during the aging process, further adding to the appropriateness of a given dose for a demented individual. In summary, one of the major concerns regarding polypharmacy is that, for every dollar spent on pharmaceuticals in nursing homes, another dollar is spent treating the iatrogenic illnesses attributed to medications. Therefore, to prevent iatrogenic illness, the clinician must consider that the development of new signs and symptoms in the elderly may be the consequence of the current drug therapy. Starting with one-third of the recommended dose is a general principle that could help eliminate potential harmful effects *(3)*.

URINARY TRACT INFECTIONS

Urinary tract infections (UTIs) are the most frequent bacterial infection as well as the most common cause of bacteremia in the elderly. Alzheimer's disease (AD) is associated with incontinence—increasing these patients' risk of developing UTIs. The usual clinical presentations, such as dysuria, urinary frequency, fever, and suprapubic tenderness, may be masked in the elderly demented patient. This poses a particular challenge in that symptoms such as nausea, vomiting, and decreased urine output must be acknowledged as possible signs of UTI in these patients *(4)*.

A positive urine culture does not confirm a UTI in the elderly. Furthermore, this possible asymptomatic bacteruria does not usually warrant nor is improved by antibiotic treatment. Most studies in the long-term-care population have documented a 50% positive urine culture representing asymptomatic bacteruria. The clinician must keep this in mind when many patients with pneumonia also have a positive urine culture that is unrelated to the etiology of the current fever. Furthermore, do not prematurely cease the clinical assessment of a febrile geriatric patient upon finding a positive culture *(5)*.

The etiology of most UTIs in the elderly includes a wide spectrum of both Gram-positive and Gram-negative organisms, which often requires broad-spectrum antibiotics, and for longer duration of time. The diagnosis of UTI in the geriatric population is now a diagnosis of exclusion, in that they already possess many of the typical symptoms of UTI secondary to co-morbid medical problems or, as in the complicating case of the demented patient, they cannot communicate these symptoms to the physician. Clinicians must first rule out pneumonia, myocardial infarction, dehydration, and a host of other conditions before diagnosing this condition accurately.

Fluoroquinolones such as ciprofloxacin and levofloxacin are the first-line class of agents for managing UTIs in the elderly. Trimethoprim-sulfamethoxazole can also be considered a first-line agent in women only, because it does not penetrate the prostate gland. Also, we must treat females for at least 10 days and males for at least 14–28 days. All oral β-lactam and nitrofurantoin antibiotics are excellent second-choice agents. The use of topical estrogen preparations among postmenopausal women has been shown to reduce the frequency of UTI by 50%. It is primarily up to the treating physician as to whether to treat asymptomatic bacteriuria. However, cost–benefit analyses have concluded that there is a greater harm brought by treating this condition due to increasing the risk of resistant pathogen selection *(5)*.

PNEUMONIA

The incidence of pneumonia increases with age and is an important cause of death in the elderly. Cognitive impairment increases the mortality risk approximately sevenfold. Clinicians must be aware that, again, some elderly patients do not display the usual set of symptoms, such as cough, fever, chills, rigor, and chest pain. Other nonspecific manifestations include confusion, lethargy, failure to thrive, headache, weakness, anorexia, abdominal pain, episodes of falling, incontinence, and a global deterioration. These atypical presentations are seen most commonly in those with cognitive impairment. Classic signs of pneumonia, such as fever and chest consolidation, may be absent in the elderly. However, the presence of tachypnea with a respiratory rate greater than 26 breaths/min is a strong indicator of the possible presence of a lower respiratory tract infection *(2)*.

The causes of pneumonia in long-term-care facilities overlap with those that are community-acquired and include *Streptococcus pneumoniae, Haemophilus influenzae*, enteric Gram-negative bacilli, and *Staphylococcus aureus*. Diagnosis of the elderly patient includes the following medical workup: chest radiograph, blood cultures, routine hematology, and routine biochemistry. Keep in mind that the chest radiograph may be normal early in the course of pneumonia. This is especially true in dehydrated patients *(2)*.

A decision based on the clinician's findings needs to be made as to whether to admit the patient to an acute-care hospital. Although there are no absolute criteria for making this decision, patients with markers of severe disease and patients who will probably have a complicated course should be admitted. However, currently available data indicate that transfer to an emergency room or hospital has significant risks and few benefits for patients with advanced dementia. Immediate survival and mortality rates are comparable for acute care vs care in the long-term facility for the treatment of pneumonia. There has been a decline in the rate of acute-care hospitalization for demented long-term-care patients, which could possibly reflect either an improved assessment of a changing treatment philosophy *(2)*.

The clinician must decide which if any antibiotic treatment to administer. If antibiotic treatment is elected, it should cover the most likely offending microorganisms. Empiric therapy is provided by amoxicillin-clavulanate and second-generation cephalosporins; long-term-care-facility-acquired pneumonia is by broad-spectrum *(6)*. Finally, the physician must decide on the route of administration as well as the duration of treatment. Intravenous therapy is extremely difficult in cognitively impaired individuals, as they cannot comprehend the need for the medical treatment. Furthermore, in patients who have very poor oral intake, antibiotics can be administered by intramuscular injections, as is the case with cephalosporins.

Some opt not to treat, as they along with the family have agreed that antibiotic administration only prolongs pain and suffering. In a given patient, studies have shown that antibiotic therapy does not prolong survival in severely demented patients. Results indicate that antibiotic therapy was not always necessary. Comfort measures such as analgesics, antipyretics, and oxygen may provide improved care for these patients without prolonging pain and suffering *(2)*.

If antibiotics are utilized, there is still limited data on the duration of treatment. Moreover, no clear-cut advantage has been noted for intravenous vs oral antibiotics as long as there is adequate bioavailability and tissue penetration. Hospitals commonly start intravenous and switch to oral as soon as the patient is hemodynamically stable *(6)*. Patients who carry a dementia diagnosis tend to develop recurrent infections. Therefore, the use of antibiotics in advanced dementia should take into account the recurrent nature of infections, the adverse effects of antibiotics as well as the diagnostic procedures, and the lack of any significant enhancement of patient comfort *(2)*.

PAIN

The International Association for the Study of Pain has defined pain as an unpleasant sensory and emotional experience associated with actual or potential tissue damage. Pain should not be considered a natural or necessary part of aging. Dementia confounds assessment and treatment of pain secondary to impaired perception and communication. Pain is quite prevalent in the general nursing home population, with estimates of 45% to 80% of nursing home residents living with untreated pain. Pain has severe consequences, including depression, social isolation, sleep impairment, decreased functioning, and increased health care costs. Unrecognized pain is the most common reason for behavioral problems in patients with dementia *(2)*.

The elderly patient with chronic pain may develop autonomic tolerance in which he or she may not display the usual autonomic symptoms associated with pain, such as tachycardia, anxiety, and increased blood pressure. Patients with cognitive impairment may develop increasing vocalization and agitation as the only signs of pain, which can often be misread as worsening dementia.

According to some researchers, a direct relationship exists between cognitive impairment and pain. Moreover, some have proposed that patients with advanced dementia have a reduced affective component of pain secondary to memory loss. However, it remains questionable as to whether the decreased pain is caused by less cognitively perceived pain or decreased ability to report pain. More important, cognitively impaired patients still suffer a great deal of untreated pain *(7)*.

Because there are no objective markers of pain, assessment relies on the patient's report and the clinician's judgment in cognitively impaired patients. At the present time, there is no single assessment tool that is useful for cognitively impaired patients. Some indicators of pain include specific facial movements such as the orbicularis oculi movements, agitation and screaming, withdrawal, refusal to eat, or refusal to ambulate. A study by Douzjjan and colleagues demonstrated that regular scheduled doses of acetaminophen allowed the discontinuation of psychotropic medications in five out of eight nursing-home residents with agitated or difficult behavior.

The goal of pain management should be to reduce pain to a more tolerable level. Medications should be started at the lowest dose and increased very slowly. Frequent reassessment is necessary. In addition to pharmacological agents, other means, such as relaxation techniques, should be utilized when possible, and for more mildly demented patients a form of cognitive-behavior therapy as well as physical therapy *(7)*.

First-line agents for pain control include nonopioid analgesics such as acetaminophen, salicylates, and nonsteroidal anti-inflammatory drugs (NSAIDs). Although there is no tolerance to these drugs, there is a ceiling effect, which involves little relief by increasing doses beyond a certain point. Doses should not exceed 4 g/day of acetaminophen secondary to hepatotoxicity. Because gastric erosion is a common problem in the elderly, the co-administration of a proton pump inhibitor or cytoprotective agent may offer some protection. Renal function must be followed while on NSAIDs. NSAIDs may potentiate digoxin and aminoglycosides while inhibiting the effects of diuretics, β-blockers, and angiotensin-converting enzyme inhibitors *(7)*.

Opioids are divided into weak compounds, which include codeine, hydrocodone, oxycodone, and propoxyphene, as well as strong compounds such as morphine, methadone, fentanyl, and meperidine. The liver metabolizes codeine rapidly; therefore, higher doses are required for analgesia. Codeine results in constipation. Physicians must acknowledge possible side effects of opiates, including sedation, confusion, respiratory depression, constipation, urinary retention, nausea, and vomiting. Adjuvant therapies for pain include anxiolytics and antidepressants. Anticonvulsants have been used successfully for treating neuropathic pain. Tricyclic antidepressants such as amitriptyline and nortriptyline work by potentiating opioids, enhancing sleep, and improving mood. This class of medications, however, has anticholinergic properties, which could exacerbate an already depleted cholinergic system. The physician should treat this very important condition with high regard to drug–drug interactions and the side-effect profile *(7)*.

DELIRIUM

Delirium is defined as a sudden disturbance of consciousness that is characterized by a change in cognition manifesting as an impairment of attention. Published studies have identified risk factors for this condition, which consist of advanced age, preexisting dementia or cognitive impairment, chronic medical illness, and psychiatric conditions. Although polypharmacy is a risk factor for delirium within any age group, it is more common in the elderly. Delirium is a multifactorial event, with the prevalence in hospitalized elderly patients in general ranging from 14% to 56%. Furthermore, of patients who are admitted without this syndrome, approximately 12–60% become delirious during their hospitalization *(8)*.

Patients may manifest delirium as a disturbance of their sleep–wake cycle, presenting in acutely agitated states to minimally responsive states. This "quiet" delirium often is clinically unrecognized. Anticholinergic delirium is a noteworthy topic, as it may result from many psychiatric medications such as benztropine, tricyclic antidepressants, and low-potency phenothiazines. Symptoms include visual hallucinations, hyperpyrexia, urinary retention, constipation, dry mouth, and anhydrosis, as well as blurred vision and tachycardia. Treatment for this condition includes reviewing all drugs with possible anticholinergic effects, stopping their use if medically safe, and substituting an alternative treatment as well as supportive measures *(8)*.

Life-threatening causes of delirium including Wernicke's encephalopathy, syncope resulting from arrhythmias, substance-induced delirium, hypoxia, hypoglycemia, hypertensive encephalopathy, intracerebral hemorrhage, meningitis, or encephalitis. Among the elderly, an infection such as a urinary tract infection and pneumonia are likely sources. Bowel obstructions and dehydration may also result in the clinical presentation of delirium *(9)*.

As with any disease process, the clinician must conduct a thorough physical examination with a focused selection of laboratory and imaging studies. This examination should focus on the cardiopulmonary, metabolic, and gastrointestinal status of the patient. The neurological exam should focus on possible focal or generalized muscle weakness, pathological reflexes, and cranial nerve abnormalities. The patient should also be observed for tremors, asterixis, myoclonus, or focal seizure activity.

Laboratory testing is individualized and should include electrolytes, glucose, renal, and liver profiles. Also, a complete blood count is to be obtained to rule out anemia and leukocytosis, as well as a urinalysis and chest radiograph. An electrocardiogram is indicated for patients with a cardiac history or symptoms suggestive thereof. Unless there is a prior history of falls, suspected trauma, or a focal neurological deficit, neuroimaging yield is quite low.

A febrile, delirious, or unresponsive patient may require a lumbar puncture with cerebrospinal fluid analysis and cultures to exclude bacterial, fungal, or viral meningitis *(8)*. For much of the medical workup of delirium, the physician may have to deal with an extremely agitated patient, who is thrashing about and pulling out intravenous lines. This is an extreme challenge to health care providers, who must ensure the safety of the patient and staff, as well as getting the necessary information to find the source of the delirium.

The physician should therefore employ pharmacological agents during severe delirium when the patient's behavior interferes with medical therapies or poses a danger to themselves or others. Low doses of high-potency agents such as haloperidol have traditionally been utilized with marked success. These agents have been preferred because they have a lower risk of anticholinergic or hypotensive side effects. Older patients may respond to doses as low as 0.5 mg. However, the new atypical agents are effective for behavioral disorders with an improved side-effect profile in that they are less likely to cause extrapyramidal symptoms or tardive dyskinesia. Benzodiazepines are not first-line agents, as they may result in oversedation, worsen the confusion, and cause paradoxical agitation. Of the medications in this class, however, lorazepam is still the agent of choice, as it has a shorter half-life and no active metabolites *(10)*. Delirium is considered a medical emergency that can be confused as a worsening dementia. Therefore, it is imperative that the clinician not dismiss increased agitation, sundowning, and other behavioral signs as a further decline in cognition.

PRESSURE ULCERS

A pressure ulcer is a localized area of necrotic tissue that results from compression of soft tissue between an outside surface and a body prominence for an extended period of time. Patients with AD frequently develop both urine and fecal incontinence. The components of urine as they act on the skin lead to maceration, weakening of tissue, and finally skin breakdown. The enzymes in stool may promote a chemical breakdown of the skin, which leads rapidly to skin ulceration. Containment devices or protective barriers must be applied to the skin of those patients who are bedridden and suffer from incontinence. If diapers are used inappropriately, this can result in tissue breakdown. If diapers are used, the caregiver must apply a moisture barrier. Petroleum jelly is considered an inexpensive yet effective product for this purpose *(11)*.

Immobility also leads to pressure ulcers. The ideal repositioning time frame is to turn the patient every 2 hours. In the management, nutrition is extremely important, as patients with suboptimal nutritional status are at increased risk of developing pressure ulcers. Diets high in protein are necessary to prevent and heal ulcers. A patient with an ulcer needs 1.25–2 g/kg of protein every 24 hours. Vitamin requirements include 1600–2000 mg retinol equivalents of vitamin A, 100–1000 mg of vitamin C, 15–30 mg of zinc, 200% of the recommended daily allowance of B vitamins, and 25 mg of iron *(11)*.

Moist wound healing is used to manage pressure ulcers. Topical management depends on the stage. All stages require a pressure-relief support surface. Stage I and II require hydrocolloid or transparent thin film dressings. Stage III requires the necrotic tissue to be debrided, then topical hydrocolloid only. Stage IV requires alginates, moist gauze with solution or wound filler. If the patient is unable to consume the amount of the above vitamins and nutrients, a feeding tube can be considered. This, however, is a very controversial subject, and if not addressed by an advance directive, the family or substitute decision maker should be educated about the risks and benefits of this procedure.

FEEDING TUBES

The utilization of artificial nutrition and hydration in the final stages of dementia is an emotional and highly debatable issue. The severely demented patient may develop an indifference to food, refusal of food, or failure to manage the food bolus once it is in the mouth. Approximately 30% of all percutaneous endoscopic gastrostomy (PEG) tubes are placed in patients who suffer from dementia. However, the majority of the data regarding the efficacy of feeding tubes in providing a greater benefit-to-risk ratio have been based on observational studies, retrospective studies, or data extrapolated from mixed populations *(12)*.

Two recent reviews examined the burden and benefit of tube feedings in patients with dementia and concluded that there is no clinical evidence to support their routine use. Several critics of this common practice have viewed AD as a terminal condition in which feeding tubes do little more than prolong the dying process. Furthermore, there is no conclusive evidence that confirms a reduction in the incidence of aspiration pneumonia or prevention of pressure ulcers in patients with advanced dementia who are placed on feeding tubes. Also, there have been no studies to demonstrate an improved quality of life or increased longevity with the utilization of feeding tubes in demented patients *(13)*.

Clinicians, however, may fear they are vulnerable to legal action if they do not place a feeding tube. The alternative to tube feeding is hand feeding. The hope is that an advance directive would already be in place to represent the patient's wishes, which should be discussed during the diagnostic and family meetings. Surrogates who are available to make this decision when no directive is available may feel that it is morally wrong to deny a demented person the provision of nutrition and hydration. In any event, the physician must be sensitive to all variables as they will influence the final decision.

FALLS

The progression of dementia is associated with the inability to recognize obstacles, and the gait becomes narrow-based and unsteady. As patients do not recognize these limitations, they walk unassisted, resulting in falls with subsequent injury. Over 50% of patients with AD lose the ability to walk independently just under 8 years after the appearance of the initial symptom of dementia. The risk of falls may be decreased by a modification of drug regimens and evaluating patients for treatable causes of gait disturbances. It is crucial for the patient to maintain independent motor activity as long as possible. Safer mobility can be acquired by physical therapy, use of safe footwear, and of devices such as the Merry Walker. Hip protectors, low beds, as well as bed and chair alarms with appropriate monitoring can reduce injury *(2)*.

For patients who still reside in the home, physicians may refer to a home health agency for a home safety evaluation, which is covered by many insurance policies. Enrollment in a "safe return" program is also recommended, and many connections and resources can be made available by referral to the local Alzheimer's Association. The access to and the effective use of the Alzheimer's programs offered in the community can extend the period of time that patients can be cared for in the home *(2)*.

NURSING HOME PLACEMENT

The combination of physical impairments, psychosis, behavioral problems, and a decreased ability to communicate effectively create obstacles in the maintenance of in-home care. There are few decisions in life that families must face that are more excruciatingly painful than deciding to place the patient in a facility. Approximately 75% of AD patients reside in a nursing home facility at some point. Most studies have concluded that baseline dementia severity was correlated with nursing home placement. Caregiver burdenals accounts for a great deal of the placement issues *(2)*. Research has concluded that agents that lessen the severity of the illness through behavioral improvements and slow the progression of cognitive decline have been associated with longer in-home care, which lowers the cost of caring for these patients.

The physician plays a vital role in the placement process in that often the caregiver is seeking permission from the physician to place the family member in a nursing home. The physician has a dual responsibility—to the patient as well as to the caregiver. The caregiver spends approximately 60—100 hours per week in caring for the patient. The most effective intervention that physicians can employ in order to assist the caregiver with this process is establishing a relationship based on trust and open communication as well as appropriate referral to support groups and the local Alzheimer's Association for other resources.

ELDER ABUSE

We must be aware that elder abuse is highly underreported. Contributing factors to patient abuse include caregiver depression, isolation, stress, financial dependence, mental illness, substance abuse, and the patient's disruptive behavior. All comments should be investigated, and the subject of any physical aggressiveness should be addressed. Some patients with AD may also fabricate regarding this issue. Appropriate referral to the adult protective services of the department of social services is necessary to investigate these suspicions.

Common signs of abuse include a lack of or an inconsistent explanation for falls, skin wounds, bruises, burns, or fractures. Physical signs of neglect include dehydration, severe weight loss, poor hygiene, pressure sores, or other untreated medical conditions.

Indeed, advanced AD is a complicated and unfortunate illness that requires continued monitoring of patient and caregiver health and evaluation of the ethical issues involved in the terminal care of the patient *(14)*.

REFERENCES

1. Shuster, J.L.: Death and dying: palliative care for advanced dementia. Clin Geriatric Med 2000; 16: 373–386.
2. Volicer, L. et al: Palliative care. Neurol Clin 2001; 19 (4): 867–885.
3. Williams, C.: Clinical pharmacology: using medications appropriately in older adults. Am Fam Physician 2002; 66: 1917–1924.
4. Mouton, C.: Common infections in older adults. Am Fam Physician 2001; 63: 257–268.
5. Shortliffe, L.M.; McCue, J.: Urinary tract infection at the age extremes: pediatrics and geriatrics. Am J Med 2002; 113 (suppl 1A): 555–565.
6. Feldman, C.: Pneumonia in the elderly. Med Clin N Am 2001; 85: 1441–1459.
7. Cutson, T.M.: Long-term care in geriatrics. Clin Fam Practice 2001; 3: 667–681.
8. Murphy, B.: Psychiatric emergencies. Emerg Med Clin N Am 2000; 18: 243–252.
9. Lagomasino, I. et al.: Emergency psychiatry: medical assessment of patients presenting with psychiatric symptoms in the emergency setting. Psych Clin N Am 1999; 22: 819–850.
10. Callahan, E.H. et al.: Geriatric hospital medicine. Med Clin N Am 2002; 86: 707–729.
11. Wooten, M.K.: Long-term care in geriatrics: management of chronic wounds in the elderly. Clin Fam Practice 2001; 3: 599–626.
12. Li, I.: Practical therapeutics: feeding tubes in patients with severe dementia. Am Fam Phys 2002; 65: 1605–1610.
13. Gessert, C. et al.: Clinical investigation: tube feeding in nursing home residents with severe and irreversible cognitive impairment. J Am Geriatr Soc 2000; 48: 1593–1600.
14. Snyder, L.: Alzheimer's disease and dementia: care of patients with Alzheimer's and their families. Clin Geriatr Med 2001; 17: 319–335.

50

Loneliness and Depression in Caregivers

Rose A. Beeson

INTRODUCTION

Loneliness as a contributing factor in the development of depression in the caregiver of a patient with Alzheimer's disease (AD) has been given little attention despite the fact that researchers have found a moderate to high correlation between loneliness and depression in persons other than caregivers for some time *(1–2)*. However, recent studies strongly suggest loneliness as a significant predictor of depression for husbands and wives caring for their AD spouse in the same household *(3–5)*. The purpose of this chapter is to discuss those findings.

LONELINESS IS A SIGNIFICANT PREDICTOR OF DEPRESSION

It is estimated that there are approximately 5 million AD caregiver households in the United States *(6)*. Living with and caring for a family member with AD is a highly stressful experience. Adverse effects on the mental health of the caregiver, especially in the form of depression, have been reported to be much higher that either age- or gender-based population norms or demographically matched non-caregiving control groups *(7–9)*. AD caregivers reporting symptoms of depression have ranged from 28% to 55%, with female caregivers more likely to experience depression than males *(9–11)*. The emotional strain of witnessing and adapting to a spouses cognitive, behavioral, and personality change contributes to these depressive symptoms.

In order to better meet the mental health needs of AD caregivers, health professionals must understand the elements of the caregiver/care receiver dyadic relationship and the complexities that lead to depressive symptomatology, including the relationship between loneliness and depression.

Although loneliness and depression are strongly related, the historical research perspective suggests that they can be viewed as two distinct constructs. In a review of the literature, it was stated that "loneliness and depression are separate but, in some way, overlapping constructs which may contribute to each other" *(12, p. 355)*. It has been implied that depression is a broader, more global concept than loneliness. Because it was thought that the features of the lonely person were almost entirely consumed within the depressed prototype, it was concluded: "To know that a person is lonely is to know that the person possesses some major features of depression. The converse, however, is not true, knowing that a person is depressed does not necessarily imply that the person possesses features of being lonely. There are other routes to depression besides the lonely route" *(13, p. 190)*

LONELINESS IS ALWAYS A NEGATIVE EXPERIENCE

Loneliness is a powerful human experience *(14)*. It is defined as a sentiment that is experienced when one's lifestyle is deprived of the relationships desired and current relationships are seen as inadequate in comparison to those of the past, to those anticipated in the future, or those possessed by other

From: *Current Clinical Neurology,*
Alzheimer's Disease: A Physician's Guide to Practical Management
Edited by: R. W. Richter and B. Zoeller Richter © Humana Press Inc., Totowa, NJ

people *(15)*. It reflects the unfulfilled need for human, interpersonal intimacy, a desire to be related to another distinct self while experiencing a feeling that one is yet separate *(16)*. "The fear of loneliness and the search and struggle for intimacy are the color and shape of human existence, they are the essence of man" *(16*, p. 49). Loneliness is not caused by being alone, but is a response to the absence or loss of a definite needed relationship of a close attachment figure *(17)*. One of the most common antecedent causes of loneliness is the loss of an important person or relationship *(18)*.

Being part of a marriage union in our society builds on these human needs. Marriage often represents the single most influential and sustained relationship in one's life. Sharing experiences with a spouse over a lifetime helps to define and maintain one's individual need for human, interpersonal intimacy, as well as defining who we are as an individual and a partner in the marital dyad. But in the caregiving process in AD, one of the marriage partners has emotionally and psychologically withdrawn. Exchanges of intimacy, goals, and social activities that were once shared with the now demented spouse are no longer attainable. Losing the element of reciprocity in the marital relationship fosters feelings of loneliness. With loneliness comes an unwelcome feeling of lack or loss of companionship, an unpleasant aspect of missing certain relationships as well as missing a certain level of quality in one s relationship *(19)*. Loneliness is always a negative experience *(16)*.

IT IS IMPERATIVE THAT RESEARCH ASSESSES BOTH THE PATIENT AND THE CAREGIVER

Family caregivers occupy a pivotal place in the care of persons with dementia. Not only do families provide the bulk of home care, they do not relinquish their caregiving role unnecessarily *(20,21)*. Furthermore, when their caregiving efforts are appropriately supported, they forestall institutionalization for their AD family member as long as possible. Caregivers commit a great quantity of time and money to the caregiving role *(22)*. As the population ages and the number of individuals diagnosed with AD or related dementia increase to the expected 14 million by the year 2050, so will the cost of their care increase past the current estimate of over $50 billion per year *(23,24)*. The need for caregivers and the maintenance of continued in-home care will become crucial to our society. It is therefore imperative that research assesses both the caregivers' perceptions and their feelings of the caregiving role as well as investigate the diversity of changes experienced in the dyadic relationship between caregiver and care receiver, including the potential link from loneliness to depression.

WHAT RESEARCH STUDIES REVEAL ABOUT THE RELATIONSHIP

A recently published study of 242 husbands, wives, and daughters providing care for family members with AD residing in the same household was conducted in order to examine the relationship among loneliness and depression and the following variables: quality of the past relationship, relational deprivation or the negative restructuring of the caregiver–patient relationship, quality of the current relationship, and distance felt due to caregiving *(4,25)*. Loneliness was significantly related to depression ($p < 0.001$), relational deprivation ($p < 0.001$), and quality of the current relationship ($p < 0.001$). AD caregivers who experienced higher loneliness and depression also experienced higher relational deprivation and a poorer quality of the current relationship.

AD caregiving wives reported significantly more relational deprivation, loneliness, and depression than AD caregiving husbands, but not AD caregiving daughters. Caregiving wives had a mean depression score of 16.7, compared to caregiving daughters at 12.9 and caregiving husbands at 9.9. The difference in means on depression reported by caregiving husbands and caregiving wives was significant at $p < 0.001$. Caregiving wives also reported significantly more loneliness than caregiving husbands, but not caregiving daughters, indicating that the relationship of caregiver to care receiver may be more important to the demands of the caregiver role than gender. Caregiving wives in this study were experiencing a more difficult time with the demands of the caregiving role than caregiving husbands or daughters, indicated by their feelings of greater relational deprivation, loneliness, and depression.

Loneliness, relational deprivation, quality of the relationship (past, current and distance felt due to caregiving), and the kind of relationship to the AD patient collectively predicted 43% of the variance in caregiver depression when depression was the dependent variable. Loneliness was the only variable significant in the prediction of depression for AD caregiving husbands, wives, and daughters. This strongly supports the consistent link found between loneliness and depression previously reported in the literature *(2,19,26–28)*.

In a community sample of 101 caregivers residing in the same household as their AD patient, 49 caregiving spouses reported significantly higher levels of loneliness ($p < 0.05$) and depression ($p < 0.001$) than 52 noncaregiving spouses *(3)*. Loneliness was significantly related to all study variables: spousal relationship, being a wife caregiver ($p < 0.05$), relational deprivation ($p < 0.01$), loss of self ($p < 0.001$), and depression ($p < 0.001$). The more loneliness reported, the greater the relational deprivation, the greater the loss of self and the greater the feelings of depression.

MORE DEPRESSION AND LONELINESS IN CAREGIVING WIVES THAN HUSBANDS

AD caregiving wives reported significantly ($p < 0.001$) higher levels of loneliness and depression than did AD caregiving husbands. Caregiving wives had a mean loneliness score of 40.8 and a mean depression score of 12.4, compared to caregiving husbands' loneliness score of 33.8 and a depression score of 5.6 (SD = 4.21). AD caregiving spouses reporting higher levels of loneliness and depression also reported more loss of self. For AD caregiving spouses, being a wife caregiver and reporting greater loss of self were associated with significantly higher levels of loneliness and depression. In the explanation of AD caregiver depression for this sample, 49% of the variance in depression was explained by loneliness. It was the only study variable to make a significant contribution to AD caregiver depression.

In a sample of 102 AD spousal caregivers, loneliness was associated with higher levels of caregiver relational deprivation ($p < 0.001$), higher levels of patients' depressive symptoms ($p < 0.01$) and disruptive behaviors ($p < 0.01$), poorer quality of the current relationship ($p < 0.001$), and higher levels of caregiver depression ($p < 0.001$) *(4)*. The results of this study showed that AD caregiving husbands and wives who experienced greater relational deprivation, greater patients' depressive symptoms and disruptive behaviors, and poorer quality of the current relationship had higher levels of loneliness and depression. Loneliness was found to have the strongest correlation to depression ($p < 0.001$) of all the study variables as well as being the strongest predictor for depression, explaining 38% of the total variance in AD caregiver depression.

IMPLICATIONS OF STUDY RESULTS

The results of these three studies strongly support loneliness as a significant predictor of depression for husbands and wives caring for their AD spouse in the same household. Future intervention studies are required for understanding the complex pathway to AD caregiver depression, improving the quality of the caregivers' mental health, and supporting them in keeping their AD spouses in the community setting. It is overly simplistic to assume that "more interaction is better". We need to support a shift from an examination of "how many" and "how often" to a more broad understanding of the meaning of social relationships and the interactive process they play in the lives of AD spousal caregivers.

SOCIAL CONTACT SHOULD BE GUARANTEED FOR THE CAREGIVER

AD caregiving problems surrounding feelings of loneliness and depression demand that research look at means of removing obstacles to social contact for the AD caregiver. It is only through the knowledge and understanding of the influence of these concepts on the well-being of the AD caregiver and the care receiver that health professionals can develop effective interventions to prevent or better manage AD caregiver depression. This is of particular importance since the caregiving role may extend to a period of 10, 15, or even 20 years.

Emphasis should be placed on the concept of loneliness and its influence on the development of AD caregiver depression. Being lonely is painful, but being married and lonely can be excruciating. Being part of a marriage union in our society engenders expectations of closeness and intimacy that can become searingly poignant when unfulfilled and lost during the caregiving process. Lack of intimacy and concomitant feelings of abandonment as well as pain can become a part of the caregiver's life. Although the marital relationship may be lost, the AD spouse remains a viable presence in the household. Additional research is needed to understand this changing relationship between caregiver and care receiver during the disease process.

Health care professionals must go beyond the known interventions and increase their assessment of AD caregivers' feelings of loss or grief, loneliness, and depressive symptoms. Maintaining the caregivers' mental as well as physical health is paramount to protecting the family caregiver as a critical resource in today's society. Clinicians need to focus and intervene on those conditions that are amenable to change in the AD caregiver's life. Loneliness and depression are treatable—they are not irreversible conditions of life *(19)*.

SUMMARY

To meet the mental health needs of caregiving spouses of AD patients, loneliness must be addressed by health care professionals. Research has found loneliness to be a significant predictor of depression for husbands and wives caring for their AD spouse. In several recent studies, loneliness was the only predictive variable for AD caregiver depression. Although certain conditions of the AD caregiver's life are not amenable to change, loneliness is treatable.

REFERENCES

1. Shaver, P.R. et al.: Measures of depression and loneliness. In: Robinson, J.P.; Shaver, P.R.; Wrightman, L.S. (eds.): Measures of personality and social psychology attitudes. Academic Press, San Diego, CA, 1991: 195–289.
2. Mullins, L. et al.: The influence of depression, and family and friendship relations, on residents loneliness in congregate housing. Gerontologist 1990; 30: 377–384.
3. Beeson, R.A.: Loneliness and depression in spousal caregivers of those with Alzheimer's disease versus non-caregiving spouses. Arch Psychiatr Nurs 2003; 17: 135–143.
4. Beeson, R.A.et al.: Loneliness and depression in spousal caregivers of persons with Alzheimer's disease (AD). Submitted 2002.
5. Beeson, R.A. et al.: Loneliness and depression in caregivers of persons with Alzheimer's disease or related disorder. Issues Mental Health Nurs 2000; 21: 779–806.
6. Family caregiving in the U.S., findings from a national survey. National Alliance for Caregiving, Bethesda, MD, 1997.
7. Haley, W.E. et al.: Psychological, social, and health impact of caregiving: a comparison of black and white dementia family caregivers and non-caregivers. Psychol Aging 1995; 10: 540–552.
8. Russo, J. et al.: Psychiatric disorders in spouse caregivers of care recipients with Alzheimer's disease and matched controls: a diathesis-stress model of psychopathology. J Abnormal Psychol 1995; 104: 197–204.
9. Schulz, R. et al.: Psychiatric and physical morbidity effects of dementia caregiving: prevalence, correlates, and causes. Gerontologist 1995; 35: 771–791.
10. Chappell, N.L. et al.: Behavioural problems and distress among caregivers of people with dementia. Ageing Soc 1996; 16: 57–73.
11. Stuckey, J.C. et al.: Burden and wellbeing: the same coin or related currency? Gerontologist 1996; 36: 686–693.
12. West, D.A. et al.: The effects of loneliness: a review of the literature. Comprehens Psychiatry 1986; 27: 351–363.
13. Horowitz, L. et al.: The prototype of a lonely person. In: Peplau, L.A.; Perlman, D. (eds.): Loneliness: a sourcebook of current theory, research and therapy. Wiley, New York, 1982: 183–205.
14. Ernst, J.M. et al.: Lonely hearts: psychological perspectives on loneliness. Appl Prevent Psychol 1998; 8: 1–22.
15. Lopata, M.: Loneliness. In: Maddox, G.L.; Atchley, R.C.;Evans, J.G.; Finch, C.E.; Hultsch, D.F.; Kane, R.A.; Mezey, M.D.; Siegler, E.C. (eds.): The encyclopedia of aging. Springer Publishing, New York, NY, 1995: 571–572.
16. Mijuskovic, B.: The phenomenology and dynamics of loneliness. Psychology 1996; 33: 41–51.
17. Weiss, R.S.: Loneliness: the experience of emotional and social isolation. MIT Press, Cambridge, MA, 1973.
18. Rokach, A.: Surviving and coping with loneliness. Psychology 1989; 124: 39–54.

19. De Jong Gierveld, J.: A review of loneliness: concept and definitions, determinants and consequences. Clin Gerontol 1998; 8: 73–80.

20. Rockefeller, J.D., IV: A call for action: the Pepper Commission's blueprint for health care reform. JAMA 1991; 265: 2507–2510.

21. Ory, M.G. et al.: Prevalence and impact of caregiving: a detailed comparison between dementia and non-dementia caregivers. Gerontologist 1999; 39: 177–185.

22. Ernst, R.L. et al.: The U.S. economic and social costs of Alzheimer's disease revisited. Am J Public Health 1994; 84: 1261–1264.

23. U.S. General Accounting Office: Alzheimer's disease: estimates of prevalence in the United States (GAO/HEHS-98-16). U.S. General Accounting Office, Health, Education, and Human Services Division, Washington, D.C., 1998.

24. Leon, J. et al: Health service utilization costs and potential savings for mild, moderate, and severely impaired Alzheimer's disease patients. Health Affairs 1998; 17: 206–216.

25. Pearlin, L.I. et al.: Caregiving and the stress process: an overview of concept and their measures. Gerontologist 1990; 30: 583–594.

26. Andersson, L. et al.: Association between elderly experiences with parents and wellbeing in old age. Gerontology 1993; 48: 109–116.

27. Green, B.H. et al.: Risk factors for depression in elderly people: a prospective study. Act Psychiatr Scand 1992; 86: 213–217.

28. Kempen, G.I.J.M. et al.: Depression, loneliness, physical disability and the utilization of professional home care among older adults. J Health Sci 1990; 1: 271–276.

51

Frequently Asked Questions About Alzheimer's Disease

Brigitte Zoeller Richter

IS THERE A PRODROMAL PHASE IN ALZHEIMER'S DISEASE?

It is very likely a prodromal phase exists in Alzheimer's disease (AD), but so far there is no diagnostic tool to prove it. With a combination of neuropsychological and neuroimaging tests, however, it may soon be possible to be able to predict AD accurately. In a longitudinal analysis conducted by Marilyn S. Albert and co-workers at Harvard Medical School, the researchers could differentiate 89% of the people who subsequently developed AD from the controls by using just four tests (three of them assessed memory, one executive functions) and with this assess a prodromal stage. Executive function decline at baseline was the strongest dementia predictor among subjects with prodromal AD, while memory loss alone did not predict dementia *(1)*.

Volume reductions in the entorhinal cortex (not in the hippocampus), when measured with MRI and SPECT (combined), are statistically correlated with test scores of executive function.

The involvement of the entorhinal cortex in the preclinical phase of AD has been confirmed by neuropathological findings. This suggests that as the disease spreads, atrophic changes develop within the hippocampus.

WHAT CAN THE CSF TELL US?

Increased levels of phosphorylated tau protein (p-tau$_{231}$) in the cerebrospinal fluid (CSF) may be a useful, clinically applicable biological marker for the differential diagnosis of AD. Phosphorylation of tau protein at threonine 231 (tau has 441 amino acids at full length) occurs specifically in post-mortem brain tissue of AD patients.

Associated with increased levels of phosphorylated tau levels as well as decreased cerebrospinal fluid levels of β-amyloid peptides appears to be a polymorphism of CYP46, the gene encoding cholesterol 24-hydroxylase *(2)*. This gene plays a key role in the hydroxylation of cholesterol, thereby mediating its removal from the brain.

CSF levels of tau protein and beta-amyloid protein (ending at amino acid 42) may have a role as biomarkers in the clinical workup of patients with cognitive impairment, especially to differentiate early AD from normal aging *(3)*.

Markers of oxidative stress are also found increased in the CSF of AD patients *(4)*. The most prominent marker of DNA oxidation is 8-OHG (8-hydroxyguanine) in the ventricular CSF. This may become a future marker for disease progression or to control the efficacy of therapeutic antioxidant intervention.

From: *Current Clinical Neurology,*
Alzheimer's Disease: A Physician's Guide to Practical Management
Edited by: R. W. Richter and B. Zoeller Richter © Humana Press Inc., Totowa, NJ

CAN THE PROGRESSION RATE BE ESTIMATED?

Progression rates are variable between subjects with AD. Particularly, newly diagnosed patients and their families want to know how fast the disease will progress. Rachelle Smith Doody and co-workers tried to calculate the progression rate based on the initial decline prior to the first physician visit. They could classify patients as rapid, intermediate, or slow progressors with good predictive value. Patients who begin with progression rates that are more rapid than average (> 5 Mini-Mental State Examination points per year) continue to experience clinically significant decline sooner than patients who begin at slow (< 2 points per year) or average rates (2–4.9 points/year). Slow progressors take the longest time to reach clinically meaningful deterioration *(5)*.

WHAT ARE THE RISK FACTORS FOR HIV-DEMENTIA?

In a prospective study in New York conducted in a cohort of nondemented subjects who were HIV-positive, the following variables were significantly associated with the time to develop dementia: cognitive deficits, the diagnosis of minor cognitive/motor disorder, depression, and female gender *(6)*.

DOES NSAID USE REDUCE THE RISK OF AD?

Evidence suggests that several commonly used medicines may delay or prevent the onset of AD. Among the most thoroughly studied of these are nonsteroidal anti-inflammatory drugs (NSAIDs). A recent analysis from the Cache County Study confirms the potential protective effect. Long-term NSAID use thus may reduce the risk of AD, provided such use occurs well before the onset of dementia. More recent exposure seems to offer little protection. The study found that increased duration of non-aspirin NSAID use was associated with stronger reduction in AD risk, whereas current use was not associated with reduced risk unless its duration had extended two years or more prior to the evaluation. The study also found that sustained use of aspirin (even low-dose) compounds for more than two years may be similarly associated with reduced risk of AD. The mechanisms are not yet explained. The protective effect, however, must be beyond the mere attenuation of inflammatory responses in the brain. Other suggested possible mechanisms include antiplatelet effects, reduction in glutamate-related excitotoxicity (thought to involve COX-2 in postsynaptic signal processing), or inhibition of free radical production by intraneuronal cyclooxygenase-2 (COX-2) *(7)*.

CAN ESTROGEN PLAY A ROLE IN THE PREVENTION OF AD?

Estrogen has well-known neuroprotective effects. Animal studies suggest that estrogen modulates neurotransmitter systems and regulates synaptogenesis. These beneficial effects occur in brain areas critical to cognitive function and involved in the pathology of AD. The question is: can estrogen replacement therapy (HRT) after menopause protect against or reverse cognitive deficits and reduce the risk for AD?

Recent large trials failed to show a beneficial effect for long-term estrogen replacement for women with AD. Also, in terms of risk reduction, HRT did not show any substantial effect *(8)*. Further prospective studies are ongoing, such as the National Institutes of Health in the Women's Health Initiative and the Preventing Postmenopausal Memory Loss and Alzheimer's with Replacement Estrogens studies to provide a better assessment of the role of estrogen for age-related health issues, including dementia *(9)*.

One mechanism to support the potentially beneficial effects of estrogen in the brain of postmenopausal women involves its ability to alter the processing of amyloid precursor protein (APP), believed to play an important role in the pathogenesis of AD. In a preliminary study it was recently shown that estradiol can serve as a β-amyloid-lowering agent for HRT-naïve women with AD *(10)*.

Given together with a cholinesterase inhibitor, no additional benefit of HRT in menopausal women with AD was reported in a French study *(11)*.

According to a recently published investigation, there is no correlation between estrogen levels and cognitive functioning in postmenopausal women treated with conjugated equine estrogens *(12)*.

In conclusion, at this time there is no evidence to state that estrogen can definitely prevent AD. Neither may the hormone have significant effect on the clinical course of AD in elderly women with this disease. A critical period for hormone use for the primary prevention or protection of AD may well exist, but cannot yet be identified.

DOES TESTOSTERONE INFLUENCE COGNITIVE SKILLS?

Testosterone may be a potential biological factor for protection against decline in memory and other cognitive skills in later life. Having higher levels of circulating free testosterone is associated with a reduced risk of certain types of memory loss. Free testosterone levels were significantly associated with higher scores on verbal and visual memory tests in a cohort of the Baltimore Longitudinal Study of Aging (BLSA). According to further data of the BLSA, as many as 68% of men older than 70 years have low levels of free testosterone *(13)*.

DOES MARIJUANA USE AFFECT COGNITIVE PERFORMANCE?

Very heavy use of marijuana is associated with persistent decrements in neurocognitive performance even after 28 days of abstinence. As the number of joints smoked increases, performance (memory, executive function, psychomotor speed, manual dexterity) decreases. These data are of interest because marijuana is the most widely used illicit drug in the Western Hemisphere and because the legalization of the drug is being heavily debated *(14)*.

DOES WINE DRINKING LOWER THE RISK OF DEMENTIA?

According to data from The Copenhagen City Heart Study, monthly and weekly intake of wine is associated with a lower risk of dementia. (This is in contrast to excessive drinking, which is associated with an increased risk, caused by a direct neurotoxicity of ethanol, indicating a J-shaped relationship between alcohol intake and dementia risk.) The suggested mechanism behind these beneficial effects: wine, especially red wine, contains flavonoids, which are natural compounds with an antioxidant effect. Another explanation might be that wine drinkers have a healthier diet than people drinking other spirits or beer. Monthly intake of beer, in contrast, in this study was associated with a significantly higher risk of dementia. Odds ratios for dementia risk were best with a weekly alcohol intake of 8–14 drinks, and worst with an intake of 22 or more drinks per week *(15)*.

DOES NICOTINE HELP?

Chronic nicotine treatment may effectively reduce beta amyloid-peptide aggregation in the brain. This is the result of experiments carried out with a mouse model of AD. Nicotinic drug treatment thus may be a novel protective therapy in AD *(16)*. If this applies to cigarette smoking also is yet to be determined. Epidemiological studies initially indicating a lower incidence of AD in smokers now suggest conflicting results. Clinicopathological findings also are mixed as to how smoking behavior affects the manifestations of AD *(17)*.

DOES STRESS PLAY A ROLE IN THE DEVELOPMENT OF AD?

Stress has a major impact on neurodegenerative diseases and mental disorders. It has the potency to exert either ameliorating or detrimental effects. Thus acute stress may even improve biological functions and performance. The hippocampus, a predominant site of the manifestations of AD in the brain, appears to be sensitive to stress, and its involvement in neurodegeneration may account for some severe clinical disabilities (for example, memory loss) *(18)*.

DOES COGNITIVE FUNCTION DECLINE AFTER CORONARY BYPASS GRAFTING?

Several studies have assessed perioperative cognitive decline after coronary artery bypass grafting (CABG). The incidence of cognitive decline in a new prospective study was 53% at discharge, 36% at 6 weeks, 24% at 6 months, and 42% at 5 years. The majority of patients thus seem to return to baseline functioning within 6 months. However, at 5 years a considerable percentage of patients may present with decline. This association remained significant even after adjustment for age and educational level. Before elective CABG, physicians therefore should discuss this potential risk with patients and their families *(19)*.

IS AD A VASCULAR DISORDER?

There is nosological evidence that sporadic AD is and should be classified as a vascular disorder. This opinion is based on epidemiological data and risk factor associations as well as similarities and overlaps in clinical findings and symptoms and in the results seen with various interventions (such as improvement of cerebral perfusion). This opinion, however, does not represent the current doctrine *(20)*.

CAN COGNITIVE STIMULATION REDUCE THE RISK OF AD?

Frequent participation in cognitively stimulating activities may be associated with reduced risk for AD. This is the result of a longitudinal study with a mean follow-up of 4.5 years, conducted with a cohort of 801 Catholic nuns, priests, and brothers without dementia at enrollment. A 1-point increase in cognitive activity score was associated with a 33% reduction in risk of AD. The study used an established composite measure of cognitive activity frequency. Frequency of participation in each named activity was rated on a 5-point scale (5 points = every day; 4 points = several times a week; 3 points = several times a month; 2 points = several times a year; 1 point = once a year or less). Common activities were viewing television, listening to radio, reading newspapers or magazines, reading books, playing games, laying puzzles, solving crosswords, going to a museum *(21)*.

The basis of the association of cognitive activity with incident AD is uncertain. One hypothesis suggests that with repetition some cognitive skills become more efficient and less vulnerable to disruption by AD pathology *(21)*.

WHICH DRUGS CAN CAUSE DEMENTIA?

Many prescription and over-the-counter drugs have the potential of producing severe memory impairment or delirium. The list includes sedative medications, such as hypnotics and benzodiazepines, as well as antidepressants, anticholinergics, anticonvulsants, and cardiological medications. An association between use of neuroleptics and accelerated rate of decline in AD has also been reported *(22)*.

WHAT IS THE TYPICAL PRESENTATION OF AN AD PATIENT?

The typical picture of an AD patient involves a progressive decline in memory function as well as a gradual retreat from, and frustration with, normal activities. Many additional clinical signs have been described, and all of these occur more than 10% of the time. They include apathy, agitation or irritability, aggression, anxiety, sleep disturbance, dysphoria, aberrant motor behavior, disinhibition, social withdrawal, decreased appetite (weight loss), and hallucinations. It must be kept in mind, however, that many other disorders may mimic the symptoms of AD *(23)*.

WILL THERE BE A VACCINE AGAINST AD?

Immunizing AD patients against beta-amyloid is a strategy that is under investigation. It has proven successful in animal models (transgenic mice). The first clinical vaccine trial in humans, however, had to be halted abruptly in 2002, after 18 of 298 immunized patients developed subacute meningo-encephalitis *(24)*. This trial, however, provided proof for the principle of immunization against AD.

Interventions geared toward reducing Abeta accumulation and inflammatory responses—the key players in the initiation of neuronal degeneration—should delay or prevent the onset of the clinical disease. Several research groups have shown that vaccination with Abeta results in a significant lowering of the Abeta burden in the brains of transgenic mice and in the prevention of amyloid plaque formation *(25)*. In some studies an improvement of cognitive deficits was reported also. The group of Denis J. Selkoe at Harvard Medical School currently is working on an intranasal mucosal Abeta vaccination *(26)*. Whether their data may have implications for the future development of an intranasal Abeta vaccine for humans is too early to say.

Several pharmaceutical companies are currently working on the development of an AD vaccine as well. None of these compounds has yet reached the stage of clinical testing. This means that a safe and effective vaccine for the immunization of humans against AD will not be available for at least 5 years more.

REFERENCES

1. Albert, M.S.: Detection of very early Alzheimer disease through neuroimaging. Alz Dis Assoc Disord 2003; 17 (2 suppl): 563–565.
2. Papassotiropoulos, A. et al.: Increased brain beta-amylosis load, phosphorylated tau, and risk of Alzheimer disease associated with an intronic CYP46 polymorphism. Arch Neurol 2003; 60: 29–35.
3. Andreasen, N. et al.: Evaluation of CSF-tau and CSF-Abeta42 as diagnostic markers for Alzheimer disease in clinical practice. Arch Neurol 2001; 58: 373–379.
4. Lovell, M.A.; Markesbery, W.: Ratio of 8-hydroxyguanine in intact DNA to free 8-hydroxyguanine is increased in Alzheimer disease ventricular cerebrospinal fluid. Arch Neurol 2001; 58: 392–396.
5. Doody, R.S. et al.: A method for estimating progression rates in Alzheimer disease. Arch Neurol 2001; 58: 449–454.
6. Stern, Y. et al.: Factors associated with incident human immunodeficiency viris-dementia. Arch Neurol 2001; 58: 473–479.
7. Zandi, P.P. et al.: Reduced incidence of AD with NSAID but not H2 receptor antagonists. The Cache County Study. Neurology 2002; 59: 880–886.
8. Seshadri, S. et al.: Postmenopausal estrogen replacement therapy and the risk of Alzheimer disease. Arch Neurol 2001; 58: 435–440.
9. Kesslak, J.P.: Can estrogen play a significant role in the prevention of Alzheimer s disease? J Neural Transm Suppl 2002; 62: 227–239.
10. Baker, L.D. et al.: 17beta-estradiol reduces plasma Abeta40 for HRT-naïve postmenopausal women with Alzheimer disease: a preliminary study. Am J Geriatr Psychiatry 2003; 11: 239–244.
11. Rigaud, A.S. et al.: No additional benefit of HRT on response to rivastigmine in menopausal women with AD. Neurology 2003; 60: 148–149.
12. Thal, L.J. et al.: Estrogen levels do not correlate with improvement in cognition. Arch Neurol 2003; 60: 209–212.
13. Moffat, S.D. et al.: Longitudinal assessment of serum free testosterone concentration predicts memory performance and cognitive status in elderly men. J Clin Endocrinol Metabol 2002; 87: 5001–5007.
14. Bolla, K.I. et al.: Dose-related neurocognitive effects of marijuana use. Neurology 2002; 59: 1337–1343.
15. Truelsen, T. et al.: Amount and type of alcohol and risk of dementia. The Copenhagen City Heart Study. Neurology 2002; 59: 1313–1319.
16. Nordberg, A. et al.: Chronic nicotine treatment reduces beta-amyloidosis in the brain of a mouse model of Alzheimer's disease (APPsw). J Neurochem 2002; 81: 655–658.
17. Sabbagh, M.N. et al.: The nicotinic acetylcholine receptor, smoking, and Alzheimer's disease. J Alzheimer Dis 2002; 4: 317–325.
18. Esch, T. et al.: The role of stress in neurodegenerative diseases and mental disorders. Neuroendocrinol Lett 2002; 23: 199–208.
19. Newman, M.F. et al.: Longitudinal assessment of neurocognitive function after coronary-artery bypass surgery. N Engl J Med 2001; 344: 395–402.

20. De la Torre, J.C.: Alzheimer disease as a vascular disorder: nosological evidence. Stroke 2002; 33: 1152–1162.

21. Wilson, R.S. et al.: Participation in cognitively stimulating activities and risk of incident Alzheimer disease. JAMA 2002; 287: 742–748.

22. Gauthier, S. (ed.): Clinical diagnosis and management of Alzheimer's disease. 2nd Ed. Martin Dunitz, London, 1999.

23. Santacruz, K.S.; Swagerty, D.: Early diagnosis of dementia. Am Fam Physician 2001; 63: 703–713, 717–718.

24. Orgogozo, J.-M., et al.: Subacute meningoencephalitis in a subset of patients with AD after Aβ42 immunization. Neurology 2003; 61: 46–54.

25. Nicolau, C. et al.: A liposome-based therapeutiv vaccine against beta-amyloid plaques on the pancreas of transgenic NORBA mice. Proc Natl Acad Sci USA 2002; 99: 2332–2337.

26. Lemere, C.A. et al.: Nasal vaccination with beta-amyloid peptide for the treatment of Alzheimer's disease. DNA Cell Biol 2001; 20: 705–711.

The following list provides the reader with selected resources that provide information about Alzheimer's disease as well as on support groups and other helpful institutions/organizations, mainly based in the United States.

Alzheimer's Association (USA)
Hotline: (800) 272-3900
www.alz.org
www.alz.org/hc (for physicians)
http://www.alzheimers.com

Alzheimer's Association (Australia/NSW)
www.alheimers.org.au
www.alznsw.au

Alzheimer Center Tulsa
Center of Excellence for Diagnosis
and Management of Alzheimer's Disease
Memory Clinic
1705 East 19th Street, Suite 406
Tulsa, OK 74104
Phone: (918) 743-4374
Fax: (918) 743-3081
www.alzheimercentertulsa.com

Alzheimer's Disease Association
Hotline: (212) 983-0700

**Alzheimer's Disease Education
and Referral Center (ADEAR)**
P.O.Box 8250
Silver Spring, MD 20907-8250
Hotline: (800) 438-4380
Email: adear@alzheimers.org
www.alzheimers.org

**Alzheimer's Disease and Related
Disorders Association (ADRDA)**
919 North Michigan Avenue
Chicago, IL 60611
Phone: (803) 772-3346
Email: pail.jeter@alz.org

**Alzheimer Disease Research Center
(ADRC), Washington University**
www.adrc.wustl.edu

Alzheimer's Disease Society UK
www.alzheimers.org.uk

Alzheimer's Disease International (ADI)
45/46 Lower Marsh
London SE1 7RG
www.alz.co.uk

Alzheimer Europe
www.alzheimer-europe.org

Alzheimer Page
www.biostat.wustl.edu

Alzheimer Research Forum
www.alzforum.org

Alzheimer Society of Canada
www.alzheimer.ca

From: *Current Clinical Neurology,*
Alzheimer's Disease: A Physician's Guide to Practical Management
Edited by: R. W. Richter and B. Zoeller Richter © Humana Press Inc., Totowa, NJ

Alzheimer's Web
www.alzweb.org

Alzheimer Web Sites—Short List
www.nm-alzheimers.org/shortlist.htm

Alzheimer Web Italia (ITALZ)
www.italz.it

American Academy of Neurology
1080 Montreal Avenue
St. Paul, MN 55116
Phone: (651) 695-1940
Email: web@aan.com
www.aan.com

American Association for Geriatric Psychiatry
7910 Woodmont Avenue, Suite 1050
Bethesda, MD 20814
Phone: (301) 654-7850
Email: main@aagpgpa.org
www.aagpgpa.org

American Association of Retired Persons (AARP)
601 E. Street, NW
Washington, DC 20049
Email: member@aarp.org
www.aarp.org

American Geriatrics Society
Empire State Building
350 Fifth Avenue, Suite 801
New York, NY 10118
Phone: (212) 308-1414
Email: info.amger@americangeriatrics.org
www.americangeriatrics.org

American Geriatrics Society Foundation for Health in Aging (FHA)
Empire State Building
350 Fifth Avenue, Suite 801
New York, NY 10118

Phone: (212) 755-6810
Email: staff@healthinaging.org
www.healthinaging.org

American Psychiatric Association
www.psych.org

Benjamin B. Green-Field National Alzheimer's Library and Resource Center
Phone: (312) 335-9602
www.alz.org/aboutus/library

Clinical Trials
www.clinicaltrials.gov

Cognitive Neurology and Alzheimer's Disease Center
www.brain.nwu.edu

Dementia Web
www.dementia.ion.ucl.ac.uk

Elder Web
www.elderweb.com

Elderconnect
www.elderconnect.com

Familial Alzheimer's Disease Research Foundation (FADRF) serving Oklahoma, USA-Central Region, USA, and the world
8177 South Harvard
Tulsa, OK 74137
Phone: (918) 631-3665
Fax: (918) 495-3760

Family Caregivers Alliance
www.caregiver.org

Institute on Aging (University of Pennsylvania)
University of Pennsylvania
3615 Chestnut Street
Philadelphia, PA 19104-6006

Phone: (215) 898-3163
Email: ageweb@mail.med.upenn.edu
www.med.upenn.edu/aging

John Douglas French Alzheimer Foundation
11620 Wilshire Boulevard
Los Angeles, CA 90025
Phone: (213) 470-5462
www.jdfaf.org

Medlineplus: Alzheimer's Disease
www.nlm.nih.gov/medlineplus/alzheimersdisease.
html

National Institutes of Health
Public Information Office, Building 31,
Room 2B10
9000 Rockville Pike
Bethesda, MD 20892
Phone: (301) 496-1766; National Institute

on Aging: (301) 496-1752
www.ninds.nih.gov/health_and_medical/
disorders/alzheimersdisease_doc.htm

Planning for Long-Term Care
www.alzheimers.org/pubs/longterm.html

Psychiatry Matters
www.psychiatrymatters.md

Senior Horizons—Alzheimer's
www.senior-horizons.net

WebMD
A reference for the latest health and wellness
information; publishes news articles and
reference materials on diverse topics.
Information is presented clearly enough
for nonphysicians to understand.
www.webmd.com

Index